THE SAFFRON SCOURGE

THE SAFFRON SCOURGE

A History of Yellow Fever in
Louisiana, 1796-1905

Jo Ann Carrigan

University of Louisiana at Lafayette Press
2015

© 2015 by University of Louisiana at Lafayette Press
All rights reserved

ISBN 13 (paper): 978-1-935754-48-0

University of Louisiana at Lafayette Press
P.O. Box 40831
Lafayette, LA 70504-0831

http://ulpress.org

To the memory of my cousin

Dr. Pinckney Bethell Carrigan (1871-1949).

While employed by the Mexican Central Railway Company,
he was honored for his "devotion to duty"
during a yellow fever epidemic in Tampico in 1903.
Returning to Hope, Arkansas in 1904,
Dr. "Pinck" spent the rest of his life there
practicing medicine and promoting public health.

CONTENTS

Illustrations ix

Tables xi

Acknowledgments xiii

Introduction to 2015 Edition xix

I
    The Disease Amd Its Early History 1

II
    The First Memorable Yellow Fever Epidemic in
       New Orleans, 1796 20

III
    A Half-Century of Pestilence 30

IV
    The Great Epidemics of the Fifties: 1853, 1854, 1855, 1858 58

V
    An Interregnum, 1859-1866 82

VI
    Return of the Scourge To Postwar Louisiana, 1867-1877 96

VII
    New Vulnerability, Local and National:
       The Pestilence of 1878 and its Aftermath 112

VIII
    The Yellow Fever Panic of 1897 141

IX
    The Last Epidemic, 1905 167

X
  *Theory and Controversy: Origin, Causation, and
  Transmission of Yellow Fever* 206

XI
  *Theory and Controversy: Susceptibility,
  Acclimation, and Immunity* 234

XII
  *Theory and Controversy: Specificity, Germs,
  and Mosquitoes* 260

XIII
  *Competing Modes of Treatment: A Century
  of Continuity and Change* 292

XIV
  Social and Cultural Impact of Yellow Jack 334

XV
  *Economic and Political Consequences
  of Epidemic Yellow Fever* 359

Notes 383

Bibliography 451

Index 485

ILLUSTRATIONS

Map: Yellow Fever on Louisiana's Waterways 57

St. Louis Cemetery, New Orleans 64

New Orleans Medical Journal 65

Charity Hospital 66

The Reverend W.T.D. Dalzell 108

Yellow Fever Epidemic at Shreveport in 1873 109

"Martyr-Priests" of Shreveport 109

1878 Epidemic at Labadieville on Bayou Lafourche 138

Mississippi River Traffic Halted at Memphis in 1878 138

Quarantine Notice, Louisiana State Board of Health, 1883 139

Public Health Pioneers:
    Dr. Samuel P. Choppin (1828-1884)
    Dr. Joseph J. Holt (1840-1922)
    Dr. Stanford E. Chaillé (1830-1911)
    Dr. Joseph Jones (1833-1896) 140

Yellow Fever Crusaders:
    Dr. Quitman Kohnke (1857-1909)
    Dr. Edmond Souchon (1841-1924)
    Dr. Joseph H. White (1859-1953) 181

Lapel Buttons to Promote the Oiling and Screening
    of Cisterns, an Anti-Mosquito Measure 182

Screened Ambulance for Transporting Yellow Fever
    Cases to Hospital During 1905 New Orleans Epidemic 182

Mississippi River Quarantine Station Under U.S. Control 204-205

Dr. Josiah C. Nott (1804-1873) 227

Dr. John L. Riddell (1807-1865) 228

Dr. Charles Deléry (1815-1878) 247

Dr. Jean-Charles Faget (1818-1884) 248

Yellow Fever Commission of the U.S. National Board of Health
    in Havana, Cuba 289

Dr. Carlos J. Finlay (1833-1915) 290

Major Walter Reed (1851-1902) 291

Dr. Bennet Dowler (1797-1878) 312

Dr. Edward Hall Barton (1796-1859) 313

Dr. William H. Holcombe (1825-1893) 314

Advertisements During Epidemics
    Londonderry Lithia Water...322
    The Terrible Scourge Yellow Fever..323
    Yellow Jack 324

Member of Howard Association Treating a Victim
    of Yellow Fever, 1878 358

Cartoon: "A Stab in the Back" 373

TABLES

1. Yellow Fever Mortality in New Orleans, 1796-1847 55
2. Yellow Fever in Louisiana Outside of New Orleans, 1811-1829..........56
3. Yellow Fever in Louisiana Outside of New Orleans, 1837-1847..........56
4. Yellow Fever Mortality in New Orleans, 1848-1858 80
5. Yellow Fever in Louisiana Outside of New Orleans, 1853-1858..........81
6. Yellow Fever Mortality in New Orleans, 1859-1866 95
7. Comparing New Orleans Epidemics.. 162
8. Yellow Fever Mortality in New Orleans, 1867-1905 165
9. Yellow Fever in Louisiana Outside of New Orleans, 1867-1898......... 166
10. Yellow Fever in Lake Providence, 1905 192
11. Yellow Fever in Louisiana, 1905 194

ACKNOWLEDGMENTS

This book would never have been finished (or even started) without the encouragement and patience of Glenn R. Conrad, Director of the Center for Louisiana Studies. More than a decade ago Glenn expressed interest in publishing a revised, expanded version of my 1961 LSU dissertation on yellow fever, and I began a task that proved more demanding and time-consuming than I had anticipated. The work of revision and additional research progressed intermittently and unevenly, halted by ordinary and extraordinary obstacles, stretching first over months, then years–through various illnesses of self and others, eyesight problems, transient typists, word processing disasters, and so on. Several times I came close to abandoning the project altogether.

The manuscript was almost completed, however, more than three years ago–except the chapter on therapeutics–Chapter 13. By that time I was learning to use a computer and relying less on typists (a succession of whom had left town, or lost disks, or used systems no one else could decipher). It took some time and effort to overcome my usual difficulties with facing the blank screen, especially in dealing with the formidable topic of a century of yellow fever treatments. Eventually, I got started and dashed off ten good pages that I promptly lost forever through some "word processing error." I made little further progress on the troublesome Chapter 13 until last summer when I finally finished it. (Friends had suggested that I rearrange the manuscript and give that chapter a different number!) Glenn Conrad has been remarkably understanding through my various misfortunes and tolerant of my procrastination and writing blocks that border on the pathological. For his interest and support, as well as the photocopies of letters and papers he supplied, I am sincerely grateful.

Others also deserve a special note of appreciation for assisting me in a variety of ways during the years I have been involved with this study. Two friends read an early version of each chapter (including the long delayed Chapter 13) and offered valuable suggestions. Linda Ray Pratt, Professor of English at the University of Nebraska, Lincoln, saved me from many errors of omission and commission and through our discussions and her insightful questions helped me to clarify my own thoughts. She now claims to know more about yellow fever in Louisiana than any other professor of poetry in the world. Wendell Oderkirk, a former student of mine, who teaches nursing history at Clarkson College in Omaha, also read the rough drafts and provided good advice on matters of form and substance. I am especially indebted to Linda and Wendell for investing their time and energy and for their constructive criticism and encouragement. Sarah Santana and Kitty Whalen also read several chapters in their earliest form; Sarah gave me the benefit of her expertise in epidemiology, while Kitty as a well-informed general reader spotted many vague or awkward constructions in need of revision. Barbara Hayhome, a friend and colleague with whom I have shared a home for many years, took photographs for me of gravestones, churches, cisterns, and other epidemic sites in Louisiana. She has lived with years of talk about this topic, when I was working on it and when I was not, and although a patient, attentive, supportive listener (for which I am most appreciative), she will no doubt be happy to see the project concluded.

Katherine Wyatt, formerly a student at the University of Nebraska at Omaha, now working toward a Ph.D. at Louisiana State University, assisted in compiling the bibliography. Jack Belsom of New Orleans checked bibliographical references for me at several Crescent City libraries, straightening out uncertainties in dates and publishers resulting from deficiencies in my ancient note cards. Winston DeVille, Louisiana genealogist-historian, called my attention to (and helped translate) a French colonial report that seems to document a yellow fever epidemic in New Orleans as early as 1739. Jack and Winston were my students at LSU once upon a time, as was Kathy more recently in Omaha. I appreciate their friendship and their assistance.

Kathleen Puglia and others at the Tulane Medical Library were especially helpful when I was doing research there on several occasions. Kathleen also answered many of my queries by long distance telephone, taking time to check some bit of information for me in the stacks. The librarians and archivists at LSU in Baton Rouge, LSU in Shreveport (especially Laura Street), Tulane University, the New Orleans Public Library, the Louisiana State Museum Library, and the Historic New Orleans Collection (Jon Kukla and John T. Magill) all offered me every kindness and courtesy during my visits to their collections. I also wish to thank the Interlibrary Loan Department at my own University Library for facilitating my research at this distance from the source.

Acknowledgments

A summer fellowship funded by the Faculty Senate Research Committee some years ago, as well as a Faculty Development Fellowship at the University of Nebraska at Omaha, provided time for travel to Louisiana libraries and for working on the manuscript. (A recent mini-grant from the University Committee on Research funded the preparation of the index.) Thanks to Marvin Barton, cartographer in the Geography Department, for preparing the map included herein that shows the major towns along Louisiana's waterways where yellow fever spread; and thanks also to Andy Barela, artist in the Audio-Visual Department, who designed the book jacket. His mosquito drawing is based on an illustration of the *Aedes aegypti* that I had obtained (Courtesy The Historic New Orleans Collection, Museum/Research Center, Acc. No. 1974.25.11.114). Placing the mosquito over the state of Louisiana was Andy's idea.

In 1988-89 Shirley Miller, then a typist at the University of Nebraska Medical Center, did most of the word processing of the final drafts, faithfully working with me on many Saturdays and Sundays. Jo Headrick, History Department secretary, helped me live through Chapter 13 last summer by typing into WordPerfect the several sections of the chapter as I wrote and revised them. She also helped me figure out how to use a new printer in the department, a skill of considerable value.

Several revised chapters or portions of chapters from the dissertation have appeared as articles on specific epidemics or topics in the following journals: *Journal of Southern History* (1959, 1970); *McNeese Review* (1963); *Civil War History* (1963); *Tulane Medical Bulletin* (1967); *Louisiana Studies* (1967); *Louisiana History* (1963, 1988). In some form or another most of this material has been incorporated into the final version of *Saffron Scourge*.

This seems to be the season for yellow fever books–two others having been published recently: John Ellis, *Yellow Fever and Public Health in the New South* (University Press of Kentucky) and Margaret Humphreys, *Yellow Fever and the South* (Rutgers). These works appeared after I had completed my manuscript (except Chapter 13), but I have benefited greatly from information and insights in various articles by Ellis and by Humphreys (Warner), as well as an unpublished paper on the 1878 epidemic made available to me by Ellis some years ago.

My 1961 dissertation at Louisiana State University was directed by John Duffy (and Edwin Davis). I have retained the chronological-topical organization of the original work. The introduction has been considerably expanded and includes some new material on what might be the earliest yellow fever epidemic in New Orleans. Other chapters have been revised and expanded, and several new chapters added, especially covering the postbellum years, somewhat slighted in the dissertation. The work has been informed by a considerable body of scholarship in medical history published since the dissertation, when the field was relatively new among historians without the M.D. degree. Additional material has been added on "theory and controversy," on therapeutics, and on social, economic, and political impact of epidemics. In retrospect, retaining the structure of the dissertation may not have been the best strategy for organizing the century-long story. And the mixture of the new and the old, narrative and analysis, anecdotal and quantitative—as a canvas one might have painted on and reworked over a period of decades—has its problems. But whatever its flaws, at last it is finished, and it is mine.

June, 1993

THE SAFFRON SCOURGE

INTRODUCTION TO 2015 EDITION

When the Center for Louisiana Studies made plans to issue a new paperbound edition of *Saffron Scourge*, originally published in 1994, I was delighted. The book has been out of print for a number of years and was only available in a few overpriced used copies and in university libraries. The possibility of a new edition always raises questions about how much revision to do, and what kind. There are, of course flaws in organization and insufficient attention to several aspects of the yellow fever story, but I have decided to let the text remain as first conceived and constructed. If I started pulling threads here and there, I am afraid the whole fabric would come unraveled. A new introduction that updates the scholarship, however, seemed worthwhile.

I can hope that the original historical study remains useful as it is: as a reference work, with detailed index, with chapters tracing the main outlines of yellow fever's appearance in New Orleans and the gradual spread of the disease through developing trade and travel; highlighting major epidemic years from the late eighteenth through the early twentieth century; and covering theories, therapies, and social, political, and economic ramifications for state and nation during the long experience with the disease.

A new survey of the field will sample some of the works concerning yellow fever published since *Saffron Scourge* appeared in 1994, not merely searching for new Louisiana material, but casting a wider net. I wanted to see what was "out there," what new questions were being asked, the extent of continuing interest and inquiry, the issues and themes in recent yellow fever scholarship. In addition to the relevant history publications, mainly through articles and book reviews in major journals, I began a preliminary search through academic databases, as well as Google Books and Amazon Books, websites which did not exist when I was doing research for *Saffron Scourge*.

The sophisticated search engine of Amazon, for example, yielded more than 700 items on "Yellow Fever History." A search for the general topic "Yellow Fever" found more than 9,000 items. An English-only search for publications between 1994 and 2012 in Google Books turned up almost 3,000 volumes; and in any language, more than 16,000. A Google Books search for "Yellow Fever History" without linguistic or temporal parameters offered 894,000 results, and for "Yellow Fever" in general, 4,570,000 items. Bibliographic databases, such as JSTOR, FirstSearch, WorldCat, ArticleFirst, Ebscohost, and ProQuest, provided lists of books, articles, and dissertations, as well as references to yellow fever in titles without any obvious subject connection.

The number and variety of references is perhaps not surprising. The history of yellow fever epidemics provides dramatic stories of heroes and villains, sickness and death, tragedy and horror, frightful scenes of community chaos, views of another place and time, as well as a compelling setting for fiction in books, or movies. People clearly like to write about this subject, and apparently people also like to read about it. Given the enormous volume of material, I have only managed to scan portions of the various lists and to select and sample the literature that seemed most pertinent to my quest.

I was surprised by the number of volumes of juvenile fiction and nonfiction using either the Philadelphia epidemic of 1793 or New Orleans's 1853 epidemic as the setting for the story, some designed for elementary and others for high school readers. One example of non-fiction for young readers is Jim Murphy's *An American Plague: The True and Terrifying Story of the Yellow Fever Epidemic of 1793*. An award-winning writer whose work has received high praise for its power to interest students in history, Murphy relates the Philadelphia epidemic to current concerns with outbreaks of new diseases such as SARS (Severe Acute Respiratory Syndrome).[1]

A charming piece of juvenile fiction set within the same Philadelphia epidemic, Laurie Anderson's *Fever 1793*, is told through the eyes of a fourteen-year-old girl. The story shows her experience of the chaos of the city and the sorrow of losing family and friends. Anderson weaves the girl's experience into the epidemic history and includes an Appendix with brief discussions of medical theories and treatments, Dr. Benjamin Rush, George Washington, the Free African Society—and the continuing presence of yellow fever in today's world. The book is a painless way to expose adolescent students to medical-social history.[2]

The New Orleans yellow fever epidemic of 1853 has also inspired a number of fictional offerings for children. A series of brief novels with illustrations directed primarily toward elementary and junior high school girls features young New Orleanian Marie-Grace and her friend Cecile, described as being from an "affluent free black family." They serve as volunteers at an orphanage and face a variety of adventures in the pestilential city.[3] Using the Memphis epidemic of 1878 as historical background, another novel designed for preadolescents spins a cemetery

Introduction xxi

ghost story about a twelve-year-old boy, a young child he rescues, and a girl who works at the graveyard.[4]

Writers of adult fiction have also been attracted by the history of a city in the throes of yellow fever as a ready-made medium into which their characters and stories can be blended. For example, Josh Russell's *Yellow Jack* is a romantic tale about a French photographer who takes memorial pictures of corpses in 1840s New Orleans during epidemic season, while involved with two women, one an "octoroon" skilled in voodoo.[5] James Brewer's *No Escape* is a mystery-detective novel about a murder on a Mississippi riverboat quarantined in Memphis during the 1873 epidemic.[6] *The Rebel Wife* by Taylor Polites is a "gothic" tale of an Alabama widow during Reconstruction, who loses both her husband and her property in the midst of an epidemic—this one also available in LARGE PRINT edition.[7]

A final example that seems in a category beyond the others is the work of Barbara Hambly, award-winning novelist and screenwriter of mysteries, historical fiction, science fiction, and fantasy. *Fever Season* is one of a series about Benjamin January, a "free man of color," trained in medicine in Paris, who returns to New Orleans years later in 1833, and is able to find employment only as a music teacher; however, he tends to the sick in Charity Hospital at night when both cholera and yellow fever strike New Orleans that year. He also becomes involved in a murder mystery. Critics have praised the work as well-written, complex, and captivating.[8] None of this fiction, juvenile or adult, adds new substance to yellow fever history, but to whatever extent the narratives remain faithful to the historical elements and insofar as distortions are minimal, such story-telling can be informative and pleasurable for young and old alike.

Nineteenth-century sources that I read in the original editions in Louisiana libraries, rare book rooms, and archives many years ago are now available as paperbound reprints or in digital format versions, accessible directly onscreen. Almost any internet search will find the yellow fever books or pamphlets of Erasmus Darwin Fenner, Edward H. Barton, J. M. Keating, Rene LaRoche, Henry Rose Carter, and many other well-known classic accounts.

Few recent scholarly works have focused specifically on Louisiana's experience with yellow fever; I found only one small book and a few journal articles. In 2005, the Center for Louisiana Studies published a brief volume recounting yellow fever's years in New Orleans, *Fearful Ravages* by Benjamin Trask, as No. 15 of the Louisiana Life Series. Concluding with a discussion of the recent concern with epidemic diseases (West Nile

Fever and SARS), and noting the terrible aftermath of Hurricane Katrina then underway in New Orleans, Trask observed that hurricanes seem to have become the new "scourge" of the Gulf and South Atlantic coastal regions.[9]

In an issue of the *Journal of American History* devoted entirely to Hurricane Katrina and "the past," an article by Henry McKiven shows how various kinds of disasters, past and present, prompt "political construction" of the event, explanations framed in diverse ways to promote one interest group or another. McKiven used the New Orleans yellow fever epidemic of 1853 as an earlier example of how the party in power in the city and the reformer politicians explained the epidemic in different ways to support their own respective positions, whether involving issues of corruption, voting rights, nativism, "good government," or sanitary improvements.[10]

Two more articles on the New Orleans epidemic of 1853 deserve mention for their complex statistical approaches to calculating differential mortality rates for the city, squeezing out some of the limitations of available raw data. Their findings reinforce the insights most historians have previously offered about susceptibilities and resistance to the "strangers disease," although their calculations did not reveal the apparent gender gap in mortality that the records suggest. These works, both by J. B. Pritchett and Isan Tonali, illustrate the approach and research of "econometrics."[11]

Other journal articles recount the Louisiana-Mississippi quarantine conflict of 1905 and the 1873 epidemic in Shreveport.[12] That terribly destructive yellow fever episode in Shreveport's history continues to fascinate local historians and journalists, and a search found several pertinent websites. A brief sketch of the epidemic by Monica Peis is posted on the "caddohistory" website.[13] On the Oakland Cemetery website, Eric Brock's "Historical Overview" calls attention to the mass grave where some eight hundred yellow fever victims were buried in 1873.[14] A five-minute video tour of the cemetery can be viewed onscreen, conducted by historian Gary Joiner of LSU-Shreveport, available via the C-SPAN Video Library and also posted on YouTube.[15] A list of names of the hundreds of fever victims is also available online.[16]

Another discovery was the recent reprint edition, with illustrations, of a Victorian novel about the 1873 Shreveport epidemic: *Angel Agnes* by Wesley Bradshaw, a Philadelphian and popular author at that time.[17] The epidemic had received widespread newspaper attention throughout its three-month siege, and this book appearing soon after became a national bestseller. In the story, the title character Agnes, from a well-to-do Philadelphia family, responds to the call for help reported in the papers

Introduction xxiii

and travels to Shreveport as a volunteer nurse, believing herself immune because of exposure to fever on a previous visit to New Orleans. The novel describes the distress of the city and Agnes's efforts to care for the sick and comfort the dying as best she could. She was considered an "Angel" by those she attended. There is also a melodramatic love story, of course, and the lover dies of yellow fever with Agnes at his bedside.

Despite the overblown sentimental 1870s prose, the work conveys a sense of what it might have been like to be a caregiver in the midst of a major epidemic, cause unknown and most treatment ineffective. The fictional "Agnes" is representative of the volunteers from various parts of the state and nation who actually did come to Shreveport to provide whatever relief they could; many of them died of the fever and were buried among those they came to serve. Shreveport's epidemic of 1873 was one of the worst yellow fever outbreaks to impact a city in the nineteenth-century United States.[18]

Recently I became aware of a nineteenth-century Redemptorist priest with a place in yellow fever history and an ongoing connection to New Orleans. Father Francis Xavier Seelos, originally from Bavaria, came to the United States in the 1840s and served in various locations as pastor, teacher, and itinerant missionary, before volunteering for assignment to St. Mary's Assumption Church in New Orleans in 1866. While attending the poor and the sick during the yellow fever epidemic of 1867, Seelos himself became ill and died of the disease (one of many clergy who died in nineteenth-century yellow fever epidemics). He had acquired a widespread reputation for the power to comfort and to heal prior to his death, a reputation which persisted thereafter as people in different parts of the country prayed for his intercession. A record of presumed cases of healing accumulated over time, and in 2000, one documented case attributed to his intercession was accepted by Rome as a "miracle," and Seelos was beatified by Pope John Paul II. His advocates submitted another case of healing in 2010, believing this to be the second "miracle" that would result in sainthood for Blessed Francis Seelos. This case was not validated by the Vatican authorities. Although disappointed, his advocates continue to believe that eventually a definitive case will result in his canonization. While this story may seem little more than a footnote in the city's yellow fever history, it is included here as a subject of enduring importance to many in the New Orleans of today.[19]

Any publication touching on some aspect of yellow fever's years in the United States almost always refers to New Orleans as the major center for the nineteenth-century importation of the disease and the focal point from which it spread inland and along the coast. For the New Orleans material, most general studies rely in large measure on prior scholarship, usually (but not always) with appropriate attribution.

Looking beyond Louisiana to other areas, I found only one book-length statewide study, Deanne Nuwer's *Plague among the Magnolias*, detailing Mississippi's experience during that most widespread yellow fever epidemic of 1878. She makes highly effective use of primary sources to present a close-up view of the devastating impact on individuals and entire families. Diaries and letters reveal the intensity of human suffering as mortality figures alone do not. Nuwer tells of many deaths within a single family, survivors taking care of friends and neighbors, burying the dead, demonstrating "self-help" and "independence." But needs soon overwhelmed resources, and Mississippians had to issue a call for outside help. There is especially good coverage of small town experience, the deaths of local officials, bankers, shopkeepers, and doctors, and the departure of large numbers of whites, leaving black majorities in many towns, with resulting racial tension. Black caregivers did what they could within their own communities and offered personal assistance to whites as well, despite the tension.

Volunteer doctors and nurses along with contributions from charitable associations and individuals poured in to Mississippi from all over the nation, providing medical assistance, funds, food, and other supplies. African Americans in Mississippi received far less than a fair share of these funds and supplies that were controlled almost entirely by local white committees or officials. According to Nuwer, black Louisianans seemed to have access to more resources than those in Mississippi because of their New Orleans leaders, their mutual aid societies, and religious institutions. (This was perhaps the case, insofar as self-help goes and mainly in the city. But black organizations there also complained, as did some religious groups, about being denied assistance by the major dispensers of relief. The depth of poverty in New Orleans was so great that the central relief organizations, lacking sufficient supplies to answer all requests for aid, decided to give the families of yellow fever victims priority, thereby excluding others who were simply unemployed and destitute, whether white or black.[20])

In response to disease and despair, Mississippi's state government offered little but advice; the federal government, on the other hand, authorized the provision of United States Army rations to those in need and organized major relief efforts, greatly benefiting the people of Mississippi and other states along the river. Nuwer identifies two major changes after

Introduction xxv

the Civil War that led citizens to expect more from state government: the suffering of "elites" in 1878 who asked for official help, and "a model of more active government" during Reconstruction in Mississippi. It takes time to develop effective institutions with adequate funding and enforcement, but the movement toward public health legislation, state and national, was set in motion by the yellow fever epidemic of 1878.[21]

Nuwer and others who have studied the epidemic of 1878 have observed that the magnitude of suffering provided the occasion for an extraordinary degree of northern benevolence and southern gratitude, which at least temporarily seemed to reconcile the sections after the bitterness of Civil War and Reconstruction. This point has been made even more explicitly and in a far broader context by Edward Blum, first in an article emphasizing the reconciliation of northern and southern whites through epidemic trauma, northern generosity, and southern appreciation, all of which helped wipe out old memories and create new, more favorable ones for both sections. In his book on *Reforging the White Republic*, Blum extends and deepens the argument, showing the influence of white northern Protestant Christian spokesmen and other cultural forces in reuniting North and South, solidifying a white nation (under God), accepting the exclusion and segregation of the black population, and abandoning any thought of racial equity and justice. The 1878 epidemic, in Blum's view, "stood as a pivotal moment in postwar national reconciliation and the marginalization of African Americans." He also links "whiteness," religion, and intense nationalism to the American imperialism of the late nineteenth century. Blum perhaps paints with too broad a brush, but there is clearly some truth to it.[22]

Destitute blacks in 1878 often encountered obstacles in obtaining food and other donated supplies from white committees, but Blum asserts further that "systematic medical negligence caused the deaths of countless African Americans."[23] There is insufficient evidence for this conclusion. While some southern white physicians might have been negligent, Blum has no convincing evidence that it was "systematic." In any case, medicine actually had little to offer as effective therapy and could even be harmful. Good nursing care by family or friends would have been more useful. And perhaps the real negligence was not so much medical but lack of food and other necessities of life.

The index to *Saffron Scourge* contains thirty-eight references to nurses and nursing, clearly the most beneficial form of care available and an important aspect of yellow fever history. Nineteenth-century yellow fever epidemics are now receiving attention as an aspect of nursing history, an expanding field of inquiry in recent decades. Epidemics are also being examined as a facet of "disaster studies," sharing similar themes with hurricanes, earthquakes, fires, and other occasions of mass destruction, injury, or illness.[24] This interest in disasters has prompted comparisons of official and popular responses to yellow fever epidemics and to hurricanes, Katrina in particular—alluded to by a number of writers.

Nurses on the Front Line, a recent edited work on the history of nursing activities during various kinds of disasters, includes a contribution by Deanne Nuwer on the demand for nurses in the 1878 yellow fever epidemic in Mississippi when the state's communities were calling for help. She describes the work of the Sisters of Charity and the Sisters of Mercy, many of whom lost their lives during the epidemic. The Howard Association, an organization designed specifically for medical and other relief work during epidemics, actively recruited in other states and sent nurses to Mississippi towns overwhelmed by the fever. Some came on their own, others came for pay—including black and white, men and women. Women received less pay than men, and blacks less than whites. Black male nurses were directly supervised by a white male or female whenever working outside their own communities. The years after the 1878 epidemic saw the gradual development of state institutions for the formal training of nurse professionals.[25]

In another anthology on *Nurses Work*, Linda Sabin authored a chapter describing the "unheralded work of male nurses in yellow fever epidemics" in nineteenth-century Mississippi towns and in Jacksonville, Florida, during the outbreak of 1888. In time of crisis, from a sense of honor and duty, men were expected to offer whatever assistance was needed, including nursing service—to family, to neighbors, to community—and many actually did. Community-wide nursing usually required the recruitment of additional outside help, both volunteer and paid, for hospitals and asylums, as well as domestic nursing service. The opportunity for good wages during the crisis (paid with donations from benevolent societies and individual contributions) attracted men and women, black and white. After 1900 few epidemics occurred that required such service, and by that time, nurse training schools were creating a profession that southern men seemed quite willing to leave to women. The role of men in the history of nursing is a topic that merits further exploration, as Sabin suggests.[26]

Sabin also contributed a chapter in another collection, *History as Evidence: Nursing Interventions Through Time*. She provides a broad overview of early nineteenth-century southern nursing practices in epidemic yellow fever cases. Using the experience acquired over time, the nurse offered bedside

Introduction xxvii

therapeutic and comfort care, sometimes under the direction of a physician (sometimes not), following traditional or alternative therapies then in use. Sabin skillfully extracted information from a variety of sources, showing the specific nursing functions implied by various recorded therapies, but rarely if ever spelled out as clearly as she managed to do. Especially useful are the tables Sabin devised, describing what the nurse might have done in coping with the patient's manifestation of fever, chills, pain, vomiting, diarrhea, coma, and death. The nurse would assist the physician in procedures of bleeding or cupping, but actually performed most other interventions, such as administering enemas, purges, poultices, cool or hot applications, and massage; bathing or sponging; preparing and dispensing cool drinks, broth, light nourishment, and stimulants; keeping patient and bed cleaned after numerous occasions of vomiting and diarrhea; communicating with the patient, dealing with patient discomfort, restlessness, and resistance; communicating with the family, and perhaps the doctor; and finally managing either convalescence or end-of-life care. These relentless tasks went on for a week or two, and the work was difficult, exhausting, messy, sad, and potentially dangerous. But the almost constant bedside care by an attentive nurse could make the difference between survival and death, and even in fatal cases, would provide some measure of comfort throughout the illness.[27]

Among the several relevant Ph.D. dissertations located through ProQuest, one seems a particularly valuable source for the history of both yellow fever and nursing: the account by Adrian Melissinos of nursing experience in the 1878 Memphis epidemic as reflected in the letters of a volunteer from Houston, Texas. Kezia DePelchin went to Memphis as a Howard Association nurse, carefully recorded her daily activities in letters from late August until her return to Houston in December, thereby offering a detailed picture of nursing work when experience served as the only training yet available in the South and individuals varied greatly in knowledge or skills. The demand for nurses and increasing awareness of their value stimulated the development of schools and professionalization in the late nineteenth-century. Melissinos also suggests that these DePelchin letters, revealing the vital role and various functions of a disaster nurse, offer significant lessons for today's nurses confronting the increasingly frequent disasters of our own times.[28]

Two other dissertations explore different facets of yellow fever history: (1) Kathryn Keller's highly theoretical discussion of the "differentials of power," "the complex and chaotic process of collective knowledge production," and "the politics of *how we choose to remember*,"[29] and (2)

Michael Thompson's study of waterfront laborers, black and white, in Charleston, South Carolina, from the late eighteenth century until the Civil War, with attention to the impact of yellow fever on competition for employment.[30] It seems that yellow fever has a place in postmodernist epistemology and labor history as well.

Scanning the various lists of books and articles revealed the enduring popularity of biographies of heroes in the "conquest of yellow fever"—Carlos Finlay, Walter Reed and his associates, William Crawford Gorgas, and others. Histories of the construction of the Panama Canal and the scientific work of the Reed Commission are favorite topics for narrating again and again. One recent well-written, carefully documented volume, *Yellow Jack: How Yellow Fever Ravaged America and Walter Reed Discovered its Deadly Secrets*, by Dr. John R. Pierce, retired colonel, U.S. Army Medical Corps, with Jim Writer, a journalist, presents a story well-known in general outline. Based on a large collection of primary sources and thorough use of secondary works, the book manages to offer an absorbing, detailed account of the Reed Commission's work in Cuba, the day by day results of yellow fever experiments, individual personalities and relationships, and some basic yellow fever history before and after Walter Reed as well.[31]

Journals and magazines continue to publish both scholarly and popular articles about specific yellow fever years in specific cities—Philadelphia, Charleston, Savannah, Memphis, Mexican and Cuban ports, and various places in Africa and Central and South America. There always seems to be room for one more epidemic or one more retelling.

Recent popular interest no doubt has been stirred by the news of emerging and reemerging infectious diseases, including mosquito-borne viruses causing West Nile, dengue, and dengue hemorrhagic fever. Yellow fever, caused by a related mosquito-borne virus, is still endemic in many parts of Africa and in Brazil and other South American countries, with occasional serious outbreaks. According to the World Health Organization's estimate, some 30,000 deaths among 200,000 cases of yellow fever occur annually.[32] Other current concerns include the risk of importing old or new diseases via rapid international travel and trade, the potential threat of disease as a bioterrorist weapon, and the likely effect of global warming on the northward movement of certain insects that transmit deadly microbes.

Numerous general works on the major infectious diseases in human history have appeared recently, aimed at this popular interest and sometimes designed to capitalize on preexisting public curiosity and anxiety—with yellow fever as one among the several pestilences covered. Some volumes,

Introduction xxix

of course, are based on careful research with solid documentation; others are loosely compiled from secondary works and contain errors from careless misreading or misunderstanding of sources, with unorthodox citation style, if any at all.

Two books by award-winning journalists, specifically on yellow fever, both published in 2006, exhibit some of the features professional historians and public health scientists find troubling: James L. Dickerson's *Yellow Fever: A Deadly Disease Poised to Kill Again*, and Molly Caldwell Crosby's *The American Plague: The Untold Story of Yellow Fever, the Epidemic That Shaped Our History*. The titles themselves are a bit hyperbolic.[33] As other critics have pointed out, both works are plagued with making or repeating errors of fact or interpretation, exaggerating the originality of their findings, and overstating the potential of yellow fever as an imminent threat to the United States.[34]

Dickerson narrates the frequently-told tales of a century of yellow fever epidemics, blurring the complexities of nineteenth-century public health issues and policies. After discussion of U.S. military research programs on biological warfare, ostensibly now "limited" to defensive purposes, he explains in detail how he thinks yellow fever virus could easily be used against us by bioterrorists as a "weapon of mass destruction." This is unlikely, according to various experts, because the virus is unstable and not very effective in aerosolized form; and if involving infected mosquitoes, pesticides are available for control.[35]

In a chapter titled "Global Warming Casts Ominous Shadow," Dickerson also contends that the United States is at great risk for resurgence of yellow fever from climate change, while acknowledging conflicting scientific opinions on the matter. CDC physicians discount any immediate threat of yellow fever to the United States, suggesting greater potential for major outbreaks in Puerto Rico and Mexico, mainly because of socioeconomic factors. Given the complexity of mosquito borne diseases, "the interplay of climate, ecology, vector biology, and many other factors defies simplistic analysis."[36] Some researchers, on the other hand, argue that higher temperatures by expanding the range of mosquitoes do pose a threat and point out that dengue, malaria, and West Nile are already affected by climate change. Dickerson concludes with this dire warning: "America's survival as a nation, at some point in the not too distant future, may depend on its understanding of its worst enemy, *yellow fever*."[37]

Molly Crosby's *American Plague* is a well-told and much publicized account of the 1878 Memphis epidemic and the work of the Reed Commission. Her narrative derives much power from letters and diaries of Memphis doctors, nurses, nuns, clergy, and others, but Crosby's subtitle, "The Untold Story of Yellow Fever, The Epidemic that Shaped Our History," is an overreach, to say the least. Many of us have been telling and retelling much of this story for years, as she seems to acknowledge in her unconventional discussion of sources; and the epidemic of 1878, although of considerable significance, was certainly not the only force "that Shaped Our History" (unless she is referring mainly to the history of Memphis, but the title *American Plague* and context suggest otherwise).

Both Crosby and Dickerson give special attention to two yellow fever cases that appeared in the United States in the 1990s and one in 2002. Each case involved travel to Brazil or Venezuela, and all died, in California, Tennessee, and Texas, their disease unrecognized and misdiagnosed initially, but eventually determined by autopsy. Given that airlines can transport infected persons and mosquitoes vast distances in a short time, both writers saw such cases as the potential "spark" for a major epidemic. Crosby, like Dickerson, also suggested the possible bioterrorist use of yellow fever virus, as well as the threatened recurrence of North American yellow fever epidemics from global warming and vector migration.

Southern states are indeed to some extent "at risk" with a large *Aedes aegypti* vector population, plus an aggressive newcomer mosquito relative, *Aedes albopictus*. If the virus were imported in an infected person (whether by accident or design), and other appropriate circumstances of precise timing and exposure to vectors converged, a yellow fever outbreak could *possibly* occur, especially if not recognized right away. Public health experts say this is not likely, given the prevalence of air-conditioning, screening, and pesticides, as well as the knowledge of epidemiology. Once diagnosed, the isolation of cases and mosquito control measures would be effective public health responses. The resurgence of dengue fever, also transmitted by *Aedes* mosquitoes, is occurring now in many parts of the world, and may become a more likely threat to the United States than yellow fever, especially in Florida.

Renewed attention to mosquito control measures is probably called for (and a well-funded, well-prepared public health system), as protection against West Nile, dengue, or any potential yellow fever import or other mosquito-borne *new* virus intruder as well. While a recurrence of yellow fever is not impossible, it seems unlikely to be introduced by bioterrorists as there are much simpler and more effective means of creating biological chaos. Although who knows what old or new diseases and disasters may befall us in the future, yellow fever outbreaks, if returning to our shores, would probably be more manageable than other likely effects of climate change.

Introduction xxxi

Among numerous recent general works on major diseases in history (including yellow fever), two should be noted here because they are reliable and especially appealing. Edited by Kenneth Kiple, who also wrote on some of the diseases, *Plague, Pox & Pestilence* is a collection of succinct, highly informative essays by prominent medical historians, covering twenty-six diseases from ancient times to the present, with bibliographical references for each. Filled with well-captioned illustrations such as paintings, drawings, cartoons, posters, photographs, and engravings, this oversized volume could grace a coffee table and be a conversation piece for its title and cover alone. The stated theme of the book is that "human progress breeds disease and has always done so." According to Margaret Humphreys, who contributed several of the chapters, yellow fever is not a "serious threat" to us today, but dengue "may well become a major public health problem in the United States in coming years." While not as likely to be lethal as yellow fever, dengue can be a miserably painful illness with social and economic consequences, and in its hemorrhagic form, highly fatal.[38]

The other volume in this "major diseases" category that has great appeal is a forty-eight-page illustrated book, designed for young readers (but fun for ages seven up to almost eighty), published more than a decade after the work just discussed, with exactly the same title—except for the addition of an "s"—*Plagues, Pox, and Pestilence*.[39] An excellent elementary introduction to the history, microbiology, and epidemiology of major infectious diseases (including yellow fever), the booklet offers much information in small doses, scattered about in boxes among the colorful cartoon-images of ugly little microbes dashing about a lab. There are also huge mosquitoes with blood-filled red bellies and arrow-like noses, and similar comical illustrations of large fleas, flies, and ticks, plus a giant rat with big ears and nose, dressed in a lab coat and looking through a microscope. Also included are pictures of how protists, bacteria, and viruses actually appear under the microscope. Both *PP&P* books are informative and delightful, each in its own special way.

With few exceptions, scholarly books and articles since the mid-nineties have treated yellow fever not as the main focus but as a facet of a larger subject, such as diseases in history, nursing, disaster studies, the American Civil War, African American health, railroad development and quarantine, Caribbean colonial wars, European and American imperialism, and environmental history. These studies have explored previously neglected topics, offered new perspectives, or delved more deeply into related areas other historians had skimmed over.[40]

It has long been well-known that Yankee and Rebel armies both lost far more lives to disease than to battle wounds in the American Civil War.[41] Despite the continuing scholarly and popular interest in Civil War history, research on the extent and influence of specific diseases is not one of the overworked fields. In *Mosquito Soldiers,* Andrew McIlwaine Bell has undertaken a careful study of the impact of the mosquito-borne diseases, malaria and yellow fever, on Civil War troops and military operations. He viewed mosquitoes as "a third army" that could help or hurt either side depending on the circumstances. Troops on both sides were most at risk in theaters west of the Mississippi River.

Malaria actually posed the greater illness threat, but yellow fever was more frightening. Yellow fever outbreaks in Texas, Florida, and the Carolinas, among troops and on ships along the coasts, sometimes caused Confederates to abandon their mission of protecting port cities, sometimes disrupted Union blockade activities, and at times influenced both the planning and outcome of military operations. In a chapter on "biological warfare," Bell details a Confederate plot to introduce yellow fever into Washington, D.C. in trunks of "infected" clothing and blankets taken from fever victims, based on the mistaken belief that the disease was transmitted in this fashion. The plan was discovered and came to naught (but could not have worked anyway). Bell's contribution to the medical-military history of the Civil War offers much more than the summary statements noted here. All medical historians and many others would agree with his view that "Epidemiological history may never receive the same popular acclaim given to biographies and crisp military narratives, but it demands the attention of those who are dedicated to understanding the messy realities of life in previous centuries."[42]

Sick from Freedom by Jim Downs attracted my attention because it dealt with African American illness experience after slavery, and I was curious to see what might be said about yellow fever. The book is "not only a study of disease and death as consequences of emancipation but of the expansion of federal power during the mid- to the late nineteenth century." Although yellow fever was not one of the important diseases in the book, one epidemic was mentioned that "tore through New Orleans in 1862." This outbreak, according to Downs, "tore through the region, infecting hundreds of people, both black and white." And because New Orleans had no "established system of privies and a quarantine area, people turned to the city's streets when they became ill, which were soon filled with black vomit, which is symptomatic of yellow fever infections."[43]

This item immediately called for further investigation: an 1862 New

Orleans outbreak that I had missed? And streets filled with black vomit? The source cited was Benjamin Butler's memoir, which I had used years ago. Reexamining *Butler's Book*, I found his report of only two cases of yellow fever in New Orleans in 1862. Numerous cases and deaths occurred among ship crews at the Quarantine Station about seventy miles downriver from the city, but the fever never spread beyond quarantine. In 1864, Butler was concerned with a yellow fever outbreak in New Bern, North Carolina, which, he said, affected about half the population there, both black and white, as well as many troops.[44] This is probably Downs's "New Orleans epidemic." I was unable to find in the pages cited any reference by Butler to city streets "filled with black vomit."

A relatively new field called evolutionary, ecological, or environmental history involves a convergence of natural sciences, social sciences, and humanities in the broadest possible multidisciplinary arena. *Yellow Fever, Black Goddess: The Coevolution of People and Plagues*, by the eminent biologist Christopher Wills, offers a strong example of the "evolutionary theme, a dance between survival and extinction in which both host and parasite take part." Each infectious disease is a variation of this process. Both humans and microbes have evolved through "an endless war that has shaped not just the diversity of our own species but that of the entire living world," a diversity that is important to our own long-term survival on the planet. Despite the book's title, there is little about yellow fever itself, but much about plague, cholera, malaria, AIDS, and other human-microbe relationships. Having noted the recent resurgence of malaria and dengue fever in Latin America and other areas, Wills suggests that yellow fever, also a mosquito-borne disease, may be "another epidemiological time bomb." The interaction between environmental factors and human activity, deliberate or inadvertent, is the complex multidisciplinary subject some medical and other historians now study.[45]

J.R. McNeill, son of noted historian William McNeill, also offers new perspectives on environmental and medical history with his impressive work, *Mosquito Empires: Ecology and War in the Greater Caribbean, 1620-1914*. In this book, he tracks the influence of malaria and yellow fever during three centuries of colonial and revolutionary wars and imperialist ambitions in "the Greater Caribbean" (an area he defines as an ecological unit that includes the coastal areas of the southern United States, Mexico, Central America, the islands, the northern coast of South America, and the Atlantic coast from Brazil to Virginia). McNeill brings together and makes sense of an enormous amount of history in this large geographical area during a long period of time using an ecological lens and focusing on the various consequences of interrelationships among the environment, mosquitoes, microbes, and human ambitions and actions.

Survivors of yellow fever gain life-long immunity against the disease (and repetitive experience with malaria provides a measure of resistance). This process within a few generations after conquest and settlement gave rise to local (mainly Spanish) colonial populations that possessed "differential immunity," which served as a military advantage against rival European armies. Lacking prior exposure to yellow fever, invading troops confronted not only the defenders, but also destruction by disease. McNeill shows how this "differential immunity" enjoyed by most local, native-born populations meant that outsiders, newcomers, military or otherwise, were the ones most vulnerable to the "Stranger's Disease" (well-known in nineteenth-century New Orleans). This insider advantage worked repeatedly through many decades, among the several European nations competing for power and wealth in the Greater Caribbean. "Differential immunity" also facilitated Haitian success in "world history's largest slave revolt" with the devastation of French troops by yellow fever as they attempted to suppress that revolution. As a result of this decisive defeat, Napoleon abandoned his imperial plans for the Americas and sold France's vast Louisiana colony to the United States. Although yellow fever was the more important military factor in the Greater Caribbean, it appears that malaria served as a potent ally of the American revolutionaries by crippling the British troops at Yorktown.

By the early nineteenth century, Latin American revolutionaries fighting for independence found yellow fever working for their side against the armies sent from Spain to suppress rebellion. For almost two centuries, the immunity difference had helped Spain defend its empire, using mainly creole (native-born) forces; later the differential immunity helped the creole revolutionaries win their independence from Spain. A final important point from the book is that during the twentieth century, with expanding knowledge of preventive medicine, population differentials in disease vulnerability came to depend more on wealth or poverty than on previous disease experience or ancestry. Rich, well-developed societies had the means to provide pure water, sanitary facilities, vaccinations, and effective medicines for many diseases. As a result, "the rich got healthier and the healthy got richer (and more powerful)," but, as McNeill points out, this situation can change, and probably will. His ground-breaking study is perhaps the most important new work relating to yellow fever that I have encountered in my explorations.[46]

In contrast to McNeill's wide-angle, far-ranging view, although with

Introduction   xxxv

similar interest in disease and imperial power, Mariola Espinosa's *Epidemic Invasions* takes laser-like aim at yellow fever in relation to United States policies toward Cuba in the late nineteenth and early twentieth century. The eradication of the perennial threat of yellow fever to the U.S. was deemed essential for the protection of the southern states and the nation's economy, and for the pursuit of commercial and imperialistic ambitions in the Caribbean and in Panama. American interest in Cuba had earlier roots, but discussion intensified after the devastating yellow fever epidemic of 1878, and another outbreak in 1897, both apparently introduced from Havana, a major endemic center of the disease. Although the Spanish government had no interest in selling Cuba, or taking responsibility for controlling yellow fever there, it was, however, engaged in a fierce ongoing attempt to suppress the Cuban rebellion, and the U.S. found grounds for action. According to Espinosa, control of yellow fever was a principal motivation in 1898 for U.S. intervention in the Spanish-Cuban-American War, and for imposing military occupation until 1902, and again in 1906.

This U.S. domination of Cuba (despite its "independence") resembles, in many important respects, European power relations with colonies in Asia and Africa. The "benevolent" work against disease was undertaken for the benefit of the "liberating" country, not the occupied one. The Platt Amendment included a provision requiring the Cuban government to maintain the sanitary system established during occupation, which meant that any recurrence of yellow fever would be grounds for U.S. reoccupation—which did occur. Cuba was responsible, in other words, for the protection of the U.S. from yellow fever. American newspapers, medical journals, and state and federal officials repeatedly denigrated Cubans as dirty and irresponsible and unlikely to attend to the necessary measures for control of yellow fever. Espinosa documents the protests by Cuban leaders against these charges and describes their efforts to maintain mosquito control and sanitary programs.

Because of immunity acquired through mild cases in childhood, most native Cubans (similar to antebellum New Orleanians) did not consider yellow fever a problem—except for newcomers or "foreigners," or when spreading to United States territory. With their limited resources, most of Cuba's public health expenditures had to be focused on prevention of yellow fever rather than diseases affecting their own population (tuberculosis was especially prevalent). This emphasis was necessary to avoid another takeover by the U.S., and clearly unfair in Cuban eyes because vulnerable states in the U.S. failed to establish equally rigorous sanitary and anti-mosquito regimes for their own protection.

Espinosa also confronts the issue of primacy in the "discovery" of the mosquito vector and shows its relation to national power. Using archival material, she clarifies the independent role of Jesse Lazear. Influenced by Henry Rose Carter's work on "extrinsic incubation" and Carlos Finlay's mosquito hypothesis, Lazear began experimenting with Finlay's mosquitoes while Reed and James Carroll were still preoccupied with the hunt for the germ and uninterested in mosquitoes. Not until after Lazear's death from mosquito-induced yellow fever (and two other cases) did Reed lay claim to the hypothesis and devise experiments that would disprove the filth theory and confirm "Finlay's mosquito" as yellow fever's vector. From the Cuban point of view, this appropriation of Finlay's work without sufficient credit symbolized the unfairness and illegitimacy of American domination, especially with regard to public health policies, and "the figures of Carlos Finlay and Walter Reed became . . . embodiments of independence and domination, respectively." Espinosa's brief but thoroughly documented study, from U.S. and Cuban sources, brings attention to a neglected subject, and highlights the perceptions and experience of Cubans in dealing with yellow fever and their "limited independence" imposed for decades by the powerful United States.[47]

Two books about yellow fever that I almost passed by, thinking they were probably another recounting of the same old epidemic tales about Memphis in 1878 and Philadelphia in 1793. Fortunately I took a second look, and both books offer far more than a simple retelling of old stories. Jeannette Keith's *Fever Season: The Story of a Terrifying Epidemic and the People Who Saved a City*, hot off the press (October 2012), is a well-constructed narrative that reflects in fascinating detail the lived experience and the work of "saving" Memphis in 1878. Trained both as journalist and historian, Keith writes an engrossing story, broadly researched and documented, centering on "personalities" and issues of "character," showing how various individuals responded to epidemic crisis, with strength or weakness, courage or cowardice. Five persons are traced throughout the Memphis epidemic (and afterward): a doctor, a nurse, a merchant, an editor (J. M. Keating, of the *Daily Appeal*), and a former slave, plus many others who played their part in this tragic bit of history.

Courage was expected of men; as in war, so in epidemic disaster, "manhood" required that they stand and fight. Hence, people were shocked by men who abandoned their sick families, congregations, or official positions, fleeing the city for safer ground. Women who exhibited unexpected bravery, however, seemed especially impressive. Annie Cooke turned her brothel into a yellow fever hospital where she and one of her girls, from Louisiana, remained to nurse the patients, while sending the other prostitutes away to safety. Cooke herself eventually fell victim to the fever. Also risking and sometimes losing their lives, Episcopal and Catholic nuns came to Memphis to serve as caregivers, as did other female (and male) volunteer nurses under the auspices of the Howard Association.

Using material from newspapers, diaries, letters, and official documents, Keith packs into the epidemic narrative a wealth of detail about the biographies and daily activities of her major "characters" and many other participants, describing vital tasks of maintaining order, dispensing relief, caring for the sick, collecting the corpses, digging graves, burying the dead, and organizing refugee camps outside the city. She provides an account of contemporary medical theory and therapeutics, funeral rituals, the Howard Association and its doctors and nurses, the key role of black police and black militia units, community leadership, and the Citizens Relief Committee. She underscores the critical importance of telegraphers and railroad workers, who made possible communication with the outside world and who brought in food, medicine, and other supplies from nationwide donations—many also losing their lives while supporting the city.

Despite the heroic efforts of women, blacks, and working class whites, without whose contributions the city would have collapsed into chaos, none were invited to the various banquets where "heroes" were honored at the end of the epidemic, thereby forming the official public memory of the event. Elite white men were the heroes, of course, with the absent women "toasted" in appreciation for their "support." The contributions of black residents (and white workers) were rarely acknowledged at all.

According to Keith, the yellow fever epidemic of 1878 "more than any other event, made Memphis the city that it is today." By 1900, the population had become less cosmopolitan with less ethnic diversity than before, changed by the influx of poor black and white farmers from surrounding areas, characterized by segregation, intensified racism, and eradication of black civil rights previously enjoyed. An affluent black businessman (former slave and son of a white steamboat captain), Robert Church, having amassed in post-Civil-War decades a fortune in commercial and rental properties, used his wealth and influence to open a park and build an auditorium as an "oasis" for African Americans where black music and culture and community life could thrive; and there in the Beale Street area, Memphis "became the home of the blues and the cradle of rock 'n roll."[48]

The only item in this excellent book that I question is Keith's assertion that yellow fever had not been "stigmatized" or blamed on immigrants and the lower classes because northern businessmen and their families were equally susceptible on arrival in New Orleans. Because all newcomers were at risk, she says, it was difficult to blame or scapegoat any particular group, whether based on ethnicity, race, religion, or behavior. This is *not* what I found to be the case in New Orleans. The native-born and long-resident upper class (and even one recently "acclimated" northern adolescent) blamed yellow fever epidemics on immigrants, the laboring classes, the poor, for their "mode of living"—meaning alcohol use, food preferences, unhygienic habits, and so on. First, it was the American "foreigners" arriving in Spanish and French Louisiana, later the Irish and Germans, finally the Italians, and almost always the "lower orders." The nativist and "acclimated" tendency to blame the victim—the foreigner and the poor—was alive and well in New Orleans from the late eighteenth century through the last yellow fever epidemic in 1905.[49]

Filled with new questions, ideas, and approaches, *A Melancholy Scene of Devastation*, edited by J. Worth Estes and Billy G. Smith, is a collection of essays by various contributors on public responses to the 1793 Philadelphia epidemic, not merely official responses but reactions of ordinary people and particular groups. Insights are revealed with regard to medical ideas of the times, the role of newspapers as emotional outlet and unifying force, concepts of community and different "communities," Benjamin Rush's social and political views reflected in his therapies, the African American contribution to epidemic relief, the role of black nurses and importance of nursing care, negative white reaction, and black counter-response. Other chapters discuss public-private projects for sanitary improvements, political party positions on disease causation and prevention, the political dimension of medicine and public health, the social and demographic impact of the epidemic, yellow fever after 1793, and its historiography. These thought-provoking essays show that yellow fever history remains a fertile field for cultivation.[50]

In her historiographical essay, Margaret Humphreys suggests a number of directions for future research: utilize some of the strategies employed in this collection; apply the concept of "communities" to other urban epidemics and varied responses; analyze medical writing as a distinct genre; explore in greater depth the "delicate question" of racial susceptibility and resistance, which has given rise to some controversy; investigate further the influence of medicine and disease in imperialistic ventures; broaden the scope of yellow fever study to the larger geographical area within which the disease traveled and made history, from Africa to the Americas, throughout the Caribbean islands and coastal areas of North,

Introduction xxxix

Central, and South America. (J.R. McNeill's 2010 work on "mosquito empires" in the "Greater Caribbean" has since provided a comprehensive view of this broader arena in which yellow fever and malaria influenced imperialism and revolution). As Humphreys concludes, "The new student of yellow fever should take heart—yes, there is still much to be done on this fascinating and horrible disease."[51]

And more books keep coming. Two recent publications dealing with public health (and yellow fever) are *The Contagious City: The Politics of Public Health in Early Philadelphia* by Simon Finger, and *Fevered Measures: Public Health and Race at the Texas-Mexico Border, 1848-1942* by John McKiernan-Gonzalez. Although covering exceedingly different times and places, they both analyze the role of public health issues in shaping "identities," "communities," and the expansion of state power. Finger refers to Philadelphia as "a city that fever made." The very language of eighteenth-century medicine and politics was closely interrelated, and collective concern with public health was basic in "creating a political and social community" in early Philadelphia. According to Finger, throughout the eighteenth century, a "common theme" underlying the politics of health and cultural change was "the formation of shared identities through the processes of inclusion, exclusion, and regulation."[52]

In *Fevered Measures*, McKiernan-Gonzalez asserts that "Public health, as much as formal politics, shaped the encounters between people and the states that took shape in the Texas-Mexican borderlands." He provides a complex, multilayered picture of a region along both sides of the Rio Grande, with population centers once united by the river and easy movement back and forth, but cut apart in the mid-nineteenth century when the river became an international boundary after the Texas-Mexican War. The complexity of group designations and identities is illustrated by the different labels in use at different times by different parts of the population. On the Texas side of the border, who is Mexican or American, Mexican-American, Texas-Mexican, Anglo, African American, citizen, and who decides? McKiernan-Gonzalez makes clear that U.S. public health authorities not only tried to control disease, but their "deciding who to protect became key to establishing what it meant to be Mexican or American."

The Mexican-Texas yellow fever epidemic of 1882 involved the U.S. Marine Hospital Service (later renamed the Public Health Service) and the first use of military power to enforce quarantine around a large area in South Texas to contain the disease. Quarantine, forcible vaccinations, personal disinfection, house inspection, and other measures became increasingly important in the late nineteenth century both as public health policy and as an instrument of expanding federal authority.

A yellow fever outbreak in Laredo, Texas, in 1903, gave the U.S. Public Health Service its first opportunity to use the new knowledge of the mosquito-vector in an attempt to suppress the epidemic. The federal officers complained of resistance from local authorities and residents, which limited the effectiveness of their work; nevertheless, they claimed success in keeping the disease from spreading beyond the city as a victory for "American medical expertise and political authority." (Two years later, in the New Orleans epidemic of 1905, the federal health agency had the full support of state and local officials and community business and professional leaders in the "war" on the mosquito).

In the Texas-Mexican borderlands, local, state, and U.S. health authorities by the "processes of inclusion, exclusion, and regulation" (Finger's phrase) defined and labeled population groups and influenced the formation of "identities" and "communities." Breaking new ground, McKiernan-Gonzalez traces the complications in this "Borderlands" story involving issues of race, ethnicity, nationality, class, disease, health authorities, and unequal power.[53] Public health history is often told as a triumph of cleanliness over filth, man over microbe, science over superstition, enlightenment over ignorance. And that is "partial truth." But the viewpoint of the powerless, the persons objectified, defined, and dominated by the "measures," who see arrogance, self-righteousness, zeal, prejudice, disrespect, and sometimes outright error from the "health authorities"—that viewpoint and experience, that aspect of the "truth" is not often so well-represented as it is in this study, complexities and all.

A controversial issue appearing in post-1994 yellow fever historiography concerns "black resistance" to yellow fever that occurs repeatedly in the historical record of the Americas. The question is whether it is to be explained by acquired immunity from surviving a mild or subclinical attack, or whether by some genetic trait inherited from West African ancestors, who by natural selection could have developed resistance to the lethal effects of the virus. According to Kenneth Kiple and Donald B. Cooper in the *Cambridge World History of Human Disease* (1993), and in the *Cambridge Historical Dictionary of Disease* (2003), "The question remains unresolved." As they point out, however, considerable historical evidence suggests genetic selection as a possibility.[54] This judgment coincides with my own conclusion, based on historical records from more than a century of epidemics, and formed some years before the controversy erupted.

Until the mid-nineteenth century, it was widely believed that blacks

Introduction

enjoyed complete immunity to yellow fever. Physicians and others acquainted with the disease, however, knew they were not entirely exempt. Well-aware of cases (and deaths) that occurred in the black population, official reports, medical journals, and newspapers noted their greater likelihood, however, of surviving an encounter with the fever. In epidemic after epidemic, historical sources, whether general observations or official records, have shown a pattern, not of complete exemption from the disease, but of generally milder cases and lower case fatality rates among blacks than among whites.

Kenneth Kiple's publications, in 1978 and 1984, amassed the historical and scientific sources to make the case for "biological history" and "black immunities and susceptibilities." Many observers had long commented on black resistance to yellow fever throughout the "Greater Caribbean" (to use McNeill's term), and Kiple found ample historical data and evolutionary theory to support the probability of genetic resistance to the worst effects of the disease based on West African ancestry. Sheldon Watts, in 1997, in his highly praised work, *Epidemics and History: Disease, Power and Imperialism*, denounced such "disease determinism" and declared emphatically that no such inherited immunity existed. He viewed the very notion of "black immunities" as a "Construct" devised by slave owners and physicians to justify African slave labor, a falsehood further perpetrated, he argued, by misguided historians who accepted their sources uncritically. According to Watts, all instances of presumed genetic protection could be explained by acquired immunity.[55]

Lower case-fatality rates during epidemics, it seems to me, cannot be explained entirely by immunity from surviving a previous case of the disease. Those having already acquired immunity would probably not be among the cases counted during an epidemic. The significant differential was in the percentage of cases that died, or survived. How could previously acquired immunity explain the substantial difference in case-fatality rates?

The 1878 Memphis records, for example, show approximately 11,000 cases of fever among the 14,000 African Americans in the city, and of that number some 9 percent died; whereas, almost all of the 6,000 whites remaining in Memphis became ill with the disease (98 percent), and about 70 percent of white cases died. Other examples could be cited from Louisiana epidemics with greater differentials in case-fatality rates.[56] Even taking into account the flaws of early record keeping, the sheer volume of similar data throughout the southern states over a long period of time gives weight to the idea of some kind of special resistance.

In the *Journal of Social History* in 2001, Watts wrote a "reappraisal" directed at Kiple and "his followers," to which Kiple wrote a "response," and Watts a brief counter-response. The exchange presents the divergent views, as far apart as ever.[57] Kiple's evidence seems much stronger, but Watts's challenge, at least, succeeded in calling attention to the issue. And now most historians, when dealing with the black-white differential in case-fatality data, find it necessary to mention the "unresolved question" of inherited resistance. They make it clear that the difference, if genetic, is not to be viewed as "racial" *per se*, but related to ancestral connection with a particular region (not all) of Africa where centuries of selective pressure from endemic yellow fever might have conferred some survival mechanism on the indigenous population and their descendents. Historians are also quick to acknowledge that no genetic factor has yet been scientifically identified, although evolutionary biologists expect heritable resistance to develop in a population sharing a particular geographical location with lethal viruses and their vectors during many centuries.

In *Mosquito Empires*, when it comes to the question of African slave response to yellow fever, McNeill is inclined to favor "heritable" resistance (as did all the biologists he consulted). But, however obtained, whether acquired or inherited, he says, it makes no difference to his particular argument about the significance of "differential immunity" as an advantage against invading armies of non-immunes.[58]

I am probably giving this subject too much attention, but the issue almost demanded discussion because it has generated such intense disagreement. In a different light, it deserves attention for it reveals problems of definition, perception, and judgment. Perhaps there will eventually be a definitive genetic answer, but historians reach conclusions, however tentative, based on carefully evaluated historical evidence, without always waiting for scientific "proof," desirable as it may be.[59]

Margaret Humphreys in her work on black troops in the Civil War has a brief, clear (albeit indirect) response to Watts's charge against virtually all southern historical/medical sources as unreliable. As she points out, the fact that southern physicians may have been racist does not necessarily negate their observations about differences in disease susceptibilities. She also provides a common sense discussion of the broader issue of "race" and biology; the ongoing debate among scientists and social scientists about whether to dispense with the "social construct" of racial categories altogether; the difficulties encountered in doing so; and issues in defining "human groups" in terms of population genetics, geographical location of ancestry, or self-identification. Within a few pages, Humphreys supplies

Introduction xliii

an excellent summary of several highly complex subjects.[60]

I lack the expertise to deal with the extensive and complex recent scientific literature on yellow fever and related viruses, some of which I have actually read. I will only discuss several ongoing research areas that have received attention in the popular press. During the past decade or so, research using highly sophisticated molecular techniques has been able to identify and manipulate genetic factors in viruses, vaccines, and mosquitoes, with the hope of developing new vaccines or improving old ones, and of producing genetically-engineered mosquitoes whose progeny cannot survive, or bacteria-infected mosquitoes that cannot effectively serve as virus-transmitters.

Mosquito: A Natural History of Our Most Persistent and Deadly Foe (2001), by scientist Andrew Spielman and journalist Michael D'Antonio, is a useful reference for the general reader interested in mosquitoes, the diseases they transmit, and the role of trade and travel in the global spread of vectors and viruses. The book explains how in the late 1970s and 1980s the importation of used tires from Asia, for recapping and resale elsewhere, introduced the Asian tiger mosquito (*Aedes albopictus*) into the United States. From here it spread to other places through international commerce. In previous years, piles of used tires accumulating rain water provided ideal breeding sites for the resurgence of *Aedes aegypti* in the American South; today, used tires everywhere serve as incubators for *A. albopictus* as well. Not yet associated with disease outbreaks in the U.S., this newly established mosquito can function as host for viruses that cause yellow fever, dengue, Eastern equine encephalitis, and West Nile fever, among others. Unlike *A. aegypti*, its relative, it will bite birds and various animals as well as humans, which makes this mosquito a potential "epidemiological bridge" between humans and "new" pathogens in birds, deer, and rodents—a major public health concern.[61]

As protection from yellow fever, a safe, effective vaccine (17D) has been available since the 1930s, but in recent decades (and especially since the early 2000s), vaccine-associated adverse events and allergic reactions have increased in number, some quite serious, even lethal. Infants, the elderly, pregnant and nursing women, and persons with compromised immune systems are most at risk for adverse effects such as encephalitis or multiple organ failure (neurotropic or vicerotropic disease). Aside from mosquito control and quarantine, this vaccine is the only real "weapon" against yellow fever. Because of the newly observed risks (perhaps from a shift in the attenuated live virus, or changes in vaccines), molecular biologists, geneticists, virologists, and others have focused on identifying and isolating the specific viral components needed to activate the immune response, and on constructing a safer vaccine. Progress has been reported, and a more specifically designed and targeted yellow fever vaccine made from killed virus is showing great promise, but has yet to be approved for general use.[62]

Meanwhile, in light of the increased risk, new protocols have been devised with regard to those who probably should not receive the standard vaccine, unless traveling to an area where the likelihood of exposure to yellow fever is extremely high, which is not always an easy judgment to make.[63] There are large endemic areas in South America and Africa where subclinical cases of yellow fever go unrecognized and unreported. Official reports represent only a small fraction of the World Health Organization's estimate of annual cases and deaths. Serious outbreaks do occur occasionally, and vaccination is needed for resident populations and visiting travelers.[64]

Since the 1970s, dengue (yellow fever's viral cousin, also transmitted by *A. aegypti*) has become a matter of far greater concern because of its rapid spread around the globe, with almost half of the world's population at risk. There is no treatment for dengue or yellow fever except symptomatic and supportive care; unlike yellow fever, however, for dengue no vaccine exists, but a great deal of attention is now being devoted to its development in laboratories all over the world.[65]

The problems of constructing a dengue vaccine are especially complicated. There are four different strains of the virus. A first attack (painful but seldom lethal) leaves a person immune thereafter to that one specific strain. A second attack by one of the other three types is more likely to become life-threatening. Hence, the challenge is to develop a dengue vaccine that will protect against all four strains simultaneously. Otherwise, a vaccine for only one type would put the person at risk for "severe dengue" (previously known as dengue hemorrhagic fever) with a subsequent infection by a different strain. Or as Dr. Thomas Monath has stated the problem: "Moreover, our limited understanding of viral neutralization and immune correlates of protection, and the difficulty of distinguishing cross-reactions from the development of type-specific antibodies, create challenges for vaccine development."[66]

Several public-private research endeavors using varied approaches are at different stages of development. One method involves genetic engineering of a "chimera," utilizing 17D yellow fever vaccine as a base or "vehicle" to deliver a mixture of appropriate genes from the four dengue types. The result is "live attenuated dengue-yellow fever chimeric viruses

Introduction xlv

[which] elicit antibodies only to dengue." Early trials suggest that several doses of the chimeric vaccine will be required for complete and lasting immunity. Carefully monitored field trials will also be necessary, given the potential for severe dengue to occur in later infections. Research continues on many fronts, by government agencies and corporations, using various techniques in the quest for greater understanding of mechanisms at work in the interaction between viruses, between virus and individual immune responses, and between virus and vectors.[67]

While the laboratory work on vaccines and viruses goes on, other molecular-level strategies are being directed against the *A. aegypti* mosquito, principal agent of transmission of both yellow fever and dengue viruses. Receiving the most public attention and generating considerable opposition, genetically-modified mosquitoes are referred to by some opponents as "Franken-skeeters."[68]

A two-part article in the *New Yorker* (2012) by Michael Specter presents a comprehensive readable account of the research and development of transgenic *A. aegypti*. After Oxford University scientists finally succeeded in the genetic modification of the mosquito, a British biotechnology company, Oxitec (Oxford Insect Technologies) was spun out to handle the next phase of mass production and field trials, preliminary to seeking licensure and marketing the insects. The plan involves the release of vast numbers of transgenic male mosquitoes carrying a lethal gene that will kill their progeny; in time, the mosquito population could be greatly reduced or eradicated completely. The objective is to halt the spread of dengue by eliminating its vector. Previous efforts to sterilize male *A. aegypti* by radiation rendered them too weak to compete for mates when released into wild populations. But the male transgenic mosquito is able to mate and transmit the "poison pill" to its offspring, which will hatch from eggs, but will not survive to fly. The first trials took place on Grand Cayman in the Caribbean in 2009 and 2010, and Oxitec reported a reduction in the targeted mosquito population by 80 percent in a matter of months. In Brazil where dengue is prevalent and severe, a production facility has now been established, and larger field trials are underway with similar reductions of wild populations.[69]

In the first half of the twentieth century, the *A. aegypti* had been greatly reduced in the southern states of the U.S. and in much of Latin America. Mosquito control programs gradually came to a halt because of cost and awareness of the hazards of pesticides (and the absence of epidemics). By the 1960s and 1970s mosquito populations had returned and expanded greatly in number, including the sturdy new arrival from Asia. With the reinfestation of mosquitoes came the renewed risk for dengue and yellow fever. In fact, dengue has now become "one of the most rapidly spreading viral diseases in the world."[70]

Recently, dengue cases have appeared in Key West, Florida, after an absence of some seventy years. After spending a million dollars a year on insecticide spraying, which has its own potential ill effects, the local mosquito control agency asked Oxitec about a possible trial there of the transgenic mosquito. Public reaction was swift, fiercely opposed, and soon organized against the "robo-Franken mosquitoes." Nevertheless, in 2011 Oxitec submitted a request to the Food and Drug Administration (FDA) for permission to release the transgenic insects in a trial in Key West. How long it will take for the FDA decision to grant or deny permission is unknown at this time. In Brazil, Oxitec seems to have won the support of the authorities as well as the immediate communities affected, although some opposition continues to be expressed by environmental organizations and activists.[71]

Reasons for opposing the genetically modified mosquitoes include the general fear of unintended consequences from releasing these laboratory-constructed insects into the environment, perhaps some hazard that cannot be reversed. As only the males are to be released, female mosquitoes are sorted and removed from the modified batches, but a few are always missed. What is the possible ill effect of a bite from a transgenic female mosquito (only females bite humans)? Also, a small percentage of the progeny do survive despite carrying the lethal gene; do they pose a threat of some kind? Eventual destruction of this species will leave an empty ecological niche, which some other insect will fill, perhaps an even more dangerous disease vector. Dengue virus, under pressure, might become more virulent. The virus would likely find other means of replication and transmission for survival. *A. albopictus,* which has been spreading through the international used tire trade and settling in new territory, would be a suitable candidate. Already competing with and displacing *A. aegypti* in some parts of the American South, this mosquito is more aggressive and winter-hardy and is capable of transmitting dengue, yellow fever, and other viruses.[72]

Oxitec and its supporters answer the various arguments and try to quell the fears. They say the lethal gene kills only mosquitoes, not humans, and would not be spread to humans by the biting females. *A. aegypti* does not fill a key niche, is not the main or only source of food for any bird or animal, and would not be missed if completely eradicated. In any case, extreme reduction or eradication of the mosquito population by spraying with pesticides poses similar, if not greater, problems, exerting the same pressures on dengue virus to evolve another mode of replication and transmission. The mosquitoes are already developing resistance to the use of insecticide fogging; and pesticides are a matter of concern for possible ill effects on children and on the environment. Finally, the proponents argue that the use of transgenic mosquitoes would prove less costly and more benign than insecticide spraying. They admit there are always unknowns, but relative to minimal risk, they stress the benefits; that is, the reduction or elimination of diseases spread by this particular mosquito, both yellow fever and dengue, but especially dengue, of special concern at this time.[73]

Although Oxitec with its transgenic mosquitoes is the leading contender in the anti-dengue-vector contest, another strategy by a team of Australian university scientists shows promise, without stirring up as much public opposition. Their method does not involve genetic modification, nor does it aim to eradicate the *A. aegypti*. Instead, it is designed to spread a bacterial infection among the mosquitoes that does not harm them, but interferes with their capacity to serve as host and vector of dengue virus. The *Wolbachia* bacteria, common and relatively harmless in many insects in nature, were not easy to "coax" into infecting *A. aegypti* and passing through females to generations of offspring. Once these goals were achieved, however, this *Wolbachia* strain can spread easily from each generation of infected females to their progeny, and the bacteria prevent the mosquitoes from effectively hosting the dengue virus.[74]

The first trials, in two small communities in Australia, proved effective in spreading the bacterial infection to 80 to 90 percent of the local *A. aegypti* population within a few months. The next step is to undertake larger field trials in Vietnam where dengue is endemic. Opponents of the genetically modified approach tend to support this non-transgenic strategy because it is not designed to kill off the species, but to render it incapable of transmitting the virus. The Australian scientists admit that many unknowns are still in play because every kind of intervention that affects transmission puts pressure on the virus to find another path to replicate and survive. Furthermore, it remains to be seen how much effect either type of mosquito manipulation, genetic or *Wolbachia*-infected, will actually have in suppressing the incidence of disease in human populations.[75]

Thus, the laboratory work, the mathematical models,[76] and the field trials go on, and results, while encouraging, are still uncertain. Whether chimeric vaccines; transgenic, infected, or sterilized[77] mosquitoes; or antiviral drug therapies—we are always seeking new "weapons" in our never-ending "war" on diseases. With mosquito-borne diseases (yellow fever, dengue, West Nile, malaria, and others), like it or not, we are caught in this hazardous triangle of microbe, vector, and human. We win a battle now and then, but the ongoing war is certain to continue. Our insect and microbe partners in the triangle have a much greater capacity for rapid adaptation in a changing environment than we do (either biologically or culturally, it seems).

Among the numerous works I have examined in this general survey, some items added nothing new, but used yellow fever history as a framework for fiction, or journalistic recounting of well-known stories and predicting future epidemic crises; some books and articles expanded the scope or depth of themes or topics only touched upon in *Saffron Scourge*; and some dealt with yellow fever as an important element in other historical research areas—nursing, war, imperialism, labor, disasters, and environment; plus the current scientific work using molecular-level approaches. Although these expanded topics and exciting new avenues add much to yellow fever historiography (and genetic manipulation of mosquitoes, viruses, and vaccines), I found nothing so far that substantially alters my account of yellow fever's history in Louisiana.[78]

For the most part, now twenty years after its first appearance, *Saffron Scourge* seems to be holding its own, as I note with pleasure its citation in numerous studies of nineteenth-century southern (and "the Greater Caribbean") disease experience. With the publication of this new edition, I hope it will continue to serve scholars and the general public as a useful reference and worthwhile reading for years to come.

I

THE DISEASE AND ITS EARLY HISTORY

Introduction

The history of yellow fever in Louisiana from the late eighteenth century through the early twentieth century is essentially the history of yellow fever in New Orleans. The state's largest city as well as the metropolis of the nineteenth-century South, New Orleans served as the principal port of entry for yellow fever, brought in repeatedly on ships arriving from endemic centers in the Caribbean and Central America. Transported from place to place on ocean vessels, river boats, and later on trains, this urban disease, transmitted by a household mosquito, did not spread easily in rural areas where neither human nor mosquito populations were sufficiently concentrated to support a full-fledged epidemic.

After Louisiana became American property in 1803, its population steadily and rapidly increased during the first half of the nineteenth century as French refugees from the West Indies, Anglo-Americans, and European immigrants arrived in large numbers to develop New Orleans and its hinterland. In time, the towns along the Mississippi River and other waterways, engaging in trade with New Orleans, began to experience outbreaks of yellow fever as the virus spread outward from the city through infected persons or mosquitoes. The introduction of the steamboat in the early nineteenth century vastly expanded the volume of river trade and travel, and with it the spread of the pestilence. Likewise, in the second half of the century the extension of railroad transportation facilitated the dissemination of infection to many places around the state and region where the disease had never previously occurred. The impact of a yellow fever epidemic on a small or medium-sized community resulted in terror, confusion, disorder, and serious losses, perhaps to a greater extent than in New Orleans itself with a sizeable immune population and a fatalistic acceptance of the fever.

If New Orleans enjoyed a relatively disease-free summer and autumn, the interior communities had slight cause for worry. If the Crescent City experienced a severe yellow fever epidemic, other towns might or might not be affected, depending on the extent of their communication with the city as well as other contingencies involved in the production of an epidemic. New Orleans was not only the yellow fever capital of the state, it was the yellow fever capital of the Gulf Coast and Mississippi Valley because of its position as the major center of trade with Latin America. Widespread attacks of yellow fever in the southern and valley states could usually be traced to an initial epidemic in New Orleans.

Between 1796 and 1850 New Orleans suffered a few cases of the fever every year and some fifteen to twenty outbreaks of major epidemic proportions. The 1850s witnessed the climax of yellow fever activity in Louisiana when the scourge struck violently four times within a single decade, spreading more extensively beyond the city and the state than ever before. In the postbellum years yellow fever outbreaks diminished in frequency and in virulence, appearing in serious epidemic form only four or five times. The continuing threat of the disease, however, occupied the attention of public health officials, businessmen, and the residents of southern towns until the early twentieth century.

In its numerous attacks spread over more than a century of Louisiana's history, the saffron scourge destroyed thousands of lives, cost millions of dollars, and affected almost every facet of community life. The diversity of opinion regarding the fever's cause and transmission resulted in years of disagreement over methods (and costs) of prevention. As the battle raged among those who favored sanitation, quarantine, both, or neither, the concept of public responsibility for community health gradually emerged, found public acceptance, and was crystallized into such institutional forms as the Louisiana State Board of Health, quarantine measures, and other regulatory health laws. The "scourge of the South," as yellow fever was often called in the nineteenth century, also provided a strong impetus for instituting health legislation in other southern states, especially from the outbreaks of the 1870s onward. Stimulated at least in part by widespread fear of the disease and by its disruptive effects on interstate commerce, consciousness of the federal government's role in preserving the nation's health—as well as its role in protecting commercial and transportation interests—also began to develop by the late nineteenth and early twentieth century.

The abundance of references to yellow fever in almost every primary and secondary source on nineteenth-century Louisiana reflects the pervasive and long-term influence of the disease. Personal and business correspondence, diaries, and medical essays revealed individual reactions to epidemics. Newspapers, medical journals, travel accounts, board of health reports, and other state and national documents provided information about medical and lay opinion, social conditions, and institutional responses to the recurring pestilence. Sources on yellow fever in New Orleans are voluminous. For epidemics in the small interior communities, descriptive records are scarce and often lacking altogether. New Orleans possessed the population base for a concentrated articulate medical community, associated with the earliest medical schools and medical journals in the state and region. Although the periodicals, especially the *New Orleans Medical and Surgical Journal*, received and published communications about yellow fever in towns throughout the South, most of the articles dealt with disease in the Crescent City. During the first half of the nineteenth century, after all, New Orleans ranked among the top half-dozen urban centers in the Union in population and trade. Yellow fever's recurrent depredations, however, damaged the antebellum city and continued for the rest of the century to act as a drain on its resources and its capacity to compete in the contest for metropolitan empire.

This study attempts to cover the history of yellow fever throughout Louisiana, incorporating available information on the epidemic experiences of small towns and plantation communities, with an occasional reference to other southern cities afflicted by the pestilence. New Orleans, however, remains the focal point for telling the yellow fever story. Louisiana's hundred-year ordeal with the saffron scourge may be seen as an extreme case, but in most respects the inhabitants of small interior southern towns everywhere shared the same fears and responded to epidemics in similar ways. Residents of coastal ports frequently visited by yellow fever, such as Mobile, Pensacola, Savannah, and Charleston, in contrast, were likely to resemble New Orleanians in their individual and collective reactions to the disease.

Louisiana's experience with yellow fever will be examined chronologically from 1796 through 1905, with attention to the historical peculiarities of major visitations as well as similarities observed in all epidemics. The focus will then shift to a topical discussion of medical theories and controversies, changing patterns of therapy, and the social, political, and economic effects of yellow fever during its century of influence.

Epidemiology

Almost every question relating to yellow fever served as a subject of major controversy. Physicians, journalists, and others debated these issues for decades: Was yellow fever contagious or not? Was it local in origin or imported? A specific disease or the most malignant grade of a related class of fevers? Could it be transported from one place to another? If so, was it carried by persons or did it spread through the air? Should quarantine measures, sanitary reform, or nothing at all be employed against the pestilence? Which proved more costly, the economic losses occasioned by the fever or those resulting from quarantine itself? Which treatment seemed most effective in saving lives?

Despite the scientific advances of the late nineteenth century, little was clearly settled about this complicated disease until 1901 when the United States Army Commission in Cuba headed by Walter Reed demonstrated the transmission of yellow fever from person to person by the *Aedes aegypti* mosquito. That discovery made possible at last the development of effective measures to combat the disease. Until that time, yellow fever remained a mysterious malady—erratic, unpredictable, terrifying. The disease still holds many secrets. Yet in the light of present knowledge of its pathology, etiology, and epidemiology, yellow fever can be controlled to a high degree. Furthermore, armed with that knowledge, one can more readily understand at least some of the features of past epidemics that seemed inexplicable to eighteenth- and nineteenth-century observers.

A complex malady, yellow fever is an acute virus infection occurring primarily in tropical and subtropical areas and transmitted from person to person by the female *Aedes aegypti* mosquito. This domestic or household mosquito prefers residence near human populations and selects as its breeding place artificial containers of water such as barrels, casks, cisterns, cans, or jars rather than swamps, ponds, or ditches. Primarily an urban dweller in the Western Hemisphere, the *Aedes aegypti* traveled from port to port with maritime commerce, breeding on shipboard in the open casks in which sailing vessels carried their water supply. To become infected, the mosquito must feed on the blood of a yellow fever patient within the first three or four days of the illness when the virus is at a high level of concentration in the blood stream. After an incubation period of ten or twelve days, the infected mosquito is able to transmit the virus when biting susceptible persons, and it remains infective for the rest of its life, sometimes as long as a month or more. After the infected mosquito bites a person, the incubation period before onset of the disease is usually three to six days.[1]

A delicate balance of conditions is necessary for the development of an epidemic within an area where yellow fever is not an endemic disease. First, the *Aedes aegypti* must be concentrated in substantial numbers, and the weather must be warm enough to allow for mosquito activity. Further, a considerable number of non-immune persons must be concentrated in an area where the mosquitoes are active, and the virus must be introduced into that area either by a previously infected mosquito or by a person in the incubation period or the earliest stage of the disease. The introduction of one virus-bearing mosquito or one infected person, unnoticed or unrecognized, may result in a full-scale epidemic—or it may not, depending on the circumstances. If the imported mosquito bites only those who are immune or dies before biting susceptible persons, the virus will not spread. If the person arriving with the infection is not bitten by a female *Aedes aegypti* within the first three or four days of the illness, the disease will not spread.

In the usual pattern of urban yellow fever (as opposed to jungle yellow fever, which has its own pattern), the continued propagation of the virus requires constant transmission back and forth between mosquitoes and non-immune persons. Otherwise the disease will completely disappear. Only in areas where there is a "critical mass" of human and mosquito populations, where the supply of susceptibles is continually replenished by birth or immigration, and where the climate is warm enough to permit year-round mosquito activity can urban yellow fever be maintained as an endemic disease.[2] In New Orleans, with the coming of frost each winter, mosquito activity ceased, thereby terminating the life cycle of the disease-producing virus. Commercial relations with Latin American ports, however, almost guaranteed its reintroduction through trade and travel in the spring or summer of each year—and when all the conditional requirements were met, an epidemic occurred.

Unaware of the mosquito's role as transmitter, medical thinkers before the twentieth century found it impossible to account for the strange behavior of the disease as it spread from person to person and place to place. Direct contact with the sick did not consistently produce disease, and cases appeared with no obvious connection to any previous locus of infection. Yellow fever's appearance during warm weather and its cessation with the coming of frost led to the belief that climate was related to its cause and development. Native-born persons in an area where yellow fever was endemic or frequently present exhibited an apparent immunity to the disease, while strangers or newcomers always seemed particularly vulnerable. It was long believed that creoles (the native-born) had immunity because they were accustomed since birth to the extreme heat and humidity of the region. Their immunity, however, was produced by a mild case of yellow fever in infancy or childhood which had escaped notice, and one attack, no matter how mild, confers life-long immunity. The same was true for long-term residents of New Orleans who lived through several epidemics without exhibiting any sign of the disease and were therefore considered "acclimated." To acquire immunity, they must have experienced an extremely mild case of the disease which passed with little more than headache but provided lasting protection.

According to a 1987 medical reference, up to 10 percent of clinically diagnosed cases may be fatal, but because of the many "inapparent infections" the overall death rate is considerably lower.[3] Using immunity tests (sero-surveys) on populations in the endemic areas of Latin America and Africa, twentieth-century studies have demonstrated how widespread the mild and clinically undiagnosable form has been. The prevalent idea of yellow fever as a highly malignant disease appears to be incorrect; the case fatality rate is relatively low when the large numbers of inapparent cases are taken into account. Henry Rose Carter, a meticulous and perceptive investigator of yellow fever epidemics, expressed a similar judgment in 1922:

> Yellow fever is counted, and with reason, a disease of high mortality, and yet this is not true of all epidemics. The variation of different epidemics is

> so great that it is futile to speak of an average mortality, yet it is fair to say that in the past the mortality rate recorded has been decidedly greater than the truth. This comes from not recognizing mild cases which, naturally, recovered.[4]

As Carter acknowledged from his own experiences with epidemics extending back to 1879, however, the death rates occasionally could rise to extraordinary levels. Some sources have reported fatalities as high as 50 to 85 percent of recognized cases, although such rates were admittedly exceptional.[5]

From time to time New Orleans physicians tried to calculate the statistics of yellow fever, but for most of the nineteenth century the problems of incomplete records and reporting, confused diagnoses, and inconsistent disease nomenclature made it impossible to arrive at much more than an educated guess. In any event, to the average citizen in the nineteenth century (or perhaps in any century) the case fatality rate, even if properly estimated, would have seemed largely irrelevant. In the presence of an epidemic with hundreds or even thousands dying within a matter of weeks, to know that 75 to 95 percent of the sick would recover offered small comfort. It was the general extent of mortality, not the precise rate, that impressed. It was the high visibility of death within a specific community and a short period of time, the unpredictable, random occurrences of the disease and its extreme variability in effects that prompted terror. What caused it? Where would it strike next? Who would fall victim? What could be done? No one knew.

Symptoms

The symptoms of yellow fever include a long list of physical reactions that may be present in different combinations and exhibit great variance, from the case so slight as to escape attention to the severe case with all the classic symptoms and a fatal conclusion. Some of the symptoms are similar to those of malaria, hepatitis, influenza, and dengue, and confusion in diagnosis is highly possible. The illness begins with fever, together with slight or rigorous chills. Body temperature quickly reaches $102°$ to $103°F$. In the first two to five days, nausea, vomiting, constipation, headache and muscular pain, epecially in the legs and back, extreme prostration, and restlessness are characteristic. Within a few days the fever may rise to a maximum of 104°F, seldom higher. If the disease becomes acute, jaundice or yellowness of the skin ordinarily appears, along with passive hemorrhages from various parts of the body—eyes, ears, nose, mouth, bladder, uterus. A serious sign, but one which does not invariably occur, is the so-called black vomit. Blood hemorrhaging within the stomach is acted upon by stomach acids, and the resulting product is often vomited, resembling coffee grounds in appearance. This "black vomit" seems to gush forth without any effort by the patient. In terminal cases, delirium, convulsions, or coma will occur, with death resulting from damage to the liver, kidneys, heart, and blood vessels. In the majority of cases, recovery begins within a week or two after onset, and full convalescence sometimes requires several weeks.[6]

Parson Theodore Clapp, who lived through a succession of yellow fever epidemics in nineteenth-century New Orleans, remarked that he found it almost impossible to sleep during the periods of pestilence, so disturbed were his dreams by the agonizing sights of patients he had visited. His graphic description of a yellow fever victim provides some basis for understanding the terror and revulsion that epidemics produced:

> Often I have met and shook hands with some blooming, handsome young man today, and ... [later] I have been called to see him in the black vomit, with profuse hemorrhages from the mouth, nose, ears, eyes, and even the toes; the eyes prominent, glistening, yellow, and staring; the face discolored with orange color and dusky red.
>
> The physiognomy of the yellow fever corpse is usually sad, sullen, and perturbed; the countenance dark, mottled, livid, swollen, and stained with blood and black vomit; the veins of the face and whole body become distended, and look as if they were going to burst ....[7]

In the period just before death, patients may become "delirious and wildly agitated." Such scenes of "violent and uncontrollable agitation" were awesome to behold and contributed to the sense of panic often manifested during epidemics.[8]

The Fever's Many Labels

The characteristic jaundice or yellow tint of the skin gave rise to the now universally accepted name of the disease, yellow fever. In his classic

The Disease and its Early History

work on the disease, George Augustin collected a list of 152 synonyms for yellow fever from American, English, Spanish, Italian, and Portuguese sources. In his opinion, no other malady had so many different terms applied to it. Several commonly used labels were American fever, American typhus, ardent fever, bilious putrid or bilious malignant fever, black vomit or *vomito negro, maladie de la saison, maladie du diable, mal de Siam*, Yellow Jack, and Stranger's Fever.[9] Residents of New Orleans and other towns along the Mississippi River and the Gulf Coast began to think of the pestilence in anthropomorphic terms as the disease became a common occurrence. Hence, popular names developed, and newspaper editors and other commentators often referred to yellow fever as "Bronze John on his Saffron Steed," "His Saffron Majesty," "the Saffron Warrior," and "the Saffron Scourge."

Nineteenth-century observers of epidemics portrayed the disease metaphorically, endowed it with an identity, called it the "enemy," the "visitor," the "invader." They spoke of "attacks" on cities and persons—sometimes "indiscriminate," sometimes "selective." The "King of Terrors" was said to "claim" victims, "levy tribute," "cut down the ranks," and during winter to "retreat from our shores." In another common metaphor, the "scourge"—perhaps in the hands of God, or wielded by some unknown material force—"lashed" at the populace, "cut down" victims, brought great suffering, and implied punishment or chastisement for violating the laws of God or the laws of nature.

Dr. John S. Billings of the United States Army Medical Service, one of the nation's leading nineteenth-century public health advocates and outstanding medical bibliographer, commented in 1880 on this tendency to personify the disease. A yellow fever epidemic was perceived, he said, as the presence of "an invisible entity presenting so many peculiarities in its results that it was the most natural thing in the world to imagine it as being endowed with the attributes of purpose and will, and to speak of it as 'Bronze John' or 'Yellow Jack.'" Billings also observed that this approach to the malady was especially common among those most familiar with it. Physicians and nurses, keenly aware from experience of the vagaries of the disease, were likely to discuss Yellow Jack "in much the same terms as they would speak of a highly disreputable but very interesting acquaintance—a sort of Bohemian among diseases."[10]

It still seems "the most natural thing in the world" to personify yellow fever and to write about epidemics in a metaphorical way, especially after extensive exposure to nineteenth-century sources. In fact it seems necessary in order to convey a sense of the way epidemics have been experienced. Yellow Jack sometimes appears as a villain in a mystery, sometimes as an invading enemy to be fought and driven out. The complex ecological interaction of virus, mosquitoes, humans, and environment defines the parameters of epidemics; the physical response of a human host to the parasitic activity of the virus constitutes an instance of disease; yet the phenomenon of epidemic disease also assumes another dimension in subjective human experience and as a social reality with wide-ranging effects. In that respect, "it" seems to require some measure of reification and metaphorical expression.

Personification and metaphor in nineteenth-century accounts of the disease provided a framework for describing epidemic "visitations" and gave some sense of understanding through familiarity. Labels can function in many useful ways. Repeated references to yellow fever throughout the nineteenth century as the "strangers' disease," in describing its seeming preference for the "unacclimated," served to diminish its importance, to set it apart from those who considered the city their own, to make it a disease of the foreign, the poor, the negligible. New Orleans newspaper editors often insisted that "our" city was the healthiest in the Union—*except* for the strangers. While recent immigrants did serve as yellow fever's principal victims, natives were not always exempt and New Orleans was not otherwise generally healthy. Nevertheless, for years the "strangers" served as a scapegoat for epidemics, and the "acclimated" New Orleanians could view the problem as something other than their own.[11]

In her provocative essay, *Illness as Metaphor*, Susan Sontag explored the ways in which certain illnesses have been used as metaphors in cultural and social description, and conversely how imagery is borrowed from economics, science fiction, the military, and other areas in discussing disease processes—all of which she viewed as a deplorable, false way of dealing with disease. Illness, after all, is not a metaphor. Sontag did make a distinction between the relatively benign "premodern" medico-social imagery and the "modern" use of metaphor in which the "master illness" (tuberculosis in the nineteenth century and cancer in the twentieth) becomes a symbol for the fears, weaknesses, evils, and corruptions of the times. Such associations, she argued, make the illness seem even more frightful or hopeless than it may actually be, and in the absence of etiological knowledge or therapeutic control, blame may be projected upon the sick for bringing their illness upon themselves through a particular temperament or life style.

In a projection not entirely unlike that which Sontag described for tuberculosis and cancer, yellow fever's "victims," the strangers or newcomers, especially the poor, were sometimes seen as the architects of their own misery. And the "strangers' disease" image, with the associated belief in creole or native immunity, did serve to sustain a nativist, exclusionist, upper-class, laissez-faire bias. Nevertheless, most of the metaphoric expressions associated with yellow fever served mainly as a way of "explaining" a mysterious, frightening phenomenon in terms of a more familiar set of images. As profound an impact as yellow fever had on nineteenth-century New Orleans, it did not itself become a metaphor for the problems and discontents of the day.[12]

Whatever name it was called, yellow fever continued to baffle the doctors in their attempts at treatment. From the late eighteenth to the mid-nineteenth century physicians tried to "subdue" the disease by bloodletting, cold baths, huge doses of quinine, calomel or other mercurial compounds, and a variety of heroic measures. Before the end of the nineteenth century they had generally abandoned harsh remedies in favor of a moderate supportive therapy. Observers often remarked that some patients died and others recovered whatever the form of treatment, including none at all. A therapeutic approach that seemed to work well during one epidemic might fail completely in the next, and in various cases the same regimen had different results. There is still no specific drug to cure yellow fever. Complete bed rest and good nursing care are considered of vital importance, and therapy is designed primarily to alleviate the symptoms. According to one yellow fever expert writing in 1951, most patients recover "no matter what is—or is not—done for them," but nothing whatsoever seems to help in certain cases of severe infection.[13]

Origin and Early History

Many of the long-standing medical questions about yellow fever have been answered in the twentieth century, though increasing knowledge has also revealed additional unknowns relating to the virus and its sometimes inexplicable activity. Aside from the medical questions, some historical problems encountered by early researchers continue to the present. The origin and early history of the disease are by no means clear. It was almost certainly unknown to Europeans before the discovery of the New World. Because the disease was first observed and recorded in the Western Hemisphere, nineteenth-century medical chroniclers generally considered Latin America the fever's native clime.

In his massive *History of Yellow Fever* published in 1909, George Augustin concluded that the evidence pointed to Mexico, Central America, and the West Indies as "the original cradle of the awesome scourge." He rejected the opinion that Africa was yellow fever's place of origin, a hypothesis advanced at various times in the nineteenth century. Twentieth-century medical and historical studies, however, indicate a high probability that yellow fever originated in Africa and that both the virus and the *Aedes aegypti* mosquito were gradually introduced into the Western Hemisphere by vessels engaged in the slave trade. Although never experimentally tested, it has long been observed that yellow fever in black people generally exhibits mild effects and very low fatality rates. This racial tolerance or resistance may be attributable to the ancient African origin of the disease.[14]

Transplanted to the New World from Africa, the yellow fever mosquito and virus eventually gained a foothold in their new tropical habitat. The first epidemics of yellow fever clearly recognizable from descriptive records occurred in Yucatan, Havana, and Barbados in the 1640s. By the late seventeenth century the disease was established at various points in the Caribbean; in the 1690s it began to appear in North American ports. Intermittently during the eighteenth century, ships from the West Indies brought yellow fever into Atlantic port cities, causing serious outbreaks in Charleston, New York, Boston, and Philadelphia.[15]

In French Colonial Louisiana

Possible outbreaks of yellow fever in early colonial Louisiana, as well as the date of its first appearance in New Orleans, long have been subjects for historical speculation and disagreement. The difficulties arise in part from a scarcity of medical records for the colonial period. Letters and documents reporting disease ordinarily provided a few brief statements, using vague terminology for the ailments that plagued the inhabitants—

such as the "fever," the "malady," the "pestilence."[16] The task of the medical historian who attempts to trace a specific disease is complicated not only by the absence of uniformity in disease nomenclature and the limited diagnostic procedures of past times, but more directly by the prevailing medical theories that emphasized the essential unity of all disease.[17]

Joseph Jones, an eminent nineteenth-century Louisiana physician, health official, and prolific medical historian, examined the records available to him and concluded that the disease had been transmitted occasionally during the early eighteenth century to French settlements on the Gulf Coast through contacts with the West Indies where yellow fever prevailed. But he noted several factors that probably served to postpone its appearance as an epidemic in New Orleans: the long and tedious trip (about 100 miles) up the Mississippi River to the town, the sparse population, and the limited commercial activity during the French colonial period. Nevertheless, Dr. Jones refused to declare positively that yellow fever had never visited New Orleans under French rule. No medical journal or native medical work describing the local maladies ever appeared in French colonial Louisiana. Jones wisely concluded that the mere absence of medical records failed to demonstrate the total absence of yellow fever.[18]

Writing in the early twentieth century, Alcée Fortier, one of Louisiana's major historians, admitted that little could be learned from the records about eighteenth-century epidemics. He believed tht yellow fever first appeared in French colonial Louisiana as the cause of Commandant Sauvolle's death near Biloxi in August, 1701.[19] But it is also possible that the commandant died of "tertian fever" (malaria) or some other malady among the various complaints reported in the settlement that summer. The recorded evidence is simply too vague to allow a conclusive retrospective diagnosis.[20] Epidemics later presumed to have been yellow fever occurred at Biloxi in 1702 and 1704 and Mobile in 1704 and 1705.[21] According to virtually all accounts, there is no further record of yellow fever activity in colonial Louisiana for almost six decades, and the evidence for the 1760s is suggestive rather than conclusive.

"Mal de Siam" in 1739

Eighteenth-century sources regularly described summer and fall as the "sickly season" in the colony. It seems that malaria was one of the common chronic and debilitating maladies, which in conjunction with a variety of unidentifiable hot weather "fevers and fluxes" augmented French Louisiana's seasonal death list. Standard histories of Louisiana mention a severe outbreak of "autumnal disease" in 1739 among Bienville's troops concentrated at Fort Assumption on the Mississippi (near the present site of Memphis) for a campaign against the Chickasaw Indians. Troops recently arrived from France and from Canada were especially hard hit by illness, whatever it might have been, and large numbers died. According to Charles Gayarré's account, approximately 500 of Bienville's 1,200 white troops died of disease that fall and winter.[22]

A French officer who had arrived in Louisiana in June, 1739, with reinforcements for the Chickasaw expedition reported in his journal that many were sick when they first landed at the Balize, an outpost at the mouth of the Mississippi. During several weeks spent in New Orleans, 70 men died and 75 others were too sick to travel when the companies were finally dispatched to Fort Assumption. As the transport vessels continued upriver, sick soldiers had to be left behind at various posts along the way, and some were sent back to New Orleans. Throughout the months of the campaign, the officer occasionally noted in his journal the number of sick troops and officers returned to New Orleans, including himself in March, 1740. But he offered not a single descriptive clue to the nature of the prevailing sickness.[23]

Such fragmentary evidence raises and leaves unanswered a number of questions. Was "the sickness" one disease or several? Was it principally malarial fever, as several historians have suggested? Did the French troops bring the disease with them, or did they encounter an infection present in Louisiana, or both? It is safe to assume that the soldiers suffered from a variety of disorders, universally the case whenever men were transported long distances and concentrated for military ventures, especially in hot and humid regions unfamiliar to them. Malaria was almost certainly one of the maladies affecting the newly arrived troops. Intestinal infections of various kinds usually plagued military expeditions because of unsanitary habits and conditions of camp life. Scurvy, a vitamin-deficiency disease, was a common ailment among soldiers and marines during long periods when fresh fruits and vegetables were altogether missing from their diet. In addition to all these afflictions, it now seems that yellow fever was also present among the troops in Louisiana that sickly season of 1739.

A document filed in the *Archives Nationales* in Paris, apparently escaping the attention of previous researchers, provides strong indications of a yellow fever outbreak in New Orleans and vicinity in 1739. Henri de Louboey, one of the king's lieutenants in Louisiana, wrote a ten-page letter to the minister of marine, October 12, 1739, reporting on the state of affairs in the colony, including the Chickasaw campaign, ship arrivals and departures, crop prospects, weather, and disease, among other matters. This letter is probably the strongest direct evidence yet found for the presence of yellow fever in the city prior to the well-documented epidemic of 1796. Louboey reported that *"La contagion"* continued to "ravage" New Orleans, and victims of both sexes and every age were buried daily. The number of French troops lost since arrival in the colony totaled almost 150, counting a few soldiers still hospitalized in New Orleans whom the physicians did not expect to recover. The disease had claimed many victims at the Balize as well as in New Orleans. "There is no doubt that the King's vessels brought us the malady from St. Domingue," he wrote. The troopships had stopped there when *"le mal de Siam"* was prevalent.[24]

In his lengthy report Louboey devoted far more attention to a controversy involving officers' ceremonial rights and privileges at burial services than he did to the epidemic itself, which received only a few lines. He did, however, link the disease with Saint-Domingue, where French vessels on the way to Louisiana usually stopped for water and supplies, or for commerce, and where yellow fever was well known, and he used the label "mal de Siam," an explicit reference to yellow fever. Although a misnomer, that term was one of the common names for the disease in the French West Indies.[25]

There is ample evidence from other sources that Saint-Domingue had numerous outbreaks of yellow fever in the 1730s and 1740s. The disease prevailed in various sectors of the Caribbean from the 1690s through the 1760s, especially in those areas undergoing rapid population growth and commercial development, and especially during colonial wars. After some twenty years of virtual absence or quiet endemicity during which the disease was considered unusual, or almost forgotten, the French, Spanish, and British West Indies again experienced the eruption of violent yellow fever epidemics during the 1790s. Revolution and war provided the conditions for transforming sporadic infection into raging epidemic disease and spreading it around and beyond the islands.[26] Thousands of non-immune European troops concentrated in the Caribbean served as fuel to the fever, and shiploads of refugees in flight from slave uprisings or from war and occupation transported disease and mosquitoes from place to place—including Philadelphia and New Orleans.

Yellow fever outbreaks in British North America exhibited a pattern reflecting the periods of greatest prevalence in the West Indies. Introduced into Charleston, Philadelphia, and New York on several occasions between 1699 and 1706, the disease appeared again as a frequent visitor to the Atlantic ports in the 1730s and 1740s. Thereafter, except for a brief recurrence in the 1760s, the pestilence seems to have been absent from British North America until a new wave of epidemics struck the shores in the 1790s. This chronological pattern closely coincides with the years of European and colonial wars, from "King William's War" in the 1690s intermittently through the wars of the French Revolution in the 1790s.[27]

Colonial Louisiana's experience with yellow fever epidemics followed a similar pattern: a few occurrences on the Gulf Coast around the turn of the eighteenth century at the beginning of French settlement; an epidemic in New Orleans in 1739 (and possibly in 1740[28]); several outbreaks in the 1760s which might have been yellow fever; and the virulent pestilence of the 1790s, finally recognized as yellow fever, and beginning a century of continuing visitations, disruptive and costly in their impact upon the Crescent City.[29]

There are reasons to believe that yellow fever appeared in colonial New Orleans from time to time in years following the 1730s, producing sporadic unrecognized cases among the *habitants* and mild, inapparent cases among their children. The regularity of contact with the West Indies almost guaranteed the recurrent presence of the disease, even as the slave ships from West Africa assured the continuing presence of the infection in the West Indies. Frequent reintroduction of yellow fever in a fairly stable or slowly growing population would have functioned as virtual endemicity, providing the opportunity for occasional infection (and the lasting immunity which it conferred on the survivor). Lacking a large concentrated susceptible population, however, and perhaps also lacking a sufficiently large vector population, early colonial New Orleans did not ordinarily provide the optimum conditions for a few cases of yellow fever to expand to epidemic dimensions. What made 1739 a special situation and created the conditions for a notable outbreak was the large number of French troops—at least 700 non-immunes, crowded on vessels, bringing mosquitoes and virus with them from Saint-Domingue, and sharing the disease with other susceptibles in New Orleans.

The Disease and its Early History   17

New Orleans' population in 1739 was probably at least 2,000, with slaves constituting perhaps 20 to 30 percent of the total.[30] The port's commerce was increasing by the 1730s with many ships arriving from Saint-Domingue, Martinique, and Guadaloupe. A royal decree in 1737 encouraged commercial activity by exempting from customs for a ten-year period all products exchanged between Louisiana and the West Indies. During the 1720s, several thousand African slaves had been imported to Louisiana by the Company of the Indies, probably twice as many as arrived during the next four decades.[31] Whether the yellow fever mosquito was introduced to Louisiana from Africa in the slave trade or by Caribbean commerce cannot be determined; probably both sources contributed pioneer stock which eventually established a well-entrenched creole *Aedes aegypti* population in Louisiana by the late eighteenth century.

Other Eighteenth-Century Outbreaks

Associated with the arrival of Spanish troops from Havana, New Orleans' epidemics of the 1760s were probably yellow fever, but the disease was not clearly described in contemporary records. In 1796, although established residents were less affected than newcomers, indicating previous exposure, local observers considered the yellow fever a strange and puzzling new pestilence. Until the 1820s, although increasingly common in New Orleans, yellow fever continued to be described by some as a new disease each time it reappeared. Residents of the Caribbean islands behaved similarly. When long periods passed without epidemics, they tended to forget the virulent form of the malady. When a sudden influx of newcomers sparked an epidemic, the local populace, although exhibiting immunity, considered yellow fever something altogether new and strange. One may assume that during the interim, the infection continued to affect native children as a mild fever and that the occasional adult cases received some common label such as bilious remittent fever. Whether yellow fever was truly endemic or only virtually so, regular opportunities for children and susceptible adults to contract the disease would have had the same result.[32]

Various dates have been suggested in Louisiana's medical and historical literature for the arrival of yellow fever in New Orleans: 1765, 1766, 1769, 1791, 1793, and 1796. Most authorities have agreed that 1796 was the year of the first unquestionable large-scale yellow fever epidemic in New Orleans. Whether that epidemic was also the initial appearance of the disease in the city has been the open question. On the basis of Louboey's letter and other evidence regarding patterns of prevalence elsewhere, a strong case can now be made for 1739 as the year of the first identifiable yellow fever outbreak in New Orleans. Of course, Louboey might have been wrong in describing the disease as "mal de Siam," but as an experienced colonial official, he must have known something about disease in the West Indies, and if familiar with the label, he was probably familiar with the disease. If 1739 was indeed the first epidemic year, it was probably not the first time yellow fever cases had been present in New Orleans, and it was almost certainly not the last appearance prior to the 1760s, or the 1790s. Contemporary confusion about the nature of fevers as well as selective and collective amnesia on certain matters compound the problems of reconstructing the early history of this disease.

Mobile and Pensacola suffered yellow fever attacks in 1765, and New Orleans was described as exceedingly unhealthy that year. Yellow fever was probably present, but there is no record to confirm it. In 1766, the year Antonio de Ulloa arrived with troops from Cuba to take possession of Louisiana for Spain, New Orleans suffered from an epidemic later said to have "closely resembled" yellow fever.[33]

A sketch of epidemics appearing in *DeBow's Review* in 1846 stated that "The Yellow Fever, according to tradition, was first introduced into New Orleans in 1769, by a British vessel from Africa with slaves." Dr. Joseph Jones, however, writing in the 1870s, could find no evidence to support that tradition. Dr. Bennet Dowler, another notable nineteenth-century Louisiana physician and student of yellow fever's history, also doubted that the epidemic of 1769 had been yellow fever. He considered it impossible to identify the disease from available records. Chroniclers writing soon after the unquestionable 1796 outbreak who called it the *first* appearance of the disease could have questioned living witnesses about previous occurrences, and Dowler felt certain that the chroniclers "would have been contradicted, had they made erroneous statements as to the period of its invasion." Many witnesses of the 1790s epidemics in the Caribbean as well as in New Orleans, however, were unable to relate the disease to any they had known before. Writing some twenty years after Dowler, Jones was convinced that the disease had been present to some degree in 1791, 1794, and 1795.[34]

Around 1840 Dr. Daniel Drake, midwestern physician, educator, and medical author, visited New Orleans, made personal inquiries about the first yellow fever invasion, and decided upon 1791 as the fateful year. He based his conclusion on the testimony of "a venerable citizen" of the city.[35] Dr. Erasmus Darwin Fenner discussed the question in the 1840s with five elderly gentlemen who had settled in New Orleans between 1797 and 1804; all told him that the disease was "spoken of familiarly" when they first arrived. One said he distinctly remembered an eminent physician's remark in the early 1800s that the first yellow fever year was 1793. One commentator not so far removed in time from the events at issue, Berquin-Duvallon, who traveled through Louisiana in 1802, wrote: "This disease has now for seven years, made every summer, great ravages at New-Orleans. . . ." From his inquiries he had learned that yellow fever was unknown in the city before 1796.[36] Unknown and unrecognized does not necessarily mean nonexistent. Individual perceptions and memories have not always accurately reflected the historical reality of collective experience with disease.

Certainly some cases of yellow fever occurred in New Orleans in the years before 1796. Under Spanish authority since the 1760s, New Orleans had experienced remarkable population growth and greatly expanded opportunities for the importing of infected mosquitoes and persons, especially through an increasing volume of trade and frequent communication with Havana, Santo Domingo, and other Caribbean areas where the disease was common. That the 1796 epidemic affected newcomers so much more severely than natives and long-term residents indicates an extensive period prior to 1796 during which some New Orleanians acquired immunity through unrecognized light attacks of yellow fever. It is certain that 1796 saw the first well-documented visitation of the disease in New Orleans, the first to be detailed with some precision in private letters and official documents, and the first to be identified by contemporaries with the pestilence called yellow fever which Philadelphia and other Anglo-American seaports recently had suffered.

II

THE FIRST MEMORABLE YELLOW FEVER EPIDEMIC IN NEW ORLEANS, 1796

The French planted their first Louisiana settlement in 1699 at Biloxi on the Gulf Coast. Other outposts were established in the early 1700s, including New Orleans on the Mississippi River in 1718. Despite the efforts of adventurers, investors, and officials, the Louisiana colony grew very slowly during almost six decades of French rule. After losing Canada and the Ohio Valley to the British in the Great War for Empire, France ceded Louisiana to her ally Spain in the 1760s and withdrew for a time from the imperial competition for North America. Spain governed the province for almost three and a half decades before trading it back to France in 1800, and in 1803 France sold the vast territory to the United States.

Under Spanish administration the colony developed and prospered as never before. Its population increased from less than 10,000 when the Spanish took control to more than 50,000 at the close of their tenure. New Orleans, the colony's capital, had maintained a population of some 3,000 from 1744 until 1769; under Spanish influence its population had almost tripled by 1800. The Spanish government encouraged immigration to the province by offering land grants, and in the case of Acadians and Isleños (from the Canary Islands), additional subsidies as well. Land and commercial opportunity attracted Anglo-Americans, and during the turbulent 1790s Louisiana received a large influx of French refugees from the West Indies in flight from revolutionary turmoil and slave insurrection.[1] These French colonials brought with them a knowledge of sugar culture and probably some cases of yellow fever.

Plantation agriculture and the slave labor system expanded and became more firmly established as the foundation for an affluent planter-merchant aristocracy. In the 1790s sugar and cotton replaced tobacco and indigo as Louisiana's staple crops. As agricultural productivity in the colony and in the developing American backcountry stimulated commercial activity, the Spanish government altered its restrictive policies to allow a brisk trade with imperial rivals. After the Mississippi River and the port of New Orleans were opened to American use by treaty in 1795, the aggressive entrepreneurs of the new republic soon succeeded in bringing Louisiana into their economic orbit, a development which led to American political absorption as well.

The 1790s brought a series of crises to Francisco Louis Hector, Baron de Carondelet, Louisiana's governor for most of the decade (1791-97). The French Revolution had widespread repercussions not only in Europe but throughout the various colonial empires. Faced with the possibility of invasion by France, or Britain, or the United States, or some combination thereof, Carondelet worked to strengthen Louisiana's frontier defenses, to stabilize Indian relations, and to keep order in the Spanish province among rebellious pro-French elements and among the increasingly restless slaves. At the same time, the governor initiated policies to promote commercial and agricultural expansion and arranged for municipal improvements such as a drainage canal, street lamps, and night watches for New Orleans. Several hurricanes struck the area in 1794, and a major fire that year destroyed about one-third of the buildings in the city. Carondelet undertook relief measures, arranging for special shipments of flour from Havana, Vera Cruz, and the United States. In 1795 the governor managed to abort a slave revolt which was planned in the Pointe Coupée district.[2]

Adding one more disaster to Carondelet's agenda, yellow fever arrived in New Orleans in the summer of 1796 and quickly became a full-fledged epidemic. This outbreak was the city's first clearly recognized encounter with yellow fever and the first to supply historians with several contemporary records containing more than the usual simple declaration that disease prevailed in the vicinity. Brief official reports filed by the Spanish attorney-general and the intendant, together with a series of letters written by a prominent resident, Baron Joseph Xavier Pontalba, to his wife, provide revealing glimpses of that extensive visitation and its impact on the city. Fragmentary and blurred as these glimpses may be, they are still a great deal more enlightening than any previous references to New Orleans' epidemic fevers.

Although it seems fairly certain that the yellow fever virus had been present earlier in the 1790s, in the 1760s, and probably in 1739, the experience of 1796 can be described as the first *memorable* yellow fever epidemic in New Orleans. That year the disease was perceived as something entirely new—in New Orleans and in several Caribbean centers, including Saint-Domingue, where yellow fever had been recorded on many previous occasions. Allowing for the possibility of an especially virulent form of the virus, one can still say that it was probably the scope as well as the intensity of the outbreak which shocked and impressed itself on memory. In New Orleans the disease attacked hundreds of newcomers, and in the Caribbean it wiped out recently arrived European troops by the thousands. One historian has referred to the renewed Carribean outbreaks of yellow fever in the 1790s as a veritable "pandemic," stirred and spread widely by the large-scale movements of military and refugee populations associated with revolution and war. Refugees from Saint-Domingue transported the infection that sparked the devastating yellow fever epidemic in Philadelphia in 1793, and undoubtedly they also helped to disseminate the disease wherever they fled to safety, including other North America ports and islands of the Caribbean, especially Cuba and Jamaica.[3]

Like a powder keg waiting for a spark, New Orleans in 1796 possessed the necessary elements for a major epidemic explosion: a white population that had grown rapidly, with many adult newcomers never before exposed to yellow fever, living in close communion near the river front; and a mosquito population which by this time had certainly developed a permanent local base. The numbers of *Aedes aegypti* might also have been increased by a vastly expanded local food supply—not only from the blood of the human population, but from the recent successful cultivation and processing of sugar in the vicinity, making ever-increasing quantities of sugar and molasses available for shipping from New Orleans docks.[4] Given a concentrated human population of susceptibles surrounded by a large population of *Aedes aegypti*, actively biting and breeding during the hot months of summer and fall, a yellow fever epidemic can be sparked by the arrival of one infected mosquito or one recently infected person. There was ample opportunity for the introduction of the infection as numerous ships arrived in New Orleans loaded with people and mosquitoes along with other cargo from the Caribbean islands.

According to Intendant Juan Ventura Morales, the epidemic appeared in late August, continued to prevail at the end of October, and "has terrified and still keeps in a state of consternation the whole population of this town." Early in September Baron Pontalba wrote his wife that "the maladies are increasing here, and they are now more dangerous than ever." Throughout September, October, and early November his daily letters were filled with commentary on the pestilence afflicting the city. From the beginning Pontalba noticed that the fever singled out the unacclimated, the newcomers—especially the Americans and English—in preference to the creole and long-resident population. In several letters he reassured his wife that the disease presented little danger except to strangers. Morales also observed the fever's peculiarity in so clearly preferring foreigners to the natives, especially attacking "the Flemish, the English, and the Americans, who rarely recover."[5] Such an obvious distinction in vulnerability is a reliable indication that yellow fever was not entirely new to the area, even if not previously recognized.

New Orleans residents, including physicians, engaged in considerable discussion and disagreement about the nature and origin of the fever, as if confronting an essentially new problem. Their uncertainty suggests that the appearance of yellow fever in epidemic proportions was indeed something new. Pontalba believed that "the maladies" resulted from an overflow of the river on the opposite shore, causing "subsequent fetid exhalations to be given off by the earth" as it dried out. Attorney General Don Gabriel Fonvergne, in a report to the city council, blamed "the stagnated waters that remain in the gutters of the streets, the little cleanliness and care given to them, the dead animals abandoned on them, and on the margin of the river" for the contamination of the atmosphere and the spread of infection. He recommended that the council take action to improve the drainage and sanitary condition of the city to prevent future epidemics.[6] The idea that epidemic diseases could be caused by "fetid exhalations" from animal and vegetable decay was a common epidemiological tenet of the times. For almost a century thereafter, the association of filth and disease would be echoed in both medical and lay opinion, usually accompanied by appeals for sanitary reform—and usually with limited results because of the expense.

In mid-September Pontalba reported the opinion of New Orleans physicians that the sickness was "the yellow fever of Philadelphia," but said he disagreed. A few days later he wrote: "In common accord, people now believe that it is the same yellow fever that had been breaking out every year in Philadelphia, and which the Americans have brought along with them." Pontalba remained unconvinced, and as late as October 30 he expressed his continuing uncertainty: "I do not understand the nature of that deadly malady, but I think it to be a kind of pestilent fever." In an official dispatch of October 31, Morales summed up the several views of the epidemic: Some called it "a malignant fever," some, "the black vomit," and others believed it to be the yellow fever of Philadelphia.[7] The reference to black vomit as a symptom provides almost certain evidence that the disease that year was genuine yellow fever. Philadelphia had experienced a devastating yellow fever epidemic in 1793 which literally decimated its population.[8] Traffic between Philadelphia and Spanish New Orleans had been active since the 1780s, with American agents stationed in New Orleans to handle the business. Although possible, it hardly seems likely that yellow fever was imported from Philadelphia; the source of disease for both cities was probably the West Indian "pandemic," spreading from points with which both commonly traded.

Confronted with what appeared to them a new and terrifying malady, the residents of New Orleans employed a variety of measures in the hope of staving off the disease. Pontalba told of the great fear among the people, especially the women, who carried bits of garlic in their clothing and burned animal skins, horns, hoofs, and tar to ward off the pestilential effluvia in the atmosphere. Baronne Carondelet, the governor's wife, placed her faith in the preventive powers of herb-tea compound and sarsaparilla.[9]

Pontalba assembled his own package of precautionary measures: "I always had camphor on me, and also much vinegar; two demi-johns of the latter were used to sprinkle my apartments . . . ." His servants were entirely soaked with vinegar, and he himself "often chewed the *quinquinia*." He solemnly informed his wife, "I was doing all this for you . . . since I was too affected mentally to give thought to myself." Pontalba later attributed his immunity and that of several friends to their regular chewing of "quinquinia" or cinchona bark.[10]

A recipe by a Dr. Masdevall, physician to the king of Spain, was published and circulated among New Orleanians as a cure for the sickness. According to Pontalba, some persons used it also as a preventive measure. The recipe consisted of various medicines to be taken over a period of several days, including "emetic wine," cream of tartar,

"Peruvian bark" (cinchona), and a mild laxative. In his official report, the Spanish intendant credited the regimen with "marvellous effects," especially among the Spaniards and the blacks who exhibited remarkable resistance to the disease. In contrast, Pontalba considered it useless, whether as preventive or cure.[11] He also expressed a lack of confidence in the local physicians' opinions and their efforts at treating the fever victims. When it seemed on one occasion that the epidemic was abating, he wrote: "The doctors pretend having found a remedy . . . ." The declining force of the disease, he believed, actually resulted from "the change in the weather," as several days of heavy rain had cleared away the infection. Although the doctors contended that only their use of emetics and blisters had arrested the "ravages" of the epidemic, Pontalba was unwilling to give these therapies much credit. He knew of several persons who had recovered completely without any of the "so-called succors" of the doctors. Attorney general Fonvergene later reported to the city council that the "most up-to-date care and remedies" had been without results.[12]

By September 19 the rains had ended, the good weather returned, and "the maladies . . . returned with it." Again in late September Pontalba thought the epidemic was finished because the winds from the north had "entirely purified the air." But in early October he had to report new cases of the fever among the English who had remained in the city. As late as November 6 the disease was still causing "some ravage," but the next day Pontalba announced that "we are now predicting the near end of the epidemic." Thereafter, he made no further mention of the disease in his letters.[13] The arrival of cold weather in November must have halted the activities of the yellow fever mosquito.

The few extant contemporary descriptions show the severity of the epidemic of 1796 in its impact on the city from late August until early November. The total mortality can only be estimated; no board of health, vital statistics bureau, or systematic secular measures existed at that time for keeping such records. A few available figures reveal the scope and magnitude of the outbreak and provide the basis for a reasonable estimate of mortality.

With several weeks remaining before the infection actually subsided, the attorney general reported on October 21 that the "cruel epidemic" had already "led to the grave more than 250 persons, almost all in the flower of their youth." Ten days later the intendant stated that the mortality had not been "excessive"; the parish registry had listed less than 200 deaths among the white inhabitants from all causes since the start of the epidemic. Upon further reflection he admitted that the loss of life was considerable. The number recorded in the registry was two-thirds greater than the mortality during the same time period "in ordinary years." Furthermore, the parish records did not include deaths outside the town limits or "the protestants who perished (and they were numerous)."[14]

The population of New Orleans in 1796 was probably about 6,000, or twice the size it had been only twenty-five years before.[15] An estimated 30 to 40 percent of the total was black, mainly slave. At least 75 or 80 percent of the white population was native born, largely French, with the remaining 20 to 25 percent made up of English, Americans, and other recent arrivals.[16] The black population seems to have been little affected by the epidemic. Most had probably acquired immunity from experience with the disease in Africa, in the West Indies, or even in New Orleans on some earlier occasion. Those attacked by yellow fever in 1796 probably exhibited mild symptoms which might not have been recognized as the same disease manifesting such a violent character in the "unacclimated" whites. Obviously the French and Spanish creole population had also acquired some measure of immunity from prior experience with the disease. Even so, some were susceptible and died of the fever, as shown by the parish registry of Catholic mortality and by a few deaths among Pontalba's close associates.

The city contained an adequate supply of susceptibles, both strangers and natives, to fuel an outbreak of yellow fever lasting ten to twelve weeks. On several occasions, Pontalba noted a death count of eight to ten persons daily—for an unspecified period of time. On September 15 he wrote that "The doctors and the monks had been keeping the true number of deaths secret...." The toll had actually been as high as fifteen to seventeen deaths each day, he said, although only for a brief time at that level. By mid-October it was estimated that more than 150 of the English inhabitants had died of the pestilence. Even as the epidemic was declining, Pontalba observed that "a few are still dying every day."[17] On the basis of these scattered figures, which are themselves imprecise, a total of 350 to 400 yellow fever deaths in and around New Orleans during the epidemic of 1796 is a fair estimate. Further calculations based on population estimates show this loss as almost 6 percent of New Orleans' total population, 10 percent of the whites, and more than 25 percent of the non-creole whites, the most susceptible element.

First Memorable Yellow Fever Epidemic

This first notable invasion by yellow fever had a drastic and dramatic impact on the community and set certain patterns that would become repetitive during a century of epidemics to come. A general exodus from the city, great mortality among "strangers," a moratorium on business, a vain appeal for sanitary reform, and the expression of depravity as well as humanitarianism invariably accompanied Yellow Jack's ravages in New Orleans.

As the disease gradually spread through the city in 1796, many persons hoping to escape an attack fled the scene. The *émigrés* sought refuge in the back country or left the province entirely for regions far to the north. According to Pontalba, more than 300 of the English residents had left by mid-October "for the country, or else to go outside the colony altogether." In commenting on their flight, he also revealed the sorry state of business in New Orleans: "The city is almost deserted; my storehouses, which had all been rented, are now left vacant."[18]

Those who did not wish to leave New Orleans entirely but desired some measure of safety for themselves and their families, or simply wanted a temporary respite from the depression of the stricken city, retired to resorts across Lake Pontchartrain or to homes in the country or across the Mississippi. Along with his account of the grim aspects of the epidemic, Baron Pontalba also described his social activities during the pestilence of 1796, including frequent house-parties at a friend's plantation across the river. Escaping from the sickness of the city, a large group of people amused themselves with pranks, jokes, and games. It is all somewhat reminiscent of Boccaccio's ten who sought diversion in the telling of bawdy tales while hiding from the Black Death. In one letter Pontalba described a party so wild and boisterous that on retiring to his room he found it necessary to barricade the door with a large table to keep the crowd from dragging him out. He justified the pranksters by pointing out that they "needed the air of the country, the maladies in town having driven them all into a state of deep melancholy." In New Orleans one heard nothing but talk of the epidemic. Across the river "all news of that sort is taboo, and they give themselves up to play," which included riding, racing, and "other extravagant things."[19]

In another letter Pontalba described more specifically some of the amusing pranks and "pleasantries" at one lively gathering across the river: "The ladies, on one side, found pleasure in knotting my bed sheets together, [and] in throwing water at me . . . while I, on the other, smudged their bed clothes with lamp-black, so that they became smeared all over with it." In further retaliation he applied a foul-smelling drug powder to their pillows, threw water at them, dropped pieces of wood down their chimneys at night, made holes in their chamber-pots, and engaged in other forms of mischief. Probably realizing that such carrying-on with the ladies might provoke a spark of jealousy in his wife, the Baron added that after paying them back in kind he had become bored with such things and ceased to participate—"since all such pranks, *mon-amie*, cannot fill the void of my days, being only amusing for a time."[20] In the course of every epidemic, individuals must have joined together in groups seeking relief from fear and desolation—drinking, joking, or playing lively games. Certainly no other account of such diversion in Louisiana's epidemic history is as detailed (or as delightful) as Pontalba's.[21]

Epidemics always offer opportunities for rising to the heights of generosity and heroism or sinking to the depths of callousness and depravity. In 1796 as in later years there were examples of both extremes. Pontabla referred to an incident which can be scored to the dark side of human nature; he told of the discovery of five dead Protestants "in the backways merely covered with leaves, the trouble not having been taken to even bury them." In his judgment, "Such terrible negligence is enough to bring on the plague...."[22] Abandoned bodies of yellow fever victims were sometimes found in later epidemics as well. Nevertheless, the social order held together, and one searches in vain for reports of widespread looting, debauchery, violence, or other signs of social dissolution so often associated with catastrophe. In later years of pestilence in New Orleans one can find official negligence, public indifference, profiteering, the priority of commercial values, and personal irresponsibility. Except for the chaos and confusion associated with the hasty departure of hundreds (later thousands) of residents, however, and the unavoidable problems of widespread sickness and death, the community continued to function and to cope with disaster.

On the positive side of the ledger in 1796, Pontalba inadvertently recorded examples of strength and humanitarianism. In attending to the needs of several friends sick with the fever, he himself demonstrated great courage and benevolence. Governor Carondelet, believing that it might intensify the panic if he left the city, bravely resisted for a time the demands of his wife and his friends that he take refuge across the river.[23] There is no evidence of any special measures by officials in 1796 for the isolation of the sick or provision of medical care such as that arranged by the Spanish governor Gálvez during a smallpox epidemic in 1779. Smallpox, obviously and indisputably contagious, prompted such action; yellow fever seemed to spread, not directly from person to person, but by "atmospheric contamination." In 1796 the indigent victims of yellow fever probably received care at Charity Hospital, at that time under the patronage of a private philanthropist rather than the government.[24]

The epidemic of 1796 was "memorable" because of its scale and its impact, and because it was attributed to a particular malady with a distinctive and descriptive name, known to have attacked Philadelphia in the recent past and believed by some to have been brought to New Orleans by the Americans. Other epidemics followed in rapid succession, reinforcing the memory of 1796 as the first in a series of similar experiences. Using available records and oral testimony, early nineteenth-century chroniclers and historians preserved and perpetuated the significance of the 1796 episode for social or collective memory. Through writing and publication they gave the epidemic a place in historical knowledge. Without repetition or emphasis by chroniclers such events can be lost in unexamined manuscripts and individual forgetfulness, which seems to have happened to the scattered outbreaks prior to 1796.

Yellow fever's earlier presence in the city must have been perceived only as individual encounters with an illness and not as a group experience consciously shared. Perhaps an epidemic could be recognized and remembered as a community experience only after New Orleans had come to view itself as a separate community with its own identity, rather than simply an undifferentiated part of the province.[25] Because the disease itself was peculiar in its apparent selectivity, yellow fever could have contributed to the self-definition of the white creoles and "the acclimated" as a privileged, relatively immune group—in contrast to newcomers, strangers, outsiders who readily succumbed to the illness. (How it might have affected black identity and sensibility is an open question.) Finally, yellow fever could be recognized as a distinctive disorder with its own name and identity only because it exhibited certain clearly discernible characteristics, especially when affecting large numbers at the same time and different groups in different ways.[26]

However memorable the experience might have appeared at the time, New Orleanians could scarcely have suspected in 1796 that the pestilence they suffered would mark the beginning of a century of recurring yellow fever epidemics. Soon to become a familiar summer and fall phenomenon, the disease would earn for the Crescent City a nationwide reputation as the "Necropolis of the South."

III

A HALF-CENTURY OF PESTILENCE
1799-1849

During the first half-century of yellow fever's history in Louisiana, the pestilence seemed to gain in virulence with each succeeding epidemic. Physicians were scarcely able to cope with a disease whose nature, causation, and transmission they failed to comprehend. As the fever was reintroduced into New Orleans summer after summer in the years following 1796, a fatalistic acceptance of its frequent recurrence became the prevailing attitude among the inhabitants.

New Orleans physicians, commercial interests, and newspaper editors fostered the illusion that their city, in comparision with others, was relatively healthy. In the absence of accurate mortality records, that misconception gained widespread acceptance among the dominant political and economic elements of the community. Under the circumstances, one could hardly expect an enlightened program in the interest of public health. With such limited knowledge, however, even the best efforts then conceivable probably would have had little effect in controlling yellow fever. Nothing short of an absolute ban on tropical commerce for six months of the year would have been likely to keep out the disease, and such a drastic step was unthinkable, especially when most physicians believed yellow fever originated in the filth of New Orleans. Even when physicians favored quarantine, the commercial interests of the city made it difficult to enforce any kind of quarantine restriction on trade. Sanitary improvements could have diminished some of the other common diseases of New Orleans, such as those spread by contaminated water, but

A Half-Century of Pestilence, 1799-1849

would have had little effect on yellow fever. Cetainly the ignorance and apathy of the times placed no obstacle whatsoever in the path of the disease, and "Yellow Jack" periodically ruled the city in a summer and autumn carnival of horrors.

New Orleans Epidemics, 1799-1809

Some cases of yellow fever probably occurred in New Orleans every year from 1796 to 1817, and no year between 1817 and 1861 passed without a few recorded cases. After 1796, New Orleans' next major outbreak seems to have come in 1799, while Louisiana was still a Spanish colony. Attorney general Pedro Dulcidio Barran in a message to the city council in January, 1800, reported that the public had been terribly frightened the previous summer and continued to worry about the recurrence of the disease. Calling for action to prevent or "to minimize the dreadfulness of the calamity that justly terrifies this community," Barran recommended certain "pressing and essential" precautions, including sanitary reform, drainage improvements, and quarantine measures.[1] No mortality figures have been found for the "calamity" of 1799.

The records of yellow fever outbreaks in the early 1800s are scattered, brief, and sketchy. During the first two decades of the century, New Orleans experienced at least five serious outbreaks: 1804, 1809, 1811, 1817, and 1819. Various writers have cited seven additional years when the fever "prevailed," but these were mild invasions and not in the same league with the "violent" attacks.[2] Even so, twelve outbreaks in twenty summers claimed more than 3,000 lives, enough at that time to populate several small towns.

New Orleans, nevertheless, continued to grow in area and population, as well as volume of trade handled through the port. More and more flatboats came down the river from the 1790s on, bringing the produce of the developing hinterland to the city for marketing and shipping—grain, flour, meat, whiskey, tobacco, hemp, cotton, sugar, and molasses. Spain returned the Louisiana colony to France by treaty in 1800, and France sold it to the United States in 1803, at which time the New Orleans population was about 10,000. By 1820 it had almost tripled in number, with a census count of more than 27,000.[3] With the continuing growth of trade and population came increased opportunities for the introduction and spread of yellow fever and more "unacclimated" persons to fuel an epidemic.

Located between the Mississippi River and Lake Pontchartrain, surrounded by cypress swamps, New Orleans became a quagmire during rainy weather. Water was never more than a few feet and sometimes only inches beneath the ground. The unpaved streets, often a foot deep in mud, animal manure, human waste, and refuse, were almost impassable at times. Only the levee, an embankment built up along the river, and several canals and drainage ditches protected the city from regular flooding when the Mississippi rose above street level. Because of climate and topography, New Orleans' special problems of drainage and sanitation were not effectively solved until the twentieth century. These features could hardly fail to catch the eyes of travelers who often responded negatively, as did Perrin du Lac, a French visitor in the years just prior to the American purchase of Louisiana:

> Nothing equals the filthiness of New Orleans unless it be the unhealthfulness which has for some years appeared to have resulted from it. The city, the filth of which cannot be drained off, is not paved. . . . Its markets which are unventilated are reeking with rottenness. . . . Its squares are covered with the filth of animals which no one takes the trouble to remove. Consequently there is seldom a year that the yellow fever or some other contagious malady does not carry off many strangers.[4]

In August, 1804, the first summer after the American acquisition of Louisiana, yellow fever again appeared in New Orleans. Finding a bountiful supply of unacclimated persons, the disease subjected the city to a three-month period of death and desolation. In his official letters, territorial governor William C. C. Claiborne traced the course of the epidemic, providing the most thorough contemporary account available. Some cases had appeared by August 10, but the city was not considered to be "generally unhealthy." The malignant disease called yellow fever was "particularly fatal" to Americans and other strangers. Having suffered and survived a violent attack early in the epidemic, Claiborne wrote President Jefferson on August 30, ". . . I am represented as the only American who has yet recovered." Not only did he suffer a debilitating attack of yellow fever himself, but in late September he lost his wife and his young daughter to the scourge.[5]

Claiborne estimated that "more than a third of the Americans who emigrated thither in the course of the last 12 months have perished, and nearly every Person from Europe who arrived in the City during the Summer Months." A physician of New Orleans wrote to a friend in Mississippi that "almost every person arriving from the country" experienced an attack. Another urban resident reported seven deaths among a group of nine persons who had come downriver to the city.[6] On a brief excursion into the country Governor Claiborne had noticed "the Humanity of several Planters who by detaining at their Houses several Americans destined for this City . . . probably rescued them from sudden death."[7] The disease did not confine itself solely to strangers, however, for in mid-September New Orleans physicians began to observe cases among the "old Inhabitants." During the last days of October the epidemic still raged in New Orleans, but by November 4 the governor reported that "the Fever has entirely Abated in this City, and Industry & Commerce seem to have revived."[8]

Perhaps as a result of the distress and disorder occasioned by widespread disease, white fears of slave revolt surfaced. Claiborne wrote President Jefferson in September that the anxiety of the city was "considerably heightened by an alarm of Insurrection among the Negro's." Slaves had exhibited a "general Spirit of Insubordination," and several armed blacks had been found traveling about at night, intensifying the fears already present in New Orleans. Although the governor did not believe there was adequate basis for alarm, he strengthened the night patrols and ordered the city militia and volunteers to be prepared for action. The insurrection apparently failed to materialize as the letters contain no further reference to the subject. Some blacks might have considered revolt during several outbreaks of this disease that seemed to affect them less than whites. Whether their advantage in an epidemic situation occurred to them or not, it did occur to whites, who claimed to see evidence of slave conspiracies on several later occasions during yellow fever epidemics.[9]

Throughout most of the nineteenth century, newspapers, not only in New Orleans but also in any town stricken with epidemic disease, generally adopted a policy of ignoring its presence as long as possible, then minimizing its importance, and sometimes prematurely declaring the epidemic ended. In the early 1800s New Orleans journals usually avoided direct commentary altogether, indicating the existence of disease only through published bills of mortality and obituary notices. This practice prevented or at least hindered the isolation of the community by other towns, which ordinarily cut off communications and commerce with the infected center as soon as the news leaked out that an epidemic might be in progress. Usually it was only a matter of time until the word spread through the city, whence it was carried to other areas by fleeing émigrés, who sometimes carried the disease as well.

In time, the subterfuge of the journals created a widespread reputation of hypocrisy and unreliability for the editors and for the city's leaders. Editors argued that a few cases were bound to occur each season and that epidemics did not invariably develop from a handful of cases. Physicians and editors agreed with merchants that there was no need to generate unnecessary panic among residents or neighboring communities as long as a chance existed that an epidemic might not happen. Sometimes the season did pass without an epidemic; sometimes Yellow Jack struck with full force and the journals would eventually admit the epidemic, provide some coverage, continue to warn strangers and "our absent friends" not to return too soon, and finally announce the decline of fever with the coming of frost.[10]

What constituted an epidemic depended on one's point of view as well as the customary health conditions of a community. Epidemics, even now, are defined as a deviation from the normal or customary incidence of a disease.[11] In the nineteenth century, when morbidity and mortality statistics were not easy to obtain, defining epidemics was even more subjective. New Orleans gradually came to accept as "normal" an extremely high level of disease and death. Outsiders were astounded by the extent of mortality required before the city's physicians, health officials, and journalists considered the disease epidemic.

The *Louisiana Gazette* during the sickly season in 1804 gave little attention to the city's pestilence. From August to November the newspaper occasionally noted in the obituaries that someone had died of "the Prevailing sickness" and published a few poems dedicated to the memory of fever victims. In the issue of September 28, which reported the death of the governor's wife, the editors explained the temporary suspension of the journal, attributing it to "sickness" and expressing the hope that as the healthy season returned the publication could be resumed on a regular basis.[12]

In December, 1804, Governor Claiborne presented to the legislative council of the territory a plan for the prevention of future epidemics suggested to him by President Thomas Jefferson. Because of New Orleans' location as the gateway to the Mississippi Valley, Jefferson believed it was destined to become "the greatest city the world has ever seen." Epidemic disease, however, could constitute a serious drawback to its growth and prosperity. Having observed that disease usually prevailed along the waterfront and the "solid-built parts" of cities, but rarely spread into the "thin-built parts," Jefferson proposed that the development of New Orleans proceed in the pattern of a checkerboard with the white squares left open and planted with trees. The president was convinced that yellow fever would not spread in a city so designed for open space and low density of settlements, and he believed that all American cities should be built in such a fashion. Although never put into effect by New Orleans developers, Jefferson's proposal shows that the city had a reputation for pestilence by the time it was acquired by the United States.[13]

Another commentary on the Crescent City's growing notoriety came in 1805 from a resident of a small town on the Mississippi River about a hundred miles above New Orleans, who declared that he would not even consider moving with his family to the city: "The Yellow Fever which annually has visited that place forbade an idea of that kind."[14] The disease was becoming known throughout the United States as a regular hazard in New Orleans. Despite the dangers, the lure of the city as an economic frontier continued for many years to attract large numbers of "strangers" from other parts of the Union and from other countries as well.

Between 1803 and 1810, the population of the territory (soon to become the state of Louisiana in 1812) increased from approximately 50,000 to more than 76,000, and that of New Orleans from 10,000 to an official count of 17,000, although some sources provide a much higher estimate. Population increase in New Orleans at this time came not so much from American or European arrivals as from an influx of French refugees from the West Indies, once again dislocated by the repercussions of European conflict within the various colonial empires. Previously in flight from revolution in Saint-Domingue in the 1790s, the exiles had scattered to Louisiana, Cuba, and other points in the Antilles. With Spain and France again at war, those who had settled in Cuba had to seek aslyum elsewhere in 1809. In June and July of that year thirty-four ships from Cuba brought almost 6,000 persons to New Orleans: French-speaking whites, slaves, and free persons of color— in almost equal numbers. Still more displaced French colonials arrived shortly thereafter from Cuba, Jamaica, Guadeloupe, and other islands, making a total of approximately 10,000, according to some estimates, and almost doubling the population of New Orleans in a matter of months. As a result, French language and culture for a time were reinforced and American influence diluted.[15]

Yellow fever also arrived in New Orleans the summer of 1809. Although the Caribbean French and blacks brought the virus with them, they were less likely than the American newcomers to provide a mass of susceptibles for an outbreak of yellow fever. Many of them probably had already acquired immunity in the islands. In contrast, some 2,000 United States troops concentrated in New Orleans that summer suffered greatly from disease, especially in August and September, and nearly 800 died, some no doubt from yellow fever.[16] According to one American residing in New Orleans, "people die here this year without almost any warning," including several persons he knew who had fallen prey to yellow fever—all Americans.[17] The outbreak of 1809 was relatively mild in its overall impact on the city. Perhaps the disease was hindered by an expanded population of non-susceptible residents, reducing the probability for extensive propagation of the virus.

Reporting the death of the second Mrs. Claiborne in 1809 to the "same dreadful malady" that had taken the lives of his first wife, his daughter, and his secretary in 1804, Governor Claiborne complained to President Madison about the unhealthy location of the governor's residence. It was near the river front, he wrote, where accumulations of filth along the water's edge contaminated the atmosphere with offensive and pestilential fumes. In addition to his own personal losses, Claiborne pointed out that Governor Gayoso and Governor Carondelet's brother had also died of yellow fever at the official residence in the 1790s. All these fatalities, he thought, clearly demonstrated the need for a healthier location.[18]

1811-1829

When the next epidemic struck in 1811, few contemporaries used the yellow fever label in writing about it. Despite New Orleans' repeated experience with yellow fever in the early 1800s, both medical and non-medical observers continued to exhibit much uncertainty about the nature of the seasonal "fevers" that plagued the area. Doctors, officials, and journalists applied vague general designations to the prevailing disease: "the autumnal fevers," "the prevalent and contagious disease," "the sickness," and "the yellow or some other Malignant Fever."[19]

In August Claiborne noted that the "Fevers of New-Orleans" had commenced with "Symptoms which forbode much mortality." Eventually he recognized the illness that had cost him so dearly and informed President Madison that New Orleans was again "Visited by that dreadful Scourge, the Yellow Fever, and many Good Citizens have fallen Victims." As usual the "Strangers" suffered the greatest losses.[20] Claiborne reported to the secretary of the navy that the fever had proved highly destructive to the Marine Corps, having carried off two valuable officers and more than a third of the privates by late October. Reports from the city recorder, the manager of Charity Hospital, the Protestant sexton, and Father Antoine added up to a total of more than 700 deaths during the three-month epidemic in 1811. Probably 500 or more were victims of yellow fever.[21]

Newspapers gave little attention to the epidemic in 1811. After nearly two months of extraordinary sickness, the *Louisiana Courier* briefly mentioned the "autumnal fevers which now rage over our unfortunate country." Both the *Courier* and the *Louisiana Gazette* in early November acknowledged the continuing presence of the disease when reporting on the delay in the work of the convention elected to draft Louisiana's first state constitution.[22]

Reflecting the medical opinions of his professional circle, a French physician advised the mayor of New Orleans in 1811 that the prevailing fevers were seasonal in character, produced by the intense summer heat, and not at all contagious. The doctor further explained "that these fevers became dangerous in Certain individuals from their mode of living, [and] the fears which they entertain of the Malignancy of the disease . . . ." He also criticized "the mode of Curing" which employed "Strong and irritating medicines."[23] Thus an ordinary seasonal ailment became a fatal disorder in certain individuals and groups because of their imprudent or intemperate "mode of living," or by an excess of fear that literally scared them to death. New Orleans physicians, parroted by journalists, continued to set forth this judgment for decades, directing it first against American newcomers of whatever rank, later applying it to other "strangers" such as the Irish, German, and Italian immigrants, and to the laboring poor, whatever their nationality. The French physician's criticism of "Strong and irritating medicines" was obviously aimed at the standard American medical practice which then emphasized bloodletting and purging with large doses of mercurial compounds. In contrast, the French practice in

Louisiana relied on mild remedies and nursing care, which ultimately proved to be the wiser course.

Yellow Jack's next big performance in 1817 gave rise to New Orleans' first association of physicians, *La Société Médicale*. At the first meeting in August, the members shared their observations and opinions on the "diseases . . . extending their ravages throughout this city, and exciting inquietude among the people." Description of symptoms by various members provided a classic picture of yellow fever, including jaundice and black vomit. The organization of French Louisiana physicians unanimously agreed that the "acute fevers" observed in recent weeks were cases of the "American Typhus" (one of the synonyms for yellow fever), appearing almost exclusively among individuals not accustomed to the extreme heat, "those undergoing imprudent fatigues, or intemperance or melancholy."[24]

At the close of the epidemic, Drs. Adrien Armand Gros and N. V. A. Gérardin presented a report on "la fièvre jaune" to the medical society. As causes, they listed the city's topographical situation, abundant rainfall, stagnant water, excessive summer heat, and an aggregation of unacclimated strangers. They observed that frost and cold weather seemed to destroy the deleterious effluvia in the atmosphere. In an enlightened conclusion, Gros and Gérardin recommended that the state of Louisiana, with its population and trade increasing daily, assume responsibility for screening out "morbific fluxes" likely to be introduced by commerce, and intensify its efforts to maintain the public health, without which there could be no lasting prosperity.[25]

Increasing sentiment in favor of state action against the pestilence led to the passage of an act by the state legislature early in 1818, creating a board of health for New Orleans and providing for quarantine regulations. When cases of yellow fever appeared in the summer of 1818 despite the quarantine, a reaction set in and the legislature repealed the law in March, 1819. The severe outbreak in 1819 and a moderate one in 1820 occasioned another experiment with health regulations and quarantine, established by state law in 1821. Again the defenses proved inadequate to stem the pestilential tide that appeared regularly each summer. Having lost all faith in quarantine, and under pressure from commercial interests, Louisiana lawmakers repealed the measure in 1825.[26] The theory of importation fell into disrepute, and the idea of local causation dominated medical philosophy until the 1840s and early 1850s when yellow fever spread more extensively than ever and forced a reevaluation of medical explanation.

After the epidemic of 1819, a committee of *La Société Médicale* again prepared a report on "la fièvre jaune," comparing the recent experience with that of 1817. Both years witnessed the first cases in May, but in 1817 the epidemic period extended from July to late October, and in 1819 from August to mid-December. In both epidemics the fever had attacked mainly Europeans and Americans fresh from the North, but its victims each time included some long-time residents and a few creoles as well. No black person was affected by the fever of 1817, but some died in 1819.[27]

Conflicting sets of figures exist for yellow fever mortality in 1817 and in 1819. Even when fairly complete burial lists are available, it is almost impossible to determine the mortality from any one particular disease. Burial certificates often failed to state the cause of death, and even with stated causes, one must cope with the problems of uncertain diagnosis and variety of disease labels. From records of the various cemeteries, reports of the medical society, and other data available to him, Dr. Bennet Dowler in the mid-nineteenth century conservatively estimated at least 800 deaths from yellow fever in 1817.[28]

Similar obstacles arise when calculating the death toll of the even more destructive epidemic of 1819. Benjamin Latrobe, the great American architect, commented during the epidemic that "no exact register is any where kept of deaths and burials, & uncertainty on this subject is inevitable on many accounts." He estimated the fatalities from August to mid-September as ranging from ten or twelve to forty-six per day, and considered a report he heard of fifty-three in one day as not improbable.[29] The *Louisiana Courier*, rising to defend the city's reputation, attempted to counteract the "exaggerations" circulating both inside and outside New Orleans. The editor denied the report of more than fifty burials in one day and asserted that days with as many as twenty-five burials were hardly common. Except for a few cases, he said, the disease attacked only those persons having recently arrived in the area (as if this fact greatly lessened the seriousness of the situation).[30] Throughout much of the nineteenth century, newspapers, medical journals, and other defenders of New Orleans' inherent salubrity often employed this kind of reasoning to explain away the "seeming" unhealthiness of the Crescent City. Estimates of the yellow fever mortality in 1819 range from 425 to 6,000. A cautious conjecture based on the total mortality that year within the incorporated limits of the city would place the number of yellow fever deaths at less than 1,000.[31]

During the 1820s yellow fever appeared in New Orleans every summer. In seven of the ten years epidemics occurred, including mild outbreaks killing only 100 to 400 victims. An annual yellow fever mortality of a mere 100 or so came to be expected as one of the inexorable facts of life in New Orleans. Two epidemics of this decade stand out as unusually severe: 1822 and 1829, each causing at least 800 to 900 fatalities and probably more.[32]

A French Louisianian residing near the city believed the malady of 1822 had been brought to New Orleans from Pensacola by the Americans. "The foreigners who can are leaving," he wrote, and in the absence of fuel for the fever, he expected the epidemic to subside.[33] At the outset of the epidemic, the New Orleans mayor recommended that those who could afford to should leave the city; for unacclimated strangers lacking resources but wishing to leave, funds would be provided to send them to the other side of Lake Pontchartrain until the end of the sickly season. The principal victims, as usual, seemed to be the newcomers, this time mainly German and Irish immigrants.[34] In mid-September the *Louisiana Gazette* published a report of the local health board advising all strangers to leave town until the fever declined.[35]

Although continuing the standard policy of delayed reporting and understatement, some newspaper editors began to recognize that when an epidemic was well under way and could no longer be ignored, a diminution of the unacclimated in the city meant fewer potential victims, hence a more rapid decline of the epidemic. Sometimes, however, the dispersion of the émigrés after a certain point only served to spread the disease. In 1829 the *Louisiana Courier* incurred the wrath of other New Orleans newspapers by printing as early as July 10 a letter to the editor announcing the appearance of yellow fever in the city and advising strangers to evacuate. A journalistic battle developed as the *Price-Current* and the *Mercantile Advertiser* both insisted the city was unusually healthy in spite of attempts to discredit its salubrity. Undaunted, the *Courier* editor continued his frank reporting on the pestilence which "threatens entire desolation to our city," warning the unacclimated to disperse. On October 12, proclaiming that the early arrival of cool weather had terminated the epidemic, the *Courier* assured absent citizens they might return home in perfect safety.[36]

1830s and 1840s

After some twenty-five years of residence in New Orleans, the Reverend Doctor Theodore Clapp, Unitarian minister, remarked in the 1850s that he had "passed through the same scenes of toil, anxiety, and suffering, at least twenty times," including Asiatic cholera as well as yellow fever epidemics. "There is a wonderful sameness," he wrote, "in the sombre realities of the sick room, the death struggle, the corpse, the shroud, the coffin, the funeral, and the tomb."[37] After researching a dozen or more epidemics and attempting to write about them, the historian begins to see and feel something of that "sameness" Dr. Clapp described—deadening, desensitizing, predictable, even boring. Certainly the attitude of the "acclimated" city-dweller who had lived through many epidemics becomes understandable: another epidemic, the usual summer complaint, how dull.

There are patterns, however, that begin to take shape from the repetitions: similarities can be observed in the timing of Yellow Jack's arrival and termination, the curve of rising and declining mortality, the reactions of denial, indifference, or flight by various groups of New Orleanians, the journalistic techniques for "containing" epidemics within a familiar framework and reducing panic responses, ritualistic controversies between New Orleans newspapers and others outside the city or the state regarding the presence and extent of the fever, the standard explanations of disease in terms of "outsider" groups affected and how through "imprudence" and "intemperance" they brought it on themselves, disagreements among physicians regarding causation and therapy, and other uniformities or recurring themes in more than a century of yellow fever epidemics. There are differences as well, distinctive elements that marked each visitation as singular and some with greater significance than others.

In the 1830s and 1840s the scourge of New Orleans followed the same general pattern of the three preceding decades: no year passed without at least a few cases; five to seven years of each decade witnessed outbreaks ranging from mild to violent; and of the five to seven outbreaks in each ten-year period, at least two or three must be classified as severe epidemics. Major visitations during the two decades occurred in 1833, 1837, 1839, 1841, and 1847, with estimated fatalities of 1,000; 1,300; 800; 1,800; and 3,000, respectively.[38]

Although not particularly severe, the yellow fever epidemic of 1832 is noteworthy for its association with the first appearance of Asiatic cholera in New Orleans. In late October and November the city suffered the simultaneous effects of both pestilences. When frost arrived, yellow fever subsided, but cholera continued throughout the winter. According to Dr. Joseph Jones, the combined force of the two plagues raised the total mortality of New Orleans in 1832 to more than 8,000 in a population of 55,000: one-seventh of the entire population died. Of the 8,000 deaths that year, cholera caused more than 4,000 and yellow fever about 400.[39]

The following year, 1833, New Orleanians again suffered the two deadly maladies, each claiming about 1,000 victims. Dr. Edward H. Barton described it as the "most violent and malignant of the Epidemic Yellow Fevers with which this city had ever been visited." He also noticed the unusual quantity of flies and mosquitoes in New Orleans before the outbreak and remarked that "the latter continued throughout the season."[40] Others before and after Barton observed this phenomenon, but not until the early twentieth century was the connection between the mosquito and yellow fever clearly established.

Founded in 1837, the New Orleans *Picayune*, in its first summer of publishing news and opinion, optimistically reported the city free of any widespread sickness in July and predicted that the season would pass without an epidemic. "At present no city in the union is more healthy or more pleasant than New Orleans," the editor proudly declared.[41] This statement became part of a litany, a summer ritual, which could be found in almost any New Orleans paper, repeated many times between June and August, every year.

Despite the editor's prediction, Yellow Jack did arrive in 1837, and by late August and early September New Orleans newspapers finally acknowledged the epidemic proportions of the disease and reported from seventy-five to one hundred deaths per day. The recurring and vexatious problem of obtaining accurate mortality statistics attracted the attention of the *Picayune* editor, who considered the graveyard reports of doubtful accuracy and noted that five or six cemeteries in the city did not issue reports at all. On September 13, he complained, "Until a Board of Health is organized, and regular reports kept . . . we may expect a wide difference of opinion as to the mortality of our city at this season, and with that difference no little exaggeration."[42] Journalistic complaints about the lack of a health agency, or the deficiencies of whatever temporary board happened to exist at the time, would be another recurring motif in newspaper coverage of New Orleans health conditions—especially during the first half of the nineteenth century.

Other repetitive features of epidemics included the disruption of trade and the lengthy delay in opening the business season based on the harvest. The *Picayune* set forth a graphic description of the unhappy situation in September of 1837:

> The levee is dull, dreary and lifeless at this time. No business doing, and the few ships in port are losing money for the want of cargoes. Steamboats arrive but seldom, and bring neither news, money or goods. Every person feels like sleeping or running away for the next three weeks and a half—but most of those now in the city are bound to stay, to fulfill engagements, live or die. We make out to bury our dead, drink juleps, or brandy toddies . . . talk to each other, read letters and the news of the day. . . .[43]

Also noting the dullness of the market that September, the New Orleans *Price-Current* announced optimistically that the scourge would eventually cease, crops would seek the great market of the southwest, and the wheels of trade would move again.[44] Most epidemics did in fact come to a halt by early November. Years of observation had demonstrated that the arrival of frost somehow meant that the end of the epidemic was in sight.

The epidemic of 1841 was declining in early October when an influx of strangers furnished new fuel and the disease flared up again. Finally in late October the *Picayune* proclaimed: "The Yellow Fever is dead-dead-dead!" Joyfully, the editor noted that only nine fever deaths had occurred the day before. All persons might now come to the city in safety as frost had arrived; the enemy "has been driven from among us by the unseen power that controls the revolving seasons."[45] The New Orleans *Bee* waited until November 3 before reporting the conclusion of the epidemic. Depicting the city in the act of casting off its blanket of gloom and despair, the editor wrote this vivid passage—a typical description of post-epidemic New Orleans whatever the year:

> Business dawns once more upon us; strangers begin to arrive, old friends are flocking in; the streets are refilling; the thorough-fares wear a busy and thronged aspect; the cares, bustle, pleasures of the present, and anticipation of the future, occupy every mind, and the horrors of the past will soon be remembered no more. *Forgetfulness is sometimes a beneficent faculty.*[46]

November always found the Crescent City a lively scene with citizens returning and newcomers arriving, steamboats and ocean vessels at the wharves, ready for a resumption of active commerce and society.

Population growth can account for some of yellow fever's increased depredations during New Orleans' first fifty years as an American city. Almost doubling in the 1820s and more than doubling again in the 1830s, the city's population reached a total of 102,000 by 1840, making New Orleans the third largest city in the Union. The growth rate declined during the 1840s but rose again in the 1850s to 45 percent. Not only the absolute population increase but also two specific demographic trends contributed to the increasing prevalence and high mortality levels of epidemic yellow fever: (1) the decline of the black population in number and percentage, and (2) the increasing proportion of foreign immigrants, mainly Irish, German, and French. Until the 1830s the city's population was 40 to 60 percent black. In the next twenty years their numbers were drastically reduced by the sale of urban slaves for plantation labor and by the departure of many free blacks when their status worsened and economic opportunities diminished. During the same period foreign immigration soared. By 1850 almost 80 percent of New Orleans' population was white, of which the foreign born constituted nearly half.[47]

A rapidly growing population with many susceptible newcomers and large numbers of *Aedes aegypti* provided a fertile field for epidemics whenever the yellow fever virus was introduced into the community. In earlier decades (from 1810 to the 1830s) with a black majority in New Orleans, and many immunes among both white and black creoles, the probability of extensive outbreaks was limited by the large proportion of immunes to susceptibles. Even when visibly affected by the disease, few blacks died from it; hence, yellow fever mortality levels did not reach the heights of later outbreaks when European immigrants and other strangers constituted a near majority in New Orleans. The volume of Louisiana sugar and molasses shipped through the port of New Orleans also increased greatly from the 1830s through the 1850s—with enormous potential for promoting a population explosion among the *Aedes aegypti*.[48]

From the earliest epidemics yellow fever's special preference for strangers was obvious to all, but not until the 1820s did New Orleans observers gradually begin to notice class distinctions in vulnerability. A report on the 1820 epidemic published by the New Orleans organization of American physicians considered the fever about equal in "malignity" among Europeans and northern Americans, especially the recently arrived "Northern sailors, western country boatmen, and German Redemptioners." Dr. Pierre Thomas in his account of the epidemic of 1822 reported that the Germans and Irish had suffered great losses and that the mayor had offered financial aid to indigent strangers wishing to depart the city. Robert Randolph, United States naval surgeon, also observed that the "labouring classes, particularly the poor Irish and Germans, were the chief victims" of the most serious form of the fever in 1822, with at least two of every three cases among them resulting in death.[49]

By the 1830s and 1840s, with rapid growth and heavy immigration, poverty became more common and more visible, as did also its association with disease, especially yellow fever. In August, 1837, when yellow fever was raging but New Orleans had no board of health to declare an epidemic in progress, the *Picayune* argued for a "legally constituted authority" to investigate and report on the health of the city, "to apprise strangers, and especially the poor and illiterate, of danger—to influence them to have early recourse to efficient medical aid," especially since foreigners usually provided the "first subjects of attack."[50] The poverty of the class most liable to the disease intensified the suffering and distress occasioned by epidemics. The Howard Association, a benevolent society first organized in New Orleans during the pestilence of 1837, served until the late nineteenth century to alleviate the misery of destitute victims whenever epidemics occurred.[51]

In August, 1839, when reluctantly acknowledging the presence of yellow fever after weeks of vehement denial, the *Picayune* emphasized that victims thus far had been confined to the laboring class and that persons following a program of moderation and prudence had little to fear. A few days later the newspaper again reassured its readers that the pestilence preferred strangers, sailors, and laboring men: "To those who live regularly and pay attention to cleanliness, we think there is little cause for apprehension." The *Bee* also reported that the strangers and laboring classes were bearing the brunt of the current attack.[52] Yellow Jack, no respecter of persons, seemed class-conscious because the more settled, well-to-do portions of the population for the most part belonged to the ranks of the acclimated. Furthermore, many who could afford to do so left New Orleans during the hot and humid "sickly season" for resorts with a more comfortable climate.

The yellow fever outbreak of 1841 set a new record in causing an estimated 1,800 deaths in New Orleans. Newspapers gave much attention to newcomers, complaining that despite all warnings "fresh arrivals"—both American and foreign—continued to pour into the city providing additional fuel for the epidemic.[53] Little or nothing was said about class differences among the victims. In contrast, the extensive visitation of 1847 intensified awareness and led to the explicit articulation of class as a significant epidemiological variable, although not always as consistent a category as nativity or "acclimation" in predicting differential effects.

In August, 1847, the *Picayune* announced that yellow fever had not yet become epidemic despite the presence of large numbers of the unacclimated, including volunteers returning from the Mexican War and immigrants "of the poorer sort." Two days later the journal reported that the fever was "now prevailing in nearly every part of the city" and the board of health had declared "that we are on the eve of an epidemic."[54] The disease attacked "the lower class" first, but by late August its influence had extended to "all ranks of society." On August 31, when five "gentlemen of the community" died, the editor of the *Bee* commented that "neither rich nor poor can now claim exemption." The *Picayune* also reported that the disease had begun to affect "classes at first almost exempt." Nevertheless, yellow fever usually claimed most of its victims among newcomers, the lower classes, and working-class males, especially whites between the ages of twenty and forty. Nearly three-fourths of the yellow fever fatalities in 1847 were in the age category twenty to forty years.[55] Whenever a substantial number of creoles, children, blacks, or the "better element" was visibly affected by yellow fever, that aspect of the epidemic received attention as an unusual, noteworthy deviation from the customary pattern.

Observers considered the visitation of 1847 the most widespread epidemic that had ever occurred in New Orleans. One resident wrote in late October: ". . . we have had a season of deep distress—& in all my experience I never saw the like." Members of the Howard Association attended some 1,200 fever patients among the poor that year and provided sustenance for their families as well.[56]

According to Dr. Erasmus Darwin Fenner, the older physicians of New Orleans agreed that the fever of 1847 was "the most extensive that ever prevailed" in the city, but believed it less "malignant" than the pestilence of 1839 or 1841. He cited Charity Hospital statistics showing the case fatality rate as less than one-third in 1847, whereas ordinarily it ran as high as one-half or more. The "poorer classes" suffered most from the disease, in Fenner's judgment, because of their "imprudent manner of living." An estimated 20,000 to 25,000 cases occurred in New Orleans; if so, at least one of every five New Orleanians experienced the disease that season. Yellow fever deaths reported by sextons of New Orleans cemeteries totaled 2,306, not including the 613 interments reported by late October from the suburban community of Lafayette. Even as late as December some cases and deaths continued to occur. Fenner considered 3,000 a reasonable estimate of mortality for New Orleans and Lafayette. Only twenty-three deaths were recorded as native New Orleanians, mostly children.[57]

The widely accepted theory of blending fevers undoubtedly added to the ordinary difficulties of medical diagnosis and contributed to the problem of determining the exact yellow fever mortality. According to this medical concept, various kinds of fevers could be explained as gradations of one basic fever. It was believed that milder grades blended together during an epidemic and sometimes merged with the most malignant form, yellow fever. The editor of the *New Orleans Medical and Surgical Journal* observed the presence of all forms and grades of fever which blended in a variety of combinations during the epidemic of 1847: mild intermittent, remittent, dysentery, congestive, and pernicious intermittent, as well as mild and grave yellow fever.[58]

The terms refer to vaguely understood symptom-complexes rather than to specific diseases with specific causes. Diagnoses based on superficial symptoms, quite similar in a variety of disorders, could not always define the precise nature of a patient's illness. Many cases of mild or severe yellow fever might have been recorded under another label. The historian's problem of interpreting diagnosis and nomenclature in terms of modern disease concepts can be well illustrated by a list of twenty-seven "fevers" in addition to yellow fever compiled from the New Orleans Board of Health mortality reports for 1847: "Fever," adynamic, ataxic, bilious, bilious remittent, congestive, idiopathic, gastric, hectic, icterodes, intermittent, intermittent pernicious, intestinal, malignant, malignant putrid, nervous, pernicious, pernicious congestive, puerperal, remittent, putrid, scarlet, scarlet malignant, traumatic, typhoid, typhoid congestive, and typhus.[59] Some of the 600 deaths attributed to these varieties of fever undoubtedly belonged in the yellow fever column. On the other hand, it is somewhat less likely that deaths were mistakenly attributed to yellow fever because many physicians insisted on the appearance of the "black vomit" (which did not invariably occur) and other obvious symptoms of jaundice and spontaneous hemorrhage before pronouncing a case yellow fever.

In discussing the scope of the 1847 outbreak, Dr. Fenner and others observed that no major epidemic had occurred since 1841, and that the population increase since then had provided new supplies of the unacclimated. More than 20,000 Europeans had settled in New Orleans in the four or five years prior to 1847, and immigration that year was said to have been particularly heavy, consisting mainly of the destitute. In addition, large numbers of discharged soldiers returning from the Mexican War stopped in New Orleans.[60] The *New Orleans Medical and Surgical Journal* reported that yellow fever prevailed in Vera Cruz, but only a few cases had been brought from there to the Crescent City.[61] One imported case or one infected mosquito, however, could have set the epidemic in motion.

Necropolis of the South

A half-century of regular visitations established for yellow fever an accepted role in New Orleans. It was viewed as an inevitable scourge to be endured, but fortunately limited to two or three major appearances per decade. As the disease carried off hundreds of victims, a constant stream of immigration furnished more than sufficient replacements, and the population of New Orleans continued to grow in spite of the hazards. Most citizens only saw absolute numbers and failed to consider the declining rate of increase—even as they noted only the absolute growth of shipping and failed to perceive their declining share of the expanding upper Mississippi Valley trade, which increasingly went by rail to the northeast. Although the business season was delayed during epidemic years, the vigorous renewal of trade always dimmed the memory of earlier distresses.

As the population increased and the fever raised the death count year by year, acclimated New Orleanians experienced a diminishing sensitivity to its ravages. The definition of a mild epidemic changed as the outbreaks became more severe. The epidemic of 1843, for example, claiming only about 700 victims in a population of more than 100,000, was moderate in comparison with the previous epidemic of 1841 which killed 1,500 to 2,000.[62] But in 1817, 800 deaths in a population of 24,000 had constituted a major disaster. The worse the epidemics became, the more loudly editors, physicians, and others protested that New Orleans was the healthiest city in the Union—except during occasional epidemic years. Unfortunately, that claim was simply not true. Even in non-epidemic years New Orleans had the highest mortality rate in the country.[63]

Yellow fever was the most widely known cause of New Orleans' high death rate, but it was simply one among many diseases contributing to the mortality lists. Epidemics always attract attention because they are by definition the unusual, sudden, dramatic occurrence. In the nineteenth century, they were also mysterious and terrifying. Nevertheless, the common, ordinary, endemic maladies, although little noticed, killed more New Orleanians over the years than the highly publicized saffron scourge.

The delusion regarding the salubrity of the city was generally accepted in New Orleans (with a few notable dissenters), but failed to gain credence in other parts of the country. Regardless of protests to the contrary, New Orleans, largely because of yellow fever, acquired a national reputation as a center of pestilence and death, the "Necropolis of the South." There can be no doubt that this reputation and the reality behind it had a significant long-term negative effect, posing obstacles to the city's achieving its potential population growth and economic development relative to other nineteenth-century urbanizing centers.

In the early decades of the nineteenth century New Orleans physicians were divided by language and culture as well as theoretical and therapeutic perspectives. Two professional medical associations functioned separately, one almost entirely French or French Louisiana physicians, the other mainly American and other English-speaking practitioners. Such division further limited professional influence in sanitary reform or other public health concerns at a time when the medical profession had little strength, effectiveness, or unity anywhere. Physicians engaged in post-epidemic analyses of each outbreak, and debated the issues of treatment, probable causes, and possible measures to prevent future epidemics. They published their views in pamphlets, reports, newspaper articles, and after its inception in 1844, the *New Orleans Medical and Surgical Journal*.

Since the late eighteenth century, medical philosophers in New Orleans and elsewhere had attempted to rationalize and explain the nature, causes, and transmission of yellow fever. Unaware of the mosquito's role, physicians found it difficult to account for the fever's unpredictable spread. The inconsistencies of the disease seemed to defy all efforts at generalization, and medical controversy until the late nineteenth century generated more heat than light. "Who shall decide when doctors disagree?" was a common nineteenth-century expression.[64] The popular response to conflicting medical views was that anyone and everyone could have an opinion, but few would support health reform measures in the face of such uncertainty among experts—especially if the action required public funding.

Since both French and American physicians generally believed that epidemic yellow fever resulted from filthy conditions, sanitary reform was an obvious objective. During the first half of the nineteenth century boards of health existed intermittently in New Orleans, several created by the state legislature, others by the city council, usually including city officials and physicians as members. Not one operated with any degree of efficacy. Dependent upon an uncooperative city council for funds and enforcement of health regulations, the boards, no matter how enlightened, could draft but not implement a comprehensive sanitary code. Although willing enough to appoint a board, the council was seldom willing to appropriate funds to carry out the board's recommendations.[65]

Complicating matters further, between 1836 and 1852 New Orleans was divided into three separate municipalities, each functioning as an independent corporate entity in charge of its own finances and most other urban functions. The three municipal councils met as a General Council to handle matters of broad policy and common interest, and a mayor elected at-large presided over the General Council. Conflict between French and American interests, which gave rise to the division, had been largely resolved by mid-century with the consolidation of an elite leadership representing both ethnic groups. Debt and inefficiency attributable to the ill-functioning tripartite monstrosity became a threat to the city's prosperity, and in 1852 state legislation reunified New Orleans and added to it the suburban community of Lafayette.[66] City finances improved, but the new arrangement had almost no effect on urban sanitation. Neither the commercial elite nor the ethnically diverse voting masses yet espoused the cause of public health. The sanitary reform movement was just beginning at mid-century in the cities of the northeast. Although New Orleans also had a few physicians calling for reform by 1850, the development of public support for sanitary reform and health regulations required many more years, more epidemics, and more pressure from the outside world. Even then, implementation and enforcement were no easy matters in the Crescent City.

Yellow Fever in Other Louisiana Towns, 1811-1847

The disease does not seem to have spread much beyond New Orleans before 1811, when it first appeared in St. Francisville, a small but important trade center about a hundred miles up the Mississippi from the Crescent City.[67] Within the next few years the developing hinterland of cotton and sugar plantations began to supply bountiful crops and interior markets, while improvements in steam navigation made possible an expanding volume of traffic along Louisiana's waterways. When yellow fever prevailed in New Orleans, it was likely to be carried with travelers and commerce to some of the villages and steamboat landings along the rivers and bayous.

With the passage of time, more and more communities along the waterways acquired the necessary concentration of human and mosquito populations for a yellow fever outbreak to be set off by an infected person or mosquito arriving on a steamer from New Orleans. During the epidemic in 1817, the disease traveled upriver and landed in Baton Rouge for the first time and in St. Francisville for the second time, then proceeded as far north as Natchez, Mississippi. In 1819 the scourge again hit the previous targets as well as a new one, Alexandria on Red River. Thereafter, the disease appeared in some or all of these river towns whenever a major epidemic was under way in New Orleans. During the 1820s yellow fever traveled beyond the city almost every year, sometimes attacking Donaldsonville on the Mississippi, Thibodaux on Bayou Lafourche, and Opelousas, as well as the most frequently visited points—Baton Rouge, St. Francisville, and Alexandria.[68]

Following the same self-serving impulses as the New Orleans journalists, small town newspaper editors also engaged in attempts to deny, discount, or discredit early "rumors" of epidemic disease in their midst. Controversies between journals developed within the same town or in neighboring towns, with charges and countercharges of propagating lies— saying, for example, that yellow fever prevailed where it did not, or calling the disease negligible when it was actually quite serious. Eventually, however, as in New Orleans, when the disease reached a certain level of undeniable prevalence, newspapers acknowledged its presence, urged strangers to leave town for a time, and cautioned those who had fled not to return until the disease had been terminated by frost.[69]

In early September, 1822, the editor of the Alexandria *Louisiana Herald*, feeling his responsibility as a "public sentinel," announced the presence of yellow fever, but hastened to add that it was not likely to continue except for cases that might be imported. He advised against alarm, insisting that the disease, although transportable, did not become contagious. Admitting that "about" five deaths from yellow fever had occurred the previous week, the editor proceeded to explain each one in a manner clearly designed to allay local fears:

> The first that of a gentlemen, whose death is announced today, a seafaring man recently returned from the south. The second was a young lady but a few days arrived from New Orleans; the third a lady, an ancient inhabitant, whose case was greatly aggravated, if not produced by an excessive indulgence in green unwholesome fruit. The fourth was a youth of 17, who brought on his disease by unnecessary exposure to the sun, and extravigant [sic] indulgence in immature and pernicious fruit. And the fifth was a man of long confirmed habits of intemperance.[70]

The editorial reported that the doctors strongly urged those who were alarmed to leave town because fear was one of the most potent predisposing causes of yellow fever.

Demonstrating its unpredictability, yellow fever did not spread beyond New Orleans during most of the 1830s, except in 1837 and 1839 when it visited old spots and added several new ones. All contemporary sources agreed that the epidemic of 1839 was Louisiana's most extensive visitation yet to occur, affecting New Orleans, Donaldsonville, Plaquemine, Baton Rouge, Port Hudson, Bayou Sara, and St. Francisville along the Mississippi; Thibodaux on Bayou Lafourche; Alexandria and Natchitoches on Red River; Franklin, St. Martinville, and New Iberia on Bayou Teche; and Washington on Bayou Courtableau.[71] In November, 1839, a New Orleans resident wrote: "The sickness has not been half so bad this Season as in 1837 (when I had it)—not in the City but the country has been more troubled with it than ever it was before, & in most of the Towns on the coast and Rivers it has been very fatal."[72] River and coastal towns outside Louisiana stricken with yellow fever that year included Vicksburg, Natchez, Biloxi, Houston, Galveston, Mobile, Tampa, Savannah, Augusta, and Charleston.[73]

Most of Louisiana's river and bayou towns had only a few hundred inhabitants when yellow fever first attacked them, and most had less than 1,500 residents as late as the 1850s. Small town doctors and officials exhibited even less concern with recordkeeping than those in New Orleans, and mortality figures are rarely available. Occasionally a physician wrote up his observations for publication in the *New Orleans Medical and Surgical Journal*, providing a glimpse of yellow fever's impact on interior communities. Dr. T. A. Cooke, for example, reported that Opelousas suffered 250 cases of yellow fever in 1837 in a population of about 1,400. In 1839, the disease "spared none who remained in town, except only those who had previously had it. . . ." So many had contracted yellow fever in 1837 and 1839 that only twenty-five cases and eight deaths occurred when the disease reappeared in 1842. Although he did not believe the fever contagious, Cooke found much evidence to indicate its transportation from New Orleans to Opelousas. Epidemics exhibited great diversity in different places at different times, he thought, because the yellow fever "poison" was affected by a wide variety of purely local influences and conditions.[74]

Only two outbreaks in the 1840s spread extensively beyond New Orleans, those of 1843 and 1847. In 1847 the disease spread to Lafayette and Carrollton, suburban communities adjoining New Orleans; to Algiers across the Mississippi; and to Covington, Madisonville, and Mandeville across Lake Pontchartrain—the latter places having been considered safe resorts from the city's plague in earlier times.[75] The transmission of yellow fever through the channels of trade and travel was always facilitated by émigrés fleeing New Orleans, many carrying the pestilence with them. In 1847 several German and Dutch families left New Orleans for Covington to escape the fever. Three persons became ill and died shortly after arriving in Covington. From that beginning yellow fever eventually infected the townspeople, resulting in 160 to 180 cases of which about ten died. One Covington physician later said he doubted the outbreak was "genuine yellow fever."[76]

St. Francisville, Natchitoches, and the bayou towns had suffered the disease in 1839 but apparently escaped in 1847. Some cases appeared in Plaquemine, Baton Rouge, and Bayou Sara on the Mississippi. Alexandria on Red River suffered a serious visitation. On October 9 the editor of Alexandria's *Red River Republican* attempted to discount the severity of the outbreak. He complained that local physicians had alarmed the populace by declaring an epidemic in progress, causing many persons to leave town. A number of cases had occurred, especially among the "poor and destitute," but the editor insisted that the fever was generally mild in its effects, and he expressed the hope that no more sickness would develop. His wishful thinking was no match for the doctors' judgment; yellow fever continued to spread, and by mid-October the town was desolate as many families left the area. Not until early December did the epidemic completely run its course, as in New Orleans. Cool weather must have come later than usual in 1847, permitting a continuation of mosquito activity and disease transmission for several more weeks than was customary.[77]

Some small-town doctors and other non-medical observers found it increasingly difficult to believe in local causation (and its corollary, non-contagion) as they repeatedly witnessed the introduction of first cases from New Orleans. Within a small community where the comings and goings of each person were known to all, one could identify the earliest cases and their travel histories, an impossible task in the large, impersonal setting of the Crescent City. Although not an annual visitor in the river and bayou towns, yellow fever appeared often enough to provide immunity to some, while others left during an outbreak. In the absence of rapid growth or a large immigrant population, fuel for the fever was limited and relatively scattered, diminishing the probability of large-scale disaster, although not eliminating it altogether as demonstrated by the Great Epidemic of 1853.

Table 1.

YELLOW FEVER MORTALITY IN NEW ORLEANS
1796-1847

Year	Estimated Deaths	Population (Approx.)
*1796	350-400	6,000
*1799	?	
*1804	?	
*1809	?	
*1811	500	18,000
*1817	800	24,000
1818	115	
*1819	1,000-2,000	26,000
1820	400	
*1822	800-2,000	32,000
1824	108	
1827	109+	
1828	130+	
*1829	900	48,000
1830	117+	
1832	400	
*1833	1,000	58,000
1835	284+	
*1837	1,300	68,000
*1839	800	74,000
*1841	1,325-1,800	79,000
1842	211+	
*1843	500-700	84,000
1844	148	
1846	100-160	
*1847	2,300-3,000	109,000

*Major epidemics. Other years listed are those with at least 100 reported deaths.

+For many years, the only figures available for yellow fever mortality in the city are the figures for yellow fever deaths in Charity Hospital, indicated by a plus after the number. Presumably there were other deaths in New Orleans in private practice during those years.

Table 2.

YELLOW FEVER IN LOUISIANA OUTSIDE OF NEW ORLEANS
1811-1829

	1811	1817	1819	1822	1827	1829
Alexandria			X	X	X	
Baton Rouge		X	X	X	X	X
Donaldsonville					X	
Opelousas						X
St. Francisville	X	X	X	X	X	X
Thibodaux						X

Table 3.

YELLOW FEVER IN LOUISIANA
OUTSIDE OF NEW ORLEANS
1837-1847

	1837	1839	1843	1847
Alexandria	X	X		X
Algiers				X
Baton Rouge	X		X	X
Carrollton				X
Covington				X
Donaldsonville		X		
Franklin		X		
Lafayette (N.O.)				X
Madisonville				X
Mandeville				X
Natchitoches		X		
New Iberia		X		
Opelousas	X	X		
Plaquemine	X	X		X
Port Hudson		X	X	
St. Francisville		X	X	
St. Martinville		X		
Thibodaux		X	X	
Washington	X	X		

Major points affected; not a complete list.

A Half-Century of Pestilence, 1799-1849

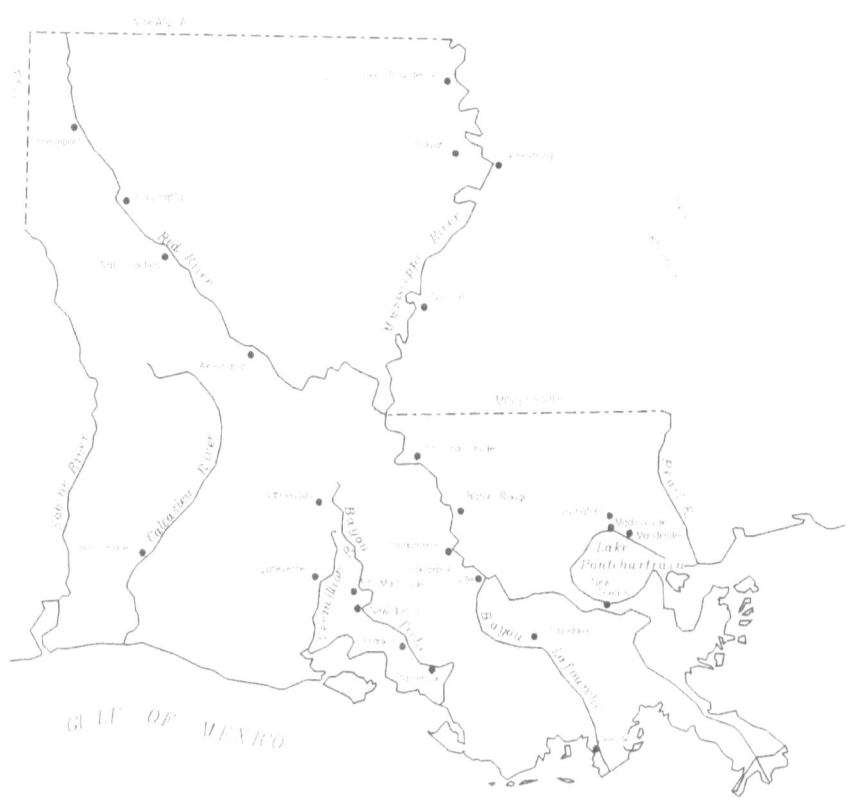

Yellow Fever on Louisiana's Waterways

IV

THE GREAT EPIDEMICS OF THE FIFTIES
1853, 1854, 1855, 1858

Yellow fever reached its peak of virulence in Louisiana in the 1850s, striking four severe blows within a six-year period. In 1853 New Orleans suffered "probably the worst single epidemic ever to strike a major American city."[1] "The bloodiest battle-fields of modern-time scarcely can compare with the New Orleans epidemic of 1853, which *destroyed five times more* than the British Army lost on the field of Waterloo," wrote Dr. Bennet Dowler. By his calculations, in 1853 the disease claimed some 8,400 lives in the Crescent City.[2] Yellow fever returned in serious epidemic form in 1854, 1855, and 1858. Survivors scarcely had time to forget one epidemic before another occurred. In the four widespread attacks of the 1850s, the pestilence killed more than 18,000 persons in New Orleans alone.

Between the extensive outbreak in 1847 and the most malignant of all epidemics in 1853, New Orleans had not been entirely exempt from the fever. During that five-year period the total yellow fever mortality had amounted to more than 2,000, but the largest number of victims in any single summer was only about 800. With a population increase of almost 50,000 during the same period, the city's losses from yellow fever seemed negligible. In the absence of an outbreak destructive enough to meet the local standard, no "epidemic" was recognized or declared, and New Orleans journalists and physicians allowed themselves to hope and then to believe that yellow fever was no longer a disease to be feared. By general consent the doctors and health officials considered a disease *sporadic* rather than *epidemic* until the number of deaths from that particular malady exceeded the number from all other causes in the weekly mortality record.[3]

In May, 1852, the *New Orleans Medical and Surgical Journal* confidently announced that "the Yellow Fever—the dread of the stranger and sojourner in our midst, has long since been banished [from] the city . . . ." In November the same medical editor noted considerable improvement in New Orleans' health record which he attributed to the recent municipal efforts at street cleaning, paving, and drainage of swamp land surrounding the city. Five years had passed without the occurrence of epidemic yellow fever, and the editor felt certain that the disease could be completely eliminated by a large-scale program of sanitary improvements.[4]

1853: New Orleans' Worst Epidemic

The ideal of urban cleanliness and the reality of achieving such a condition in New Orleans remained unreconciled, and in that fateful summer of 1853, when frequent rains alternated with blistering heat, the sanitary condition of the city steadily worsened. Gutters and drains were open sewers, clogged with every imaginable kind of waste, while streets and alleys were filled with garbage, manure, the rotting, reeking carcasses of dogs, and "festering nastiness of every description." Newspapers complained of the filthy conditions and repeatedly denounced city officials for neglecting their duties. In view of the unsanitary state of the city, Dr. Erasmus Darwin Fenner thought it strange that anyone should look beyond New Orleans for the cause of the pestilence. "Indeed it was so bad," wrote Fenner, "that if it had given rise to *Egyptian Plague* instead of yellow fever, it ought not to have surprised anyone."[5]

Several cases admitted to Charity Hospital in May were pronounced yellow fever by the attending physicians, but other doctors who viewed these cases rejected the diagnosis. Similar cases near the waterfront in the Fourth District and at various points around the city also prompted diagnostic uncertainty. According to Dr. Fenner's description of the discussion and debate,

> Some thought the subjects were too yellow, others that the yellowness was not exactly of the right hue . . . some said what was pronounced black vomit was not dark enough, others that it was too black; others, again that it was not

black vomit because it was of a reddish hue; whilst others, admitting a resemblance, still could not find "the old fashioned Black Vomit." Some would not admit the cases were Yellow Fever, because they occurred "too early in the season,"—they had never known Yellow Fever to break out so early in this city, and therefore did not think it possible.

Finally, on June 10, an "unquestionable case" entered Charity Hospital: an Irish female from Tchoupitoulas Street who turned quite yellow, and before she died the following day produced large quantities of "unmistakeable, old-fashioned, coffee-grounds black vomit," thereby ending the medical controversy. "The skeptics all gave it up after seeing this," said Fenner.[6]

From late May onward the disease continued to spread but received little publicity until mid-July. New Orleans had no board of health at the time. Lacking sufficient authority to enforce its regulations and denied support by the city council, the last board had adjourned *sine die* in 1852, leaving only a secretary who continued to issue the weekly interment reports under the mayor's direction. "This was all the *correct* information that was published," Fenner stated, "and even this was complained of by some who thought it better to suppress the truth than cause a panic." Although some of the early cases occurred in scattered locations, yellow fever first appeared and became prevalent on the waterfront in the Fourth District and in the adjacent neighborhood, populated by the laboring poor, mostly Irish and German immigrants. Highly susceptible to the disease, they lived in crowded, deteriorating wooden huts and tenements, the floors often covered with water and mud. Rains kept the unpaved streets in a marsh-like state and the culverts overflowing with filth that steamed under the hot sun following the summer showers.[7]

The customary departure of the well-to-do for summer resorts in the North or the upper South was well under way when the first cases of yellow fever began to surface. As rumors of fever spread about the city, the mass exodus quickened, reaching high tide when the disease was finally acknowledged by the press in mid-July. Estimates of the number of émigrés that summer ranged from 36,000 to 75,000, or one-fourth to one-half of the city's population.[8]

As always, New Orleans newspapers tried to ignore or to minimize the early signs of Yellow Jack's presence in the city. The *Daily Delta* apologized on June 12 for having previously included "by accident" a report from Charity Hospital listing two deaths from the black vomit. Without interpretation, such a fact might give the "wrong impression, here and abroad." With unknowing irony, the editor explained that the cases had come in from Havana, and since yellow fever was not an importable disease, there was no reason to fear its spread from a few imported cases. Assuring his readers that New Orleans was "one of the healthiest cities of the Union," the editor declared it necessary to interpret all reports with great care "so that nothing calculated to mislead persons abroad or citizens at home, should have publicity."[9]

While the pestilence made further inroads and must have been a subject for discussion, speculation, and anxiety in many quarters, New Orleans journals filled their editorial columns with clever commentary on such topics as the "Can't Get Away Club," meaning those persons who found it necessary, for whatever reason, to remain in the city during summer. The *Daily Crescent* glorified the pleasures and benefits of the lazy season enjoyed by "club" members and cast doubt upon the wisdom of the émigrés who thought they had to go north "in pursuit of health, comfort, and recreation," especially since "yellow fever had become an obsolete idea in New Orleans."[10] Other articles facetiously dealt with the mosquitoes "which serve to remind us that New Orleans, in summer, is not quite Elysium." The *Weekly Delta* declared, ironically, "We have never known the mosquitoes to be half so severe as they are at present," and despite the prophecies of certain pessimists, "we don't believe Yellow Jack will favor us with his grim presence this year, for the simple reason that Providence does not afflict us with two curses at one and the same time; and, to add yellow fever to the present terrible visitation of mosquitoes, would be too much for human endurance."[11]

During the last weeks of June and early July, the newspapers carried without comment occasional reports from Charity Hospital and interment figures from the cemeteries. The press did begin to pay more attention to the filthy streets, charging the city council with negligence and calling for the creation of an effective board of health.[12] Dr. Fenner later said he realized by the first of July that an epidemic was on the way if not already in progress. On July 13 the *Orleanian* admitted the presence of the infection but discounted the significance of the outbreak. On the same day several newspapers printed a notice calling a meeting of the Howard Association, the organization that cared for the sick poor during epidemics. This item should have furnished a clue to many readers that the situation had become more serious. By July 16 the pestilence had claimed more than 300 lives, and as the word spread, the ranks of the *émigrés* swelled as citizens fled by the thousands. During the week ending July 23, more than 400 persons died of the fever.[13]

At last the newspapers began to discuss the pestilence openly, blaming the city government for allowing unsanitary conditions to develop, conditions which, according to the best medical opinion of the time, gave rise to disease, yellow fever included. Under public pressure and with the urging of Mayor A. D. Crossman, the bicameral council finally reached agreement and established a temporary board of health on July 25.[14] In the last week of July, after appointing the members of the new health board, the New Orleans City Council delegated its powers to the Finance Committee and adjourned until October, leaving the city virtually without a government for two months in the midst of a disaster. Some council members fled to places of safety in the North, some to resorts along the gulf where the epidemic pursued them, and some stayed on and offered their services during the crisis. One New Orleans journal commented disgustedly: "What a humiliating position! A City Council, in the midst of an unprecedented epidemic, adjourning for their own health, convenience, and comfort . . . . What a burlesque on municipal government!"[15]

Describing the plague-stricken community in August, one "samaritan" wrote: "The whole city was a hospital, and every well man, woman, and child were instrumental, in one way or another, in relieving the sick." The streets were empty except for "the hasty pedestrian on an errand of mercy" or physicians charging along in their gigs. Morning and evening, funeral processions lined the roads to the cemeteries. The usual noises of activity, the sounds of shoppers, sellers, and workers, were silenced by disease, death, or fear as New Orleans economic activity came to a halt. Most shops closed, and the wharves were all but deserted.[16]

The coroner's records listed dozens of yellow fever victims, some of them "unknown," found "lying dead" in houses, in stores, near the levee, and at the gates of Lafayette Cemetery in the Fourth District. Most were described as natives of Ireland and Germany; some had come from other parts of Europe or the northern states.[17] By early August, wrote one observer, the pestilence "clothed itself in all its terrors, striking down everyone who came in its way—sparing neither man, woman nor child who had not had it before, or been here more than six years." When the disease went beyond "the emigrant army" and began to attack "the citizens," it quickly spread throughout the city.[18]

Entire families fell victim to the fever, and "tenants for the cemeteries" multiplied faster than graves could be provided. In August the burial count in the city's cemeteries ranged from 150 to more than 250 per day. Eighty to 90 percent of deaths were attributable to the epidemic as the mortality from yellow fever climbed to record heights that month: 900 the first week, 1,200 the next, and two full weeks of more than 1,300 each.[19]

Long-term residents had cause for alarm during the terrible month of August. Up to this point they had felt relatively secure, believing that only the newcomer, the imprudent, and the unclean fell to the raging fever. When several of New Orleans' oldest citizens succumbed to the pestilence, a new dread seized the city. Even the French creole inhabitants, the last to fear the disease, grew anxious. French-language newspapers attributed the fever's increasing virulence to the noxious effluvia emanating from the gutters and from graveyards filled with rotting, half-buried corpses.[20]

Burial in New Orleans was complicated by topography and climate. Situated between river and swamps, drained only by a few ditches and canals, the city was drenched by rainfall averaging sixty inches per year. Digging a grave in such marshy soil meant opening a water-filled pit, two to three feet deep at most. From the city's early years the dead had been buried above ground in tombs or vaults of brick or stone. Row after row of such structures, many covered with plaster and painted white, made the cemeteries appear to be what they were often called, "the cities of the dead." Only those whose families could not afford vaults or those buried at public expense were laid to rest beneath the ground in watery graves.[21] A foreign visitor once remarked that the dead were "immersed" rather than "interred."[22]

Older cemeteries in the center of the city sometimes caused complaint when the brick vaults along the walls, often hastily constructed and not well-sealed, released fumes from decaying corpses and polluted the air for some distance around. Since most yellow fever deaths came from the ranks of the laboring poor and the destitute, thousands of graves in designated "Potter's Fields" had to be provided by the city. In some cases friends and family dug the grave and buried their own dead so that the coffin would not be left in soaking rain and blazing sun, waiting with dozens of others until a grave was ready to receive it.[23] To speed up burials, gravediggers resorted to long ditches, no more than two feet deep, into which they tossed the coffins and threw on a "few shovelfuls of dirt." Sometimes the coffins floated in the water, and some workmen had to stand on them

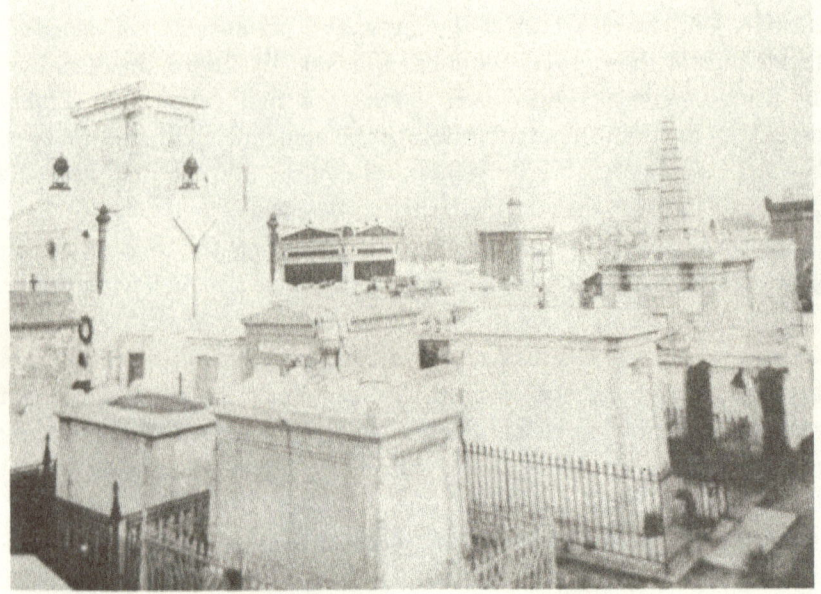

St. Louis Cemetery, New Orleans.
From *Art Work of New Orleans* (1895).

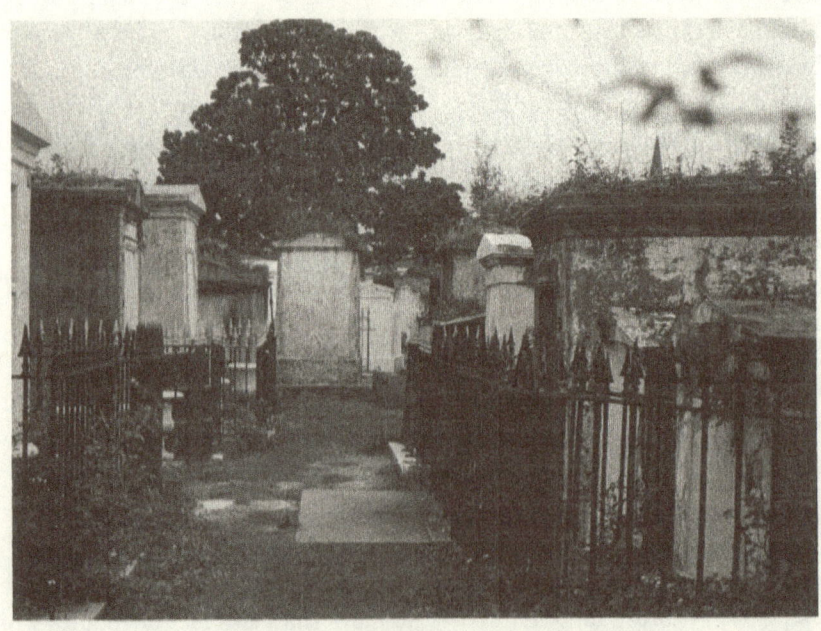

St. Louis Cemetery, New Orleans,
Courtesy B. A. Hayhome, Photographer (1979).

NO. I. **THE** VOL. I.

NEW-ORLEANS MEDICAL JOURNAL,

DEVOTED TO

THE CULTIVATION OF MEDICINE,

AND THE

ASSOCIATE SCIENCES.

(*BI-MONTHLY.*)

ARRANGEMENT.

1. ——Original Communications, Cases, and Surgical Operations occuring in Private Practice.
2. ——Health of the City, with Reports from the New-Orleans Hospitals.
3. ——Periscope of Practical Medicine — or Spirit of the Medical Journals, Foreign & Domestic.
4. ——Brief Notices of Recent Medical Literature.

EDITED BY

ERASMUS D. FENNER, M. D.

AND

A. HESTER, M. D.,

One of the Physicians to the New-Orleans Charity Hospital.

"*Summum bonum Medicinæ Sanitas.*"
(GL.)

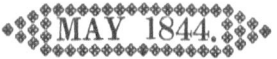

NEW ORLEANS,
PRINTED BY J. DOE.

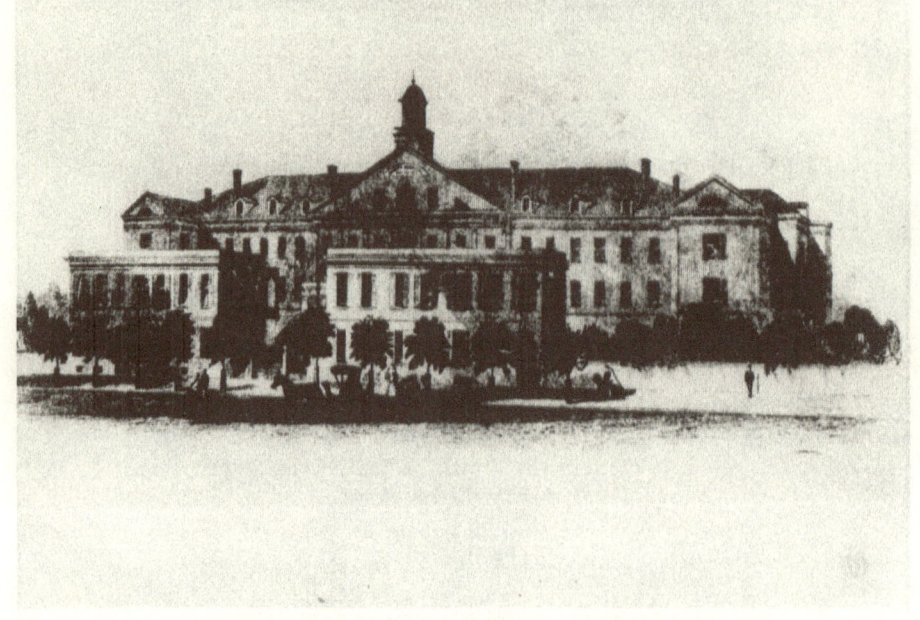

Charity Hospital of Louisiana, New Orleans, 1855.
Courtesy Rudolph Matas Library, Tulane University Medical Center.

while others piled on a layer of soggy earth, barely covering the flimsy boxes that were almost level with the surface of the ground. The daily rains soon washed away this thin covering and exposed the coffins to the blistering heat of the sun after each brief downpour. Often the putrefying bodies burst through the poorly built pine boxes and filled the air "far and near, with the most intolerable pestilential odors."[24]

Under the circumstances it was no easy task to keep enough gravediggers at work to cope with the numbers of dead delivered to the cemeteries by the city carts, Charity Hospital wagons, and private hearses. On one occasion so many coffins accumulated at the cemetery gate in the Fourth District that several dozen bodies remained unburied for more than twenty-four hours, "piled on the ground, swollen and bursting their coffins, and enveloped in swarms of flies." To remedy the problem, the mayor set the black "chain gang" to work digging graves and hired additional gravediggers, black and white, at the enormous wage of five dollars per hour.[25]

On the recommendation of the board of health, Mayor Crossman ordered that four hundred rounds of cannon be fired daily at sunset in the various public squares in an attempt to purify the atmosphere and subdue the disease. With the same purpose he ordered the burning of barrels of tar in the streets and in the cemeteries during the night. The effort to fight the fever with smoke from burning tar and gun-powder explosions was based on the widely accepted theory that a peculiar "epidemic constitution of the atmosphere" in conjunction with effluvia from local accumulations of decaying matter provided the conditions that generated disease and facilitated its transmission over an extensive area. The smoke and explosions were intended to neutralize the effluvia and alter the atmospheric conditions conducive to disease. According to one newspaper, "The smoke of the burnt powder and tar, wherever it appears, is a killing dose to the mosquitoes. This fact alone is proof that the concussion and smoke act as powerful purifiers." The mayor halted the cannon-firing after two days when the noise was found to be disturbing the sick, but the tar-burning continued for some time.[26] The roar of the guns and the fires in the night together with the terrors and odors of the pestilence, which spread so insidiously and so mysteriously, must have presented a truly hellish spectacle to those who were forced to endure it.

Most people believed that filth and offensive odors had something to do with the production of disease, although the process was a mystery. One New Orleans physician, however, in the midst of the epidemic startled his colleagues and the community at large with his theory that filth was a factor *retarding* the development of yellow fever. Dr. J. S. McFarlane argued that the city's filth in previous years had drained into the swamps and produced an atmosphere favorable to malarial and congestive fevers but antagonistic to yellow fever. Although his theory was more subtle and complex than it first appeared, journalists had a fine time ridiculing McFarlane's strange idea. The *Daily Crescent* proposed that a public laboratory be funded to produce a supply of nauseating vapors which could be given to the citizens of New Orleans in nose bags for their protection against yellow fever.[27]

The debate about causes reflected political and ideological perspectives. The New York *Tribune* suggested that yellow fever was a consequence of slavery, having been introduced from Africa, and that the scourge continued as a punishment of the South for its peculiar institution. The New Orleans *Weekly Delta* responded that yellow fever was not an imported disease and that black resistance to the disease was an argument in favor of slavery.[28] On another occasion the *Delta* explained the majority of yellow fever deaths as the result of white laborers violating nature's laws by "doing the work in hot noon-day summer sun that negroes ought to do." Later that year Dr. Samuel A. Cartwright outlined a similar theory in the pages of the *New Orleans Medical and Surgical Journal*.[29]

The traditional speculation among physicians concerning the mysteries of yellow fever had to be postponed until the epidemic was over. Their most immediate concern was treating extraordinary numbers of the sick. No therapy seemed consistently effective in dealing with the fever that year. Patients recovered and patients died under every possible form of treatment. When the old heroic measures such as bleeding, blistering, purging, vomiting, and dosing with large quantities of calomel and quinine proved useless, physicians became somewhat more cautious and moderate. The widespread southern experience of failure with such traditional therapies probably provided the death blow to the old methods that many had already begun to question and modify. Relying more on the body's natural recuperative powers, physicians prescribed warm or cool drinks, mustard footbaths, enemas, warm or cold sponging, and attentive nursing, measures recommended for decades by Louisiana's French creole doctors.[30]

Charity Hospital was soon filled beyond its capacity, and many patients had to lie on the floor as daily admission reached 100 or more. "The sick were almost constantly being brought in, and the dead carried out," wrote one journalist.[31] Usually during epidemics about 50 percent of the yellow fever patients at Charity died. In 1853 the fatality rate was closer to 60 percent with more than 3,000 cases and almost 1,800 deaths during the four months of the epidemic. As it was impossible for Charity Hospital to take care of all the destitute victims, the newly appointed board of health moved quickly to establish four temporary infirmaries as well as two places of asylum for children orphaned by the epidemic.[32]

The Howard Association also opened four temporary hospitals for the indigent sick, one specifically for convalescents, and a temporary orphan asylum in each district of the city. Association members divided the city among themselves, as they had done in the past, and took responsibility for locating destitute yellow fever patients and calling on them daily; arranging for home medical and nursing care; paying for medicines, ice, groceries, and bedding; and, when necessary, transporting patients to hospitals and orphans to asylums, and arranging for burial of the dead.

Whenever possible, they tried to provide a doctor and nurse of the patient's own nationality, or at least persons able to speak the patient's language.[33]

The Howards obtained wet nurses for the orphaned infants and hired nurses and servants to care for the homeless children gathered in each district asylum. The board of health also gave the Howard Association supervisory authority over the two shelters the city had established. Some 250 to 300 orphans received care during the epidemic and eventually were placed in families or divided between Catholic and Protestant groups, each vying for the children. Whenever their religion could be determined, the orphans were distributed accordingly. In dealing with small children when there was no way of knowing the parents' religion, the representatives of Catholic and Protestant asylums divided the little ones "by alternate choice." Some small children were brought in by persons who found them on the street or crawling about houses where all the adults had died. In such cases, neither the name, nationality, nor religion of their parents was ever to be known.[34]

Contributions exceeding $200,000 poured in to the Howard Association from individuals and groups throughout the Union. The long list of contributors from Washington, D.C., included the name of President Franklin Pierce. Before Baton Rouge developed its own epidemic, a deputation of its citizens came to aid the New Orleans Howards in nursing the poor and attending to the needs of their families. As the epidemic in New Orleans declined, the Crescent City Howards looked beyond the homefront and supplied physicians, nurses, and medicines to other fever-stricken communities in Louisiana, Mississippi, Alabama, and Texas.[35] In New Orleans the association had attended to 11,088 yellow fever patients, 5,203 males and 5,885 females. Of the total number, 2,942 died—almost 27 percent. Approximately 5,800 of their cases were Irish immigrants, and 2,900 were German.[36]

At a time when municipal governments gave minimal attention or aid to the poor, the Howard Association filled the need as well as it could, performing a wide range of vital social services for the indigent sick and their families, collecting funds, and distributing goods and medical services during epidemic emergencies. Numerous ethnic benevolent associations functioned as mutual insurance societies, assisting sick members during the epidemic and providing relief to widows and orphans. Labor unions, firemen, and other occupational organizations had their own relief committees. Dozens of associations, religious and secular, large and small, came to the aid of their members as well as others who needed help in those desperate times.[37] Residents who did not flee the city operated a dense network of voluntary associations which responded to the needs of epidemic victims, within and across class lines.

Ordinarily the New Orleans papers took issue with reports and editorials appearing in upstate, out-of-state, northern, and foreign journals. On at least one occasion in August, however, a New Orleans editor was delighted to publish an excerpt from the *Philadelphia Ledger* praising the Crescent City's populace for their calm, unruffled approach to the disease in their midst. The Philadelphia journalist commented upon the difference between New Orleans newspapers and those of the North in the measure of attention accorded the pestilence. In Philadelphia, he said, everyone discussed the New Orleans epidemic and anxiously awaited the daily telegraphic reports in the newpapers telling the progress of the disease and the increasing mortality. New Orleans journals, on the other hand, avoided "creating unnecessary fear and excitement in the public mind." Business, never active in summer, proceeded in its customary slow fashion; courts continued in session; and politics remained a subject for discussion. "When an entire population can take up an epidemic thus cooly," the Philadelphian declared, "they rob it of half its terrors, and are in the best possible condition for reducing its malignity." In Philadelphia or New York, he said, the announcement of 200 yellow fever deaths per day "would cause a general stampede of the inhabitants."[38] The northern journalist overlooked the fact that the stampede in New Orleans had already occurred at least a month before this time, that commerce was at a standstill, and that most members of the city council had left town. Nevertheless, there was some truth to the observation that the population remaining in the city exhibited little of the panic, disorder, or extraordinary criminal behavior often associated with disaster.

The week ending August 27 witnessed the peak of the epidemic; yellow fever had claimed almost 1,400 victims in seven days. By the first of September the pestilence was beginning to decline, "deaths from it now only amounting to about 100 a day." Through September and early October, the weekly death count decreased steadily: 700, 400, 200, 125, 85, 42. On October 13 the board of health declared the epidemic at an end and assured absentees and strangers a safe entry to New Orleans.[39] Although a few scattered cases occurred after that date, the crisis was over, and the city could begin the work of regeneration for the delayed business season. Physicians could start the task of explaining New Orleans' most virulent plague, one which had spread throughout the gulf states and the lower Mississippi Valley, covering more territory than ever before.

Established by resolution of the New Orleans Board of Health and appointed by the mayor, the Sanitary Commission of New Orleans was given the task of investigating and reporting on the facts of the recent calamity. Dr. Edward H. Barton, head of the commission, made an extensive statistical study of the epidemic, limited, however, by the inconsistencies and uncertainties of the available records and by a simple methodology yielding crude results. Yet his figures do provide a general outline of the demographic catastrophe.

Estimating a total population of almost 159,000 in New Orleans in 1853, including some 5,000 transients, and taking into account the flight of almost one-fourth of the population when yellow fever appeared, Dr. Barton arrived at a figure of approximately 125,000 persons remaining in New Orleans throughout the epidemic. By Barton's calculations, total cases in New Orleans numbered 29,000; total deaths from yellow fever, 8,101, or about one of every fifteen persons remaining in the city; the case fatality rate, almost 28 percent. Among the deaths from yellow fever, 68 percent were male; 42 percent, aged 20-29; 58 percent, aged 20-39. Only forty-three blacks were recorded as yellow fever deaths. Blacks constituted almost 20 percent of the city's population but only one-half of one percent of the yellow fever mortality. In other words, the death rate among whites was sixty-three per thousand; among blacks, 1.4 per thousand. Place of birth for many victims was unknown, but Irish and German immigrants furnished the highest totals of any groups recorded, and by all accounts the majority of the victims came from the ranks of the foreign-born. Only eighty-seven native New Orleanians appeared in the death list.[40]

Assuming a smaller "at risk" population and a larger number of cases and deaths, other estimates made by contemporaries yielded a worse overall picture of the epidemic in both absolute and proportional terms. Dr. Fenner believed that only 100,000 persons remained in New Orleans during the epidemic; of that number, 8 percent (or one in twelve) died of yellow fever and more than one-fourth fell sick with the disease. John Duffy's study of the epidemic shows about one-third of the population in flight, leaving 100,000 in the city, among which 40,000 cases of fever developed and almost 9,000 died—possibly more.[41]

1853: Scourge of the South

In 1853 yellow fever affected a much wider area than before, in Louisiana itself and throughout the lower South. Yellow Jack attacked every town along the Mississippi River as far north as Napoleon, Arkansas, at the mouth of the Arkansas River; practically every village in Mississippi and Louisiana south of Vicksburg; and almost every plantation along the Mississippi south of Natchez. In 1853 for the first time many plantation slaves were affected by the disease. Some died, but commentators invariably noted that most cases among blacks were relatively mild and the case fatality rate extremely low.[42] Pensacola, Mobile, Biloxi, Galveston, and Houston also experienced severe epidemics, and from each place the fever spread to hinterland communities where it had never been seen before. Posing new problems for medical theorists, the disease raged with equal force in clean and unclean areas, in high and dry regions and low and wet localities, in piney woods as well as filthy streets, in slave quarters of sugar plantations as well as crowded centers of river and gulf port towns.[43] Some physicians held firm to the doctrines of local causation and "epidemic constitution of the atmosphere" in explaining the fever's origin and transmission. Others were converted to the concept of transportability, and some even adopted the contagionist position.

In many Louisiana towns where the first cases were directly traceable to a previous center of infection, it was difficult to avoid the conclusion that the disease had been imported. Even so, local causationists could always point to imported cases that failed to set off an epidemic, or local cases that had no prior contact with an infected person or location. Despite the efforts of town and parish officials to protect their territories by quarantine measures, no barrier seemed to work against the invisible enemy. St. Mary Parish, a densely populated sugar-growing region west of New Orleans, established strict rules to prevent the entry of steamboats and to detain passengers from infected centers for several days at a quarantine station. Armed with shotguns, citizens of Franklin, the parish seat, demonstrated on one occasion their willingness to use force if necessary to compel boats to stop at the quarantine line. Standing their ground on Bayou Teche, they forced a contrary steamboat captain from New Orleans to turn back and follow the rules.[44]

Eventually yellow fever appeared in the parish at Centreville, reaching epidemic proportions in September with some forty to fifty cases in a population of about 200. The town council of Franklin established a quarantine barrier attended by armed guards on the road a half mile below town. Persons from Centreville, some five miles to the south, could enter Franklin on business for several hours during the day. Franklin citizens leaving town were warned not to visit infected places or they would not be readmitted until after a nine-day detention period. Not always consistently enforced, the restrictions were never applied to physicians. When it appeared that Centreville's epidemic was over, the barrier was removed for several days in October. When the Centreville epidemic flared up again, Franklin's authorities decreed absolute non-intercourse. Four or five cases did develop in Franklin, but they were all in one household, and the disease spread no farther.[45]

Yellow fever spread from New Orleans along the state's waterways to all the usual places and some new ones: Algiers, Donaldsonville, Plaquemine, Baton Rouge, Bayou Sara, St. Francisville (and nearby Clinton), Vidalia, and Lake Providence along the Mississippi River; Alexandria, Natchitoches, and Shreveport on Red River; Cloutierville on Old River, a branch of the Red; Washington on Bayou Courtableau; Pattersonville, Centreville, and Franklin on Bayou Teche, and Opelousas nearby; Thibodaux on Bayou Lafourche; Trenton on the Ouachita River; Covington and Madisonville across Lake Pontchartrain from New Orleans; and other small towns in close proximity to the infected centers.[46]

Some of the small towns suffered losses proportionally greater than New Orleans. In Baton Rouge, according to Dr. Bennet Dowler, in a population of about 2,000, at least 200 died of the fever; a later estimate set the figure as high as 400.[47] A report from Thibodaux described a desolate situation there in early September. The town had been largely abandoned, and almost every person remaining had the fever. In one day twenty-two persons had died and about 160 new cases had developed. According to Dowler's figures, yellow fever claimed nearly 150 persons, or 15 percent of the resident population of Thibodaux. In his well-known account of travels through the "Cotton Kingdom," Frederick Law Olmsted mentioned the effects of the disease on Alexandria, where he visited soon after the epidemic. The community ordinarily had a population of 1,000, but had been almost entirely deserted by its citizens when the pestilence struck. Olmsted was told that 120 deaths occurred among the 300 persons remaining in town. Dr. Dowler estimated that one-fifth to one-sixth of Alexandria's population had been wiped out by the disease. Lake Providence, where yellow fever had never appeared before, lost more than half of its small population.⁴⁸

1854

An experience such as the Great Epidemic of 1853 could scarcely be forgotten by those who lived through it, not even by New Orleanians long accustomed to epidemic disease. This time, however, no intermission followed, no summer or two in which the memory of epidemic yellow fever might begin to fade. The very next year the disease again appeared in New Orleans and carried off almost 2,500 additional victims.⁴⁹ Although costly in terms of total mortality, the outbreak of 1854 killed less than a third of the number lost the year before. A resident of New Orleans wrote in his diary in September; "This is considered among the old residents one of the bad 'epidemic years' yet coming after the frightful pestilence of last summer it seems to excite but little attention—such is the power of 'contrast.'" In November he noted that "the epidemic just closing is pronounced the worst that has ever existed in New Orleans except those of 1847 and 1853."⁵⁰

Not once throughout the entire 1854 season did the *Picayune* admit the existence of an epidemic. While publishing the weekly interment figures and Charity Hospital reports, the editor repeatedly declared the city free from anything resembling epidemic disease, apparently taking the disaster of 1853 as the new standard. Others were willing to call the outbreak an epidemic but considered it a mild type of disease. One doctor reported in the *New Orleans Medical and Surgical Journal*, ". . . in no former epidemic for eighteen years has yellow fever yielded more readily to timely medication."⁵¹

Once again in 1854 the city had no board of health as the previous one was purely temporary, and once again the city council recessed during the sickly season. When the members reassembled in October, the mayor informed them, with some sense of outrage, that in the absence of a board of health he had been unable to obtain any precise information to present them regarding the epidemic, which he said "was similar to the awful calamity of the previous year." Denouncing the "lamentable inefficiency" of a city government that failed to act in the interest of public health, one citizen of New Orleans felt that "the ever patient, enduring public has had enough of it—a change must come, and that soon."⁵²

In 1854 yellow fever was less virulent in New Orleans and less extensive than the year before in its spread through the state, although it did revisit St. Mary Parish and a number of other settlements in South Louisiana. Coastal cities of Norfolk, Charleston, Savannah, Mobile, Pensacola, and Galveston were also visited by the fever that year, and some cases even appeared at the quarantine station in Philadelphia and the Marine Hospital in New York, as had also happened the year before.[53]

The Quarantine Question

The first two major epidemics of the 1850s resulted in an intensified investigation of the facts relating to yellow fever in an attempt to shed light on its cause, means of transmission, and possible methods of prevention. Thousands of words filling hundreds of pages poured forth from the pens of physicians, journalists, and others. With so much new empirical data, the old theoretical fight became more intense than ever. Many still considered yellow fever non-contagious, locally caused, and spread by that indefinable essence, the "epidemic constitution of the atmosphere." Others had come to believe that the disease was brought into New Orleans from Latin America and spread from there to other communities, if not by infected persons then by goods or baggage infected in some unknown manner.

The old attitude of fatalistically accepting the inevitable recurrence of the pestilence was shaken by the unparalleled impact of the disease in 1853. In the midst of the Great Epidemic, the *Picayune* published a letter to the editor expressing the beginning of a change in public opinion. The writer complained that New Orleans had suffered too long without exerting any real effort to thwart the recurring disease. Although many medical men ridiculed quarantine measures and commercial interests opposed such restrictions, this citizen said he knew that some reliable physicians favored inspection and quarantine of incoming vessels as a possible means of keeping out yellow fever. Furthermore, he believed that "public opinion is daily growing more and more strong in favor of such . . . regulations."[54]

The *Picayune* itself presented a stream of editorials demanding both quarantine and sanitation measures for protection against the scourge. While the importationists and the local causationists carried on an interminable argument, both quarantine and sanitation might be tested. "Amid all the uncertainty . . . we think it may safely be assumed, that either they [the epidemics] are of local generation, or they are of foreign importation; or they are both," the editor reasoned. Therefore, both internal and external sanitary measures should be established "to meet all the postulates."[55]

The Louisiana legislature considered the quarantine issue early in 1854, but reaching no agreement, postponed the final resolution of the matter until the following session. The return of yellow fever in the summer of 1854 strengthened public demand for protective measures, and finally on March 15, 1855, the lawmakers passed "An Act to Establish Quarantine for the Protection of the State." The statute also created a board of health to administer the quarantine—Louisiana's first state board of health and the first in the country as well.[56]

1855 and 1858

Unfortunately, Yellow Jack arrived in New Orleans again in the summer of 1855 before the new board of health was able to make the necessary arrangements for establishing the quarantine stations.[57] For the third consecutive summer the city experienced a severe yellow fever epidemic. In its September issue the *New Orleans Medical and Surgical Journal* announced that "The Yellow Fever of 1853-4-5, a triune or triennial epidemic, though temporarily suspended during the winter season, rages still in New Orleans." At the close of the epidemic, the editor with his best rhetorical flourish offered a eulogy: "The beleagured city, after a three years' pestilential siege, stands forth like a scarred veteran, yet strong, hopeful, undismayed, unconquered and ready to meet the inexorable decrees of fate quietly and without retreating." The Louisiana State Board of Health reported 2,670 yellow fever deaths in New Orleans during the outbreak of 1855.[58]

One resident of New Orleans thought the "worst feature" of the 1855 epidemic was "its general diffusion thro' this State and Lower Mississippi." In previous years "the timid found a safe retreat from the scourge of the city in the country towns and on the Plantations of the coast—[but] now the country is no longer safe." Since the epidemic of 1853, he observed, "the whole Southern portion of the United States seems to have become the home of 'the fever,' [especially] . . . along the water courses and in the marshy Bays and inlets of the sea and Gulf Coasts."[59]

The state board of health reported only seventy-four yellow fever deaths in New Orleans in 1856, and 199 deaths in 1857.[60] In 1858, however, the city again experienced another violent epidemic, second only to the Great Epidemic of 1853. According to the *New Orleans Medical News and Hospital Gazette*, some cases first appeared in mid-June, but at that stage the disease was almost entirely confined to the working classes, especially along the waterfront, and had not yet become "anything like epidemic." By early August an epidemic was clearly in progress and had been for some time. One New Orleanian wrote in his diary: "The subject of Yellow Fever is beginning to excite attention. The rapid increase of deaths in the Hospital . . . shows its epidemic character, and there is no doubt that it bears the genuine West Indian type." Later he described the fever as "a very vicious type" and out of control: ". . . it is everywhere!—in the houses of the rich and the houses of the poor."[61]

Through September and early October the fever carried off hundreds of victims weekly. Despite repeated warnings in the newspapers, a steady stream of strangers poured into the city, "furnishing fresh food to the destroyer." By mid-November, as usual, the worst was over.[62] Although disseminated widely throughout the South in 1858, yellow fever seems to have spared most of Louisiana outside of New Orleans. Perhaps the disease had exhausted the supply of susceptibles in many small towns. Outbreaks were recorded for Plaquemine, Baton Rouge, Franklin, and the New Orleans suburban communities of Algiers, Gretna, and McDonoughville. Beyond Louisiana that year the scourge struck Galveston, Houston, Brownsville, Pass Christian, Biloxi, Vicksburg, Natchez, Woodville, Mobile, Savannah, and Charleston.[63]

Louisiana's Quarantine System and State Board of Health

Having failed to prevent a highly malignant epidemic in 1858, Louisiana's quarantine system and its managers came under increased attack from many quarters. The quarantine had enemies from its inception, including newspaper editors reflecting commercial priorities, shipping interests opposed to inspection fees and costly delays, and physicians who insisted that yellow fever was not and could not be imported. The epidemic of 1858 undoubtedly turned many other New Orleanians against quarantine, many who had counted on the new system to protect the city from yellow fever's regular invasions. The editor of the New Orleans *Bee* declared the quarantine both useless and costly and insisted that yellow fever was clearly "of indigenous origin."[64]

Operating under the legislative act of 1855, the state board of health had established three quarantine stations: the most important, on the left bank of the Mississippi River, seventy-two miles below New Orleans and thirty-four miles from the river's entrance; one near the mouth of the Atchafalaya River; and a third at the entrance from the gulf to Lake Pontchartrain. At the Mississippi Quarantine Station the board arranged for the construction of two hospital buildings, a warehouse, and quarters for the resident physician and other personnel. The law required that all vessels entering the river be inspected. Only those found in a clean condition, without cases of cholera, yellow fever, or other infectious diseases aboard, could be cleared to proceed upriver to the port of New Orleans.

If a ship arrived from a port known or believed to be infected (and so declared by the governor or the board), the quarantine office was required to detain the vessel for at least ten days. Ships found to have cases of infectious disease on board were also subject to detention. The sick were removed to the quarantine hospital, and cargo was sometimes unloaded prior to cleaning and fumigating the vessel. All expenses of these procedures had to be paid by the ship's owners. All vessels were charged a fee for inspection and certification whether detained or not. The board of health had the authority to extend the period of detention at its discretion. Captains of vessels refusing to stop at the station or to comply with the regulations could be fined or imprisoned.

Because of the great outcry by commercial interests, the legislature came close to repealing the quarantine act in 1856 but decided that the system deserved a longer trial period. Complaints and challenges continued, however, and in March, 1858, the legislature altered the requirements of the original act, allowing a vessel to count the days spent in traveling from an infected port as part of the ten-day detention period. The new law also gave a considerable amount of "discretionary power" to the board and to the resident physician. Healthy, "acclimated" persons could be allowed to go on to New Orleans even though the ship on which they arrived from an infected port had to remain in quarantine.[65]

In its annual report for 1858 the board of health defended its work and attempted to explain the epidemic. Insisting that yellow fever was an imported disease, the board argued that quarantine had failed because legislative amendments to the original act rendered it ineffectual. The detention period required of vessels from infected ports had been reduced for those ships that seemed to be free of sickness on arrival. Denouncing this change as a dangerous concession to commercial interests, the board recommended a series of new amendments to strengthen quarantine regulations.[66]

The epidemics of the 1850s mark the peak of yellow fever activity in the South and a turning point in Yellow Jack's history. The Great Epidemic of 1853, together with three additional outbreaks within the next five years, led to a revived interest in the old etiological and epidemiological issues surrounding yellow fever. Was it caused by a gaseous substance generated from filth and spread through the atmosphere? Was it influenced by heat and humidity? Was it caused by a specific living entity transmitted from person to person? Why were some people more susceptible than others? Could the disease be prevented by cleansing the city, by quarantine measures, or both? A journalist summed up the problem in 1853: "The truth is, that nothing—absolutely nothing—is known of . . . [yellow fever's] cause, although it has been studied attentively for more than a century, with all the aids that modern science could afford."[67]

The battle between local causationists and importationists raged fiercely through the decade of the fifties. Although a quarantine system was instituted in 1855, and continued with various modifications from then on, the issue was by no means settled, and for the rest of the nineteenth century quarantine methods continued to be a subject for debate. Absolute non-intercourse with tropical ports during the hot months might have excluded the disease. Or perhaps a lengthy detention period for all passengers and ships, in conjunction with a fumigation process thorough enough to destroy the yet unsuspected mosquito, might have succeeded. Almost all local interests would have opposed an absolute quarantine, however, and such a measure could never have been enforced. Even a short detention period was difficult to enforce with any consistency because of the protests of shipping interests and some medical experts as well. Nevertheless, Louisiana's board of health, operating under tremendous handicaps, continued its quest for effective measures to protect the health of the Crescent City and the state.

The Louisiana State Board of Health itself was a byproduct of the Great Epidemic, and with the gradual expansion of its powers and duties, the board in time would evolve into a vital state institution. The epidemics of the fifties shocked some New Orleanians into a reevaluation of their mortality statistics and brought greater awareness of the city's terrible health record relative to other urban centers, even in years without epidemics. Still the sanitary revolution was a long time coming.

Table 4.

YELLOW FEVER MORTALITY IN NEW ORLEANS
1848-1858

Year	Estimated Deaths	Population (Approx.)
1848	872	116,000
1849	769	
1850	107	
1851	17	
1852	456	
*1853	8,400	154,000
*1854	2,500	157,000
*1855	2,670	159,000
1856	74	
1857	199	
*1858	4,855	166,000

*Major epidemics.

Table 5.

YELLOW FEVER IN LOUISIANA OUTSIDE OF NEW ORLEANS
1853-1858

	1853	1854	1855	1858
Alexandria	X	X	X	
Algiers	X			X
Baton Rouge	X		X	X
Bayou Sara	X	X		
Carrollton			X	
Centerville	X		X	
Clinton	X			
Cloutierville	X	X		
Covington	X			
Donaldsonville	X			
Franklin	X	X		X
Grand Ecore	X			
Gretna				X
Harrisonburg			X	
Lake Providence	X			
McDonoughville				X
Madisonville	X			
Natchitoches	X			
New Iberia			X	
Opelousas	X			
Paincourtville			X	
Pattersonville	X	X	X	
Plaquemine	X		X	X
Plaquemines Parish		X		
Pointe Coupee Parish			X	
St. Francisville	X			
St. John the Baptist	X			
St. Martinville			X	
St. Mary Parish	X	X		
Shreveport	X			
Thibodaux	X	X		
Trenton	X		X	
Vidalia	X			
Washington	X	X		
Waterproof			X	

Based on reports in newspapers and official publications.

V

AN INTERREGNUM, 1859-1866

After the succession of epidemics in the fifties, unparalleled both in frequency and malignancy, epidemic yellow fever subsided in New Orleans for the first time since the 1790s. In the eight years between the major outbreaks of 1858 and 1867, Yellow Jack claimed only about 300 victims. In 1861, for the first time in more than a half-century, no death from yellow fever was reported in the Crescent City. During the period in which yellow fever seemed to have abdicated its throne, the Union was challenged by the Civil War, and New Orleans itself was occupied by Northern troops.

Yellow fever had earned for New Orleans a reputation as the most insalubrious city in the Union. It was widely known that newcomers, especially European immigrants and Northerners, always bore the heaviest burden of yellow fever mortality, while native and long-resident New Orleanians exhibited considerable resistance or immunity to the ravages of the "strangers' disease." Ironically, at the very time the city might have considered Yellow Jack more friend than foe, the disease remained conspicuously absent. Had New Orleans experienced an epidemic during the period of Union occupation, the Northern forces undoubtedly would have suffered severe losses and disorganization.

The relationship between the Civil War and the health status of New Orleans attracted the attention of the Louisiana State Board of Health even before the Yankees captured the Crescent City. In its 1861 report the board calculated a total mortality of about 5,500 for the entire year, a figure much lower than usual for New Orleans. The board also announced that not even one death from yellow fever had been recorded during the year. This extraordinary phenomenon was attributed to the Federal blockade, "partial though it may have been," which together with Louisiana's quarantine restrictions had diminished the possibilities of introducing disease from foreign ports. Someone suggested that the reduction of the usual summer population by the numbers away in military service might explain the decrease in mortality. The board of health, however, considered this theory fallacious, pointing out that the wartime conditions that had drawn off some to the army had also kept in New Orleans many persons who ordinarily spent the summer in the North or in Europe.[1]

At least one New Orleans resident agreed with the board's position on the indirect advantages resulting from the Federal blockade, for he wrote in his diary in July of 1861 that "the *impudent* 'Lincoln blockade' is acting in our favor by keeping out the yellow fever, and stimulating our heretofore dormant industry and self-reliance."[2] This year of complete exemption from the pestilence marked the beginning of a brief interregnum in yellow fever's long reign in New Orleans, while Yankee troops moved in to dominate the city.

In late April, 1862, the city fell to Union forces and remained under military occupation throughout the war. Particularly during the first year of wartime occupation, yellow fever was much on the minds of both conquerors and conquered—a source of great fear and dread to the one, of hope and encouragement to the other. General Benjamin F. Butler, in command of the Federal occupation forces during the first year, later wrote: "I learned that the rebels were actually relying largely upon the yellow fever to clear out the Northern troops, the men of New England and the Northwest . . . whom they had learned from experience were usually the first victims of the scourge." Furthermore, he had also heard "that in the churches [of New Orleans] prayers were put up that the pestilence might come as a divine interposition on behalf of the brethren."[3]

Although he found this reported attitude difficult to believe, Butler had noticed "many things that render[ed] it almost probable." It seemed to him that New Orleanians deliberately cultivated a "condition of perfect nastiness" as if in the hope of generating the fever. If they did go so far as to offer up such prayers, he wrote, they did not pray aloud in the churches because Federal soldiers attended their services. But "in the course of the liturgy the clergyman always gave out at a certain point . . . an opportunity for silent prayer," the general noted, "and then the people either prayed for the yellow fever, or Jefferson Davis to come there victorious; neither of which was comforting to the Yankee worshiper...."[4] These observations, although perhaps somewhat exaggerated, were not entirely a product of Butler's imagination. A New Orleans physician, writing after the war, remarked that "the hostile population of New Orleans ... [had] confidently anticipated that if the enemy should take New Orleans, the yellow fever would take the enemy."[5]

The hopeful expectation of an epidemic that would wipe out the Yankees in New Orleans was apparently not confined solely to its residents. One newspaper in Virginia consoled the people of the Confederacy over the Union capture of New Orleans with this thought: "They have got the elephant, it is true, but it is a prize which will cost them vastly more to keep than the animal is worth, if his Saffron Majesty shall make his usual annual visit to the city and wave his sceptre in the hospitals there."[6]

Northern soldiers, aware of the terrors of yellow fever, were often reminded of its obvious preference for the unacclimated stranger. On one occasion, two New Orleanians, wishing to intensify the fear among the troops, armed themselves with measuring tape and notebook and set off on a sardonic mission. Approaching a group of Federal soldiers, the pranksters began to measure the height of the Northerners and jot down notations of the same. They explained that a contract had been obtained for making 10,000 coffins that would be needed for the 2,500 soldiers in the city plus the steady stream of Union replacements sent in as yellow fever carried them off, one by one. New Orleans children also participated in the harassment of the United States troops. In late May and early June of 1862 they jeered at the soldiers in the streets:

> Yellow Jack will grab them up
> And take them all away.[7]

For once it seems that the citizens of New Orleans would have welcomed the arrival of the saffron scourge to aid them against the new adversary from the North. According to General Butler, all conversations of New Orleanians in the presence of his officers included descriptions of past epidemic horrors, especially the disaster of 1853 when yellow fever had claimed at least 8,000 victims in the city. Under a constant barrage of this demoralizing propaganda, Butler's men soon began to evidence its effects. Many of the officers were panic-stricken, depressed; some requested transfers to different areas; others offered every conceivable excuse for leaves. But the general held firm and proceeded to study the problem of yellow fever with the idea of forestalling an epidemic.

First, he asked an old New Orleans physician about ways to prevent the fever. No means existed, he was told, and no way to prevent its spread once under way. The physician admitted that quarantine of incoming vessels might be useful, but he pointed out that the presence of unacclimated troops together with the city's unsanitary condition made it likely that the disease, if it broke out at all, would rage with great fury. Butler obtained books on the subject and a New Orleans map indicating the localities where yellow fever usually prevailed. Upon investigation of those places, he found them uniformly "filthy with rotting matter."[8]

After much research and thought, General Butler developed his own theory of fevers. He concluded that exhalations from putrid animal matter produced typhus fever and exhalations from rotting vegetable matter produced congestive fevers. Yellow fever, however, was not indigenous to New Orleans but had to be imported. Once its "seeds" were introduced yellow fever would spread throughout that portion of the atmosphere contaminated by *both* animal and vegetable effluvia. It was possible, he thought, for these seeds to last through the winter hidden away in woolen clothing and protected from the frost. Without the dual contamination of the atmosphere, however, he believed the seeds of disease, whether imported fresh or preserved through the winter months, would be unable to propagate.

Having settled upon three indispensable factors involved in the production of an epidemic, Butler set out to deal with them without delay. Since he believed yellow fever to be imported, he decided to enforce a strict quarantine on the Mississippi River below New Orleans. Because of the dense vegetation around the city, Butler realized it would be impossible to dispose of all decaying plant matter. But if a *combination* of animal and vegetable elements was required to produce an epidemic atmosphere, the disposal of either one of the two elements would suffice. He was convinced that putrid animal matter and filth could be cleared away. With this outline in mind, General Butler set out to institute an effective quarantine system and clean up the city of New Orleans.[9] Interestingly enough, his theory represented a composite of most of the epidemiological concepts available for centuries, and his preventive program combined the two suggestions so long debated by yellow fever philosophers: quarantine *and* sanitation.

Although previous attempts had been made to institute such measures, never before had sanitation and quarantine been so rigorously enforced as under Butler's iron hand. He established a firm, uncompromising guard at the state's regular quarantine station seventy miles below New Orleans where, in his words, "thirty-two and sixty-eight pound shots should be the messengers to execute the health orders." His quarantine regulations and means of enforcement stood in striking contrast to the lax, inconsistent, and easily evaded system previously attempted by Louisiana health authorities. By Butler's order, all vessels entering the river were required to stop below Fort St. Philip (about five miles downriver from the quarantine station), for initial inspection by a specially appointed health officer, who reported to the general the condition of the vessel, its passengers, crew, and cargo. If the physician gave a clean bill of health and Butler in turn telegraphed his consent, then and only then could the vessel proceed upriver to the city. "If any vessel attempted to evade quarantine regulations and pass up without being examined," recalled Butler, "the vessel was to be stopped if there was power enough in the fort to do it." Unlike Louisiana's lawmakers who had drafted the state's quarantine legislation, Butler accepted the literal meaning of the term "quarantine" and required any ship with an infectious sickness on board to remain at the detention station for forty days, after which another thorough inspection was necessary. All vessels from ports where yellow fever had been reported were required to spend forty days in quarantine, even when they arrived with a clean bill of health.[10]

Butler obtained the services of a competent physician and paid him well to administer the inspection and to report on the condition of incoming vessels. The general threatened to invoke the death penalty, however, should this physician make false reports or allow an infected ship to proceed upriver to New Orleans. According to Butler's own account, only on one occasion during his command in 1862 did yellow fever slip through the stringent quarantine, and not because of negligence on the part of the appointed physician. Butler himself had allowed a tug carrying much-needed provisions from New York to come upriver without undergoing the forty-day detention, accepting the captain's oath that only coal had been taken on at the Nassau stop where yellow fever prevailed. Several days later two cases of fever appeared in the French Quarter: two passengers from Nassau who had come in on the tug. The military took over immediately and surrounded the square where the cases were located.

Under Butler's order several acclimated persons went in to attend the patients and came out only after being thoroughly cleansed. Fires fed with tar and pitch burned day and night at the four corners of the square. When the two patients died, everything in and around the building that Butler thought might harbor "yellow fever seeds" was burned; even the bodies were cremated. No other cases developed, but the deceitful captain of the tug spent three months in jail and paid a fine of $500.[11]

On first assuming control of New Orleans, General Butler had intended to leave the administration of ordinary civil functions, including sanitation, in the hands of the municipal government. He soon realized, however, the necessity of action on his part against what he considered the causative forces of yellow fever.[12] After establishing quarantine regulations, Butler proceeded to the "Herculean task" of cleaning up the city early in June, 1862. In a message to the military governor and the New Orleans City Council, General Butler directed that the city employ a force of 2,000 men for at least thirty working days and provide the necessary tools and supervision to clean the city's streets, squares, and unoccupied lands. Seeking the full cooperation of the council members, Butler played on their sentiment: "The epidemic so earnestly prayed for by the wicked will hardly sweep away the strong man, although he may be armed, and leave the weaker woman and child untouched." Reminding them of the presence of many women and children who ordinarily left New Orleans during the summer months, he suggested that "The miasma which sickens the one [the troops] will harm the other."[13]

One squad from the cleansing force was sent to the French Market with an order, "accompanied by a few bayonets," that the area be cleaned. The superintendent in charge of the market said he could not have it done; nevertheless, the clean-up crew proceeded with the task, scraped up the filth, sent it down the river, and charged him with the expense. It is not at all surprising that General Butler gave top priority to the cleansing of this particular area. On first inspection he had been shocked by its filthy state. "In the French market," he wrote, "the stall women were accustomed to drop on the floor around their stalls all the refuse made in cleaning their birds, meat, and fish." Furthermore, he added, "Here it was trodden in and in. This had been going on for a century more or less." The remaining sanitary detail then went through the streets, clearing away all putrefying animal matter, scraping and sweeping out every drain and ditch in the city. The city waterworks was ordered to flush the streets with all its pumps, and as the water flowed through the freshly scraped drains and ditches into the canals leading to Lake Pontchartrain, the accumulated filth was forced into the lake and eventually into the gulf.[14]

Butler issued detailed orders to the people of New Orleans on the subject of cleanliness. The head of every household was required to have the premises cleaned inside and out to meet the approval of military inspectors. All refuse from each household was to be deposited in a box or barrel acceptable to the inspector, and on two or three specified days a week the receptacle had to be placed at the end of the street. From that point the refuse would be hauled off in wagons drawn by mule teams. Those in charge of the wagons were instructed to disinfect the containers with chloride of lime. In addition, all persons were expressly forbidden to throw anything into the streets, alleys, or any open spaces, including their own back yards. One might suppose such regulations difficult to enforce. But according to Butler it was a fairly simple task, and he provided several examples to illustrate his point.

One citizen, deliberately testing the orders, walked along the street and called a policeman to watch him throw down a small piece of white paper. Informed of this willful disobedience, Butler sent for the man, who freely admitted the act and insisted it was his privilege to toss paper on the street. The general replied that "the streets were made to pass through, and when he took his privilege I would take mine and pass him through the streets into the parish prison to stay three months." Another case involved a "high-toned woman" who tried to ignore the sanitary regulations. This "fashionable lady" of New Orleans adamantly refused to clean her back yard, which contained a box of excrement not yet hauled off from the privy. She informed the military inspector that her back yard was "as I choose to have it, and it won't be altered at the order of any Yankee." When the inspecting officer told her to gather up whatever clothes and articles she wanted to carry to jail, she burst into tears and agreed to accept another opportunity to comply with the regulations. By the next afternoon, "the yard was in apple-pie order."[15]

Despite his efforts, Butler was unable to attain a perfect state of urban purity. In August, 1862, the editor of the *Daily True Delta* complained of the filthy gutters. Having observed several gutters with green scum on the water "thick enough to bear the weight of a small-size bird," the *Delta* editor recommended that the authorities attend to the removal of all such pestilential influences.[16] Nevertheless, General Butler must be given credit for forcing New Orleans into what was perhaps the best sanitary condition that it had ever enjoyed. In November of 1862 the *Picayune* declared that only once before had the Crescent City been so clean: a relatively pristine condition had prevailed for a short time immediately after the epidemic of 1853 when the city government had been aroused temporarily to action. After the Civil War even the most acrimonious Rebel was willing to admit that General Butler had been "the best *scavenger* we ever had among us."[17]

When the Union forces occupied New Orleans in the spring of 1862, none of Butler's surgeons had ever seen a case of yellow fever or possessed the vaguest notion of how to combat the "hideous foe." In July, after the inauguration of sanitation and quarantine measures, a pamphlet was prepared with the assistance of several New Orleans physicians for the instruction of the Union surgeons in the Department of the Gulf. It outlined in detail the diagnostic and prognostic indicators as well as specific treatments for yellow fever. The pamphlet stated that every precaution had been taken to prevent the fever's occurrence but emphasized the ever-present possibility of an outbreak, as well as the duty of an army surgeon to be prepared for all emergencies.[18] Fortunately for the Yankees, the first year of the Federal occupation of New Orleans passed with only two known deaths from yellow fever—the two passengers from Nassau who had slipped in on the tug. The mortality records are imperfect, however, and it is entirely possible that other cases occurred. The significant fact is that in spite of the appearance of a few cases the pestilence did not spread to any noticeable extent.[19]

In November of 1862 General Nathaniel P. Banks was appointed to replace Butler as Major-General Commanding the Department of the Gulf. When Butler left New Orleans in December, he stated in his farewell address to the citizens: "I have demonstrated that the pestilence can be kept from your borders. . . . I have cleansed and improved your streets, canals, and public squares. . . ."[20] One creole of New Orleans took a different view of the matter, according to a story in the *Picayune* several years later. When asked to admit that "Beast" Butler had demonstrated great ability in preserving the city from the pestilence while in command there, the New Orleanian reportedly said: "By gar, vat you take me vor? You no believe in God? You no believe zere is mercie? Yellow fever and G-e-n-e-r-a-l Butler at the same time!!!"[21]

During the remainder of the occupation, sanitary regulations were administered and enforced through the cooperative efforts of General Banks, the military governor, the mayor of the city, the provost-marshal, the medical director of the department, and specially appointed sanitary inspectors. Quarantine regulations continued in force, although never quite as strictly administered as under General Butler.[22] Among the civilian population of New Orleans, two yellow fever deaths were reported in 1863, six in 1864, and one in 1865. In 1863 and 1864 disease broke out on several vessels of the United States river fleet and spread to the Naval Hospital—approximately 100 cases in 1863 and 200 in 1864. But, although clearly present in the New Orleans vicinity, Yellow Jack strangely failed to develop into an epidemic.[23]

Under wartime occupation, Louisiana's board of health had been converted into a military bureau with the medical director of the Department of the Gulf serving as president. Not until April, 1866, was the Louisiana State Board of Health reorganized on its prewar basis, with six members appointed by the governor and three by the New Orleans City Council. Almost immediately the board encountered its traditional problems: no power, no funds, and no cooperation from the municipal authorities.[24] These problems had not existed for the military command. In July of 1866 the *Picayune* editor commented on the need for more energetic enforcement of sanitary measures to remove potential sources of disease. The editor felt that the authorities should pay more attention to "this cause of complaint and of danger."[25]

Provost-Marshal James Bowen, who served in New Orleans for two years during the war, had predicted that with the return of the "usual lax administration" of sanitary regulations by the civil authorities New Orleans would again be visited by pestilence.[26] As if to fulfill his prophecy, both yellow fever and Asiatic cholera appeared in New Orleans in 1866. While cholera claimed more than 1,200 victims, the saffron scourge struck lightly that year, causing only 185 fatalities. In 1867, however, the city suffered a two-fold increase in its total mortality and a yellow fever epidemic causing more than 3,000 deaths.[27]

New Orleans physicians reviewed the health measures of the war years in an attempt to reconcile prevailing theories with the facts, or vice versa. Dr. Erasmus Darwin Fenner in 1866 examined the record of health in New Orleans under military rule to see what lessons might be learned. He praised the tremendous efforts of the army authorities to bring about sanitary reform. "Such efforts were never made here before," he declared, "although so often urged by the medical profession in previous years." But, Dr. Fenner added, "perhaps, it may be said *such motives* were never presented before." In spite of the war and the dark side of its balance sheet, he felt that New Orleans should be thankful for "this great sanitary experiment." Compared to its previous condition, the city had been kept unbelievably clean throughout the period. "It was a Herculean task," said Fenner, "and, in our humble opinion, nothing short of military despotism would have accomplished it."

To Dr. Fenner the great lesson of the wartime experience was the validation of his own theory of fever causation. He had long held the opinion that filth and atmospheric contamination produced diseases of all sorts, including yellow fever. From the premise of local causation, he had always reasoned that sanitary measures would best serve to prevent disease. In contrast to this view, many persons attributed the freedom of New Orleans from epidemic disease during wartime occupation to the rigorous quarantine measures. Fenner disagreed. Although quarantine had been strictly enforced through much of the period, Fenner said that he knew definitely of one case imported from Key West and believed there were others as well. Admitting the likelihood of several imported cases of yellow fever each year during the war, he thought it extraordinary that the disease had not become epidemic in the city. It could only be explained by the consistent enforcement of sanitary regulations, Dr. Fenner insisted. And, as he reasoned further, how could quarantine be expected to afford complete protection against a disease so clearly indigenous to New Orleans?

The "sanitary experience" of the period between 1862 and 1866 had provided "useful instruction," and Fenner felt it should not be overlooked by the citizenry. Suggesting that Generals Butler and Banks deserved much credit for their achievements, he maintained that "We may yet have occasion to mingle some thanks among the many curses that have been heaped upon their heads for their unnecessary severity upon the citizens of New Orleans." For twenty years or more, some physicians of New Orleans had preached the gospel of cleanliness without appreciable effect. But, said Fenner, "In the mysterious course of events the hand of the tyrant has been brought to our aid, and the results are marvelous." Now that the true path of sanitary reform had been clearly demonstrated, not only by logic but also by the Yankee experiment in not-so-gentle persuasion, Dr. Fenner hoped that New Orleanians would not revert to antebellum practices.[28]

Dr. Stanford E. Chaillé, eminent New Orleans physician, editor, and medical educator, studied the facts relating to yellow fever and sanitation during wartime occupation and arrived at conclusions different from those of Dr. Fenner. Writing in 1870, Chaillé observed that many of his colleagues attributed the relative freedom from yellow fever during the war to Yankee sanitation measures. Although a strong believer in the desirability of sanitary reform, he argued that the conclusion about the effect on yellow fever was "not logically deducible from the true premises." The faulty syllogism went something like this: For years New Orleans had been visited by yellow fever epidemics which carried off thousands of victims, and during those years the city was incredibly filthy. During the four-year period from 1862 through 1865 no epidemic occurred, and New Orleans was one of the cleanest cities in the country. Therefore, the exemption from epidemics was due to the unusually clean condition of the city. Chaillé then stated his version of the "correct syllogism with the true premise" in this manner:

> New Orleans enjoyed during eight years, 1859-66, an exemption, unexampled in her history, from yellow fever epidemics. During four of these eight years, viz., 1859-60-61-66, the city suffered notoriously with its habitual filth, and during the four remaining years, viz., 1862-65, it enjoyed an unusual degree of cleanliness. Therefore, — — — what?

If sanitary measures protected the city during the war years, what factors operated in the other non-epidemic years before and after the war, when New Orleans was as filthy as ever? Chaillé's study of available mortality records also revealed that despite the absence of major epidemics New Orleans' average annual mortality during the war years was higher than the average for 1856-60 and for 1866-69 when epidemics had occurred. Diarrhea and dysentery, consumption, malaria, smallpox, typhus, and typhoid fever were common causes of death during the war among both military and civilian populations in the New Orleans area.[29]

More skeptical than most, Dr. Chaillé was not willing to concede that the military health measures coinciding with a period of exemption from yellow fever epidemics had really proved anything. He could only say that there were many unanswered questions about the irregularities of the disease. And so the arguments continued among both medical thinkers and laymen. Some saw quarantine as the decisive factor; others gave sole credit to the clean-up campaign; others compromised and allowed that it was the combined effect of the two; still others argued that the war efforts proved nothing whatsoever.

It is impossible to determine precisely how much the rigid enforcement of quarantine and sanitary measures had to do with the city's freedom from a yellow fever epidemic during the war. Quarantine, when literally and absolutely enforced, would have held out the disease, but after Butler the detention period was reduced (from forty days to ten) and other regulations became less severe. Moreover, yellow fever was definitely imported on several occasions, but failed to spread extensively. Sanitary regulations might have reduced the incidence of certain endemic diseases and certainly eliminated some of the offensive, if not pestilential, odors of the city. Such measures would hardly have affected the yellow fever mosquito, however, which chose cisterns and indoor water receptacles as breeding places in preference to gutters, stagnant pools, and swamps. Many factors, some affected by chance, are necessary for the production of a full-scale yellow fever epidemic. In addition, there is the mutable nature of the virus itself, which can exhibit great variability in virulence from year to year and even from case to case. For whatever reason, yellow fever had already begun its gradual retreat from the New Orleans sector after reaching a peak of activity in the 1850s. Although the disease continued to excite much interest through the rest of the century, except for two or three major outbreaks its appearances were relatively mild in nature.

It could be argued that without Butler's careful isolation of the two imported cases in 1862 they might have sparked a great epidemic in the city. On the other hand, they might not have resulted in another single case, even without the special attention he devoted to them. Wartime conditions and the blockade, by diminishing the normal extent of Latin American trade and travel, also reduced the numerical possibilities for yellow fever's introduction. Yet when all the circumstantial factors are present in the required space-time arrangement, one imported case of yellow fever or one imported virus-ridden mosquito can initiate a devastating epidemic. In spite of the several cases that did appear in New Orleans, no epidemic materialized. Given the presence of yellow fever mosquitoes in large numbers and the introduction of the virus to an area, a crucial variable in the making of an epidemic is the proportion and concentration of susceptibles in the population. No doubt the four extensive outbreaks of the

1850s left a large proportion of the city's surviving population immune to yellow fever. Furthermore, the war had disrupted the heavy flow of foreign immigration to New Orleans, thereby limiting the supply of newcomers and transients usually most susceptible to the disease. Despite the presence of Northern troops, the proportion of susceptibles in the city's wartime population was probably smaller than that of previous decades. Whether or not a yellow fever epidemic would have occurred without the conscientious efforts of the Union commanders to prevent such a development remains an open question.

In any case General Butler deserves considerable credit for his comprehensive sanitation and quarantine programs, a kind of double-barrelled shotgun fired at Yellow Jack's mysterious causes. By combining the prophylactic measures advocated by the two competing schools of yellow fever theorists (the local causationists and the importationists), Butler did everything possible, given the limited epidemiological and etiological knowledge of the time, and he accomplished a great deal more than had ever been attempted before. His successor, General Banks, for the most part followed his example, though with neither the same degree of consistency nor ostentation.

The long-term significance of the military health regulations can be seen in the impact on medical and lay opinion in New Orleans and the future development of public health activity. If New Orleanians were somewhat disappointed that Yellow Jack had not saved them from Yankee domination, they were nevertheless impressed by the simultaneity of three factors during the war years: strictly enforced sanitary measures, rigid quarantine, and the absence of a yellow fever epidemic. As a result, many were convinced that either quarantine or sanitation, or both, had prevented the occurrence of an epidemic. Medical opinion, although still divided, inclined toward an acceptance of quarantine, at least as an adjunct to sanitary reform.[30]

Retrospectively, the experience gave credence to the view that yellow fever might be a preventable disease after all and not the inexorable destiny of New Orleans. In spite of the faulty logic employed in evaluating the circumstances, the coincidence was a striking one, and public opinion moved one step closer to recognizing the validity of regulatory measures consistently enforced to preserve the health of a city. Although the general apathy and official negligence that characterized the first half of the nineteenth century would recur as obstacles again and again, and the public health movement by no means progressed in an even line without setbacks, an attitude more receptive to positive governmental action for preventing epidemics and improving health conditions had been engendered by the wartime occupation of New Orleans.

Table 6.

YELLOW FEVER MORTALITY IN NEW ORLEANS
1859-1866

Year	Estimated Deaths	Population (Approx.)
1859	92	167,000
1860	15	
1861	0	
1862	2	
*1863	2	
*1864	6	
1865	1	
1866	192	178,000

*During 1863 and 1864, some 100 and 200 cases, respectively, occurred in the United States river fleet, resulting in a number of deaths, but the disease failed to spread to the city.

VI

RETURN OF THE SCOURGE TO POSTWAR LOUISIANA, 1867-1877

Yellow Jack's activity in Louisiana in the last third of the nineteenth century was remarkably different from its antebellum pattern. During thirty-three years, from 1867 through 1899, New Orleans experienced eleven years with no yellow fever deaths reported and seventeen years when the annual yellow fever mortality ranged from one to sixty. Five epidemics occurred, but only two, in 1867 and 1878, could compare with earlier visitations in magnitude. Relatively mild outbreaks, in 1870, 1873, and 1897, affected interior communities more severely than New Orleans. As in previous years, when yellow fever became epidemic in the city, it usually spread to other places along rivers, bayous, and railroad lines within and beyond Louisiana's boundaries. Except for a few outbreaks in the 1870s, the disease exhibited a less virulent character than it had in the antebellum years. But the impact on towns of the interior was greater than ever before.[1]

Medical explanations, public health measures, and popular attitudes and reactions also underwent striking changes, although some features of the previous era persisted. Controversies over quarantine and sanitation policies became more intense, with variations on old themes and the introduction of new ones. Interstate quarreling about quarantine barriers eventually led to a measure of cooperation among southern states for the protection of commerce as well as health. In the early 1880s fierce opposition by the Louisiana State Board of Health contributed to the failure of the National Board of Health, an experimental federal agency established in the wake of the widespread yellow fever epidemic of 1878.[2]

Dr. Carlos Finlay of Cuba in the 1880s virtually solved the puzzle of yellow fever transmission by correctly identifying the mosquito vector, but his inconsistent experimental results failed to attract the interest of the international scientific community. His work received little attention until the U. S. Army Commission in 1900 decided to test his theory and succeeded in transmitting indisputable yellow fever with Finlay's mosquitoes. The germ theory, on the other hand, emerging from the work of Louis Pasteur, Robert Koch, and other European laboratory scientists, gained widespread acceptance in the 1870s and 1880s and led to an intensive search for the yellow fever germ in the blood and excreta of patients.[3] Influenced by germ theory, health officials became more interested than ever in disinfection. Chemical germicides as well as age-old practices believed to neutralize "noxious effluvia" were now used to disinfect premises and materials contaminated by the sick and to destroy the *germs* believed to be carried on trains and ships in bedding, clothing, luggage, and other cargo.[4]

New Orleans, 1867

New Orleans' first yellow fever epidemic after the Civil War occurred in 1867 during Reconstruction. Although the last of the federal troops were not removed from Louisiana until 1877, the state board of health returned to civilian control in the spring of 1866, and the execution of sanitary and quarantine regulations again became the responsibility of Louisiana authorities. Almost two hundred deaths from yellow fever were recorded in New Orleans in 1866, far more than the total during the war years but not enough by the city's standards to be considered epidemic.[5]

Without the incentives provided by bayonet and military arrest, sanitary regulations were ignored by officials and citizens alike, and New Orleans reverted to its customary state of filthiness. In May of 1867 the *Picayune* called attention to the crowded and unsanitary tenement houses and the drainage canals and gutters filled with garbage, giving off "a stench so rank it smells to heaven." Believing that decomposing matter produced disease, the newspaper editor urged the state board of health and city council to attend to sanitary matters *before* an epidemic occurred.[6] When several yellow fever deaths were reported in July, the board of health provided for the cleansing and disinfecting of the premises wherever cases had appeared. For a time it seemed that the disease had been halted, but early in August a malady said to resemble yellow fever erupted "with great violence" at military headquarters. The pestilence apparently made slow progress for on August 14 the board of health reported only a slight increase in cases and declared the city relatively healthy. To limit the spread of disease, the board strongly recommended the use of carbolic acid and sulphur as disinfectants.[7]

On August 22 General Philip S. Sheridan, commanding officer of the federal forces in Louisiana, telegraphed his superiors in Washington that yellow fever had become epidemic in New Orleans and requested that his chief surgeon be authorized to employ nurses for the stricken troops in the city. His request was granted immediately. In contrast to General Sheridan's expressed concern, neither the state board of health nor local physicians and journalists considered the disease epidemic. According to the city's accepted usage of the term, a disease became *epidemic* only when its victims exceeded the total number of fatalities from all other causes during a specified time period, usually a week. In addition, many New Orleans doctors and journalists measured the seriousness of yellow fever outbreaks against the absolute mortality in previous epidemics and in terms of classes affected. In late August the *Picayune* editor declared that "Seventy-seven deaths in a week does not create much alarm in a community that has suffered in the same space of time to the number of nearly twelve hundred." Readers were probably also relieved to be informed that most of the cases had occurred, as usual, among the unacclimated Europeans and northerners.[8]

The *New Orleans Medical and Surgical Journal*, reporting on the fever's spread in August, admitted that an epidemic might yet develop because of the high percentage of unacclimated persons in the population. Although the malady thus far had been unusually mild, the editor remarked that "New Orleans has long enjoyed the distinction of preeminence in sickliness, as well as wickedness, among the cities of this happy country, and we are not disposed now to take these points up for controversy." Not until September 3 did the state board of health finally declare that a "mild type" of yellow fever had reached epidemic proportions in the Crescent City.[9]

Despite all hopes to the contrary, "Bronze John on his Saffron Steed" continued to advance across New Orleans, visiting virtually every street and leaving "the evidence of his malevolence" strewn about the city in

September and October—200, 300, 400 fatalities per week. On September 22 a local journalist lamented the city's unhappy lot: "How sad to think, laboring for months as we have pertinaciously to recover from our political adversities, that the trying ordeal of a terrible plague as we are now suffering from should be inflicted upon us." Military occupation, reconstruction politics, and Yellow Jack seemed bitter potions to swallow simultaneously. But within another month the fever cases and deaths declined, and on November 5 the state board of health declared the epidemic over.[10]

The 1867 epidemic claimed 3,107 victims in New Orleans, to which should be added the 213 fatalities among the United States troops stationed there, making a total of 3,320 yellow fever deaths. According to the board of health, the case fatality rate was unusually low, only 8 percent, but the disease had attacked some 41,500 persons, or one-fourth of the population remaining in the city during the outbreak. Yellow fever deaths had amounted to only 2 percent of the city's estimated population, but among the northern soldiers in the vicinity the pestilence killed almost 20 percent.[11]

As the West Indies trade had revived after the war, yellow fever was most likely brought to New Orleans in 1867 in the shipping from Havana or some other Caribbean port. Precisely when and how it arrived remains a mystery to historians as it was to nineteenth-century observers. The first case in Charity Hospital in early June was linked to a sugar-laden ship from Havana that had been certified as clean and healthy upon arrival at the quarantine station. Several other cases in July were associated with another vessel arriving from Havana with a cargo of sugar; the *Florence Peters*, although apparently clean and healthy, was detained at the quarantine station for ten days, disinfected, and then allowed to proceed upriver to New Orleans. Within two or three weeks the ship's captain, the second mate, the captain's wife, and her sister fell sick with the fever.[12]

Having failed to prevent the fever's entry, the board of health tried a new and more aggressive approach to limit its spread within the city, exhibiting concern for "internal" sanitation as well as quarantine. Motivated by the fear of cholera the previous year, the board had proposed and the city council approved an ordinance providing for the appointment of a health inspector for each of the city's four districts. The health officers reported cases of infectious diseases to the state board and assisted in the enforcement of sanitary regulations. Having worked diligently during the Asiatic cholera epidemic in 1866-67, they continued to function under the board's direction when yellow fever replaced cholera as the prevailing disease in 1867. Whenever a fever case was reported, the board placed the house under the authority of the appropriate district health officer with instructions to cleanse the premises and fumigate the residence with sulphurous acid gas and carbolic acid.[13]

Significantly, these measures represent the board's first systematic effort to combat yellow fever in a house-to-house campaign of disinfection. Actually, the first systematic effort to deal with yellow fever in New Orleans had been undertaken by General Benjamin Butler when he arranged for the isolation of cases and the cleaning and disinfection of premises during wartime occupation. The absence of a full-blown epidemic during the Civil War was accepted by many as evidence that the measures employed by military authorities had been an effective deterrent against the spread of disease. The civilian board of health in the postwar era seems to have been following the procedures previously introduced by the military, not striking out in an entirely new direction. The board's work of disinfection expanded considerably, however, in the escalating war against disease.[14] In 1867 the board had fortuitously chosen a weapon against infection that also destroyed mosquitoes: the fumes of burning sulphur. While these efforts unintentionally would have reduced the mosquito population to some extent, the health officers could not have attended to every infected house during an epidemic involving more than 40,000 cases, many of which were never reported. The best efforts of the fumigators could not arrest the progress of this epidemic, later said to have been the most extensive outbreak the city ever experienced.

No class was exempt from the fever. A considerable number of blacks and native white New Orleanians, ordinarily less likely victims, appeared among the fatalities. The board of health later tried to account for the extraordinary number of cases relative to deaths, pointing out that the absence of an epidemic since 1858 had rendered all children of the city under eight years of age susceptible to yellow fever. Furthermore, while foreign immigration had contributed relatively little to the city's population since the late 1850s, the influx of freedmen from the hinterlands to New Orleans after the Civil War had augmented the pool of non-immunes. Both blacks and children usually experienced mild and rarely fatal attacks of the fever, a phenomenon that would help explain the large number of cases and low case fatality rate.[15]

The city's poor suffered terribly during the summer and autumn of 1867, and the extent of postwar poverty itself probably reduced the resistance of many to the ravages of disease. One witness called that period "one of the most distressing to those of limited means ever experienced in New Orleans." The pestilence disrupted summer commerce and delayed the fall business season about two months. High rents and high prices for the necessities of life intensified the distress of the indigent. When one of the New Orleans banks failed during the epidemic, many among the laboring classes lost whatever small savings they had at their time of greatest need.[16]

As in previous epidemics, the Howard Association came to the aid of destitute fever victims and their families, and many physicians freely offered their services to those who could not pay. The New Orleans Howards cared for 4,192 yellow fever patients, of whom only 340 died. The association also provided relief to more than 6,000 others in the families of the sick. Despite the sectional bitterness from war and the turmoil of Reconstruction politics, northern contributors provided generous assistance to the city during the epidemic. In November of 1867 the *New Orleans Medical and Surgical Journal* expressed "the gratitude of this impoverished community" to all those friends in the North who had "with free hand and open purse, promoted the efforts of our self-sacrificing citizens." The editor of the New Orleans *Bee* also gave thanks "to our friends of the North," noting especially a number of New York firms that had contributed to the Howard Association, and concluding that "Charity is the noblest and most effectual means for our reconstruction."[17]

Other Louisiana Towns, 1867

Other afflicted Louisiana towns in 1867 included Plaquemine, Alexandria, Shreveport, Jeanerette, New Iberia, St. Martinville, Opelousas, Washington, Lafayette, and Lake Charles, as well as several other hitherto unaffected communities in the southwestern part of the state.[18] The fever was highly variable in its effects, some towns escaping with only a few cases, others losing large numbers of citizens. Two of the worst visitations occurred in New Iberia and Washington.

New Iberia, a small town in south Louisiana on Bayou Teche, about fifteen miles from the coast and a hundred miles west of New Orleans, was in the throes of a serious outbreak long before the fever reached epidemic proportions in the Crescent City. Believed to have been introduced from Galveston (although New Orleans could also have been the source), the disease appeared in late July and raged violently for well over a month. In the second week of August the mayor of New Iberia reported the illness of several of the town's physicians and requested that nurses and doctors be sent from New Orleans. Two faculty members from the New Orleans School of Medicine, a resident medical student from Charity Hospital, and several Sisters of Charity went to New Iberia and immediately established a temporary hospital in the desperate community. The New Orleans, Opelousas and Great Western Rail Road and the Attakapas Navigation Company both offered to transport nurses and supplies without charge. E. F. Schmidt, president of the New Orleans Howard Association, went to New Iberia and helped organize a local Howard Association which immediately employed a number of nurses from the Crescent City.[19]

Business dwindled in New Iberia, about half of the townspeople were unemployed, and "the most complete destitution" prevailed. Contributions to the newly formed Howard Association for the relief of the sick and the destitute arrived from Franklin, Lafayette, Opelousas, and New Orleans. The Shakespeare Club of New Orleans gave a benefit performance to raise funds for New Iberia. One New Orleanian shipped two casks of ice weekly. The New Orleans City Council even appropriated a thousand dollars as a contribution to the afflicted community. In a population of 1,600 to 1,800, considerably reduced by the departure of many residents, no less than 700 cases and seventy deaths had occurred in New Iberia by August 31. The fever began to decline in late August and early September, mainly for lack of new subjects, and the worst of New Iberia's epidemic was over when the disease in New Orleans developed into a serious outbreak.[20]

The devastation of a small community represented a tragedy far more intensely personal than the large-scale epidemic disaster in the metropolitan center. One New Iberia observer wrote: "It is heart-rending . . . to see and realize the affliction and desolation of our community—scarce a family but is in mourning, and in many instances almost entire families have been swept to the grave by the 'fell destroyer.'"[21] Dr. Robert Hilliard, writing from the scene of the epidemic, confided to his son-in-law in a letter of August 25: "I am so enfeebled by loss of sleep, constant and laborious practice that I can scarcely stand. I trust in God to weather the storm. The disease is less violent . . . and there is an evident diminution in the number of cases." On September 1 he wrote that he had "treated 134 cases and lost ten," and on September 3 he estimated the total cases in the town as 700, with eighty-one deaths. The doctor himself fell victim to yellow fever and died on September 10. Various sources, including church records, indicate a death toll of at least one hundred during the course of the epidemic.[22]

Another small Louisiana town experienced an epidemic of catastrophic proportions in 1867. During September and October more than 500 persons fell sick and seventy-three died of yellow fever in the community of Washington, about forty miles north of New Iberia. In late October a resident wrote: "All business is suspended. . . . Our town has a deserted appearance. Provisions are getting scarce, and sometimes are not to be had." Among the citizens taking flight when the disease appeared were three of the four town council members and two of the town's three physicians. New Orleans, by this time fighting its own battle against the fever, was unable to provide as much aid to Washington as it had given New Iberia. The city's Howard Association did manage, however, to spare one thousand dollars from its funds to assist the small village.[23]

Following 1867, Louisiana was almost completely free of the pestilence for two summers. Only three yellow fever deaths were reported in New Orleans in 1868 and three in 1869. During those years, the newspapers gave little attention to health, except for an occasional remark on the city's unusually good health status. Most reporting was concerned with politics, riots, and elections, while Radical Reconstruction continued in high gear. Nevertheless, the journalistic tendency was to look forward to a bright future, and the *Picayune* editorialized in July of 1869: ". . . commercial prospects were never more flattering. The indications point to a trade which will rapidly restore the lost prosperity of the city, and make New Orleans what she certainly should become, one of the most important shipping and commercial points in the country."[24]

1870

In the late summer and autumn of 1870, New Orleans had a small-scale yellow fever outbreak, resulting in only 587 reported deaths in a population of more than 190,000.[25] The quarantine period required of all vessels entering the Mississippi River from infected ports was fifteen days that year rather than the customary ten, counting days at sea as part of the detention period. Because the quarantine had been strict, the editor of the *New Orleans Medical and Surgical Journal* believed that yellow fever had originated in New Orleans in 1870. By this time many medical and lay observers had combined both of the old opposing views into a belief that yellow fever was imported in some years and indigenous in others. The disease first appeared and for a time remained in the Second District behind the French Market. Within a month, however, it began to strike down Italian and Sicilian immigrants employed in the French Market area "whose hygienic condition in their domiciles is about the most unfavorable in the whole city." From there yellow fever spread to other parts of New Orleans, affecting "nearly all classes and nativities" to some extent. Although the epidemic of 1870 was moderate by local standards, one medical journalist expressed regret that "this hostile incursion has brought dismay upon our unacclimated population, has revived the evil reputation of our city, and has done incalculable damage to its commercial interests." The fever did not spread to any considerable extent in the state that year. New Iberia, Ville Platte, and Port Barre were the only points outside New Orleans to suffer noteworthy visitations.[26]

New Orleans, 1873

In 1871 New Orleans recorded only fifty-four yellow fever fatalities; in 1872, only thirty-nine.[27] Then came an unusual occurrence in 1873 when Shreveport suffered a more serious epidemic than New Orleans, outranking the metropolis in the total number of yellow fever deaths as well as percentage of the population affected. In New Orleans the disease claimed ony 226 victims, but in Shreveport, 759 died. With a population almost twenty times the size of Shreveport, New Orleans had less than one-third the yellow fever mortality of the north Louisiana community.

The state board of health attributed the difference in severity between the two outbreaks to the widespread use of disinfectants in New Orleans, a doubtful hypothesis, but one giving the board credit for "limiting" the Crescent City's mortality by its vigorous local measures. From the first week of August the board of health provided for the systematic disinfection of yards, alleys, drains, and sidewalks throughout any square block in New Orleans where a yellow fever case had been reported. Carbolic acid was applied by hand from sprinkling pots. Surrounding streets and roads also received a heavy sprinkling of crude carbolic acid from tanks carried on wheeled carts, and the sprinkling was repeated several times in the following weeks. Privy vaults on the premises were treated with zinc-iron chloride solution. After a patient died, recovered, or was relocated, the board ordered the infected quarters fumigated with sulphurous acid or chlorine gas and all clothing and bedding soaked in dilute carbolic acid or boiling water. In its annual report the board declared that "chemical science" had finally supplied a means of "neutralizing all noxious and malarial gases." The phrasing indicates that the board members still thought in terms of miasmatic influences rather than germ theory.[28]

On the other hand, Dr. Alfred Perry, one of the board's sanitary inspectors, in an article prepared for the *New Orleans Medical and Surgical Journal*, explained that the disinfection procedures served to destroy "disease germs," thus preventing their spread from the infected premises. He believed the large-scale effort had been effective in limiting the impact of yellow fever in New Orleans in 1873, while the disease had been rampant in Shreveport and Memphis where disinfection had not been practiced. The board's activity generated heavy opposition in New Orleans from those who complained that carbolic acid fumes caused nausea, headache, and eye irritation. One physician insisted that carbolic acid sprinkled in a nearby yard had caused his patient to die. Dr. Perry dismissed such complaints of discomfort and even a few deaths as having insufficient weight to counteract the obvious benefits of disinfection in protecting the healthy.[29]

The aggressive program of the state board of health was facilitated in 1873 by the purchase of "a complete telegraphic apparatus," an important innovation. Set up in the board's office in New Orleans, and connected to the central office at City Hall, the equipment provided immediate contact with the state capitol, Charity Hospital, and all the police stations in the city. The new mode of communication proved valuable to the health officials, saving time and the cost of messengers, and allowing the prompt reporting and handling of cases.[30]

Yellow fever probably caused more deaths in New Orleans in 1873 than the reports indicate. According to the board of health, about half the population suffered cases of "Dengue" during the epidemic season, some of which finally "assumed the appearance" of yellow fever and terminated in death.[31] Although seldom fatal, dengue fever is easily confused with yellow fever in its early stages. Some of the cases and especially the deaths reported as dengue were probably yellow fever. The New Orleans epidemic—whether largely dengue, yellow fever, or both—was soon completely overshadowed by the outbreak in Shreveport in 1873.

Shreveport, 1873

Numerous cases began to develop in late August, and by the first of September the scourge was extending its influence throughout Shreveport. More than half of the town's population of 10,000 left at the beginning of the outbreak, and most business establishments closed down. Shreveport was completely quarantined by all neighboring towns, the telegraph serving as its only means of communication with the outside world.[32]

With the assistance of a physician and several nurses sent by the New Orleans Howard Association, the Shreveport Howards established an infirmary for the indigent sick in mid-September. Contributions soon arrived, not only from New Orleans but from Philadelphia, Cincinnati, and many other locations around the country. The Western Union Telegraph Company offered free use of its lines for the transfer of financial aid to Shreveport. Because the town was isolated by its neighbors' quarantine measures, railway service was disrupted, and special arrangements had to be made to channel nurses, physicians, and supplies into the stricken center. The Southern Express Company contracted with the New Orleans Howards to ship without charge all supplies destined for Shreveport as far as its terminus in Monroe. The company agent in Monroe promised that the goods would be forwarded as soon as possible, presumably by whatever means were possible.[33]

The Texas and Pacific Railroad provided relief trains twice a week throughout the epidemic to carry poultry, eggs, other provisions, and medical personnel to a point outside Shreveport where they could be picked up and transported into town by persons from within the infected area. New Orleans in particular empathized with Shreveport's plight. Since their own small outbreak was eclipsed by the suffering of the Northwest Louisiana town, New Orleans residents, commercial firms, and the Howard Association provided generous assistance. The Shakespeare Club and the Orleans Dramatic Association, as on previous occasions, offered special performances to raise funds for the relief of Shreveport.[34]

In late September as the death toll increased, the editor of the *Picayune* remarked that Shreveport's mortality rate if applied to New Orleans' population would amount to about a thousand deaths per day. The destitute circumstances of the citizenry caused as much suffering as the disease. Shreveport's Howard Assocation attended to yellow fever patients, fed the poor, and opened an asylum for children orphaned by the epidemic. Toward the end of September the expenses of the association totalled $1,000 to $2,000 per day.[35]

By September 28 the New Orleans *Picayune* considered the "terrible fever in Shreveport" at least four times worse than the "fearful epidemic that scourged this city in 1853." On the last day of September the news telegraphed from Shreveport read: "We no longer have funerals. The hearses, followed by one or two carriages, dash through the streets like a section of artillery in a battle seeking a position . . . [;] the coffins [are] shoved in the hearses and driven rapidly to the cemetery. This is the case even with the most prominent citizens." By this time the Howard Association was feeding about two-thirds of the resident population, black and white alike. Hundreds of citizens had no money, no work, no prospects. Rapidly going through their resources, the Shreveport Howards on September 30 made an appeal to the country at large for additional aid, declaring, "the well are broken down, the poor are threatened with actual starvation, the sick and dying are about to be deprived of the commonest comforts humanity can offer them." The commander of the United States troops in New Orleans, General W. H. Emory, telegraphed President U. S. Grant on October 3 requesting permission to send 5,000 rations to the Shreveport victims. A quick reply directed the general to send the supplies at once.[36] Without regard to the bitter struggles of Reconstruction then in progress, the northern "enemy"—civilian and military—again responded with benevolent impulses and material assistance to a southern population afflicted by epidemic disaster.

The disorder of the disease-ridden, poverty-stricken community must have provided an unusual opportunity for the criminally inclined, or at least some Shreveport residents feared this would be the case. In early October, reports of robberies led to the formation of a citizens committee which posted notices stating:

> The committee of citizens on the safety of the town hereby warn all parties concerned, that any persons found depredating upon the property of our citizens will be summarily dealt with. It is our purpose to protect our city at all hazards, and evil disposed persons are warned to leave.

Although unable to prove the charge, the committee suspected four persons from New Orleans of having robbed a Catholic priest who was "on his deathbed." Of the four, two men were driven out of town and warned to stay away; the other two, a man and his wife, were allowed to remain in the city under guard until the woman, who had come down with the fever, could recover.[37]

As cold weather arrived in late October and early November, the pestilence gradually subsided. Stores began to reopen, cotton trickled in by the wagonload, and a sense of hope returned to the survivors. Still the Howard Association continued to feed the poor until more jobs developed in the reviving community. By November 4 all quarantine barriers against Shreveport were lifted, and after a suspension of two months the trains of the Texas and Pacific Railroad once again ran freely to and from the town.[38]

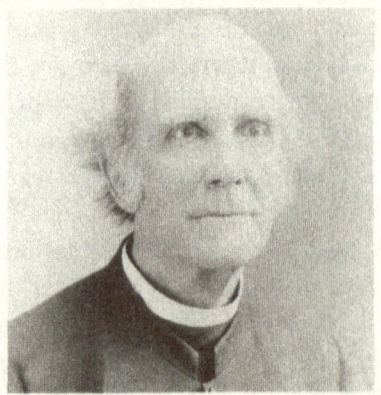

The Reverend W. T. D. Dalzell, rector of St. Mark's Episcopal Church of Shreveport. Credited as the only Protestant minister who stayed on the job and cared for the sick during the 1873 Shreveport epidemic, he had also nursed yellow fever victims in Savannah, Georgia, in 1857, and during the 1878 epidemic he went to Memphis to serve the sick. Lilla McClure and J. Ed Howe, *History of Shreveport and Shreveport Builders* (Shreveport, 1937), 256; Courtesy LSU-Shreveport Archives.

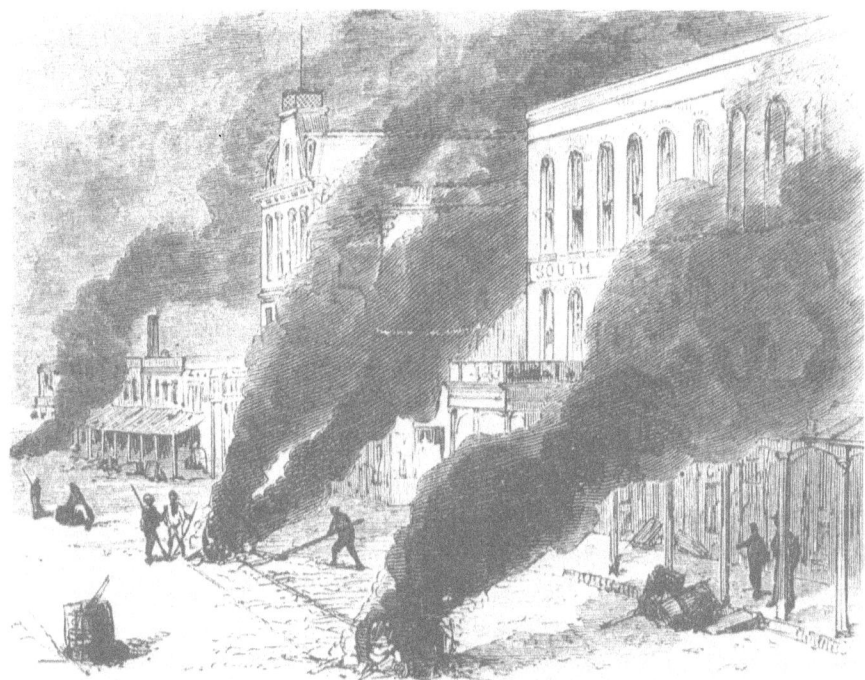

Yellow Fever Epidemic at Shreveport in 1873. Smoke from burning tar or sulphur was believed to purify the infected atmosphere. Courtesy The Historic New Orleans Collection, Museum/Research Center, Acc. No. 1974.25.11.179 (detail).

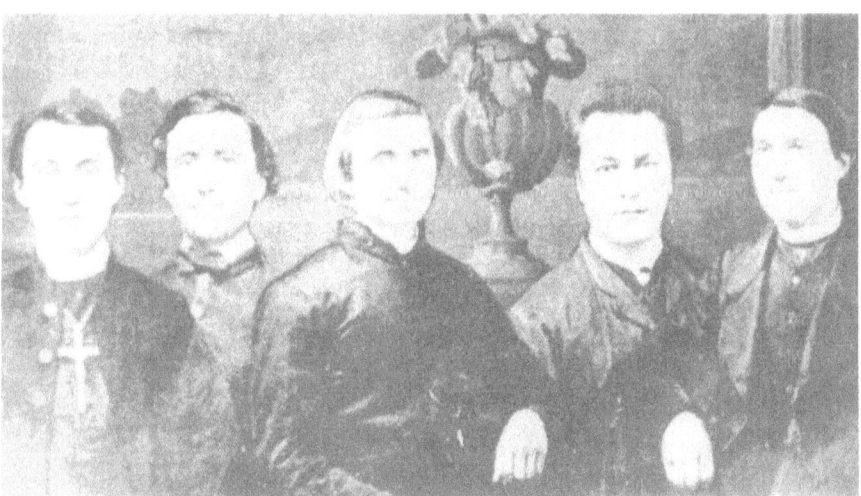

"Martyr-Priests" of Louisiana.
From Roger Baudier, *The Catholic Church in North Louisiana: A Historical Sketch of Pioneer Days and of the Diocese of Natchitoches and Its Successor, the Diocese of Alexandria* (centennial pamphlet, 1953), 36.

Serious obstructions to railroad transportation posed by town, parish, and out-of-state quarantine regulations became an increasingly acute problem from the early 1870s throughout the remainder of the nineteenth century. Previously, quarantine was mainly a concern of coastal and river ports. Sometimes local authorities had attempted to exclude persons and goods from infected areas, but seldom had these regulations been strictly enforced. After the Civil War, however, railroad lines extended across state and nation, breaking down isolation and linking the nation's communities. As the belief in yellow fever's transportability gained widespread acceptance, persons throughout Louisiana and neighboring states came to fear its spread from New Orleans or other infected communities by railroad passengers, baggage, and freight.

As news of the Shreveport epidemic spread in early September, a train from the infected city was halted at the Dallas city limits by a posse of policemen and citizens who threatened to shoot the engineer if he tried to proceed. After detaining the train until the following morning, the posse allowed it to return to Shreveport. Temporarily, the Texas and Pacific obtained permission from the mayor of Marshall, Texas, to make regular trips to that town from Shreveport provided that a physician attested to the passengers' freedom from yellow fever. On that occasion, a Dallas newspaper commented: "Things have come to a pretty pass when the Texas Pacific Railroad corporation have to apply to the Mayor of a one-horse town for permission to run their trains."[39] Such commentary seems strange coming from a city where a posse had denied permission for trains to enter.

Railroad companies either complied with the quarantine demands of towns (large or small), or ran the risk of burned bridges, torn tracks, and dead engineers. By late September of 1873 there were only two mail routes out of Shreveport, both by stage: one to Monroe and another through Trenton.[40] Problems of intrastate and interstate quarantine and the railway transportation of passengers, freight, and the U. S. mail would become more and more complex and controversial during the next three decades.

At the close of Shreveport's 1873 epidemic, the local medical society appointed a committee to investigate and report on the origin and course of the recent disaster. The committee concluded that the disease had been imported from Havana to New Orleans and from there transported to Shreveport on the Red River packets. Because the population of Shreveport had tripled since the town's last epidemic in 1867, most citizens were susceptible to the disease. It was estimated that only about 4,500 persons remained in town during the epidemic; of that number, 3,000—two-thirds of the population—experienced attacks of the fever, and at least 759 (17 percent) died. The case fatality rate was almost 26 percent. In the opinion of the medical committee, "No epidemic in America has yet occurred to show more plainly that we are not yet masters of this fearful disease, its proper treatment and the laws that govern it."[41]

Yellow fever spread that year to Marshall, Texas, about forty miles west of Shreveport, and to Mansfield and Coushatta, Louisiana, south of Shreveport.[42] According to a resident of Coushatta, the pestilence made "sad havoc" in the entire area of the Red River Valley. "The country looks desolate," he wrote; "worse than ever it looked during and after [General Nathaniel P.] Bank's raid through Red River." For a distance of at least fifty miles through the valley south of Coushatta, the area was practically deserted.[43] Yellow fever also traveled up the Mississippi River as far as Memphis, Tennessee, striking that city in a destructive epidemic comparable to Shreveport's bitter experience. Only twice before had Memphis suffered yellow fever epidemics, in 1855 and 1867. In 1873, of its winter population of 50,000 only some 15,000 persons stayed in the city during the epidemic; 7,000 fell sick with the fever and approximately 2,000 died.[44]

1874-1877

From 1874 through 1877 the pestilence claimed a few victims in New Orleans each year, but so few that the disease received little public notice. Louisiana felt the impact of a severe nationwide economic depression and a violent contest for political control of the state. Radical Reconstruction came to an end in 1877 when the last federal troops were withdrawn and the Republicans lost the state government to the Bourbon Democrats, the southern white planter-merchant elite that would control Louisiana for decades to come. In 1878, the year following the return to "home rule," Yellow Jack also returned, scourging New Orleans, the gulf states, and the entire Mississippi Valley in the most extensive yellow fever epidemic the United States had ever known.

VII

NEW VULNERABILITY, LOCAL AND NATIONAL: THE PESTILENCE OF 1878 AND ITS AFTERMATH

By 1878 yellow fever had been killing people in New Orleans for more than three-quarters of a century, sometimes by the thousands in severe epidemics. Yet the city's leadership over the years believed that long-term residents, the native-born, and members of the upper classes—such as themselves—were generally immune to the disease. They resisted expenditures for sanitary improvements, opposed a strictly enforced ship quarantine as harmful to the city's commerce, and comforted themselves with the thought that Yellow Jack was a problem mainly for the poor and the outsider, as it had long appeared to be.

The pattern of the 1878 epidemic, however, altered that kind of thinking and became the occasion for the most comprehensive measures to control the disease yet undertaken. In New Orleans, the 1878 epidemic took many of its victims from the traditionally "safe"—the natives, the upper classes, the blacks, and most shocking for many, from the white children of the "better element." Not only were the leading citizens not insulated from the fever's ravages; New Orleans, now part of a rapidly developing national commercial system, could no longer protect its economy by subverting maritime quarantine. The city was subjected to quarantine by communities throughout the state and region, and its trade suffered accordingly.

The most widespread yellow fever epidemic in the nation's history, the 1878 pestilence cut across class lines and spread to interior states not previously in Yellow Jack's sphere of influence, disrupting the nation's trade and transport system. The staggering financial and human costs provided the impetus for long range protective measures such as the National Board of Health, formal communication between state health authorities, urban sanitation, improvements in disinfection techniques and quarantine facilities, and increased scientific investigation of yellow fever. Although yelllow fever's causative agent and precise mode of transmission continued to elude researchers, and the disease occasionally slipped past quarantine officials, the systematic approach to public health regulation that came in the aftermath of the 1878 epidemic established the basis for a more effective national and local health policy.

New Orleans, 1878

On July 24, 1878, the New Orleans *Picayune* published the first announcement from the Louisiana State Board of Health that yellow fever had appeared in the city: fourteen cases of a virulent type, among which seven had died. The *Picayune* editor offered reassurance that no cause for alarm yet existed, pointing out that the board intended to halt the fever's spread by disinfecting each area where cases had appeared. In the past, he admitted, the health authorities and the press "generally refrained from specially mentioning" sporadic cases of yellow fever because exaggeration and unwarranted panic usually followed any such report. Nevertheless, information about yellow fever cases had always been transmitted by letter-writers and by persons traveling from the city. "Hence what is not announced here has been known abroad, and the very precaution taken to avoid needless alarm and to prevent exaggerated and injurious reports has had a result the reverse of what was intended." The editor declared himself in favor of publishing all infermation relative to the city's health, including every death and every disease.[1]

When the "sporadic cases" soon developed into an extensive epidemic, not only in the city but throughout the South, the *Picayune* and other New Orleans newspapers provided comprehensive coverage of the disaster, the fullest reporting on any epidemic thus far. From late July to mid-November their columns were filled with yellow fever news: reports and statements from various boards of health, reports on activities of the Howards and other benevolent associations, lists of charitable contributions from around the country, letters from readers, reports of the fever in various towns in Louisiana and neighboring states, accounts of quarantine entanglements disrupting commercial exchange, and editorial commentary. The eyes of the country were focused on the South as the regional pestilence invaded many quarters hitherto unaffected and threatened to spill over its customary northern boundaries. Yellow fever in 1878 was a matter of nationwide concern, and no newspaper, certainly no New Orleans newspaper, could afford to treat it otherwise.

According to the annual report of the state board of health, prepared after the epidemic, yellow fever had been imported to New Orleans in 1878 by the steamship *Emily B. Souder*, arriving from Havana in late May. At the time, however, board members had not diagnosed the "suspicious cases" as yellow fever; only in retrospect did they see the *Souder* as the culprit. The quarantine physician at the Mississippi River Station had given the vessel a clean bill of health, except for one crew member diagnosed as having intermittent fever (malaria) and placed in the infirmary. After disinfection, the ship was allowed to proceed upriver to New Orleans without being detained the usual ten days. Shortly after arriving in the city, several crew members sickened, and two died. The board investigated, but after some uncertainty and diagnostic disagreement, the cases were recorded as malarial fever. No additional cases of any "suspicious" fever came to the board's attention until early July, and even then, neither the board nor the press offered any public comment on the disease until July 24.[2]

That day, Dr. Samuel Choppin, board president, also sent a message to the surgeon-general of the U. S. Marine Hospital Service, informing him of yellow fever's presence in the city since about July 12: "We are endeavoring diligently to trace the origin of this outbreak, but so far find no connection with any foreign source. *It is clear that they have not resulted from the two cases which were developed two months ago on the steamer Emily B. Souder*, immediately after her arrival from Havana."[3] In later trying to reconstruct the origins of the epidemic, however, Choppin and others seemed to think that the suspicious cases had indeed been yellow fever and that the *Souder* must have started the chain of cases that eventually produced an epidemic. Dr. Joseph Jones, one member of the board, later expressed his doubts about any connection between the *Souder* cases in May and the epidemic that developed. Through his own investigation, Jones discovered that the *Souder* had made a second trip to

New Orleans in early July with a load of sugar from Havana, and on that occasion had been one source of the imported malady.[4]

In his work on the epidemic, historian John Ellis found it impossible to determine exactly when and how yellow fever first arrived in New Orleans in 1878. (For that matter, the same is true for almost any epidemic year, regardless of the "official" explanation devised *ex post facto* by the board of health.) There were many opportunities for the introduction of the fever in 1878: ships arriving from Brazil where the disease was prevalent as early as February; ships from Havana where yellow fever was reported in March; Cuban refugees arriving in New Orleans by the hundreds in April and May after the end of their unsuccessful ten-year war for independence; and numerous vessels from Central America and the West Indies that passed quarantine after fumigation without being detained.[5]

In late July the reading public first became aware of yellow fever's presence when the disease suddenly erupted in a relatively clean, middle-class neighborhood, mainly afflicting small children. From the first, this outbreak was perceived by the articulate elements of the community as significantly different from the customary New Orleans epidemic. It was especially terrifying because the first reported cases of yellow fever came from comfortable areas of the city among classes and ages usually considered exempt from its early ravages.

Unaccountably, children of the middle and upper classes were dying like foreigners of the "strangers' disease"! Within a matter of days after the first report of pestilence, thousands of families left New Orleans for safer territory. Departures had actually begun a week or so before the published announcement when many persons, already aware of the disease by personal knowledge or rumor, booked passage for themselves and their families on the outbound trains and steamers. From a population of 211,000 an estimated 40,000 took part in this extraordinary exodus. Nothing like it had occurred since 1853, and some considered this flight reaction the worst panic ever to occur in response to yellow fever in New Orleans. As in years past, some of the refugees carried the disease with them to other communities throughout the region.[6]

As the news—and the fever—spread in late July and August, quarantines were instituted against the Crescent City by towns and parishes within the state and by various state and local authorities beyond Louisiana's borders.[7] The letters of Thomas C. Porteous, a New Orleans merchant, to a Paris business associate in 1878 described the disruptive effects of the disease on commercial activity. On August 3, Porteous wrote: "I regret very much to say that the health of the city continues to give much uneasiness as to its effect on the fall trade. . . ." Even in ordinary times August was the dullest month of the year, but in 1878 "the yellow fever panic has driven nearly all our customers away and caused a rigid quarantine to be enforced all around us, which must almost paralyze the general trade of New Orleans while it lasts."[8]

Several days later Porteous complained that the streets seemed almost empty. Quarantine had been imposed by every village in every direction from New Orleans, and "in the store we are having the dullest time I ever remember, no cash sales & collections almost impossible." Even if the fever died out within a few weeks, he was afraid that quarantines would not be removed nor would families return to the city until October, "so that our trade will be bad in September as well as August." Porteous viewed these circumstances as a "great drawback & a bitter disappointment . . . as I anticipated a fair business in August & September, based upon the fine condition of the crops & good prospects of our planters."[9]

On August 23, he wrote: "At present . . . the city seems dead & one does not know what to do, I fret myself that here with a store full of goods & with prices advancing in New York, we cannot sell anything. . . ." To make matters worse, "with plenty of good accounts on the books, . . . we cannot get any money, almost all our city people are away & with the quarantine we do not know if our letters to the country reach their destination." The following week Porteous complained that retail trade was negligible when so few persons ventured into the streets or the stores. In early September he reported that his children were on their way to recovery, but one of his salesmen and a business associate had just come down with the fever.[10]

By October 15, as the epidemic was subsiding, Porteous happily noted that "ladies who have been staying in doors a great deal for the past 2 or 3 months, now begin to venture out & visit the stores & although not yet asking for fine goods, buy small articles which they see." Trade continued to improve, and cash sales increased each day. Finally, by late November, there was "no longer any sickness here & our absentees are returning daily by the hundreds, all we want now is a little cool weather & our trade will become quite active."[11]

For more than four months, the pestilence swept through New Orleans, resulting in a death toll of 4,046, according to the board of health. Estimates of the number of cases ranged from 15,000 to 27,000.[12] Dr. Joseph Jones believed the official mortality figures understated the actual number because many yellow fever deaths had been reported under other labels. He attributed this problem to "the differences of views as to the nature, origin, pathology and symptoms of the various forms of tropical and sub-tropical fevers."[13]

Another doctrinal difference was also at work in shaping diagnostic judgments. Many "creole physicians" still firmly believed in the immunity of native-born New Orleanians, refusing to recognize any sickness among them as yellow fever and reporting thousands of cases and deaths among their patients as bilious, remittent, pernicious, malarial, congestive, and hemorrhagic fever. Some French-speaking New Orleans physicians later swore they had not seen one single case of yellow fever in 1878. Aside from the difficulties of diagnostic labeling, the official mortality and morbidity figures were also limited by the failure of many doctors to report their cases, despite the board's best efforts to collect the data.[14] These problems of data-gathering were by no means new, but they seemed to provoke more than the usual comment and concern in 1878. Some physicians and journalists had come to accept numerical data and statistical analysis as essential instruments of modern science and society, a necessary requirement for understanding, probing, and comparing problems as well as for measuring improvement.

From mid-July to mid-November of 1878, New Orleans had suffered its worst scourge since the 1850s. Estimates of what the epidemic cost the city varied, depending on the values assigned to such factors as the potential economic worth of lives lost and labor diverted from productive endeavor by illness or attending to the sick; losses from derangement of business and unused capital; the cost of physicians, medicines, nursing, funerals, and disinfection; and funds spent for charity.[15] The Louisiana State Board of Health calculated a cost to New Orleans of about twelve million dollars:

Estimated number of cases	25,000
Cost of ten days' sickness of each one, at $3.00 per day	$ 750,000
Cost of 4,500 funerals at $25.00 each	$ 112,500
About 2/5 of 4,500 victims represent each a capital value of $1,000, amounting to	$ 1,800,000
Remaining 3/5 at $300, amount to	$ 810,000

Loss of time of half the industrial population, say 20,000 people for 90 days, at $2.00 per day	$ 3,600,000
Values destroyed by the epidemic	$ 7,072,500
Commercial losses by interruption of intercourse with the surrounding country and diversion of trade to other cities	$ 5,000,000
Total Losses	$12,072,500

Noting that the estimated annual profits of New Orleans' summer trade with yellow fever ports in the tropics usually amounted to only $1,500,000, the president of the state board wondered if that paltry sum was sufficient to justify the risk of importing a disease that cost the city more than twelve million dollars.[16]

At Risk: Children, Natives, the "Better Element"

In 1878 Yellow Jack seemed different from the old epidemic malady that New Orleanians had known, or known about, for years. Yet the "unusual" features that struck observers as noteworthy were not entirely new. They had been present to some extent eleven years before in the epidemic of 1867, although perhaps forgotten by many: (1) the large number of cases among groups considered immune or resistant in the antebellum era—young children, white adults native to the city, and blacks; (2) the appearance of the disease among the well-to-do; and (3) the magnitude of the city's poverty intensified by the epidemic.[17] Yellow fever was no longer as selective as it had once appeared to be when concentrated among newcomers and outsiders—especially the foreign poor.

While the poor were perhaps more numerous than ever, the foreign-born steadily declined in number and percentage during the postwar decades, from 38 percent in 1860 to 19 percent by 1880.[18] When yellow fever ceased to appear each year, the native-born lost their regular opportunities for a mild, often inapparent childhood case and thus joined the ranks of susceptibles whenever the disease returned—as it did in 1867 after an absence of nine years, and again in 1878 after eleven years (except for several minor outbreaks). After 1860 the growth rate of the New Orleans population was much lower than in the prewar decades, mainly because of the decline in foreign immigration. With its annual mortality exceeding the number of births, New Orleans' growth came not from natural increase but from black and white migration to the city from other parts of the state and nation and from a continuing small stream of foreign immigration. Despite a high infant mortality rate, the majority of the newborn survived, and children under sixteen years of age made up 34 percent of New Orleans' population in 1880.[19] In a sense, the children might be viewed as newcomers, little "strangers" who became fresh fuel for the fever whenever it revisited New Orleans.

Most of these demographic observations and explanations had been made by the board of health in 1867 in an attempt to explain that year's "new" and unexpected aspects of yellow fever epidemiology. Not many New Orleanians would have read the board's report, however, and probably few gave much thought to generalizing about the epidemic once it was over—not in the midst of the political and social turmoil of Radical Reconstruction during the late 1860s and most of the 1870s. But in 1878, when Yellow Jack's anomalous pattern of 1867 was repeated on a larger scale—with children, native white adults, and blacks coming down with the fever—many among the "better element" seemed to recognize for the first time that they too were vulnerable to what had once been called the "strangers' disease." Others, especially among the French creoles, denied the reality altogether, and many went to their graves recorded erroneously by their physicians as victims of some other fever. After 1878, few could still seriously defend the theory of "creole immunity."

Why was 1878 perceived by some as being profoundly different from prior epidemics, including the most recent major outbreak in 1867? First, the newspapers in 1867 described the early cases as occuring among the "unacclimated" outsiders, the northerners and Europeans. Only later did the disease spread throughout the city, and although extensive in scope, it was apparently less virulent than the 1878 pestilence, exhibiting a much lower case fatality rate (to the extent that available case estimates reflect the situation). By contrast, from the earliest published accounts in 1878, one would have thought that yellow fever had first appeared in a clean, comfortable section of the city among native-born middle-class children, an exceedingly different beginning from any previous outbreak.

Children under sixteen years of age, about a third of the city's population, constituted 58 percent of the yellow fever deaths reported in 1878; the toll was especially heavy among those from two to five years of age. The virus in 1878 must have been an unusually virulent strain, for this phenomenon was remarkably different from past experiences when childhood cases were common but mild in effect. In a study of the mortality records after the epidemic, Dr. C. B. White found the greatest concentration of deaths in New Orleans among four-year-old males, black as well as white. Some doctors had tried to explain this phenomenon by pointing out that "quiet manageability" was indispensable to recovery, while four-year-old boys were almost impossible to manage, being "more intractible" at that age than at others. It was also hypothesized that four-year-old males probably spent more time than younger or older children in playing and crawling about on the ground where they might have been more exposed to the germs of yellow fever, which were now believed to live and multiply on the surface of the soil.[20]

Some of the "better element" persisted in viewing the epidemic as mainly ravaging their class and their children. Perhaps the middle and upper classes did contribute more than their usual share to the list of deaths, especially the devastating loss of their children. They were shaken by their unaccustomed vulnerability to this fever of 1878, which according to one account repeatedly carried off victims from the "mansions of the rich" while passing over the "idler or vagrant, whose death would be a benefit . . . ."[21]

Poverty and Charity among Black and White New Orleanians

Despite these upper class perceptions, yellow fever, as always, worked its greatest devastation among the poor. The Howard Association, having engaged in its customary task of providing medical aid to the indigent sick, reported at the conclusion of the epidemic that more than 21,000 cases had been cared for by its members, volunteers, and physicians. The association's figures clearly indicate that the disease was prevalent among the lower classes which provided the bulk of the cases and deaths—as they always had. The foreign-born accounted for less than one-third of the Howards' case load, whereas in years past they had usually been an overwhelming majority. According to records of the board of health, foreigners constituted less than half of the city's total yellow fever mortality.[22] It was not just the strangers' disease anymore (not that it ever really had been).

Reporting on the epidemic in its October issue, the journal of the American Missionary Association noted that the disease "pays no regard to race, color or previous condition." The old idea that blacks enjoyed immunity against this pestilence "seems to have been ill-based. . . . At any rate, it is not true of this year's scourge," the *American Missionary* declared.[23] Yellow fever among New Orleans blacks in 1867 had attracted attention as an unusual phenomenon, but in 1878 the black population suffered an "unprecedented" number of cases. The Howard Association reported that its agents provided medical care to some 5,000 black patients with yellow fever. As in previous times, however, relatively few died of the disease. According to the report of the board of health, only 183 (4.5 percent) of the 4,046 yellow fever deaths in the city were "colored." At the time, more than one-fourth of the New Orleans population was black.[24]

Despite their apparent advantage over whites in surviving an attack of yellow fever, black New Orleanians suffered greatly from other diseases closely associated with poverty. The city's annual black mortality rate was extremely high, sometimes almost twice the white rate. If all yellow fever deaths are subtracted from the 1878 mortality record, the black death rate in New Orleans greatly exceeded that of the white population.[25]

There is no way to tell how many unrecorded yellow fever cases and deaths occurred in 1878 among blacks in New Orleans, many of them newcomers to the city. During the chaotic and stressful days of September, a black minister wrote to the American Missionary Association expressing thanks for a fifty-dollar contribution, which he used to assist "several of our sufferers" from the prevailing disease. "None but they who are here," he said, "can fully know the terrible suffering to which our people are reduced . . . ."[26] Black organizations, including the churches, were hard at work in 1878 offering aid and comfort to the sick and attempting to obtain contributions for the relief of their destitute people. Other ethnic and occupational mutual aid associations were similarly engaged.[27]

The New Orleans Howard Association began its work on August 16, although the board of health still refused to issue an official declaration that a yellow fever epidemic was in progress. The Howards attended to more than 21,000 yellow fever patients in the city, sent medical assistance to dozens of other towns, and dispensed almost $400,000 contributed to the association for epidemic relief in 1878.[28] In past epidemics the Howard Association had provided medical attention to yellow fever sufferers and general relief to their families and others. In 1878, so many persons were affected directly and indirectly by the epidemic that a division of labor in the relief work became necessary. While the Howards focused on attending to indigent yellow fever patients (providing doctors, nurses, and medicines), an auxiliary group, the Peabody Subsistence Association, was organized to receive donations, purchase food, and dispense rations to the destitute.

Although originally intending to offer general relief to the New Orleans poor, the Peabody group was soon overwhelmed by the needy and decided to restrict its offerings to those presenting requisitions authorized by the Howard Association, the Young Men's Christian Association, and the Ladies Physiological Society, organizations dealing specifically with yellow fever sufferers and their families. From August 31 to October 26 when it ceased operations, the Peabody Association issued 921,501 rations to 131,643 persons who would have otherwise faced starvation. Rations consisted of flour, meal, grits, rice, meat, coffee, sugar, tea, molasses, and salt.[29]

Both the Howard Association and the Peabody Subsistence Association were charged with racial and religious discrimination in dispensing relief. The Howard Association report for 1878 referred to these and other "false and mendacious" charges, including the mishandling of funds. The association strongly denied such accusations and provided a full accounting of receipts and expenditures. The report also explained that the Howards had rejected all appeals from societies representing a particular race or sect. They had refused to provide funds for other groups to distribute that had been donated specifically to the Howards, but they offered medical attention to "any needy sufferer of whatever tongue, color, or sect."[30]

In early September, the Mutual Benevolent Relief Association, a black organization, wrote a letter of protest to the Peabody Subsistence Association, which the *Picayune* published along with a reply from the Peabody Executive Committee. The black protesters complained that the Peabody Association had refused "to honor our requisitions or those of any other colored association." For that reason, they asked that donations be made directly to the Mutual Benevolent Relief Association, which would focus on assisting "our people." The Peabody Association replied that a misunderstanding had occurred because of its decision to limit aid to those with requests endorsed by the organizations working specifically with indigent yellow fever patients. Donations had been sent to New Orleans to relieve those suffering from the pestilence. The sick poor and their families and those widowed and orphaned by the epidemic had first priority; funds could not be stretched to take care of all the able-bodied unemployed of New Orleans. According to the Peabody officers, their decision to provide rations only to those approved by three groups working exclusively with destitute fever cases had eliminated the Hebrew Benevolent Association, St. Vincent de Paul, and all other relief organizations in addition to the black society. "Your charge, therefore, that we have discriminated against your color is unfounded," the letter declared. The indigent sick among the black population were directed to apply to the Howards or the YMCA for medical care and relief.[31]

Aside from the general references to religious discrimination, no specific examples have been found to clarify this charge. A brief item in the *Picayune* on September 22 reported the formation of the Catholic Relief Association, described as "catholic" in the most general meaning of the term. This group planned to offer relief to "all sick, suffering and destitute persons regardless of any consideration of race, or creed." This seems to suggest that some groups were discriminatory, or at least were believed to be.[32]

Another important source of general relief during the 1878 epidemic, especially for the black population, was the federal government. The U. S. Army Commissary in New Orleans, acting under orders from the secretary of war, offered forty thousand rations for distribution to the destitute population of New Orleans. The rations (bacon, flour, grits, rice, coffee, sugar, and tea) were transferred to the collector of customs, who called on the various relief associations to arrange for distributing the supplies. Organized as a supervisory agency for this purpose, the Orleans Central Relief Committee consisted of a representative from seven organizations—the Howard Association, the Peabody Association, the YMCA, St. Vincent de Paul, the Grand Army of the Republic, the Army of Tennessee, and the Mutual Benevolent Relief Association (for blacks). The central committee arranged for staffing various centers where government rations would be available, and it accepted private donations for the purchase of additional food supplies. In early October the secretary of war was persuaded to provide another forty thousand rations because of the serious destitution facing the city's unemployed, both black and white. In September the Orleans Central Relief Committee issued 60,000 rations to 2,680 families; in October it issued almost 165,000 rations to 4,296 families and several orphan asylums. The committee worked with at least forty-four different charitable groups in distributing the provisions.[33] According to some sources, the Army rations went mostly to the indigent blacks of New Orleans who had difficulty obtaining relief from the Peabody Association and other private agencies.[34]

From time to time, newspapers published reports on the relief work of various New Orleans occupational, ethnic, religious, and neighborhood associations. The Steamboatmen's Relief Association, the Firemen's Relief Committee, the Homeopathic Relief Association, *L'Union Française* and other ethnic societies, the Pickwick Dispensary which offered tea and soup, and many other groups supplemented the key activities of the Howards, the Peabody Association, and the Orleans Central Relief Committee.[35]

Responding to the nationwide appeals for assistance, individual donors, communities, churches, and organizations of all kinds sent contributions of clothing, provisions, and money to relief groups in New Orleans, and other towns in the pestilence-ridden South. In Washington, D.C., the clerks in several executive departments subscribed a certain amount each month during the course of the epidemic to send to the yellow fever zone. On August 27 the *Picayune* reported that a special citizens committee had been organized in Cincinnati to raise money for the suffering South. A prominent beer garden in that city pledged its receipts for one evening, and its patrons paid from one to five dollars a glass for the beer. The band played "Dixie" and other southern songs, according to the report, and the place was packed. Small communities within the southern region also came to the aid of their afflicted urban neighbors. In September the citizens of New Iberia, Louisiana, established a relief committee to collect funds and supplies for the sick poor of New Orleans. A picnic, a baseball game, and other fund-raising activities were sponsored by various groups. In all, the committee collected and sent to relief groups in New Orleans and Morgan City almost $1,600, 24 calves, 37 sheep, 7 hogs, 729 chickens, 80 dozens of eggs, 26 barrels of cornmeal, 3 barrels of potatoes, and 13 barrels of corn.[36]

On September 4 the *Picayune* estimated that the families of at least two hundred members of the police force required assistance. The editor commented on the patience and loyalty of the city police who had worked without pay for about two months. Because of the epidemic and hard times, tax collection was difficult, if not impossible, and available city funds dried up. The editor was pleased to report that the Peabody Association had agreed to provide the "necessities of life" to officers lacking resources.[37]

According to one New Orleans physician, the 1878 epidemic revealed the "depth of poverty" in the city. The "laboring classes" suffered from lack of work as well as sickness, and "genteel pauperism" was far more common "than anyone could have imagined."[38] In early September, the Peabody Subsistence Association published an appeal to "the People of the United States," describing the desperate situation in New Orleans and calling for donations of supplies and money since local resources were inadequate. In its first few days of operation, the relief association provided rations to 1,800 families for about 9,000 persons. The recipients included "every nationality, every color, every creed; and although the great mass of sufferers are from the humbler classes there are among them representatives of almost every grade of society, such is the condition of this plague-stricken city."[39]

Regional Disaster

Along the Gulf Coast and throughout the Mississippi Valley, the pestilence of 1878 extended from Louisiana to Mississippi, Alabama, Florida, Arkansas, Tennessee, and Kentucky. Cases also appeared in Cairo, Illinois; St. Louis, Missouri; Cincinnati, Ohio; and New York City. The disease spread extensively in southern Louisiana, moving outward from New Orleans to the suburbs and neighboring parishes and in all directions along rivers and bayous, especially in the southeastern section of the state. Places reporting yellow fever outbreaks included Gretna, Buras Settlement, Port Eads, St. Bernard Parish, St. John the Baptist Parish, Ponchatoula, Hammond, Tangipahoa, Clinton, Port Hudson, Bayou Sara, Plaquemine, Baton Rouge, Donaldsonville, Paincourtville, Napoleonville, Labadieville, Thibodaux, Pattersonville, and Morgan City. Apparently the only towns in north Louisiana visited by the disease were Lake Providence and Delta on the Mississippi and Delhi which was linked by rail to Delta and to Vicksburg across the river in Mississippi where yellow fever also prevailed.[40] In 1878 the railroad as well as the waterways helped spread the fever through the Mississippi Valley and the gulf states.

Remembering the earlier attacks in Shreveport and the Red River Valley in 1873, citizens of several Northwest Louisiana parishes applied rigorous quarantine measures in 1878, which probably had some effect in keeping the fever out of that part of the state. Similar memories motivated New Iberians, who had suffered greatly in 1867 and 1870, to establish a strict quarantine. From early September until mid-November, persons coming from an infected district were denied entry to the parish by a company of volunteers serving as quarantine guards. Although the fever struck several villages and plantations on Bayou Teche below New Iberia, the parish escaped the disease altogether in 1878. The town government of Vermilionville (Lafayette) to the west of New Iberia instituted quarantine against New Orleans and all other infected places as early as July 30, declaring its intention to avoid a repetition of the local experience with yellow fever in 1853 and 1867.[41]

In September, 1878, from a small town in Southwest Arkansas, a physician wrote his brother of "the fear and excitement that pervades our entire community" since one case of yellow fever had occurred. "Over half our citizens ran off . . . and have not yet returned." In between paragraphs of family news, the doctor kept returning to the subject of the epidemic:

> It makes the heart sick to read of the suffering in the yellow fever districts. The desolation in Memphis is only equaled by the wails of anguish that reach almost every part of our land. May God in mercy spare us from such a fate. It has now been 7 days since the negro, who had been in town, died, & we have had no new case, unless my partner Dr. K. has had a light attack. He thinks he had, but I don't think so. None of the negroes who nursed him or that visited him have been sick. We had them all quarantined and guarded.
>
> We have raised a little money, & sent to Memphis & indeed nearly every town in our state has sent more or less. Little Rock sent one Dr. & 25 nurses. One of the nurses have died, & yesterday 8 of them were sick.

In early October, he wrote his brother again to report that the community was enjoying good health since "the yellow fever scare," which apparently led to no other cases but caused the town to be quarantined by its neighbors.[42]

Dr. Samuel Choppin, Louisiana's chief health officer, concluded that firmly enforced local quarantine measures in 1878 succeeded in protecting a number of places from the fever, such as Galveston, Mobile, Natchez, Shreveport, and Monroe. "There must be no mediocrity in the organization of a quarantine," Choppin declared. "If it does not interpose an insurmountable barrier between the healthy and infected localities, it is worse than useless." The state's ship quarantine and disinfection system on the lower Mississippi had obviously failed to screen out the pestilence, and Choppin believed that major changes had to be instituted.[43]

Like Choppin, Dr. Joseph Jones, his successor as board president, was convinced that the 1876 legislative revision of quarantine policy had opened the gates to yellow fever in 1878. At the urging of the New Orleans Chamber of Commerce, many prominent physicians, and the state health board itself, the Louisiana legislature in 1876 had weakened the quarantine law. Although still providing for disinfection of vessels from infected ports, the new policy left the matter of detention to the board's discretion. Previously, a ten-day detention period was required of vessels from infected ports before they were allowed to proceed upriver to New Orleans. Both Choppin and Jones considered detention a necessary part of an effective screen against yellow fever, and both attempted to strengthen the rules of maritime quarantine to protect the health and commerce of the city and the valley.[44]

Appearing in at least eleven states in 1878, yellow fever affected more than two hundred communities. Estimates of the fever mortality throughout the region ranged form 13,000 to 20,000; total cases, 100,000 to 120,000. The New Orleans death count was 4,046; all other points in Louisiana, 1,000 to 1,500. The "board of experts" authorized by Congress to investigate the epidemic calculated the expenditures and losses throughout the country and arrived at a sum exceeding thirty million dollars. Beyond that, the experts also considered and tried to assess some of the "incalculable" costs, such as the disturbance to business conditions and loss of capital investment in lands, houses, boats, railroads, machines, and other property unused and unproductive because of the epidemic. By their final estimates, New Orleans alone suffered a loss of more than fifteen million dollars; the nation as a whole, between one hundred and two hundred million dollars.[45]

Not only was the visitation of 1878 the most extensive and the most costly epidemic the country had ever known, but it was also the last "Great Epidemic" of yellow fever in the United States. John Ellis has called it "one of the great disasters in American history."[46] As a great disaster, precipitating large-scale social and economic crisis, the epidemic had several important results. It stimulated a widespread public demand for the national government to enter the arena of quarantine management, to protect the public against yellow fever, and to facilitate the flow of commerce. Under pressure, Congress created a National Board of Health in 1879. Although the board functioned only about four years, it set important precedents for federal assistance to states in sanitation, quarantine, and inspection service, as well as federal support for scientific research.[47] The epidemic stimulated scientific interest and led to intensive studies of yellow fever, coming at a time when germ theory and the methods of laboratory science were opening up new paths to explore.[48]

The disaster of '78 pushed the Mississippi Valley and gulf states toward some measure of regional cooperation and agreement that state health authorities *should* provide prompt notification to each other whenever yellow fever appeared. The Sanitary Council of the Mississippi Valley, organized after the epidemic, would soon evolve into the National Conference of State Boards of Health. New associations and institutional structures were formed in response to the epidemic experience and the continuing threat that yellow fever posed to a large section of the country— the interior as well as the southern coast.[49] An increasingly interdependent national economy and national transportation network felt the effects of an epidemic that disrupted interstate commerce, tied up the lines of travel and transport, halted the flow of the U. S. mail, and brought drastic levels of unemployment and destitution at a time when the nation had not yet recovered from the economic depression and other tensions of the 1870s.

The epidemic of 1878 also heightened the fear of yellow fever in a more extensive area than ever before. The railroads had to cope with many local quarantine barriers, hastily erected at the first hint of a suspicious case of fever somewhere. Although eighteen years passed before another widespread epidemic occurred, the memory of '78, stimulated by an occasional case or minor outbreak anywhere in the South, kept the anxiety level high and popular interest in yellow fever keen, awaiting the next outbreak.[50]

Southern urban business leaders, in New Orleans, Memphis, and elsewhere, took steps to improve the health conditions—and the image—of their respective communities. Organized by New Orleans businessmen in response to the 1878 epidemic, the Auxiliary Sanitary Association raised funds to finance street and gutter cleaning, drainage, and other sanitary projects; supported the activities of the National Board of Health; and advocated the free exchange of health information and a rigorous maritime quarantine as the only means by which to retain the confidence and the commerce of the interior valley, so vital to the city's prosperity. Their motto was "Public Health is Public Wealth."[51]

The Pestilence of 1878 and its Aftermath 129

Citizens of other states had lost faith in the capacity of Louisiana's health officials to enforce a quarantine adequate for the protection of the Mississippi Valley, having seen that they often yielded to the pressure of New Orleans shipping interests to bend the rules. Companies involved in international trade had long opposed maritime quarantine as inconvenient and costly and would continue to appeal to the state board of health for special favors and exemption from quarantine restrictions.[52] Merchants, brokers, steamship and railroad companies, bankers, and other groups dependent upon inland trade, however, represented the major economic interests of the postbellum city. The economic losses of the 1870s led these groups to part company with the minor segment of shipping interests which opposed quarantine—those involved in foreign commerce, especially the summer tropical trade. As one historian described the situation, "Protecting the domestic trade took priority over the question of maritime quarantine in the Crescent City's public health movement and the battle against 'Yellow Jack' after 1878."[53]

1879 and After

The outbreak of yellow fever in the summer of 1879 was mild in its effects, probably having exhausted most of the supply of susceptibles during the previous year. New Orleans was again temporarily cut off from the interior by quarantine measures as various state and local governments acted swiftly to sheild themselves from the pestilence. Although twenty-six different points in Louisiana, mainly in the southern part, reported cases, the disease in 1879 resulted in only 162 deaths, nineteen of them in New Orleans. Memphis suffered the worst epidemic that year, hardly having had time to recover from the 1878 calamity.[54]

It was generally believed in New Orleans that the cleansing and disinfection performed by the state health board and the newly-formed Citizens Auxiliary Sanitary Association had limited the virulence of yellow fever in 1879. In October, the editor of the *New Orleans Medical and Surgical Journal* suggested optimistically: ". . . our profession should feel hopeful that the day is near at hand when we will be able to effectually banish this great arch enemy to our public health, commerce and prosperity."[55] The editor's hopes seemed almost realized during the 1880s and much of the 1890s when Louisiana enjoyed an unprecedented exemption from the saffron scourge. From 1880 through 1896, yellow fever claimed a total of only ten victims; in eleven of those seventeen years not one yellow fever death was reported.[56]

Although Louisiana was almost free of yellow fever during that seventeen-year period, the state was not free of its influence. One case was enough to set off a chain reaction of local quarantines. And during the 1880s, New Orleans had at least one reported death in six of the ten years. Almost every year of the eighties a few cases appeared somewhere in the South—in Texas, Louisiana, Mississippi, or Florida. At no time did the disease spread to any great extent, but every time it was reported or suspected anywhere, panic set in and quarantine barriers went up. Louisiana health authorities, like those elsewhere, established quarantine against infected points in other states to protect its citizens against the entry of the disease by land or water transport.[57]

Regional and National Responses

Even when absent, yellow fever remained the focus of much significant activity in southern urban sanitary reform, in the expansion and technical improvement of quarantine facilities, in scientific research, and in national health policy. The disease continued to provoke controversy on a number of fronts. Health officials engaged in bitter diagnostic disputes as they attempted to distinguish early cases of yellow fever from other diseases such as malaria. At various times, disagreement erupted among members of a local or state board examining the case; or between the agents of the National Board of Health and the state board; or among the representatives of several state and local boards sent into an area to investigate suspicious cases. Local physicians tended to resist the yellow fever diagnosis, often seeing the disease in question as dengue or malaria (which in some cases it might have been). Health authorities from other states or from the National Board usually decided that the slightest suspicion justified the assumption of yellow fever—to err, if necessary, on the safe side.[58]

Under the tense circumstances, an honest difference of opinion often led to hostility and recriminations on both sides. The local diagnosticians were seen by outsiders as deliberately practicing deception, trying to hide the presence of the disease from their neighbors. Investigators from other states, as well as the agents of the National Board, were accused of creating a panic as an excuse for quarantine to suit their own political or commercial purposes. State and local health officers from the yellow fever areas held conferences, established certain rules and regulations for quarantine, and agreed upon the free exchange of information to prevent unnecessary interstate quarantine based on rumor. Despite the efforts at regional cooperation, fear and distrust persisted.[59]

The 1880s saw the rise and fall of the National Board of Health and the continuing debate in Congress over the proper federal role in maritime and interstate quarantine, public health, and medical research. Various groups had advocated federal control of quarantine and other national health measures since the early 1870s, but with little result until the epidemic of 1878 generated a level of public demand that Congress could no longer ignore. Two lengthy and complex congressional measures, passed in 1879, established and defined the powers of the National Board of Health (NBH). Because the legislation was difficult to interpret and to implement, it was easily misunderstood by state and local officials and by the general public. The NBH was assigned large responsibilities but limited powers. Its functions included gathering information on all public health matters, providing information and expert advice on health concerns to federal and state authorities, and drafting a plan for a permanent national health agency. In addition, the NBH was assigned certain tasks in maritime and interstate quarantine for a period of four years. Specifically, it was authorized "to cooperate with, and, so far as it lawfully may, aid State and municipal boards of health" in the enforcement of regulations to prevent the importation and interstate transmission of infectious diseases.[60]

In its data-gathering capacity, the NBH subsidized many special investigations—technical, legal, statistical, and scientific. Projects included basic research in university laboratories as well as field surveys of urban sanitary conditions, water analysis methods, and engineering design in drainage, sewerage, and water supply systems.[61] In attempting to help state health authorities provide a more effective quarantine, the NBH established several supplementary quarantine stations along the Atlantic and Gulf coasts where infected vessels might be sent for treatment. The board also organized an inspection service for steamship and railroad lines leaving New Orleans and at several points farther up the Mississippi. Although not required by law, NBH certification of passengers and cargoes as free of infection facilitated trade and travel through quarantine lines because officials of the interior states had confidence in the national inspectors. During an outbreak, the National Board provided direct aid wherever it seemed necessary to prevent the interstate spread of the disease (as in Memphis in 1879).[62]

NBH operations provoked opposition from the Marine Hospital Service, a rival federal agency with considerable influence and the ambition to become the only national health bureau. Health officers in coastal states with established quarantine systems also resisted what they considered the encroachment of the NBH into their territory. Among the many obstacles encountered by the National Board, the institutional resistance posed by the Marine Hospital Service and the Louisiana State Board of Health—orchestrated by their respective directors, Surgeon-General John M. Hamilton and Dr. Joseph Jones—proved insurmountable.

As president of the Louisiana health board from 1880 through 1883, Dr. Jones fought the NBH on every point. He refused to cooperate with the national agents and engaged in disputes with national inspectors over the diagnosis of suspected fever cases. He also rejected the opportunity to use the NBH station at Ship Island off the Mississippi coast to supplement Louisiana's quarantine facilities. Jones never missed a chance to denounce the NBH inspectors as "federal spies" and troublemakers who set the rest of the country against Louisiana and represented a threat to the legitimate power vested in the state board of health. While the principle of states rights was often invoked by Jones and by quarantine officials in other coastal states, the struggle was far more complex. Matters of traditional local autonomy and professional integrity and competence were also at stake. Health officers of interior states found that NBH assistance enhanced their performance in the protection of health and the promotion of commerce. Coastal health authorities, on the other hand, felt their performance called into question, compromised and undermined, their power and influence usurped by outsiders.[63]

The intensity of Jones's relentless attack on the National Board may also be attributed in part to his combative and hypersensitive temperament. He had not always opposed the idea of national quarantine, and before he became president of the state board, he had been interested in an appointment as NBH inspector. The appointment failed to go through, presumably because of limited funds. Thereafter, Jones was an implacable enemy of the NBH and its New Orleans representatives, first Dr. Samuel Bemis and later Dr. Stanford Chaillé.[64]

When the quarantine powers of the NBH expired in 1883, Congress did not renew the grant of authority. For a few more years the board continued to engage in various research projects with its small appropriations, and then it faded from view. The NBH had won the support of the major medical and health organizations, railroad and steamship lines, and boards of trade in the interior states, but it had also accumulated powerful enemies. When yellow fever failed to spread in the years after 1878, public demand for federal action vanished. Despite its failure to survive, the National Board of Health was an important step in the gradual expansion of federal responsibility and power in quarantine and health protection. As a regulatory administrative agency, it provided the first direct federal aid to states for public health purposes. The NBH also exemplifies an early federal effort to use centralized administration, uniform rules and regulations, and research expertise to achieve order, economy, and efficiency—in this case, for health and commerce.[65]

The Civil War and Reconstruction had demonstrated the power of centralized government to accomplish large purposes. Various forces and interests in the postbellum era called for the expansion of federal power to deal with an increasingly complex, interdependent, modernizing society in the throes of industrialization and urbanization, with problems that transcended state boundaries. Other competing interests and traditions such as localism, diversity, laissez-faire attitudes, and resistance to outside authority placed limits on the development of national controls. Bureaucratic structures and administrative capacities evolved by trial and error at both state and national levels. Compromises were made between national and local interests, old and new values, as a new framework was gradually constructed, "patchwork" and piecemeal though it was.[66]

The U. S. Marine Hospital Service (MHS) had been reorganized in 1870 as a permanent quasi-military agency within the Treasury Department to provide a more effective administration of the federal program of medical care for merchant seamen, in effect since 1798. In 1878, prior to the epidemic, Congress authorized the MHS to assist state quarantine authorities, but in 1879 reassigned that function to the new National Board of Health. When the National Board's quarantine authority expired in 1883, the federal government did not retreat completely from the field. The Marine Hospital Service resumed its authority under the 1878 law to assist state and local officials when necessary to prevent the entry or limit the spread of epidemic disease. Little by little, Congress expanded the health and quarantine functions of the MHS and in 1912 changed its name to the U. S. Public Health Service to reflect its enlarged scope of activity. During the widespread panic engendered by the 1897 yellow fever epidemic, the MHS rendered valuable service in providing for inspection, detention, and certification of railroad passengers and fumigation of merchandise. Their work helped to restore at least some of the flow of interstate commerce bottled up by "shot-gun" quarantines.[67]

In the 1870s, 1880s, and 1890s, the federal government provided some small-scale support to important scientific and epidemiological research concerned with yellow fever, funding special commissions, NBH research projects, and the laboratory and field work of the Marine Hospital Service and the Army Medical Department.[68] American expansionist interests in trade, investment, and empire in the Caribbean and Central America were associated with and limited by the threat yellow fever posed to the people and commerce of the United States. These concerns made yellow fever research seem worth supporting, at least to some extent. Meanwhile, less exotic ailments such as tuberculosis, typhoid fever, and infant diarrhea, which killed more Americans in any given month than yellow fever killed in years, received little or no attention.

The bacteriologists of the U. S. Marine Hospital Service and the Army Medical Corps were among the few Americans who participated in the search for the yellow fever germ in the 1880s and 1890s. Their research, however, was sporadic, occasional, and mainly concerned with investigating the alleged discoveries of other scientists rather than an ongoing systematic search of their own. In the midst of all the interest in microorganisms and disinfection, the mosquito hypothesis advanced in 1881 by Carlos Finlay, a Cuban physician, was largely ignored until 1900 when the U. S. Army Commission headed by Major Walter Reed set up a camp and a laboratory in Cuba (under American occupation since the Spanish-American War) and proceeded to demonstrate the validity of Finlay's mosquito theory.[69] Government-funded research by uniformed, salaried government scientists clarified the specific process of transmission and made possible the prevention and control of the disease.

Louisiana's Quarantine Improvements

The Louisiana State Board of Health acquired additional duties and powers in the 1880s and pursued a more vigorous program of sanitation and disinfection in New Orleans. A lengthy court battle with several shipping lines over their refusal to pay quarantine fees was finally settled in the board's favor in 1886. In the case of *Morgan's Louisiana and Texas Railroad and Steamship Company v. the Board of Health of the State of Louisiana*, the United States Supreme Court declared state quarantine fees a proper compensation for ship inspection, disinfection, and care of the sick. These valuable services were provided by the state while exercising its police power to protect the public health against the introduction of disease. The Court ruled that the quarantine fees were neither a tax on commerce nor an infringement on congressional power to regulate commerce, as the shipping companies had argued. The decision effectively upheld the legitimacy of state quarantine authority against those who sought to undermine it.[70]

Quarantine regulations went through various revisions after the 1878 epidemic. Dr. Choppin, state board president, favored an absolute ban on summer commerce with the tropical sources of yellow fever but found little or no support in 1879 for such an extreme measure. The board agreed to a twenty-day detention period for vessels from infected ports but soon yielded to protests and retreated to the traditional ten-day detention period. While Joseph Jones was head of the board (1880-1883), the detention period was usually ten days. When a dangerously large number of infected ships accumulated at the Mississippi Quarantine Station in 1883, Governor Samuel D. McEnery, at the board's request, ordered all infected ships to depart Louisiana's waters and proclaimed non-intercourse with Vera Cruz, Havana, Rio de Janeiro, and all other ports infected with yellow fever. This action produced a great hue and cry from various shipping companies, some threatening to sue the board for assuming the right to exclude commerce altogether. Jones replied that some sacrifices were necessary to protect the nation against pestilence. Within about six weeks, however, the board abandoned the non-intercourse policy and restored the ten-day detention period, accompanied by the usual fumigation and disinfection procedures.[71]

Dr. Joseph Holt, Jones's successor as board president in 1884, applied a detention period of forty days (the original meaning of quarantine) and got the attention of the New Orleans business community. His talents for persuasion must have been remarkable, for he convinced a large gathering of business representatives to support his request for legislative funding to "revolutionize" Louisiana's quarantine system, replacing detention with modern methods of ship disinfection. He argued that a ten-day detention was as destructive to commerce as forty days, but the longer period might provide at least some protection against disease. Without better quarantine facilities and proper equipment for disinfection, Holt believed the board had no choice but to protect the state and the entire Mississippi Valley by imposing a forty-day quarantine—the equivalent of non-intercourse with most Latin American ports. Holt got his $30,000 from the legislature to implement an expanded and improved quarantine system, including an elaborate process of disinfection and fumigation that Holt called "Maritime Sanitation."[72]

The new system went into effect in 1885 and quickly attracted international notice as an effective way to prevent the entry of disease with a minimum of inconvenience to commerce. Disinfection and fumigation had been employed before, but never so thoroughly and systematically as in "Maritime Sanitation."[73] The health board spelled out elaborate rules and regulations to deal with various contingencies and established two well-equipped stations and two inspection points on the river below New Orleans. Ships with infection on board underwent extraordinary treatment at the lower station (isolated on one of the unused passes to the river) where the sick and well were separated and all kept under observation for at least ten days. Ships from infected or suspected ports received the sanitary treatment at the upper station and might be detained up to five days. Vessels from non-infected ports were inspected and detained only the few hours necessary for the sanitation process, after which they received clearance to proceed to the port of New Orleans.

Special disinfection apparatus—furnace, pumps, blower fans, tanks, hoses—had been designed and installed on a tugboat. The furnace generated sulphurous oxide which the blowers and hoses forced into the tightly-sealed hold of the ship. There the gas remained for several hours in order to kill any germs lodged in the cargo. All the surfaces of the ship were washed down with bichloride of mercury solution (mercuric chloride), and all baggage, clothing, bedding, curtains, and carpets were placed in special chambers and treated with steam heat. On infected ships, the baggage, clothing, and other materials believed to harbor germs also received a soaking with bichloride of mercury.[74]

Louisiana's new quarantine system, much admired by visiting health officers, became a model program. Charleston, Galveston, Pensacola, Mobile, Key West, Tampa, and other ports soon installed similar systems, as did all quarantine stations under national jurisdiction. According to Gordon Gillson's authoritative history of the state board, "Louisiana's outstanding contribution to the American public health movement during the last quarter of the nineteenth century was the introduction by Joseph Holt of maritime sanitation as a viable alternative to detention . . . ."[75]

"Maritime Sanitation" did seem to work most of the time, but not for the reasons believed by contemporaries. The germicidal gas used in fumigation—sulphurous oxide—would have effectively killed mosquitoes carried on the vessels, thereby diminishing the probability of importing the virus in that manner. In addition, the earlier proclamation of quarantine might have helped screen out the fever; the quarantine season began in May in the 1880s, whereas in the 1870s restrictions were not activated until June.[76] Nevertheless, the system was not without loopholes. This became obvious in 1889 when a yellow fever case slipped past the medical inspector undetected; after disinfection, the ship went up to New Orleans where one of the passengers died of yellow fever two days after arrival in the city. Even so, the board was always pressured to reduce the time of detention rather than to extend it.[77]

The most serious loophole was the special exemption granted to vessels engaged in the fruit trade. They were allowed to proceed to New Orleans immediately and unload cargoes prior to fumigation, and sometimes were not fumigated at all. The board granted this exemption in the late 1880s because the tropical fruit trade was becoming more important to the New Orleans economy, because fumigation and delay damaged the fruit, and because the companies agreed to use acclimated crews, to avoid infected ports, and to comply with other special conditions.[78] Louisiana's health authorities considered the risk negligible, and the continued freedom of New Orleans from yellow fever in the 1880s appeared to justify their policies and demonstrate the effectiveness of the system.

Infected mosquitoes (or persons) from Central America arriving in New Orleans on the banana boats most likely started the city's last epidemic in 1905, and possibly the outbreak of 1897 as well.[79] Contemporaries, however, considered Ocean Springs, Mississippi, the source, and the railroad as the means by which the infection arrived in New Orleans in 1897. Not having been visited by Yellow Jack in many years, the Crescent City had an ample supply of non-immunes, including a substantial number of European "strangers," the Italian immigrants who had arrived since 1878. The stage was set for another regional disaster. Fortunately, the intensity of the disease in 1897 did not match that of the panic it inspired.

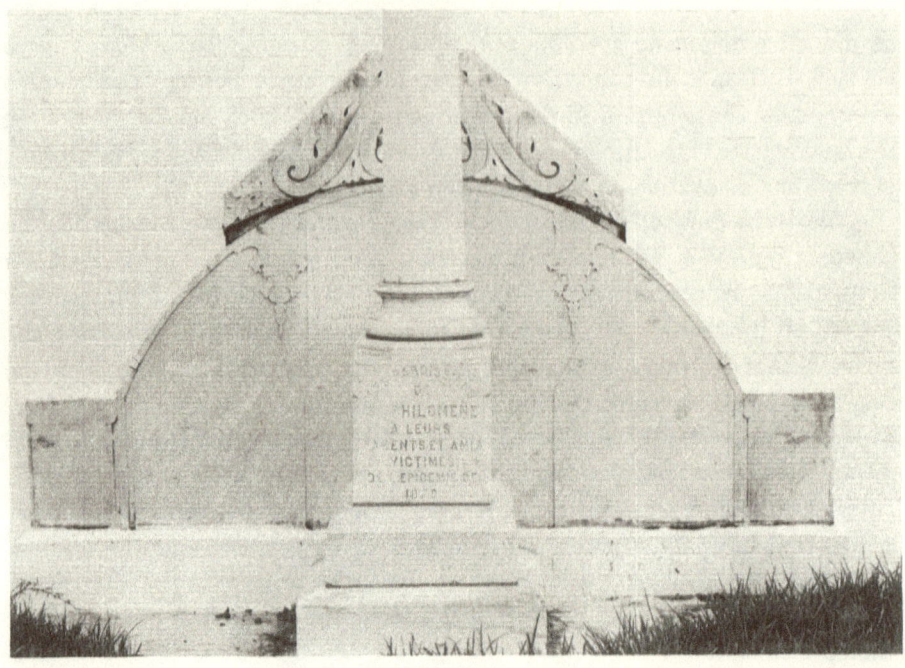

This Labadieville monument lists 163 names as victims of yellow fever in 1878.
Courtesy B. A. Hayhome, photographer (1979).

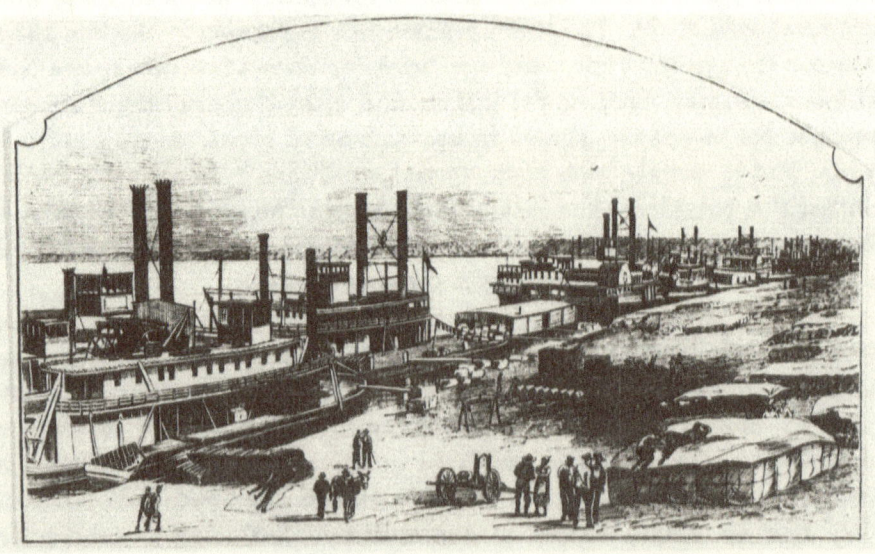

Mississippi River Traffic Halted at Memphis in 1878. Quarantine barriers throughout the South and the Valley. Courtesy The Historic New Orleans Collection, Museum/Research Center, Acc. No. 1974.25.11.178 (detail).

QUARANTINE.

OFFICE BOARD OF HEALTH,
New Orleans, April 18, 1883.

Captains and Masters of vessels, shippers and ship agents, and all parties concerned, are hereby notified that, in Accordance with official action of the Board of Health of the State of Louisiana, the Quarantine Station has been removed from Fort Pike to Rabbit Island, East Rigolets. After the 1st, of May, 1883, vessels entering East and West Pearl River and Rigolets will report at Louisiana Quarantine Station on Rabbit Island, East Rigolets.

[Signed] JOSEPH JONES, M., D.,
President Board of Health
State of Louisiana.

Quarantine Notice, Louisiana State Board of Health, 1883.
Courtesy The Historic New Orleans Collection, Museum/Research Center, Acc. No. 88-44-L.

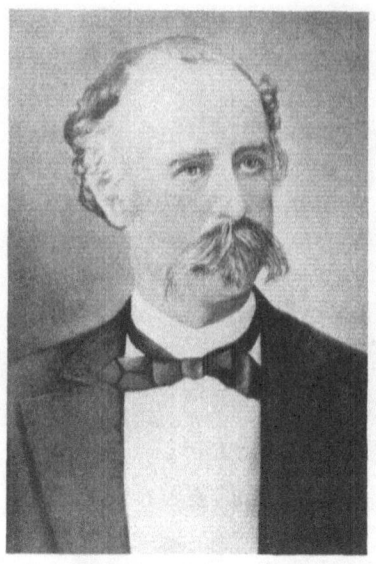

Dr. Samuel P. Choppin (1828-1884)

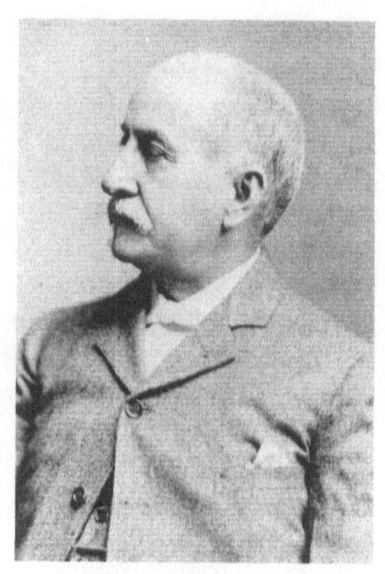

Dr. Joseph J. Holt (1840-1922)

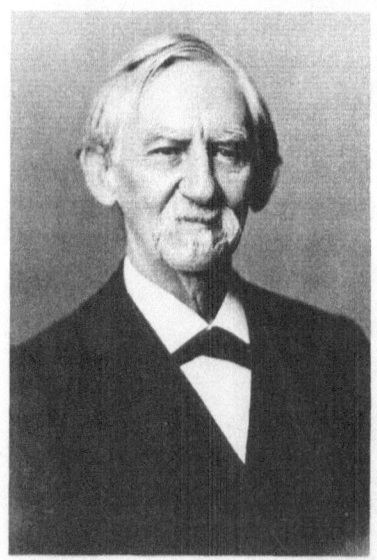

Dr. Stanford E. Chaillé (1830-1911)

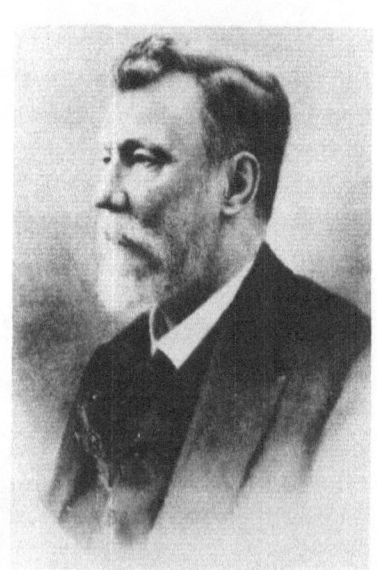

Dr. Joseph Jones (1833-1896)

Public health pioneers Choppin, Holt, and Jones served as presidents of the Louisiana State Board of Health during difficult times. Chaillé was an inspector and agent for the National Board of Health, chairing the 1879 Yellow Fever Commission sent to Havana. Photos Courtesy Rudolph Matas Library, Tulane University Medical Center.

VIII

THE YELLOW FEVER PANIC OF 1897

The yellow fever epidemic of 1897, although a minor one in terms of mortality, produced a panic in Louisiana and in other parts of the South. Never before had so much fear been manifested, and certainly never in the face of such a mild outbreak as occurred in 1897. Keeping in mind, however, the severity and extent of yellow fever in 1878 and the absence of a major epidemic since that date, one can understand the behavior of the citizens who initiated drastic measures in the hope of protecting their communities against the disease.

After the frightful experience of 1878, Louisiana enjoyed throughout the 1880s and much of the 1890s an unprecedented exemption from the saffron scourge. In 1890 the editor of the *New Orleans Medical and Surgical Journal* remarked, "it is now so long a time since the last epidemic that many of our younger medical men who have practiced in this city during the past decade have never seen a case of yellow fever in their lives." During the past twelve years, he said, the few cases that slipped through port quarantine had been discovered, isolated, and disinfected rapidly and effectively by the state board of health, thereby preventing the fever's dissemination. Although praising New Orleans for its success in combating yellow fever, the editor strongly emphasized the necessity for constant vigilance.[1] Since the germ theory had been widely accepted, it was now believed that disinfection of premises, clothing, and all articles possibly contaminated by yellow fever "germs" would prevent the spread of the disease.

1897 Outbreak in New Orleans

From 1890 through 1896 not a single case of yellow fever was reported in New Orleans. In 1897 the infection slipped in through a side door. Early in August an epidemic disease resembling both dengue and malaria broke out in Ocean Springs, Mississippi. Later in the month, after several deaths were reported there, the Louisiana State Board of Health sent a commission to investigate and identify the disease. The commission first declared it dengue. Shortly thereafter, as more deaths occurred and several cases exhibited black vomit, the Louisiana board sent a second commission to Ocean Springs. This time, in concurrence with representatives from several other state boards, the commission identified the prevailing disease as yellow fever. Louisiana then proclaimed quarantine against the Mississippi coastal resort, but it came too late to prevent many alarmed summer visitors at Ocean Springs from returning home to New Orleans.[2]

According to one estimate, some 2,000 persons returned to the city from the coast, traveling first from Ocean Springs to Biloxi by boat, then by train to New Orleans. On September 6, the Louisiana State Board of Health recorded the first yellow fever death to occur in New Orleans in eight years, a thirteen-year-old boy who had recently come from Ocean Springs. By September 10 several cases of fever, all traceable to Ocean Springs, had appeared in one city block. The board of health arranged for the isolation of the area and stationed sanitary guards in front of the infected houses with orders to permit no person to enter or to leave. The entire neighborhood was inspected and disinfected.[3]

House Isolation

As cases continued to appear in various parts of the city, the board ultimately commissioned nearly 700 volunteers as special sanitary police, paying each of them fifty dollars per month to inspect and disinfect houses and to enforce a policy of house quarantine. Infected houses were marked by red and yellow quarantine flags. Such a policy had never before been employed in a yellow fever epidemic in New Orleans. Sanitary officers were ordered to allow no one to enter or leave the infected premises without the board's explicit permission. Permits were issued to physicians, nurses, and clergymen, as well as certain persons known to be immune from having survived a case of the fever. After entering the infected premises, such persons were allowed to depart only after following elaborate procedures for bathing in disinfectant and fumigating or changing their clothing. Pedestrians were forbidden to congregate in the area, and the special officers had the authority to arrest and send recalcitrants to jail if necessary to enforce the board's orders. The guards were further instructed to remain constantly at their posts until relieved, to transmit all orders for groceries and other supplies from the infected households, and to maintain a barrier between the household and the outside world.[4]

The Louisiana State Board of Health supplied the commissioned volunteers with a "letter of authority" signed by its president, Dr. Samuel R. Olliphant, and addressed "To Whom It May Concern." The document identified the "Special Sanitary Officer" by name and confirmed in explicit terms his power to act. After "some friction" was reported over inspections of white-occupied houses by "colored" officers, an alteration was made in their letters, authorizing them to enter and inspect only those houses occupied by their own race.[5]

The house isolation policy, enforced throughout the epidemic, aroused keen opposition among many New Orleanians. Some persons even consulted attorneys on the possibility of enjoining the board or securing a writ of habeas corpus to obtain release from "enforced imprisonment" on the grounds that no one could be deprived of liberty without a fair trial. The *Picayune* editor strongly supported the position of the board, declaring that the health of the many should predominate over what he considered the unreasonable demands of the few. At a meeting of the state board, one member, Dr. Felix Formento, proposed that house quarantine regulations be modified to apply only to the sick and their immediate attendants, and not to every individual in the house. "The right of free ingress and egress of every citizen to his own home should not be denied," he insisted. Other board members did not agree; they rejected Formento's proposal and voted to retain the policy without revision.[6]

Continuing protest and violent resistance to the health measures prompted the board's attorney, B. B. Howard, to issue a public statement on the matter. The house quarantine policy was based on an ordinance dating back to 1879, he said, which provided for the regulation of entry to and departure from infected buildings, vessels, or areas, as well as for their fumigation and disinfection. Infected houses had been isolated and marked with flags many times before when dealing with diphtheria, scarlet fever, smallpox, leprosy, and other infectious diseases. The attorney thought it strange that those diseases, although less malignant than yellow fever, inspired more fear in the New Orleans populace than the saffron scourge. "Men will walk four squares to get out of the way of a smallpox flag who would not pay any attention to a yellow fever flag," he observed. Apparently the New Orleans public failed to "share the universal belief about its danger." In his opinion, their attitude toward yellow fever proved the old saying that familiarity breeds contempt.[7]

Still the opposition continued. In their determination to avoid house quarantine, many persons concealed yellow fever cases among their families and adamantly refused to call in medical aid. It was said that the inhabitants of quarantined houses often defied the guards by sneaking out through rear exits. A *New York Times* reporter in New Orleans described popular resistance to official measures in these exaggerated terms: "The masses of the people for the time being are in a revolutionary mood, because of the enforcement of the house quarantine, and are resorting to every means in their power to put obstacles in the way of constituted authorities."[8] Perhaps in the 1890s, middle- and upper-class observers—frightened by labor violence, large-scale immigration, urban poverty and disorder, and heightened class consciousness and protest—saw the threat of revolution in every act of lower class resistance to "constituted authorities." It is also possible that the article was simply the reporter's effort to write an exciting story for northern readers.

The "constituted authorities" also encountered resistance to their regulations and procedures for the burial of yellow fever victims. When a patient died, a burial crew was sent to wrap the body in a formalin-soaked sheet, and as quickly as possible to seal the corpse in its coffin and transport it to the grave—perferably within an hour or two. No one was allowed to enter the house to view the corpse, and no one from the house could leave to attend the burial. These restrictions, like other features of the house quarantine policy, were extremely unpopular and not so easily enforced. On one occasion, a large group from an Italian mutual aid society gathered outside the house where one of their members had just died. One man forced his way into the house; some in the group were armed with knives. Police had to be called out to protect the burial crew as they carried out their instructions.[9]

A letter to the editor of the *Picayune* from "an old resident of this city" denounced the health regulations as ridiculous. He had lived through "all the epidemics," he wrote, but had "never seen such tomfoolery carried on, as flagging houses and having old politicians stationed in front of doors, as if their presence could prevent the spread of fever." Furthermore, he felt that "reckoning the new cases" day by day made conditions seem even worse than they actually were. After all, he asked, "why demoralize a whole community, because a few people have fever?" The *Picayune* editor answered that "conservatism" in certain areas represented "the highest sort of civilization," but he considered it foolish to turn down the benefits of scientific advancement. After almost five weeks, only fifty-six deaths and some 500 cases had occurred; still a few "conservatives" wanted a return to the "good old days" when the fever raged in the city without obstruction.[10] This editor was convinced that the measures instituted by the board of health had limited the spread of the invisible yellow fever "germs."

At one point, the board members voted to abandon the posting of red and yellow quarantine flags at infected houses because of widespread opposition. Their attorney reminded them, however, that the flags were mandatory for scarlet fever, smallpox, and yellow fever by a state law of 1882 and a city ordinance of 1896. Continuing his vehement opposition to the policy, Dr. Formento demanded that the house guards be removed even if the flags had to remain. Other board members admitted that persons within the enclosures did indeed have to abandon their jobs for several weeks, but they believed that credit was readily available. In any case, it seemed to the board completely justifiable to inconvenience some 1,200 citizens in the interest of 260,000. Despite extraordinary pressure, the board held firm until the second week of November. When cold weather ended further danger from the disease, the board ended the house quarantines but continued to disinfect premises wherever the fever had occurred.[11]

Cleansing and Disinfection

Whatever their attitude toward house isolation, many middle- and upper-class citizens accepted cleansing and disinfection as valid preventive measures, believing that filth (associated mainly with the lower classes) provided a rich breeding ground for disease germs. An open meeting at the Chamber of Commerce resulted in the organization of a Citizens Committee on Sanitation and a proposal that the inhabitants of each block mobilize and cooperate in cleaning their premises and the streets. The board of health would be asked to supply disinfectant (chlorinated lime), and the citizens would do the work. Labor, capital, the professions, and "both white and colored races" were represented in the work of the committee, according to the *Picayune* report.[12]

The citizens committee asked the mayor to proclaim Tuesday, September 21, a general "Cleaning Day," when all regular business would come to a halt, and residents would organize and clean each block in the city. The mayor and the board of health considered this one-day cleaning campaign "inadvisable and inexpedient" because so much filth and trash could not be hauled away in one day. Furthermore, such a massive accumulation of filth and "stirring up of miasma" might be dangerous. It was recommended instead that each citizen clean and disinfect his own premises and burn all trash and rotting material. Organized effort, though less centralized than the original plan, seemed preferable to the individual effort recommended by the major. Within a week after the official rejection of the proposed general cleaning day, residents in several wards had established voluntary sanitary associations, organized by precincts and blocks, to clean and disinfect all premises in their respective areas. The associations offered to cooperate with the board in every way possible to fight the spread of the fever. In response, the board commissioned several men in each group as sanitary inspectors and provided specific instructions on the best methods for effective cleansing and the use of disinfectants.[13]

While commending these voluntary efforts, the New Orleans *Times-Democrat* called attention to the slum areas where appeals for voluntary cleansing had little effect. Long accustomed to filth, unaware of its possible dangers, and overworked to earn a bare subsistence, the slum inhabitants could hardly be expected to participate enthusiastically in a voluntary clean-up campaign. The newspaper recommended that city authorities undertake the task of cleaning up those danger spots.[14]

Isolation Hospital and Public Protest

On one occasion during the epidemic, when trying to execute a public health measure, the health officials and the mayor encountered extreme opposition in the form of mob violence. The incident seems to contradict the customary indifference of New Orleanians to yellow fever. On September

17, the board of health decided to establish a yellow fever hospital in the old marine hospital building on Tulane Avenue, offered for such use by the city government. Implementation was impossible. First, the board discovered that the building was "full of squatters." Next, the residents in the area opposed the use of the building as a hospital and presented a petition to the board requesting that some other location be selected. After reconsideration, the board decided on September 19 to use the old building as a detention center instead, where indigent persons from crowded, infected localities might be isolated; those who failed to develop the disease would subsequently be released.

The new plan was no more satisfactory to the protesting citizens than the old had been. That night "an indignation meeting" of more than a thousand persons, called by W. J. Kane, the former councilman from the Third Ward, gathered at the corner of Tulane Avenue and Broad Street. The group elected officers, listened to several "incendiary" speeches, and passed resolutions to be presented to the mayor the next day from the "voters and residents of the rear of the Third Ward." They protested the proposed detention center, which "would not only ruin all property interests in that section," but would probably spread the disease throughout the "thickly populated" area. The resolutions further warned public officials that such a project tested "the patience of many good citizens." On the morning of September 20, the mayor received the formal protest, together with the suggestion of Oakland Park as a detention area. He was able to obtain the temporary use of the park, thereby appeasing the Third Ward citizens and at the same time providing a suitable location for the detention center.[15] Thus a fortunate compromise had soothed the ruffled feelings and kept the peace, but not for long.

Although a detention camp had been provided, an isolation hospital was still considered necessary to keep indigent yellow fever cases from infecting other patients in Charity Hospital. Several days after the original crisis, the mayor secured the Beauregard School building at Canal and St. Patrick streets, a large airy structure located in the center of an otherwise vacant square, for use as a temporary hospital for destitute fever patients. The announcement of the project provoked another uproar among the residents in the Third and Fourth wards.[16] A crowd of four or five hundred persons, consisting of "some substantial citizenry" and many of the "rabble," as the *Picayune* described it, assembled in front of the school building around 6:00 p.m. on the evening of September 23. At the time, a physician from Charity Hospital and five or six Sisters of Charity were preparing the school for use as a hospital.

According to the *Picayune* account of the incident, several politicians played an important role in the gathering—just as the ex-councilman had led the earlier protest. The unruly crowd listened to speeches and heard arguments advanced against the hospital. Various speakers suggested that it was an attempt to make that portion of the city "the dumping ground for every sort of undesirable thing that came along" and that it was not only an outrage but a threat to the lives of nearby residents and their families. A committee from the assembly entered the school building to request that preparations be halted until the mayor could be consulted the next day. Attempting to placate the "indignant populace," the physician in charge and the sisters agreed to evacuate the building for the night; but even after they left, most of the crowd stayed on. Some left, others arrived, and late into the night they milled about on Canal Street in front of the school, built bonfires in the street, and continued to talk angrily about the proposed hospital. Eight or ten policemen hovered about the area, watching the demonstrators.

Comments noted by a *Picayune* reporter mingling with the crowd reflected an undercurrent of class resentment; for example, "Why don't they make a hospital out of some of those schools up in the rich and stylish neighborhood?" According to the reporter, some "responsible" persons remained in the crowd, although it consisted mainly of "toughs" of the Third and Fourth wards. Shortly after midnight, several unidentified persons set fire to two outbuildings behind the school: the residence of the "portress" and the kindergarten. Firemen rushed to the scene but encountered the obstruction of the mob, which cut the fire hoses and posed every possible hindrance to keep the fire wagons from reaching the burning buildings. Police reinforcements finally arrived, and the firemen put out the flames, but not before the two frame structures had burned to the ground. The school building itself suffered only slight damage.

On the following day when the committee of "responsible" citizens, representing the not-so-peaceable assembly of the night before, arrived at the mayor's office to register a protest against the hospital, the mayor chastised them severely for not having used their influence to call a halt to the mob activity. He concluded the interview with this statement: "Gentlemen, Beauregard School will be used." In a conference with the police chief, the mayor made special preparations to handle any further mob action. By the evening of September 26, the temporary fever hospital under the direction of Dr. Hamilton Jones, was ready for patients, guarded by police forces both day and night.

On the surface, this incident seems to reflect an intense fear of the disease motivating hundreds of people to rise up in protest. On the other hand, resentment over the use of their neighborhood as a "pest house" was probably the basis for the crowd action. It also appears that ward politicians had something to do with organizing the gatherings. Extensive unemployment might have added to the size and hostility of the crowd. Playing upon a basic fear of the fever, however great or slight, and stirring up the class consciousness of that section of the city, politicians provided an outlet for whatever tensions or frustrations existed and thus helped to create a situation that got out of hand.

Widespread Panic and Shotgun Quarantines

Outside New Orleans other incidents of violence or threatened violence occurred in maintaining local quarantines, episodes in which fear was unquestionably a factor. The year 1897 was truly the year of the shotgun quarantine. Between intrastate and interstate quarantine barriers, the railroads were caught in an incredibly complex predicament. At the onset of the epidemic, neighboring states as well as the Louisiana interior established absolute quarantine barriers against persons and merchandise from New Orleans and other infected points. Many areas would not even allow trains to run through at their highest possible speed.[17] Providing full news coverage of the exciting 1897 epidemic, the *New York Times* reported on September 15 that New Orleans was "so tightly tied up" that "there is no longer any commotion created when this, that or another town institutes quarantine." Within a radius of one thousand miles, "every town and hamlet has emphatically refused to have any intercourse with the city."[18]

The New Orleans *Times-Democrat*, like other Crescent City papers, complained indignantly of the quarantine imbroglio and recommended centralized state control of quarantine in preference to local action. By the third week in September, some interior towns had begun to suffer shortages of food and other supplies because of their self-imposed isolation. Finding it impossible to run trains profitably while complying with the multitudinous regulations of intrastate and interstate quarantines, railroad companies temporarily abandoned some of their lines. On September 18, the Texas and Pacific managed to run a train through from New Orleans to Shreveport but was allowed to stop at only a few points along the way.[19] Once it was widely believed that nothing could stop the U. S. Mail, but this belief was no longer true, according to the *Times-Democrat*, when "the pettiest village and hamlet" could exclude not only their own mail but stop other mail from passing through their limits for destinations elsewhere. By so doing, they incidentally created a "bonanza" for Western Union but a deplorable situation for everyone else.[20]

Officers of the United States Marine Hospital Service, in cooperation with the railway mail service, attempted to institute measures for clearing the mail routes. They set up a formaldehyde apparatus in New Orleans to fumigate letters, parcels, and newspapers for the purpose of killing the "yellow fever germs." This service opened up a few towns but failed to solve the problem entirely. Dr. Henry R. Carter of the Marine Hospital Service also established a federal inspection service on the railroads in an attempt to remove some of the barriers against freight and passengers from the city. In his words, "my orders are to organize train inspections to the borders of Texas, Arkansas, Tennessee and Georgia, passing through Alabama and Mississippi. It is useless to attempt anything in the latter two states, for the people are wild, panic-stricken." The Mississippi Board of Health would permit no train passenger to get off at any point within the state. Persons wanting to get on a train might do so, but once aboard they had to continue beyond the borders of Mississippi. Dr. Carter planned to appoint physicians as railroad inspectors who would indicate to local authorities at each stop along the way which passengers had been given health certificates. He hoped this measure would bring about a relaxation of the prevailing shotgun quarantines.[21]

Within a week after the inspection service started, some Louisiana towns agreed to accept *freight* from New Orleans if it was declared free of infection by the Marine Hospital Service. For the most part, *passengers* from the Crescent City continued to be rejected, despite federal certification.[22] With the lack of uniformity in local regulations, and with many towns or parishes prohibiting the passage of trains through their jurisdictions, traffic was hopelessly entangled.

President Olliphant of the state health board, Dr. John Guiteras and Henry R. Carter of the United States Marine Hospital Service, and a representative of the Southern Pacific Railroad set out from New Orleans in late September on the Southern Pacific line, hoping to clear a path westward to Lake Charles, Louisiana. They invited local health authorities to board the train as it passed through their respective towns; they also asked a health officer from Texas to join them in Lake Charles, less than thirty miles from the Texas border. The objective was to bring the various health officials together in Lake Charles and to obtain agreement for opening the Southern Pacific line for freight shipments from New Orleans to Texas, with inspection and supervision provided by the Marine Hospital Service. It was further planned that after completing the arrangements at Lake Charles, the expedition would proceed north to Shreveport and then return to New Orleans on the Texas and Pacific line in an attempt to clear away the quarantine barricades obstructing that road.

The entire project failed. From New Orleans through Lafayette, the plan worked well. Proceeding west of Lafayette, however, the train was halted at the Acadia Parish line by a party of armed citizens from the town of Rayne. They allowed no one to step off the train, they threatened to tear up the tracks, and they forced the train to return to New Orleans. Meanwhile, a message from Lake Charles declared it impossible for the health conference to meet there. Telegrams from Opelousas and from parish authorities along the Alexandria branch of the Southern Pacific also denied permission for the train's progress northward from Lafayette along that route. The well-intentioned congregation of officials found it necessary to return to New Orleans without having accomplished their mission on either the western or the northwestern railroad channels. Dr. Guiteras commented later that in all his travels throughout the civilized world he had never met "a more demented set of people," than the armed posse from Rayne. "They were scared to the very confines of stupidity," he said.[23]

Unlike many other newspapers the Baton Rouge *Advocate* did not condemn the action of the Rayne citizens as mob violence. Since the group had been led by the mayor, the Baton Rouge editor considered it a delegation with every legal right to enforce the town quarantine powers authorized by previous legislative enactment. Although upholding the legality of the action, the journalist did question the necessity of turning back the expedition; after all, the train could have "thundered through" the area at the great speed of forty miles per hour without danger of infection to any citizen of the parish, and the projected conference of health officials might have accomplished something of value to "science and commerce." According to the *Advocate*, the Rayne officials had been willing to let the train pass through until the authorities in neighboring Calcasieu Parish threatened to declare quarantine against Acadia Parish if they allowed the train to enter. Already cut off from New Orleans, Rayne could not risk losing the only other outlet for commercial exchange. To the Baton Rouge editor, this action by Calcasieu reflected the selfish, short-sighted interests of "Commerce agcinst Science." Dr. Carter, Marine Hospital Service Officer, was also convinced that commercial rather than sanitary considerations had influenced quarantine decisions in western Louisiana and probably in Texas.[24]

Continuing to support the legitimacy of local quarantine measures, the Baton Rouge *Advocate* denounced certain New Orleans firms for calling country people cowards if they refused to buy goods from the city. Early in the outbreak, Baton Rouge (with a population of about 10,000) had instituted rigid barriers against persons, baggage, and freight from all infected districts. Volunteer guards were posted on every road leading into town, at the ferry landing, the steamboat wharf, and the railroad depot. A few fever cases appeared late in October, but rigid isolation of the patients and all those exposed to them was immediately effected, and no serious epidemic materialized in the capital. House quarantine in Baton Rouge, as in New Orleans, provoked a "spirit of lawlessness and insubordination." Concealment of fever cases and resistance to guards were common responses to the policy.[25]

While such internal quarantine met with serious protest, quarantine barriers to protect towns against infection from the outside world were erected by popular demand. Even where local health officials initially opposed quarantining against New Orleans, public pressure was often such that the measures had to be instituted. For example, when news of the first New Orleans yellow fever cases reached Natchitoches in 1897, the town board of health wanted to postpone quarantine for a time, but the citizenry of that North Louisiana community, plagued by memories of 1853 and 1878, insisted that barriers be established immediately.[26] In Shreveport, mounted volunteers guarded all entrances to the city to enforce the quarantine declared by the local health board against New Orleans and all other infected places. Inspectors checked all incoming trains and steamboats and admitted only those passengers with proper health certificates from the state board or the Marine Hospital Service—when they admitted passengers at all. Quarantine arrangements were revised from time to time, but railroad traffic was generally disrupted until November.[27]

An editorial in the *Picayune* toward the end of September summed up the quarantine tangle and strongly condemned the

> ... wild and furious panic that has stopped the currents of trade, prevented the transit of passengers and the mails from one part of the Union to another, and has armed the population with deadly weapons and has set them at ferocious enmity against every man, woman, and child found outside their cordons of shotguns. . . . The entire country south of the Ohio River and the Kansas State line is dominated by madmen. They cannot be reasoned with, and there is no power on earth that can reduce them to any sense of order and common humanity. They must be left to recover from their insanity, which they will do in time.[28]

Some New Orleanians eventually began to blame the economic blockade on the detailed reporting by the city newspapers, even suggesting that business would have continued without interruption if only the journals had remained silent on the subject of yellow fever. The *Picayune* editor thought it incredible that anyone could entertain "such an erroneous and out-of-date notion in this age of telegraphing and eager search for and dissemination of news." Twenty years before, no federal health supervision had existed, "nor was the south gridironed with railways and spiderwebbed with telegraph wires as at present."[29] With the *New York Times* carrying full accounts of the various incidents of the epidemic one day after their occurrence, it is unlikely that the fever could have been concealed for long.

As weeks passed and local quarantines remained in force, the *Picayune* editor observed that the damage of the epidemic came not from the mild type of fever prevailing for the past two months, but from "the arbitrary and illegal stopping by wayside villagers of the United States mails, and the trains of great trunkline railways carrying interstate travel and commerce." Such action was clearly against the law, or so it seemed to the editor. While communities might forbid trains to unload passengers or goods in their own jurisdictions, they had absolutely no right to prevent trains from passing through to some point beyond.

Seeking a remedy, the New Orleans Board of Trade first asked the president of the United States and then the governor of Louisiana to employ force to break the quarantine blockades. Both replied that they lacked authority to use force for that purpose. The *Picayune* suggested that the first appeal should have been made to the United States courts for action against illegal obstruction to interstate commerce and the U. S. Mail. If court injunctions were disregarded by local quarantinists, then the power of the army could be used for enforcement. Reference was made to the Pullman Strike of 1894 when federal troops were sent to Chicago to enforce the court order that the strikers violated.[30] New Orleans commercial interests did not turn to the federal courts for remedy of their quarantine grievances, as the *Picayune* recommended. The disruption of trade by state and local quarantines, however, led many southern businessmen to the conclusion that federal control of interstate and maritime quarantine might be the proper solution, if not the only solution.

Cooperating with state authorities in seeking practical solutions to quarantine problems, the United State Marine Hospital Service established several detention camps in the vicinity of New Orleans. By early October, the camp at Fontainebleau across Lake Pontchartrain from New Orleans began to accept fifty persons a day, with the approval of the state board. In this manner, anyone wanting to leave the city could go to Fontainebleau, remain ten days, and if no illness developed, receive a health certificate from the Marine Hospital Service. The certificates eventually were found acceptable in Mississippi, Alabama, and Tennessee.[31]

To facilitate the transportation of skilled and unskilled laborers from New Orleans to the sugar plantations where seasonal workers were needed for harvesting and processing the cane, the Marine Hospital Service arranged for detention and certification at Camp Hutton in nearby Jefferson Parish. Many Italian laborers from New Orleans were accustomed to going to the cane fields each year to work during the harvest. Through the efforts of the federal health officers, workers with a clean bill of health began to set out by boat in October for plantations in Lafourche, Ascension, Iberville, Assumption, and West Baton Rouge parishes. As a Marine Hospital Service officer later reported, it was a remarkable achievement that no infection whatsoever was introduced by this supervised traffic, especially considering "that the sugar district on the Teche, Lafourche, Terrebonne, and the Mississippi River . . . [was] almost a continuous town, some plantations having from 800 to 1200 people on them." Had this detention service not been provided, ways undoubtedly would have been found to smuggle in workers to the sugar parishes, despite the risk. Such was the planters' need for labor and the workers' need for employment.[32]

Lack of employment became a serious problem among the working people of New Orleans during the two or three months of "overpowering disturbance to all local industries and the complete paralysis of business." The mayor, a major contractor, and a railroad representative made large contributions to start a fund that the city could use to hire the unemployed for street repair work. Wages were set at one dollar per day to spread the "charity funds subscribed by public-spirited and philanthropic citizens" among as many laborers as possible. An editorial in the *Picayune* titled "Unworthy Spurners of Charity" denounced as an "unmitigated outrage" a strike by some of the workers who demanded more pay and tried to stop others from working for the amount offered. The *Picayune* self-righteously proclaimed: "No man is compelled to work at any price, if he should choose not to do so; but such people ought to be known, so that they shall not be permitted to enjoy free benefits that are intended only for those who are worthy." The New Orleans Charity Organization Society collected and distributed funds and supplies for "the relief of the needy" until the epidemic ended and work became available with the resumption of trade and other economic activities.[33]

Quarantine restrictions gradually loosened toward the end of October. Grain, sugar, and cotton crops flowed into New Orleans, and it became possible to ship certain kinds of merchandise from the city to a number of places in Louisiana, but not before another "outrage" occurred. A bridge on the Southern Pacific Railroad line east of Lake Charles burned one night shortly after an assembly of citizens in Calcasieu Parish had resolved that Southern Pacific trains would not be allowed under any circumstances to enter the parish—"a significant coincidence," according to the *Picayune*.[34]

The Louisiana State Board of Health declared all danger of infection over on November 12 and removed the fever flags and house guards in New Orleans, setting an example for other areas to follow. On November 15 a newspaper headline read, "Quarantines Still Tumbling." Texas had removed all restrictions, and various points in Louisiana gradually followed suit. Mail disinfection was discontinued by mid-November, and the Marine Hospital Service made plans for terminating its inspection and freight fumigation service. As late as November 24, when the federal agency finally ended its work, several parishes still maintained quarantines against the railroad lines, but these too were soon ended.[35]

The officers of the U. S. Marine Hospital Service performed many valuable services for Louisiana and other states, especially for the transportation and commercial interests of the region and for the Louisiana sugar industry and its employees. The federal health officers won for themselves much popular confidence and respect in so doing.[36] In contrast, the state board, despite its best efforts, became a handy scapegoat after all the frustrations, irritations, and commercial losses resulting from the epidemic. In November the board came under heavy criticism, especially from the New Orleans commercial exchanges and the newspapers, for having failed to prevent the epidemic in the first place, and for policies that were as ineffective as they were unpopular. In early December five members of the board, including President Olliphant, resigned as a group, and the other members followed shortly thereafter. They acknowledged no fault and no misconduct in carrying out their responsibilities but decided to resign to save the governor from any embarrassment. They felt that the intense criticism from some New Orleans interest groups, although entirely unwarranted, undermined respect for the Louisiana State Board of Health. Without a change in personnel its effectiveness might be impaired in the vitally important relations with other states.[37]

Extent of the Epidemic

The pestilence of 1897 appeared in forty-one different places throughout the South, but caused only 454 deaths, a relatively slight mortality for such a widespread outbreak. New Orleans reported 1,908 cases with 298 fatalities, almost three-fourths of the total yellow fever mortality from all states. Although a few cases appeared in Baton Rouge, Clinton, Franklin, and Patterson, Louisiana, only about ten deaths occurred in the entire state outside of New Orleans. The disease had spread to almost every town along the Gulf Coast between New Orleans and Mobile; cases in Louisiana, Mississippi, and Alabama accounted for approximately 98 percent of the total number reported from the nine states where yellow fever occurred.[38]

Compared to other nineteenth-century yellow fever epidemics, this one was remarkably tame, yet the very presence of the disease in New Orleans and other coastal towns caused great alarm throughout the hinterlands. Even in New Orleans, greater fear than usual found expression—to whatever extent the crowd incidents represent fear rather than anger and other frustrations. Almost two decades had passed without the disease, and perhaps as it became a less familiar foe, it also became a more dreaded one. The opposition to quarantine flags and house isolation, however, as well as the concealment of cases to avoid the health regulations, suggest a greater dread of official measures than of the disease itself.

However New Orleanians actually felt about the disease, other parts of the state and country were clearly terrified. Small towns along the railroad lines tried to protect themselves by isolation. Total exclusion of persons and merchandise from the outside might not have been necessary; but, if absolute, it would have been effective. Absolute enforcement, however, was almost impossible to achieve. As an officer of the Marine Hospital Service commented about the unnecessarily harsh restrictions, "their very stringency well-nigh compelled their violation."[39]

An elderly physician of New Orleans, Dr. Just Touatre, called attention to another unusual feature of the 1897 epidemic—aside from the extraordinary panic it engendered. "For the first time in the history of yellow fever," he said, "it came, this year, via the railroad."[40] Always before the disease had entered New Orleans by way of the river. While the Louisiana State Board of Health maintained a close watch at the Mississippi River quarantine below New Orleans and at other south Louisiana entrances, the fever of 1897 made a landing somewhere on the gulf coast and came into New Orleans from Ocean Springs, Mississippi, by railroad. Several loopholes existed through which the fever could have entered North American territory. One possibility was the Ship Island quarantine station off the Mississippi coast which small boats from Cuba sometimes evaded; another was Mobile's lax quarantine system, allegedly so designed to attract Central and South American trade away from the port of New Orleans. Dr. Quitman Kohnke of the New Orleans health board later suggested that the disease could have entered the city in 1897 via the banana boats from Central America, which were neither detained nor fumigated.[41]

1898 and 1899

The following year, the first outbreak of yellow fever in the South was reported in Mississippi in June. States established quarantines and the Marine Hospital Service began to supervise the detention and certification of passengers and the fumigation of freight. In August a yellow fever death occurred in Franklin, Louisiana, a month before the first case was reported in New Orleans. The entire parish of St. Mary was quarantined along with

Franklin, and for a time it seemed that no epidemic would develop there, as only one other case appeared within the next few weeks. By late September the disease was raging, and according to a later estimate by the parish health officer, at least 1,250 cases and 11 deaths had occurred. State board figures were more conservative, showing only 607 cases for Franklin.[42]

When the first case was reported in New Orleans in mid-September, 1898, the Louisiana State Board of Health promptly telegraphed that information to the boards of neighboring states and to the U. S. Marine Hospital Service. Many quarantines were again declared against the Crescent City. Freight traffic was not entirely suspended because some areas had adopted the regulations agreed to earlier that year by an interstate convention of health officials meeting in Atlanta. In its mild, clinically undiagnosable form, or in "suspicious cases" which physicians simply failed to report, or in cases not seen by a physician at all, yellow fever had probably been present in New Orleans for weeks before the first official case. By the end of the outbreak, the state board had recorded for New Orleans a total of 118 cases. More than 1,000 cases were reported elsewhere; in addition to the Franklin epidemic, the disease appeared but caused few fatalities in Houma, Baton Rouge, Wilson, Clinton, Plaquemine, Lutcher, Jackson, Alexandria, Bowie, Lake Charles, Slaughter, Morrow, and other points mainly in South Louisiana.[43]

Contemporaries considered the yellow fever of 1898 extremely mild because the total mortality was so low considering the number of different towns affected. With fifty-seven deaths among only 118 reported cases, however, New Orleans' official case fatality rate was almost 50 percent, which is extremely high and almost certainly inaccurate. As usual, many additional unrecognized and unreported cases undoubtedly occurred. State board president Edmond Souchon noted that the case fatality rate outside New Orleans was only 4 or 5 percent; therefore, something was amiss with case reporting in New Orleans.[44]

In 1899 yellow fever again slipped through the state's protective barriers. Maritime quarantine had been increasingly liberalized in the 1890s to accommodate the Central American fruit trade and shipping from Havana and other Caribbean ports where the state board had stationed its own medical inspectors. Special consideration was also given to vessels from those Latin American ports where Marine Hospital Service officers were present to provide prompt and reliable notification of prevailing diseases and other on-site inspection, disinfection, and certification services.[45] Louisiana's health officials justified the revised regulations as perfectly rational and scientifically sound. The problem was that such practices did not always suffice as a shield against yellow fever.

The outbreak of 1899 caused only eighty-one reported cases in New Orleans with twenty-three deaths. Plaquemines and St. Charles parishes and Baton Rouge also had a few cases, but only one death occurred in the state outside the Crescent City. Again the familiar quarantines were declared against New Orleans, both inside and outside the state, but freight shipments, for the most part, continued under the Atlanta Regulations of 1898. Northern and central Louisiana quarantined against New Orleans, but most southern and eastern parishes manifested confidence in the state board's inspection arrangements and made no effort to impose restrictions of their own.[46]

Comparing Epidemics

The first half of the nineteenth century witnessed a steady increase in the frequency and virulence of yellow fever in New Orleans; the 1850s, a climax of epidemic activity. In the last forty years of the century, the scourge struck less frequently, and with two notable exceptions (1867 and 1878), with less virulence. Yellow fever's decline was already under way for some time before the discovery of the mosquito vector. Public health measures against the fever in the nineteenth century, no matter how rational or scientific they seemed to contemporaries, were in reality little more than a shot in the dark, which could not have consistently hit an unknown, unseen mark.

Nevertheless, the decline of the pestilence coincided with increasingly positive action by Louisiana health authorities: sanitation, disinfection, fumigation, detention, and a modified port quarantine program known as "Maritime Sanitation." The conclusion that such official measures had reduced the incidence and the intensity of yellow fever won support for even more comprehensive health measures and generally resulted in a more favorable public view of public health regulations.[47] Although a considerable amount of opposition and skepticism persisted, "experts" using "modern" methods of "scientific" sanitation were steadily gaining ground and receiving good press coverage. *Expert, modern*, and *scientific* were becoming the magic words of the day, heavy-laden with positive value.

For whatever reasons, by the 1890s yellow fever did exhibit in New Orleans a less virulent character than in previous years.[48] Alcée Fortier, writing his history of Louisiana in 1903, dismissed the visitation of 1897 with this brief comment: "There was an epidemic, called by some yellow fever, in New Orleans in 1897; but the fever was so mild and the mortalities so few that the disease was known by the name of 'yellowoid'." Fortier was recalling the outbreak of 1898 (not 1897) when Dr. Souchon, state board president, had attempted to rename yellow fever and consider it non-quarantinable. Souchon argued that the disease affecting Louisiana in 1897 and 1898 was a pale reflection of the scourge of the past and that "scientific sanitation" should be substituted for quarantine barriers. The Mississippi State Board of Health denounced his proposal and declared the label "yellowoid" unscientific, deceptive, and dangerous.[49] Despite Fortier's broad assertion, Souchon seems to have won little support for his awkward tongue-twisiting new label (except perhaps among French creole friends such as Fortier). Many New Orleanians, however, certainly agreed that the current form of yellow fever was a much diminished version of the old scourge of the city.

Dr. Felix Formento, for example, board of health member who had opposed the house quarantine policy, later remarked that the panic of 1897 had been completely ridiculous and unnecessary as yellow fever had lost much of its strength since 1853. He considered it the duty of physicians to inform the public that the disease was no longer so much to be feared. To support his point, Formento even supplied some figures—of uncertain provenance and dubious validity for they bear little resemblance to any rates that can be calculated from the extant records (which are also questionable) or from other available estimates. The "death rate" (meaning case fatality rate) in 1853, he said, was about three out of four; in 1897, one in two hundred. Although his estimates were too high for 1853 and too low for 1897, Formento was nonetheless correct in tracking the decline in virulence.[50]

Dr. Henry R. Carter, U. S. Marine Hospital Service, believed the fever of 1897 not quite so mild as some would have it. From his own observations, he concluded that the rate in 1897 was probably about 7 percent, or one death in fourteen cases—less than half the official rate, but much higher than Formento's one in two hundred. Carter said he had been told by several older New Orleans physicians that the fever of 1897 was similar in many respects to that of 1867, including the low case fatality rate.[51]

Against a background of previous epidemic experiences, physicians tended to notice similarities and differences in the disease process exhibited in cases they treated and to compare epidemics on that basis. They were acutely aware of recoveries and deaths among their own patients; that is, they were highly sensitive to comparative case fatality rates. Accepting a comparable degree of virulence in 1867 and in 1897, one is nevertheless struck by other aspects of the two epidemics in which the statistical differences seem more significant than the similar measure of virulence. In 1867, within a population of 185,000, at least 3,200 deaths occurred among an estimated 41,500 cases of yellow fever; more than a fifth of the city's population came down with the disease during the epidemic. In 1897, within a population of 260,000, only 298 yellow fever deaths and fewer than 2,000 cases were reported.[52] Yellow fever deaths per thousand population in New Orleans amounted to almost 18 in 1867 and 1.2 in 1897.

One begins to see that epidemics can be experienced directly or perceived at a distance in a great variety of ways, influenced by background, expectation, and location in society, and not simply by objective measures of relative severity. Epidemics present different facets to different observers, and much depends on which features are examined and for what purposes compared. Inasmuch as epidemic means unusual or extraordinary prevalence of a particular disease, the standard for measurement itself is based on what is considered "normal" or "ordinary," and varies from time to time and place to place. During the first half of the nineteenth century, yellow fever in New Orleans became a common cause of death. Major outbreaks raged often enough that the "normal" or expected situation included periodic epidemics killing several thousand persons in a few months, perhaps 5 to 10 percent of the population. When only four or five hundred died in a summer, yellow fever was not even considered epidemic, and judging from what had been viewed as normal in New Orleans, such numbers could not be considered "excessive prevalence."[53]

As decades passed after the Civil War with only two episodes remotely comparable with antebellum levels of severity, and after 1878 when years passed with no yellow fever at all, the standard changed. When yellow fever again appeared, the number of cases, no matter how small, was in excess of what had come to be normal—that is, none. With an expectation of the worst, based on the last bad experience in 1878, it is not surprising that many persons, especially those outside New Orleans, overreacted to the "mild" fever of 1897. An epidemic cannot be seen as mild until it is over; and "mild" in New Orleans did not always mean "mild" in small towns when the disease spread, as some villagers knew from bitter experience.

Table 7.

COMPARING NEW ORLEANS EPIDEMICS

YEAR	POPULATION (estimated)	CASES	DEATHS	YELLOW FEVER DEATHS PER 1000 POPULATION	CASE FATALITY RATE
1853	154,000	29,000	8,100	53	28%
1867	185,000	41,500	3,320	18	8%
1878	211,000	27,000	4,046	19	15%
1897	260,000	1,900	298	1.2	16% (est.7%)

Based on a variety of sources and should be considered approximations only, especially the case numbers.

Perhaps yellow fever was an insignificant disease to sophisticated city-dwellers who took a long-range view from their own experience or through knowledge of the city's history. In comparing 1897 to the 1850s rather than the 1880s they saw that the pestilence had lost most of its force. On the other hand, thousands of persons in small towns and the countryside, were tied now to the city more than ever by both rail and water transportation. They were also more frightened than ever by the prospect of having the mysterious, invisible yellow fever "germs" introduced to their communities by the very rail lines that were pulling them out of a relatively "safe" isolation and linking them into an increasingly interdependent network. Within this system they had little influence or control, and they were subject to all the ills as well as the benefits of the wider world.

Rural-Urban, Traditional-Modern in Conflict

Some elements and episodes of the "panic of 1897" may be illuminated by considering the conflicting behaviors as expressions of antagonistic sets of values: *urban* versus *rural* ways of life and views of the world. New Orleans journalists routinely referred to all of Louisiana beyond the city limits as "the country."[54] In describing and usually denouncing the interior quarantine restrictions in 1897, New Orleans newspapers condescendingly and angrily referred to the "wayside villagers" or the scared "country folk" in the "pettiest village and hamlet" who had the audacity to interfere with the U. S. Mail and interstate trade. The country folk were termed cowards. They were called stupid, backward, and irrational by the New Orleans press. Reports in the *New York Times* used similar labels.

Small town newspapers in Louisiana and neighboring states expressed little or no trust in reports from New Orleans journals, nor in the Louisiana State Board of Health itself, which was located in and identified with the city (and indeed until the 1898 reorganization the board was composed entirely of New Orleanians). From experience, the "villagers" of the interior expected the city press and the state board of health to report news and make policy in ways that best served New Orleans commercial interests, even at great risk to the health of the city and the rest of the state. And their perceptions were not altogether without factual basis. But the urban interests would have answered that there is always an element of risk to be balanced against other important considerations such as costs and profits and jobs.

Paralleling the urban-rural conflict were other fundamental differences sometimes described as "modern versus traditional": advocacy of centralized control versus local power; support for formal rules and regulations administered by bureaus or agencies (sometimes by *uniformed* personnel) as opposed to the informal spontaneous action of the armed posse, the small town volunteers enforcing shotgun quarantines. Even within the city of New Orleans, some urban dwellers remained more traditional than modern, as evidenced by the crowds that gathered, more or less spontaneously, to protest certain official decisions, and by the individual and group defiance of rules and regulations, policies and procedures.

Within the broader setting, the rural population defended traditional values. Within cities, the working-class population, including many of rural origin and enclaves of the foreign-born, sometimes resisted modern "reforms" that seemed to threaten their customary interests and old ways of doing things. Large-scale immigration from southern and eastern European villages in the late nineteenth and early twentieth centuries provided recurring infusions of traditionalism into the American urban scene where professionals of all kinds were attempting to rationalize and organize a modern social order. Conflict was inevitable.[55]

The southern Italians, including many from Sicily, constituted the largest immigrant group in Louisiana in the 1890s and early 1900s. These newcomers contributed reinforcements for traditional values and village or neighborhood identification even as they resisted large-system approaches. Defining as family affairs matters that some urban Americans had come to consider questions of public justice and public health, Italians tended to seek private revenge for insult or injury and generally refused to report cases of infectious disease to the authorities. Critical observers characterized them as clannish, secretive, and violence-prone.[56] These characteristics were certainly not unique to Italians; many Louisiana villagers, within the urban or rural setting, of whatever ethnic variety, could have been described in much the same way.[57] But such characteristics, in Italians or in others, were at odds with the "modern" world-view and the drive for an efficient, disciplined, regularized social order. Thus, many of the conflicts that occurred in New Orleans as well as throughout the state and region during the epidemic of 1897 (and to some extent in 1905) reflect the classic division between "traditional" and "modern" social forms; divergent sets of behaviors and values clashed as the new was imposed upon the old.

Despite the reappearance of yellow fever in 1898 and 1899, the people of Louisiana and other southern states did not re-enact the "panic of 1897," perhaps because the fever that year had not fulfilled their frightful expectations based on the 1878 experience. Furthermore, the regulations devised by experts for inspection and fumigation of freight and the detention and certification of travelers had *seemed* to be effective in limiting the spread of the fever. Even though the health authorities had not been able to prevent its entry to New Orleans, the old scourge now appeared to be a manageable disease. Some measure of hostility and conflict would surface again during the last yellow fever epidemic in 1905, but by that time, the experts—scientists and administrators—were more fully in charge. On that occasion, from the viewpoint of the health officials, Louisiana's Italian population posed the chief remaining obstacle to modernity.

Table 8.

YELLOW FEVER MORTALITY IN NEW ORLEANS
1867-1905

Year	Number of Deaths**	Population (Approx.)
*1867	3,320	181,000
1868	3	
1869	3	
1870	587	192,000
1871	54	
1872	39	
1873	226	199,000
1874	11	
1875	61	
1876	42	
1877	1	
*1878	4,046	211,000
1879	19	
1880	2	
1881	0	
1882	4	
1883	1	
1884	1	
1885	1	
1886	0	
1887	0	
1888	0	
1889	1	
1890	0	
1891	0	
1892	0	
1893	0	
1894	0	
1895	0	
1896	0	
*1897	298	285,000
1898	57	
1899	23	
1900	0	
1901	0	
1902	0	
1903	0	
1904	0	
*1905	452	333,000

*Major epidemics.

**From Louisiana State Board of Health figures.

Table 9.

YELLOW FEVER IN LOUISIANA OUTSIDE OF NEW ORLEANS 1867-1898

	1867	1873	1878	1897	1898
Alexandria	X				X
Baton Rouge			X	X	X
Coushatta		X			
Delhi			X		
Delta			X		
Donaldsonville			X		
East Feliciana Parish			X	X	X
Greenwood		X			
Gretna			X		
Hammond			X		
Houma					X
Jackson					X
Jeanerette	X				
Labadieville			X		
Lafayette	X				
Lake Charles	X				X
Lake Providence			X		
Mansfield		X			
Napoleonville			X		
New Iberia	X				
Opelousas	X				
Paincourtville			X		
Plaquemine	X		X		X
Plaquemines Parish			X		
Ponchatoula			X		
Port Hudson			X		
St. Bernard Parish			X		
St. Charles Parish					X
St. James Parish					X
St. John the Baptist Parish			X		
St. Martinville	X				
St. Mary Parish	X		X	X	X
Shreveport	X	X			
Tangipahoa			X		
Thibodaux			X		
Washington	X				
West Feliciana Parish			X		
Wilson					X

IX

THE LAST EPIDEMIC, 1905

The epidemic of 1905 was not only Louisiana's final bout with the pestilence but also the last yellow fever epidemic in the United States. By this time health officials had a significant advantage over their predecessors in confronting epidemic yellow fever: the puzzle of its transmission had finally been solved. After a number of inconclusive scientific investigations sponsored by the federal government during the last few decades of the nineteenth century, positive results were finally achieved at the beginning of the new century.

The Spanish-American War in 1898 and the subsequent military occupation of Cuba brought the American forces in contact with yellow fever in its own territory where it had been endemic for many years. In 1900 a commission of United States Army surgeons headed by Dr. Walter Reed went to Cuba on a special assignment to study yellow fever. Reed and his associates—James Carroll, Jesse W. Lazear, and Aristides Agramonte—followed the direction suggested long before by Dr. Carlos Finlay of Havana. Using the *Aedes aegypti* mosquitoes that Finlay made available to them and recruiting volunteers for experiment, they successfully demonstrated the role of the mosquito in the transmission of yellow fever. In October of 1900 the commission made a tentative announcement of its findings, and after further experimentation issued a full report in the spring of 1901, stating that the disease was transmitted by the *Aedes aegypti* mosquito and only in that manner.[1]

One might have expected that the announcement of this significant discovery would have stimulated the people of New Orleans and other localities with a history of yellow fever to embark immediately on an anti-mosquito crusade. Such was not the case. Many refused to believe that the small, familiar pest, although offensive and annoying, could actually be the agent of the dreaded disease. Too many theories had come and gone without result, and faith in the "scientific method" was not yet the popular religion it was soon to become. Even the medical profession was divided; many who accepted the explanation did so with reservations. The editor of the *New Orleans Medical and Surgical Journal* thought it too soon to consider the mosquito the *only* means of yellow fever transmission, although he did believe in the "urgent necessity" for eradicating the culprit, and he recommended a public campaign toward that end.[2]

In its report for 1900-1901 the Louisiana State Board of Health discussed the conclusions of the Reed Commission and acknowledged the mosquito as one factor in the conveyance of yellow fever. Nevertheless, "we Southern Health Officers, charged with the grave duty of protecting our people against this most dreaded of all diseases, are unwilling to accept the dictum of the experimenters that yellow fever can be conveyed by no other agency." They were not prepared to give up the theory of the fever's spread by fomites—substances capable of absorbing germs, such as woolen fabrics or articles of clothing.[3]

In contrast, the New Orleans City Board of Health (created in 1898) and the Orleans Parish Medical Society exhibited great interest in the mosquito theory. Shortly after the announcement of the Reed Commission, both groups made plans to investigate local breeding places of the *Aedes aegypti* as the first step toward its ultimate eradication. Dr. Quitman Kohnke, chairman of the city health board, was so impressed by the results of William Gorgas' anti-mosquito campaign in Havana that he tried to promote a similar movement in New Orleans as early as July, 1901. Circulars were widely distributed giving information on combating the *Aedes aegypti*. Through public lectures and conferences Kohnke hoped to educate householders on the life cycle and habits of the yellow fever mosquito and its favorite breeding place in New Orleans: the ubiquitous cisterns which caught rainwater from the rooftops and served as open storage tanks for household water supply.

Dr. Kohnke explained that pouring a small amount of kerosene on the water's surface where the mosquitoes deposited their eggs would destroy the developing eggs and larvae without any effect on the water because the oil would simply float on the surface. The water was drawn through a spigot near the bottom of the cisterns. Kohnke also urged that cisterns be covered with wire screening fine enough to keep out mosquitoes. In August the city health board undertook an experiment in a selected locality with the intention of visiting every house and oiling every cistern in the area. Many householders refused to participate in the program. Others allowed the oiling process once, but refused a second application, insisting that they could taste and smell kerosene in their drinking water. Hence, what was designed as a demonstration that might be repeated throughout the city failed completely. Faced with apathy and opposition, and convinced that the program could never be effected without special supporting law, Dr. Kohnke attempted repeatedly to secure an ordinance on the subject, but to no avail.[4]

Between the summer of 1901 and the summer of 1905, the *New Orleans Medical and Surgical Journal*, the newspapers, the state board of health, the city board, and the Orleans Parish Medical Association continued to recommend the screening and oiling of cisterns. Because of ignorance, indifference, or skepticism, New Orleanians failed to arouse themselves to the task. There seemed to be no compelling need; not a single yellow fever death occurred in the Crescent City in the years 1900 through 1904.[5] In the absence of the disease, few could become disturbed about a distant threat. The challenge was not met until it occurred in the form of an epidemic; only then could the health authorities stir the public to action.

In 1905 the New Orleans population numbered about 325,000 with probably less than a fourth immune to yellow fever by previous attack, according to an estimate by Dr. Rudolph Matas. Many more Italian immigrants had arrived since 1900, crowding into the old quarter near the river front. Very few houses in the city had screened windows, and most people depended on cisterns or open rain barrels for their water supply, ideal breeding grounds for a large population of *Aedes aegypti*. According to a later reconstruction of events, yellow fever apparently slipped past the quarantine station on the river below New Orleans sometime in May of 1905, escaping detection by the inspectors, carried in by an infected passenger or an infected mosquito. The state board suggested that an inapparent case from Belize or Puerto Cortez probably entered New Orleans before quarantine was established in late May against Central American fruit ports where yellow fever had been reported by the U. S. Public Health and Marine Hospital Service.[6]

Once in New Orleans, the disease spread first among the Italians living in boarding houses near the French Market, many of them employed in unloading banana cargoes from Central American shipping. Strangers in New Orleans, they were poor, unfamiliar with both yellow fever and the English language, suspicious of outsiders, and reluctant to call in medical aid. Not until July 12 did the developing epidemic come to the attention of the state and city health authorities when two "suspicious" fatalities were reported by physicians; in neither case would the families permit an autopsy. When two more suspicious cases were reported, Dr. Souchon, state board president, examined them on July 14 and found symptoms suggesting yellow fever but inconclusive. The next day he called a meeting of the board which decided that more proof was needed before making any public announcement. None of the attending physicians had been willing to state that the cases they reported were anything more than "suspicious." No one, not even the health officials, seemed willing to declare the presence of yellow fever as long as there was any chance it might be otherwise.[7]

Meanwhile, with the support of the state board, city health officials began an investigation of the district where the cases had appeared. Finding evidence of other previous suspicious cases, they proceeded to fumigate every house within several blocks for the next ten days, treating the Decatur Street area *as if it were infected* with yellow fever. Health workers with their strange anti-mosquito fumigating tactics encountered hostility and opposition from the neighborhood, but used whatever means proved necessary—in Dr. Kohnke's words, "from soft persuasion to brutal force"—to carry out their work.[8]

Dr. Souchon saw two more cases that concerned him on July 18 and called a board meeting for the following day. Finally the board agreed that the federal health service and the state health officers of Mississippi, Alabama, and Texas should be notified that some cases of disease in New Orleans were "presenting symptoms of yellow fever." Surgeon A. C. Smith, Public Health and Marine Hospital Service officer in New Orleans, had already wired the surgeon-general in Washington on July 18 that yellow fever rumors were circulating but he could get no information from the state board. After two more telegrams from Smith and a letter from Souchon on July 21, the surgeon-general sent Surgeon Joseph H. White from Mobile to New Orleans to investigate. Not until July 22 did an autopsy provide positive confirmation of yellow fever's presence in the city, and not until then did the state board issue an official public announcement. By that time, it was estimated that at least 100 cases and 20 deaths had already

Street to Barracks and from Rampart to the river. As critics later pointed out, much valuable time had been wasted while the board waited for absolute proof through autopsy. During that time, many Italians and others from the infected district had moved to various parts of the city and state, and to other states, some carrying the virus with them.[9]

Organizing the Yellow Fever Crusade: State and Local Efforts

On July 21, the day before the official acknowledgment of the fever, representatives of the local medical society, the federal health service, state and city health boards, and health officials from neighboring states, who had come to investigate, gathered in New Orleans to discuss the coming crisis that most of them anticipated. After the positive diagnosis and official recognition on July 22, the Orleans Parish Medical Society established a special committee to offer assistance to the health officials. The same day, Mayor Martin Behrman met with the presidents of the state and city health boards and several prominent citizens to make plans for an anti-fever campaign and the fund-raising to support it. The Citizens Finance Committee was established shortly thereafter under the leadership of Charles Janvier, president of the Canal-Louisiana Bank.[10]

New Orleans newspapers on July 23 published an address to the citizens signed by Dr. Kohnke and by Dr. Joseph H. White of the U. S. Public Health and Marine Hospital Service. The message proclaimed an emergency "which demands the attention of every individual, with the view to limiting and preventing the spread of epidemic disease." Since the mosquito had been "scientifically proved" to be the *only* means of yellow fever transmission, the authorities strongly recommended screening and oiling all cisterns, emptying all receptacles of stagnant water, oiling cesspools and privy vaults, sleeping under mosquito nets, and screening doors and windows. Following tradition, the *Picayune* initially minimized the extent of the outbreak, referring to the "limited area" of infection in "a section of the city occupied almost exclusively by a foreign population," and expressing confidence that the official measures then under way would quickly succeed in suppressing the disease altogether.[11]

In the days to come, as yellow fever spread and the anti-mosquito crusade went into high gear, the *Picayune* and other journals participated fully in reporting the scope of the disease and promoting the general campaign against it. No further efforts were made to deny or diminish the seriousness of the epidemic. No longer was there a need for the old false gaiety to cover the gloom and despair of past epidemic reporting; there was now an exciting campaign to emphasize and a new method available to limit the current outbreak and end the threat of Yellow Jack in the future. Accordingly, the press propagandized for "Science" and "Expert Management" which could remove all cause for "unreasoning" panic and "unscientific" quarantines against the city. An optimistic tone prevailed throughout: scientific knowledge brought power, and through systematic administration such power could be utilized to overcome the pestilence at last.

On Sunday, July 23, the Reverend Dr. Beverley Warner, rector of Trinity Episcopal Church, preached the anti-mosquito crusade from his pulpit. In the coming weeks clergymen of all denominations followed his example. On July 24 citizens of the Fourteenth Ward organized to clean all streets, yards, and gutters in the area, and to have every cistern screened. More than a hundred citizens attended the organizational meeting and made liberal financial contributions to fund the program. They divided into committees and planned to begin work the next day. As other wards proceeded to organize work forces, the city health board established a central headquarters for volunteer groups and appointed the Reverend Dr. Warner as chairman. His task was to coordinate activities in the city's seventeen wards and report to the health board, thereby eliminating duplication of work. The city board of health also established an advisory committee, composed of two board members, two representatives from the Orleans Parish Medical Society, and two from New Orleans commercial interests. Dr. Kohnke chaired the committee which met every day and directed the educational campaign against the "cistern mosquito."[12]

By Wednesday, July 26, campaign procedures were developing all over the city. The New Orleans Board of Health established a sanitary force of 100 men, organized in district divisions and gangs of five, to locate fever cases, fumigate and screen infected premises, and deal with each new focus of disease as it developed. Another force of 250 men was divided into ward squads and precinct groups and instructed to make systematic war on the mosquito. The mayor employed 100 extra workers to clean and flush out the city gutters. Not since General Butler's efforts during federal occupation, wrote a *New York Times* reporter, had New Orleans been subjected to such a thorough cleansing.[13]

The officers of the various Italian organizations in New Orleans assembled and appointed special committees to make door-to-door visits among Italians and urge them to report all cases of disease and to comply with official measures. An emergency hospital that could accommodate eighty patients was established by the city board in an old house on Dumaine Street in the infected district. It opened on July 26 and received its first patients. Under the supervision of Dr. Hamilton Jones, who had also directed the city's yellow fever hospital in 1897, every precaution was taken to keep mosquitoes away from the patients. A Catholic priest, the Reverend Paroli, assisted in persuading some of his Italian compatriots to allow the removal of the sick to the hospital.[14]

Within less than a week after the first public notice of yellow fever's existence in the city, systematic measures had been instituted by officials and volunteers for a war of extermination against the disease-bearing *Aedes aegypti*. The machinery of organization would fail in its mission, however, unless supported by public understanding and enthusiastic cooperation. To mobilize the populace, an educational campaign was a vital necessity. The New Orleans press published notices and circulars, described the activities of officials and ward committees, and provided editorial propaganda. The *Picayune* editor assured the people of New Orleans that yellow fever could be transmitted only by the mosquito. "Science has discovered its cause," he proclaimed, "and science has learned to deal with and to exterminate the cause." Day after day New Orleanians were urged to oil and screen cisterns, to sleep under mosquito nets, and to keep up the good fight against the scourge, which no longer was "the vague terror, borne on the hot winds in waves or disseminated in unknown and mysterious fashion." Federal health officers in New Orleans, observing that the "mosquito doctrine" was not "popularly accepted, nor even accepted in some instances by those in authority," prepared a circular entitled "How to prevent yellow fever—No mosquitoes, no yellow fever." One hundred thousand copies were published in late July for distribution in Louisiana and Mississippi, designed to disseminate information rapidly and "in as authoritative a manner as possible."[15]

Throughout the epidemic the Orleans Parish Medical Society issued circulars and pamphlets and tried to impress on physicians the absolute necessity of reporting immediately every case of fever, even the doubtful ones. Dr. Rudolph Matas prepared pamphlets containing instructions and advice to physicians and nurses. These booklets were distributed by the medical society and paid for by the United States Treasury Department after federal officials took charge of the campaign. Prominent physicians gave lectures on the mosquito doctrine throughout the city and in other parts of the state as well. According to Dr. Louis G. LeBeuf, Orleans Parish Medical Society president, the profession had never been so united as in the great work of propagating "the new belief." The mosquito gospel included three specific principles that "had to be taught," he said, "and practiced as the very catechism and Bible of our entire conduct": (1) the *stegomyia* mosquito (as the *Aedes aegypti* was then called) is the only means of yellow fever transmission; (2) as the mosquitoes can obtain the infection only when biting a fever patient within the first three days of illness, immediate action to isolate patients in screened rooms is imperative; and (3) as mosquitoes are unable to transmit the infection for ten or twelve days after acquiring it, there is ample time to destroy those in the infected household before their bite becomes dangerous.[16]

Almost every night during the epidemic someone lectured somewhere in New Orleans on the yellow fever mosquito. Night after night Dr. Kohnke addressed various groups, describing the life cycle of the mosquito with the aid of lantern slides, recommending that cisterns be oiled to kill the "wiggle-tails" and to keep mosquitoes from depositing more eggs on the water. Kohnke assured the people that oil could not hurt their drinking water. He also recommended sulphur fumigation of every house. Thousands of New Orleanians heard these lectures, and many were converted and enrolled in the campaign. The volunteer ward organizations issued notices, set up posters in prominent places, and sponsored educational mass meetings to inform people that extinction of mosquitoes meant freedom from yellow fever in the future. While supervising the ward committees and preparing daily reports of their work, Dr. Warner lectured almost nightly at public meetings. In a circular letter he also made a special appeal to the clergy of all denominations to promote the crusade against the mosquito.[17]

Warner and Kohnke both were instrumental in mobilizing New Orleans' black population to aid in the great war on yellow fever. In late July Dr. Warner addressed a gathering of "the leading colored men of the city" and explained that yellow fever was no longer the "bugbear it had been in former years." With reference to the traditional belief in black immunity, he expressed his opinion that if an infected mosquito should sting "a colored man" the disease would be transmitted "just the same as though a white man had been stung." The prominent black leaders present at that first meeting, including doctors, lawyers, and ministers, organized the Central Sanitary Association and made plans to establish branches among their people in the various wards of the city.[18] In mid-August, during a mass meeting of blacks at the Second Baptist Church, Professor J. L. Jones of the Central Sanitary Association appealed to the congregation: "Suppose we were immune, all persons are not, and we must help them. We are a part of the community, and our prosperity depends upon their prosperity. . . . Let's help them kill this stegomyia."[19]

Another large African-American assembly met in the First Street A. M. E. Church on the night of August 22 to hear short lectures by several black ministers as well as speeches by Dr. Kohnke and a member of the (white) Woman's League of New Orleans. A number of Woman's League members attended that meeting, and many other whites were scattered throughout the audience. Dr. Kohnke encouraged his audience to organize and assist in the crusade. "There is no difference between white and black," he said. "We live the same way, we get sick the same way, we get well the same way, we die the same way." Emphasizing the equality theme, he continued, "There is no distinction of color with the stegomyia mosquito. He is just as ready to bite you as he is to bite me. If it is an infected stegomyia, you will have yellow fever just as certainly as the white man does." Hence, it was necessary to follow the same precautionary measures. Dr. Kohnke then gave his usual lecture on the life cycle of the mosquito with stereopticon illustrations. When the black minister dismissed the meeting, he urged all persons to go forth and fumigate their houses and oil and screen their cisterns.[20] Even if the *stegomyia* did not recognize the color line, as Dr. Kohnke stated, obviously the white leaders of New Orleans did, for the black citizens were not invited to join the ward organizations but were encouraged to form separate associations instead.

Another segment of the New Orleans population, middle-class white women, worked actively with the health authorities and ward organizations although organized in their own separate groups. The Home and Education Department of the Woman's League, chaired by Mrs. W. J. Behan, sponsored numerous lectures in public meeting places throughout the city. These civic-minded women established ward clubs and undertook a house-to-house campaign, urging householders to oil and screen their cisterns and to fumigate their houses. Another "progressive" women's organization, the ladies of the Era Club, visited homes and informed housewives of the yellow fever mosquito and the proper measures to destroy it. Prompted by these female activists, women in various wards of the city formed associations to cooperate with the other (male) volunteer forces.[21]

In mid-September several prominent citizens and commercial leaders organized the New Orleans Health Association to promote the city's future health, to bring about changes in sanitary legislation along the lines of recent scientific discoveries, and to work for the enforcement of those laws. When Dr. Warner suggested to the Woman's League that they form a "women's auxiliary" to the Health Association, the members declined. The women agreed to cooperate with the new organization while continuing their own work, but if not accepted as individual members of equal standing in the society, they refused to have any formal second-class connection with it.[22] White women and blacks (both men and women) found themselves relegated to their respective segregated organizations, cooperating with, but not a part of, the central corps of white male leaders.

A new feature was introduced in mid-August at one of the educational mass meetings sponsored by the Woman's League: Dr. Felix Formento delivered a speech in Italian, explaining the role of the mosquito and requesting full cooperation with health officials. No one, he said, could be allowed to "throw obstacles in the way of the public health and safety." Many Italians attended the lecture and seemed willing to follow Formento's advice.[23] Italian-language lectures by Dr. Formento and others, the influence of prominent Italian leaders in ethnic associations, and the persuasive power of the Catholic clergy finally won the confidence and the cooperation of many previously obstructionist Italians.

As the educational campaign began to win converts, and as ward workers and city authorities went into action, the Citizens Finance Committee ordered 25,000 lapel buttons bearing the words "My Cisterns are all right: How are Yours?" around an image of the *Aedes aegypti*. To propagandize the movement, these badges were to be worn by persons who had screened and oiled their cisterns.[24] Reflecting a clever imagination, a unique advertisement for the United Hardware Company appeared in the *Picayune* shortly after the cistern-screening movement was initiated: "STEGOMYIA WIRE, in all size rolls, is one of our specialties. If you don't know what a Stegomyia is, ask Dr. Kohnke."[25]

The city-wide educational campaign was also carried into factories and school rooms. In early September Dr. Warner made arrangements with almost half the factories in the city for thirty-minute sessions with the employees. Physicians and laymen volunteered to handle the discussions and undoubtedly influenced many persons in the work place who had not been reached otherwise. During one week in October, Warner and several physicians visited fifty-one schools and talked to 43,000 children, distributing printed instructions for fumigation and other anti-mosquito measures in the hope that the children would do "their missionary work at home."[26]

At various times during the epidemic, health officials designated Saturdays and Sundays as General Fumigation Days when all citizens were urged to clean premises and to fumigate their homes and places of business by burning sulphur. Instructions were published and distributed, and the ward organizations provided sulphur free of charge to those unable to purchase their own. The Union Sulphur Company of Lake Charles contributed thirty-five tons on at least one occasion for distribution to the poor. During one fumigation day in August an estimated three hundred tons of sulphur were used throughout the city, giving the *stegomyia* "a dose of real brimstone." The volunteer groups concluded their work on October 14 and 15 with one day of general cleaning to remove all bottles and cans where mosquitoes might breed and one day of house fumigation to destroy the insects.[27]

In spite of the immediate cooperative response by some citizens, it was too much to expect unanimity of purpose in so large a city. It was recognized at the outset that many persons simply would not voluntarily screen their cisterns or follow other official recommendations unless forced to do so. An anti-mosquito ordinance was necessary to provide legal support for the crusade. Such an ordinance was introduced in the city council on July 25, authorizing the New Orleans Board of Health to treat water with oil when receptacles had not been properly screened. The ordinance also required that cisterns, tanks, barrels, or other water containers be screened or otherwise covered in a manner satisfactory to the board. Cheesecloth could be used as a temporary cover until October 1, by which time it had to be replaced with a certain kind of screen wire. The property owner or agent bore the responsibility for oiling and screening all water containers. For any single violation, there was a fine up to twenty-five dollars or imprisonment up to thirty days, or both. Failure to comply with any provision of the ordinance would be considered a separate violation for each day of noncompliance after official notification.[28]

The council passed the measure unanimously on August 1, and the mayor signed it on August 2. Copies of the ordinance were distributed throughout the city, and every property owner was ordered to comply within forty-eight hours or suffer the penalty. By mid-August a number of persons had been fined and jailed, evidencing the serious intent of the authorities. When the Orleans Parish Medical Society urged that the October 1 deadline for permanent screening be postponed because of the danger of releasing mosquitoes while re-screening the cisterns, the city council passed a new ordinance to become effective the first of the year. Present screens were to be retained; if wire screens were installed, they had to be placed over the cheese cloth without removing it.[29]

Federal Health Officers in Command

Despite the efforts of local officials and volunteer groups, the disease continued to spread, and quarantines against the city became more stringent. On August 4, representatives of all New Orleans commercial organizations, several "prominent citizens," state and city health officials, the mayor, and the president of the Orleans Parish Medical Society met and decided that the federal government should be requested to take over the management of the yellow fever campaign in New Orleans. Acting on this advice, Governor Newton C. Blanchard telegraphed President Theodore Roosevelt requesting that federal authorities assume control. Mayor Behrman dispatched a similar plea. Noting the previous success of federal health officers in combating yellow fever in Havana, the mayor appealed for "executive interposition in behalf of the people of New Orleans." President Roosevelt immediately directed Surgeon-General Walter Wyman of the United States Public Health and Marine Hospital Service to take charge of the situation. In a public announcement Dr. Kohnke informed the citizenry that the transfer of command did not mean that the epidemic was more serious or that local authorities were unable to handle the problem. "Outside communities will have greater confidence in the United States Public Health authorities," he said, "than they appear to have in the local State officers." It was hoped that quarantines against the city might ease up with federal health supervision. No radical administrative changes were anticipated; essentially the same men would carry on the work, according to Kohnke.[30]

Remarkable consensus had been readily achieved on the matter of appealing to the federal government. But several different motives led various interest groups down the same path. Certainly, as Kohnke had noted, the hope that federal supervision would bring a relaxation of quarantine restrictions against the city was an important consideration to New Orleans business interests. Another element represented by the advisory committee of the Orleans Parish Medical Society strongly favored federal control because the doctors considered the work of the city board "unorganized and unsystematic" and therefore "ineffective." The committee's letter to the city board dated August 4 called for a change:

> We regard this as the first crucial test in America [of the mosquito theory], and it must be absolutely perfect in its working to be efficient. We think that the community has lost confidence in this work [of the city board]. We know that the profession has lost faith in it. Hence, we cannot keep on upholding a system in which we do not fully concur, so we desire to strongly recommend that the system be completely reorganized, or that the entire Yellow Fever situation in New Orleans be placed in the absolute control of the United States Public Health and Marine Hospital Service.[31]

Dr. Kohnke, in an account written after the epidemic, stated that federal authorities had been invited to take command because the efforts of local health officials were "disturbed by internal bickerings, jealousies and political intrigues which endangered the final outcome." He did not explain the political problems, but he did refer to the special difficulties encountered in dealing with Italians in the originally infected district. "It is currently believed, and I think correctly so," he said, ". . . that the 'dago vote,' as it is called, is a political factor of considerable importance in that section of the city."[32]

Italian resistance to local health officials had been one point stressed by some business leaders in making the case for calling in federal authorities, who were expected to be more forceful in dealing with the "foreigners." Other political "bickerings" probably developed over matters of patronage such as control of hiring and firing the many workers then being employed by the city, organizing work at the ward level, and friction between ward leaders and health professionals. Conflicts, involving both personality and policy, undoubtedly occurred with so many diverse interests at stake: city and state health officials, the medical society and its special advisory committee, business representatives and financiers, and the politicos who ran the city. Centralized direction under an agency considered "neutral" with regard to local disputes seemed the obvious solution to those interested in efficiency and economy.

Another consideration behind the movement to bring in the federal health officers was the belief expressed by some commercial leaders that the United States government would cover the expenses of the crusade against yellow fever. Or as the *Picayune* expressed it, "dumping the entire financial burden on Uncle Sam meets with widespread approbation." This expectation was not fulfilled because the surgeon-general insisted at the start that New Orleans guarantee a fund sufficient to pay for materials and labor, estimated at $250,000.[33]

The New Orleans *Picayune* expressed editorial dismay at the decision to call in the United States government, fearing that it would result in "Federal domination" and the ultimate loss of all state quarantine power to the central government. Recalling the old fight against the National Board of Health to preserve the "sovereignty and rights of the state," the editor remarked: "Now we rush into the arms of Uncle Sam, and are only too happy if we can trade our out-of-date Democratic State sovereignty trumpery for relief from the responsibility of a plain duty, and for money enough for a temporary sanitation of the city. Truly times change." After the transfer had been effected, however, the *Picayune* considered it the citizen's "sacred duty" to support the federal authorities "so that the very best result may be obtained, a result that may be worth thousands of valuable lives and countless millions in values."[34]

From the official start of the epidemic on July 22, Dr. Joseph H. White of the U. S. Public Health and Marine Hospital Service had been at work in New Orleans, cooperating with state and local health officers and arranging for inspection and passenger detention service for trains and steamers leaving the city for "infectible territory." On August 7, as directed by the surgeon-general, Dr. White took control in New Orleans and proceeded to develop a more systematic and authoritative approach to the work already under way. Within a few days he had established a central headquarters, gathered a staff of some forty surgeons of the federal service (including regular commissioned officers and temporary medical appointees referred to as "acting assistant surgeons"), and created subdivisional headquarters in each ward. House by house, block by block, gangs of workmen proceeded each day to inspect, oil and screen cisterns, and fumigate houses. Whenever a new case of fever was reported, a squad of workers went out immediately to screen the patient's room and fumigate

The Last Epidemic, 1905

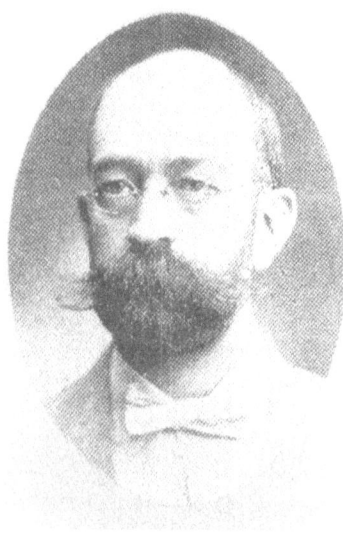

Dr. Quitman Kohnke (1857-1909)

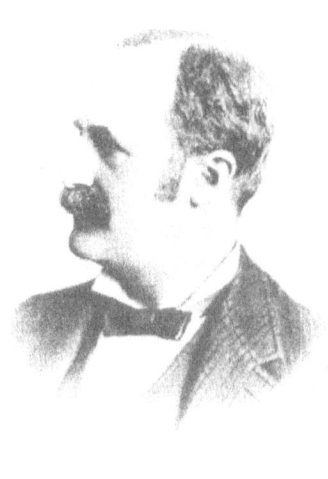

Dr. Edmond Souchon (1841-1924)

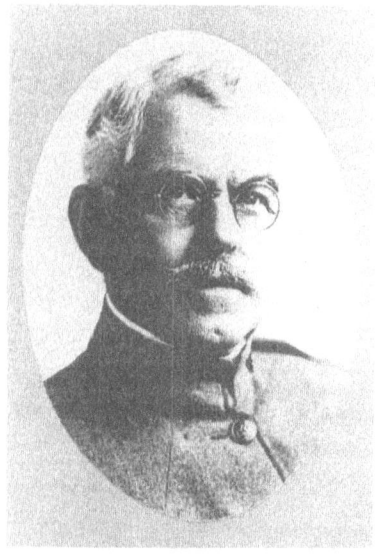

Dr. Joseph H. White (1859-1953)

Yellow fever crusaders in 1905: City, state, and federal health officials cooperated to bring the epidemic under control. Kohnke was head of the New Orleans Health Board, Souchon was president of the state board, and White was the U. S. Marine Hospital and Public Health Service officer eventually given command of the New Orleans situation. Courtesy Rudolph Matas Library, Tulane University Medical Center.

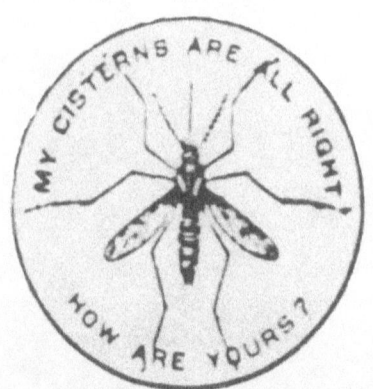

Lapel Buttons to Promote the Oiling and Screening of Cisterns, an Anti-Mosquito Measure. From Rubert Boyce, *Yellow Fever Prophylaxis in New Orleans, 1905.*

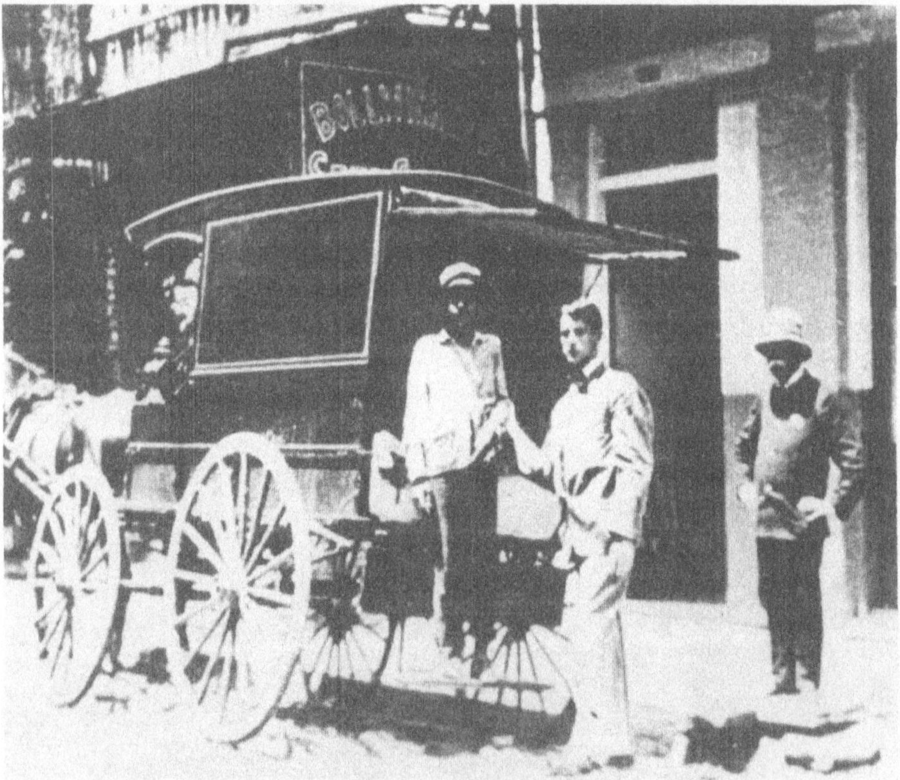

Screened Ambulance for Transporting Yellow Fever Cases to Hospital during 1905 New Orleans Epidemic.
Courtesy The Historic New Orleans Collection, Museum/Research Center, Acc. No. 1974.25.11.117.

the house. Later they fumigated all other houses in the surrounding squares to kill the mosquitoes that might have become infected. It was said that the system instituted by Dr. White became so efficient that the screening wagon usually arrived at the site and the squad began work within thirty minutes after a physician reported the case.[35]

The new command coordinated the activities of the official and the voluntary ward organizations and made a systematic survey in each ward to see where further work was necessary. Telephones were installed to link each ward office to central headquarters.[36] Dr. White worked hard to convince the citizenry that it was vitally important to obey the rules designed to prevent mosquito transmission of yellow fever. He also assured them that house quarantines would not be invoked. In a letter to every doctor in the city, he urged the immediate reporting of all cases, not only positive cases of fever, "but also any case you may be unable, even at your first visit, to say is not yellow fever."[37]

The attempt to halt, or at least to slow down, a yellow fever epidemic that had been developing for almost two months before coming to the attention of the authorities was a task of gigantic proportions, even with the knowledge of the insect vector. In a city the size of New Orleans, with almost 70,000 cisterns and millions of mosquitoes, such a task was not easy to accomplish. Since yellow fever had obtained a head start, with more than 600 cases reported by early August from various sections of the city, it was impossible for any force of public health experts, no matter how systematic or efficient, to immediately stamp out the disease. The epidemic peaked on August 12 with more than 100 new cases reported that day. Thereafter the number of cases declined daily. By early October Dr. White ordered a gradual reduction of the work forces in the wards. Although a few new cases were reported each day throughout October and early November, the epidemic had started its decline much earlier than usual. Undoubtedly, the case total was much lower than it would have been in that largely susceptible population if the fight had not been waged against the mosquito.[38]

Quarantines, Intrastate and Interstate

The first notice of yellow fever in New Orleans in late July had prompted the usual proclamations of quarantine by other southern states. Restrictions against passengers and baggage from New Orleans were common, but through-traffic and freight met with fewer obstructions than in previous years. After conferring with Dr. Souchon of the state board and representatives of the Illinois Central, Texas Pacific, New Orleans and Northeastern, and Southern Pacific railroads, Surgeon White proceeded to establish federal detention camps for all railroad lines. With five days of detention, passengers from New Orleans could secure health certificates to pass through quarantine.[39]

On July 28 the Louisiana State Board of Health proclaimed quarantine for the entire state against unauthorized passengers from New Orleans and other infected localities. Quarantine of freight was no longer deemed necessary since it had been demonstrated that yellow fever was spread by infected persons and mosquitoes, not by fomites. All railroad and transportation companies were prohibited from selling tickets to any point in Louisiana from New Orleans or other infected points, under penalty of law. Only those persons from detention camps who had received health certificates from the federal inspectors were allowed to travel from infected areas. Some parishes, although protected by the state board regulations, created even more stringent blockades. Many local boards tried to halt the passage of trains through their territory and otherwise interfered with the transportation of mail, freight, and passengers, despite certification by the federal health officers and approval by the state board. Such disruptions led the state board to issue a proclamation declaring that those persons who continued to ignore its regulations might be liable to civil action for interference with interstate commerce. The board firmly expressed its intention "to reform by persuasion, if possible, but forcibly if necessary, the present chaotic condition of quarantine matters in Louisiana." If local boards continued to pose unreasonable, as well as illegal, restraints to commerce, the state board threatened to ask the governor to call out the militia to remedy the situation.[40]

The United States Post Office Department took action against the unauthorized local quarantines by abolishing the post office in Vinton (Calcasieu Parish) when town officials, still believing that yellow fever could be carried in parcels and letters, refused to accept the mail. Hereafter, all mail directed to Vinton was to be returned to the sender or sent to the dead letter office. Postal authorities declared that Vinton would not enjoy the benefits of a post office for many weeks, perhaps months, and threatened similar action against any other town refusing mail. Observing that some railroads had halted mail service altogether to points in Louisiana, Mississippi, and Texas where passenger trains were not allowed to stop, the U. S. Post Office ordered railroads holding government contracts to fulfill their obligations to transport and transfer the mail, by freight cars or hand cars if necessary.[41]

One of the most intense conflicts over quarantine arose between Louisiana and Mississippi, a conflict in which the two states reached a point just short of war. On July 26 Governor James K. Vardaman of Mississippi accused Louisiana officials of having attempted to conceal the existence of yellow fever from neighboring states. Governor Blanchard vehemently denied the charge. Several provocative statements passed back and forth between the two governors, while tempers gradually reached the boiling point. On August 2 a New Orleans newspaper ran this headline: "VARDAMAN MOSQUITO FLEET INVADES LOUISIANA WATERS." Apparently, a Mississippi quarantine boat, patrolling the coast, had entered Lake Borgne, interfered with Louisiana fishing boats there, and tried to turn back all boats entering Lake Borgne from Lake Pontchartrain. According to the newspaper account, the Mississippi quarantine schooner had "proceeded to act as if the Louisiana lake were a Mississippi puddle in the backyard of Governor Vardaman." It was also reported that armed quarantine guards from Mississippi had crossed Pearl River and had taken their positions on the Louisiana shore. This "armed invasion" provoked an immediate protest from Blanchard to Vardaman. On August 3 Vardaman wired an ambiguous reply, stating that he had ordered Mississippi boats and guards to stay out of Louisiana territory; but, he insisted, "I am going to also see to it that the people of Louisiana are not permitted to violate the quarantine regulations of Mississippi." Upon investigation, it was discoverd that the Mississippi boats still patrolled Lake Borgne.

Governor Blanchard then ordered the Louisiana Naval Brigade to protect the state's interests and deal with the invaders. He further directed the sheriffs and district attorneys of Orleans and St. Bernard parishes to accompany the Louisiana fleet and to seize those armed vessels illegally patrolling Louisiana waters, arrest the crewmen, and bring them before the grand jury of the appropriate parish. "It is not my intention to invade the waters of Mississippi or take an aggressive course against the citizens of that State," said Blanchard. But he felt that the rights of Louisianians had been threatened by an unwarranted invasion, and "if those who were guilty of this interference put themselves in the way of the civil and military authorities of this State they must accept the consequences."

Reading the newspapers, one might think that Louisiana and Mississippi were actually at war. The bombastic description of an "encounter between the war vessels of the States of Louisiana and Mississippi" embellished a simple incident: the Mississippi boat approached the Louisiana boat and demanded its credentials and destination; when it was found to be a boat of the Louisiana Naval Brigade, the Mississippi vessel fled the scene. The highlight of the farcical war was the capture of one Mississippi quarantine vessel by the Louisiana Naval Brigade and the jailing of its crew in St. Bernard Parish. By August 6 the "War of the Waters" was over. After the United States Public Health and Marine Hospital Service took charge of the coastal area, the conflict between the two states subsided.[42]

Quarantine regulations continued in neighboring states and uninfected areas in Louisiana until late October. The state board of health finally removed the restrictions on travel from New Orleans and other infected towns in the state on October 21. Local health authorities were allowed to continue quarantine against persons but were prohibited from excluding freight or interfering with the passage of trains and boats. Early in November as cold weather arrived and the fever died out, even the most cautious could no longer justify quarantine. The last barrier in the state fell on November 10 when Lafourche Parish removed its embargo.[43]

Financing the Yellow Fever Crusade

At the beginning of the epidemic, the Citizens Finance Committee chaired by Charles Janvier had been organized to receive contributions and disburse funds to aid officials in the war against the fever. When federal forces assumed control, it was agreed that the city would pay for all labor and materials while the United States government would provide medical officers, executive direction, and inspection services. Janvier and other bankers guaranteed a fund of $250,000 so that the Public Health and Marine Hospital Service would begin its work. The state appropriated $100,000 to be used in the yellow fever campaign; the City Council provided $50,000; and the citizens committee raised $160,000 in contributions. Of the state appropriation, at least $20,000 went to aid the fight in the other infected towns of Louisiana. Federal expenditures totaled about $50,000 for salaries and expenses of medical officers, for maintenance of detention camps, and for inspecting and fumigating railroad freight cars. Additional funds collected by volunteer ward groups and used for cistern-screening and oiling amounted to $30,000. In New Orleans alone, expenditures ran well over $300,000, not including the costs to those who screened their own cisterns and houses. Thousands of additional dollars from private and government sources were spent in other parts of the state as the campaign extended to those areas where the disease had spread.[44]

The Charity Organization Society offered its services as a central relief agency for the collection and distribution of funds and supplies during the epidemic.[45] The League of Italian Societies organized an Italian Relief Committee to dispense food at an emergency kitchen and to provide physicians and medicines to the sick poor. The Italian Sisters of the Sacred Heart worked closely with the committee, offering spiritual comfort as well as material aid. For many in New Orleans, poverty was a common reality, exacerbated by the epidemic but not caused by it.[46] For some, the unemployment and destitution usually associated with yellow fever visitations did not occur in 1905. Trade continued throughout the epidemic as quarantines rarely excluded frieght. The disruption of business was minimal (by one estimate, trading was down only about 25 percent), and unemployment was correspondingly less severe than usual during an epidemic.[47]

The yellow fever campaign itself pumped at least one-third of a million dollars into the local economy, providing hundreds of temporary jobs on screening and fumigation gangs and other special epidemic activities. Such jobs in 1905 served as inadvertent work relief to many men who normally would have been unemployed during these months. Ordinarily business was slow in the summer and early fall, even during non-epidemic years, while New Orleanians waited for the crops of the interior to mature and be harvested and shipped to the city for its lively business season.

Italians and the Pestilence

As Irish and German immigrants in an earlier time had been blamed for the city's ill health, Italians were similarly singled out in 1905 and criticized for concealing the disease, allowing it to become entrenched in the city, refusing to cooperate with health officials, and speading the fever throughout the state. Although there was some truth to the charges, Italians received more attention and condemnation than they deserved. Others also traveled and spread the disease, sometimes while engaged in commercial activity, but they were not so clearly identifiable as members of a foreign group. Others also concealed cases; some physicians neglected to report their observations and suspicions until long after the epidemic was made official.

From the standpoint of the federal health service and officials of other states, Louisiana's health authorities themselves had "concealed" the existence of the "suspicious" fever past the point of reasonable doubt, thus allowing the disease to spread out of control. When Surgeon Smith, U. S. Public Health Service officer, first heard rumors of fever, he tried repeatedly to obtain information from the state and the city boards of health. Both boards responded that some suspicious cases were under investigation; they refused to let him see the cases; he was an outsider. In reporting on the New Orleans epidemic, Smith spoke of the city's tradition of concealing yellow fever:

> By a kind of common consent among the more responsible portion of the population the term yellow fever was never to be used as applied to the locality, and that physician or other individual who would publicly go contrary to this sentiment would have needed to be strongly intrenched [sic] in the esteem and confidence of the people.

Concealment by the Italians, many of them from Sicily, was also a matter of following their traditions and minding their own business. Smith perceptively and non-judgmentally described the inhabitants of the first infected district: "Such a population lives very much to itself, speaks its own language, and rarely seeks aid or sympathy for its woes outside its own circle." Describing the same phenomenon in somewhat different terms, one "prominent physician," quoted by the *Picayune* in early August, explained the "supposed high death rate" in terms of "Italian ignorance." In many cases, no physician was called in and no treatment ever administered. Some patients, he said, were unaware of the dangers of eating heavy foods while sick with yellow fever and continued to consume "bananas and macaroni, until in the last stages when a physician is notified, or the department gets word of it." In the doctor's judgment, "science has had a hard struggle with the Italians."[48] Some citizens hoped the federal health officers would be more effective than local authorities in dealing with the uncooperative immigrant population.

The *Picayune* summarized the Italian problem in a statement reflecting a common prejudice, as well as an impatience that is perhaps understandable:

> They do not speak the English language in the first place. It is impossible to reason with them. They are not submissive to modern medical treatment. When attacked with the fever they have been obstreperous, refractory and uncontrollable in many instances. When mosquito bars are placed over them they refused to allow them to remain, tearing and cutting the bars down. When convalescent, Italian patients again and again have eaten freely of macaroni, bananas, etc., which has resulted in death almost immediately. They have slipped through quarantine lines and spread disease in spite of every effort to check the infection.[49]

Eleanor McMain, a social worker and progressive activist, described several episodes in which New Orleans Italians exhibited great suspicion and fear of doctors, nurses, medicines, and everything about the Emergency Hospital where some fever patients were taken. Some Italian patients were reluctant even to drink water in the hospital. McMain said she had been told that the Sicilians had "a legend that when the cholera occurs in their country they are poisoned to death by the authorities, if they are considered hopelessly ill." Yellow fever was also a pestilence, analogous to cholera in significant ways, especially in the framework of traditional medicine. The Italians must have been especially frightened by the authoritative, forceful actions of health officials (inspectors, fumigators, oilers and screeners), strangers speaking a strange language and doing strange things, whose motives and mission initially were not altogether understood. By mid-August it was reported that Italians had become more cooperative and "amenable to reason," largely through the explanatory and persuasive efforts of the clergy and Italian leaders. Even so, some families still tried to conceal cases of fever from the officials. Italian immigrants constituted 51 percent of the New Orleans mortality until the end of August when the disease became more pronounced in other neighborhoods of the city.[50]

Yellow Fever in the Hinterland

In a number of instances, Italian immigrants spread the pestilence by moving from the original site of infection in New Orleans to Italian communities in other Louisiana towns. In Kenner, for example, the disease first appeared in the Italian section, and in Bunkie and Lake Providence the first cases of yellow fever were Italians, recently arrived from New Orleans.[51] Italians from the city also introduced yellow fever to St. Mary Parish, where the small community of Patterson and nearby sugar plantations suffered one of the worst outbreaks in the state. Suspicious of doctors, hospitals, and officials, the Italian population of Patterson proved troublesome to the authorities. The state board physician dispatched to the scene reported to Dr. Souchon that several sick Italians had been taken to the hospital where they died, and their compatriots believed the doctors had killed them. The board physician described the tense conditions in Patterson:

> We are threatened with riot from Dagoes. Several of them have died with yellow fever, and we have been warned to expect trouble. I am guarding the hospital. Fear it may be burned. Citizens are organizing for protection. Have communicated with the Governor, who tells me to do everything in my power to protect the hospital. He will send arms. The Sheriff will be here directly. Not one Dago at present in hospital. Situation looks serious. . . .[52]

Governor Blanchard sent arms and ammunition to the frightened community. On the night of September 2 a large group assembled and organized to guard the hospital and patrol the streets. Nurses and doctors armed themselves in case of an attack on the hospital. Plans were made to invite the Italians to a meeting to hear speeches by "prominent Italio-American citizens," the Italian consular agent, a Catholic priest, and others able to speak the language. Although rain prevented the scheduled gathering, the priest and some of the leading Italian citizens of Patterson met and made plans to talk with every Italian resident in an attempt to allay their fears and secure cooperation in the fight against the fever.[53]

Within a short time the situation calmed down, and many Italians agreed to allow the fumigation of their premises and the removal of their sick relatives to the hospital. Whether there had actually been a threatened riot or merely an over-reaction to rumor remains a matter for conjecture. Through the combined efforts of officials, priests, and ethnic leaders, the situation was explained to the panic-stricken Italians and their fear and distrust at least partially removed. A Benedictine abbot, Paul Schaeuble, spent several weeks in Patterson during the epidemic and worked diligently to alleviate the existing friction. As he described it, the Italians had succumbed to sheer terror. "They mistrusted everything that was being done to help them," Schaeuble explained, "and [they] believed that the medicines prescribed were poisons for the purpose of ridding the locality of the sick people."[54]

Despite all efforts, opposition to screening and fumigation and the failure to report all cases kept the fever active in Patterson. After investigating the situation, a federal health officer called it the "worst fever-ridden town in the State." Because the residents refused to cooperate with the authorities, he believed the epidemic would continue until the arrival of cold weather. By October 15 the state board had recorded more than 500 cases and twenty-seven deaths from Patterson and a neighboring plantation. A later count revealed approximately 700 cases in Patterson and vicinity (500 white and 200 "colored") with fifty-two fatalities, only one of them black.[55]

Another very bad "nest" of fever developed in Leeville, a fishing village of about 600 persons, located on both banks of Bayou Lafourche not far from the gulf. Remote from the rest of Lafourche Parish, these Cajun fishermen had regular commercial contact with the French Market in New Orleans, the city's first infected district. With the outbreak of fever in Leeville and no physician present, some inhabitants tried to get assistance from other communities but were blocked by quarantine guards. The state board heard about the distress and sent in Dr. John Devron with two male nurses. Traveling down the bayou from Thibodaux in a small "gasoline launch" to a point near Leeville, they covered the last few miles in skiffs.

The village was suffering not only from pestilence but was near starvation as well, having been isolated for about six weeks. Two other physicians came in to assist Devron and the nurses. Of the town's 104 houses, eighty-three had cases of fever. The physicians and nurses attended to the sick on both sides of the bayou and initiated the work of screening and oiling, while teaching the citizens about the yellow fever mosquito. The Wholesale Grocery Merchants Association of New Orleans donated a large supply of provisions for state board officials to distribute in the community. According to the Lafourche Parish police jury minutes, some local funds, both public and private, were also employed "to relieve the situation" in Leeville and to prevent the fever's spread throughout the parish. The state board of health reported a total of 375 cases and sixty-seven deaths; in other words, about 60 percent of Leeville's population had the fever, and more than ten percent of its people died.[56]

In North Louisiana, the hardest-hit communities were Tallulah in Madison Parish (1,040 cases with 23 deaths) and Lake Providence in East Carroll (327 cases with 23 deaths). In both of these parishes along the Mississippi River, blacks supplied the overwhelming majority of cases, and whites, the majority of deaths. The disease spread in Tallulah throughout most of the town's forty blocks. In mid-September, the state board sent a physician who organized a campaign against the yellow fever mosquito, and by the end of the month he reported that the epidemic was virtually over.[57]

Table 10.

YELLOW FEVER IN LAKE PROVIDENCE, 1905

	WHITE	BLACK	TOTALS
POPULATION	455 (30%)	1,053 (70%)	1,508
CASES REPORTED	80 (24%)	248 (76%)	327 [est. 522]
DEATHS REPORTED	15 (65%)	8 (35%)	23
CASE FATALITY RATE	19%	3%	7%
MORTALITY RATE (% deaths in population)	3.3%	0.8%	1.5%
MORBIDITY RATE (% cases in population)	18%	24%	22% [est. 35%]

Based on data from *USPH & MHS REPORT, 1906*, 147.

The *Lake Providence Sentry* on July 28 complained of the "dangerous procrastination" of the local health board which had waited several days after New Orleans' announcement of yellow fever before establishing quarantine against the city. Meanwhile, river passengers from New Orleans had been allowed to enter Lake Providence without any inspection or certification whatsoever. Within a week, the newspaper reported that an Italian woman who had recently come from New Orleans was sick in Lake Providence with yellow fever. Medical officers from the state board and from the U. S. Public Health and Marine Hospital Service went to the North Louisiana trouble-spots to investigate, to assist local authorities, and to see that appropriate measures such as fumigating, oiling, and screening were employed against the mosquito. Official figures based on reported cases show more than one-fifth of Lake Providence's population having the disease during the epidemic. The U. S. Public Health Service report gave an estimate of 522 cases in a population of 1,508, or more than one-third of the inhabitants of Lake Providence. According to the report of the state board of health, the same Italian woman from New Orleans was believed to be the original source of infection for both Tallulah and Lake Providence.[58]

Never before during a yellow fever epidemic had the state board been able to provide such effective relief and assistance to parishes suffering from the disease. Special funds were made available by the legislature and the governor for the board's use in this emergency. Physicians and nurses were sent wherever needed for diagnostic services, patient care, management of emergency hospitals, or for training and directing local citizens in anti-mosquito measures. In cooperation with state board officials, the U. S. Public Health and Marine Hospital Service also dispatched medical officers to places where the local authorities seemed unable to handle the situation and needed help in halting the spread of the fever.[59]

Some communities began educational campaigns and anti-mosquito crusades before yellow fever reached them, while others failed to meet the challenge even with the fever in their midst. Shreveport acted promptly, instituting rigid quarantine measures, careful inspection of trains, fumigation of mail and freight, and detention of all passengers lacking proper health certificates. Starting with an educational campaign, the city-wide anti-mosquito drive was made compulsory by ordinances requiring the screening of all cisterns and the fumigation of all houses. Several fever cases occurred at the detention camp outside of Shreveport, but the city itself escaped the disease altogether.[60]

Table 11.

YELLOW FEVER IN LOUISIANA, 1905

	Cases	Deaths	Case Fatality Rate
ORLEANS PARISH	3,402	452	13%
Other Parishes	5,919	536	9%
LOUISIANA TOTAL (28 Parishes)	9,321	988	11%
MAJOR EPIDEMIC CENTERS:			
1) Madison	1,040	23	
2) St. Mary	1,024	69	
3) Lafourche	891	145	
4) Jefferson	778	81	
5) Terrebonne	594	31	
6) St. John	426	44	
7) East Carroll	<u>327</u>	<u>23</u>	
Totals	5,080	416	

OTHER PARISHES AFFECTED:

Acadia	Caddo	Natchitoches	St. James
Avoyelles	East Baton Rouge	Plaquemines	St. Tammany
Ascension	Iberia	Rapides	Tangipahoa
Assumption	Iberville	St. Bernard	Tensas
Calcasieu	Lafayette	St. Charles	Vernon

Compiled from *Report of the Louisiana State Board of Health for 1904-1905*, 45-48.

According to the final report of the state board of health, the epidemic of 1905 had affected at least twenty-eight parishes, resulting in a total of 9,321 cases and 988 deaths. The statewide figures are probably too low because of the difficulties in obtaining accurate reports from numerous small towns and plantations where yellow fever reached epidemic proportions long before coming to the attention of health officials (as had also been the case in New Orleans).[61] The final count yielded a case fatality rate of almost 11 percent for the whole state and 13 percent for New Orleans. Dr. Jules Lazard, a Marine Hospital Service statistician, considered this rate too low for the city and hypothesized that many physicians during the height of the epidemic, preferring to err on the side of safety, had inflated the case list by reporting as yellow fever cases a variety of other diseases.[62]

Seven parishes—Madison, St. Mary, Lafourche, Jefferson, Terrebonne, St. John, and East Carroll—had 86 percent of all the cases outside of Orleans and 78 percent of the deaths. In praising the overworked country doctors who fought the fever, and noting that some had lost their lives, a New Orleans physician observed: "It was a different condition in the country, with infrequent trains and without necessary drugs or sulphur or with scanty resources or supplies and lacking trained assistance." Sometimes one doctor alone carried the burden in a large area, a condition considerably more difficult than that in New Orleans, "where the fight was made with the aid of the United States Government and almost unlimited money."[63]

Summing up the Victory

In the last days of the epidemic, Theodore Roosevelt made a dramatic appearance in New Orleans in defiance of advice and warnings from many quarters. Touring the South in the last two weeks of October, the president of the United States arranged his itinerary so that the Crescent City would be the last stop and he could return to Washington by boat to avoid any quarantine difficulties. On October 25, the city gave him a grand welcome, complete with parade, speech-making, and banquet. In response to Mayor Behrman's welcome address, the president praised the people of New Orleans for their battle against the pestilence, "and declared with emotion that at any moment, if he had been asked to do so, he would have come in person to assist in this fight that was being so gallantly made."[64] Some years later, recalling Roosevelt's visit to the city, Behrman said he told the president as they rode through the cheering populace, "I'm glad you won't be here long. I'd rather this city would stay Democratic." By coming to New Orleans, Roosevelt demonstrated to the nation that yellow fever was no longer to be feared. "The oiling and screening got results," said Behrman, "and Roosevelt's visit advertised the results."[65]

Sir Rubert Boyce of the Liverpool School of Tropical Medicine, who had observed the crusade in person, called it "the most brilliant demonstration upon a most extensive scale of the application of modern sanitary teaching to the arrest and prevention of Yellow Fever." The people of New Orleans had set a precedent that Boyce felt should be followed everywhere within the yellow fever zone so that the dreaded pestilence might be entirely eradicated.[66] George Augustin, historian of yellow fever, also on the scene at the time, wrote:

> The epidemic of 1905 is memorable in many ways, but what has stamped it indelibly in the minds of the great thinking public of the entire civilized world, is the grand victory which science, with the modern weapon intelligently wielded, has achieved against a disease which is foreign to this country, and which we sincerely hope, has been forever ostracised from our shores.[67]

In a similar vein, and with full recognition of the power of science as a "modern weapon," the U. S. Public Health Service report on the 1905 campaign proclaimed: "The great triumph at New Orleans, under the immediate supervision of Surgeon White, has already established confidence in human mastery of the yellow scourge."[68]

The words "scientific" and "modern" appeared with striking frequency in medical and popular journalism from the 1890s onward. In bold headlines and detailed accounts, newspapers announced that *Science* (usually with a capital S) had "declared" some new truth, or had "provided" some "modern method" to combat disease. In 1897 "scientific sanitation" (isolation, disinfection, fumigation) was set forth as the modern, rational, civilized way of limiting the spread of the fever, as opposed to the unreasonable, unnecessary, uncivilized, and unscientific quarantine barriers. In 1905 the journals informed their readers that science had demonstrated the truth of the mosquito doctrine and had thereby provided a precise and effective method to combat yellow fever. Science and modernity dominated virtually every page of reporting and commentary on the epidemic of 1905.[69] As one New Orleans journalist expressed it, despite considerable ignorance and prejudice against new ideas, "*modern thought prevailed*, and while prejudice paid its price in lives and suffering, that price was not nearly as great as it would have been if the *men of science* had failed in their duty."[70]

During the 1905 epidemic, Surgeon Joseph H. White and the other federal health officers in New Orleans served as missionaries for modern social order. They exemplified the authority of professionalism and scientific expertise, especially in conjunction with the legal power to act and direct. They wore uniforms and were described as "business-like and determined." One medical observer found the work of the federal officers a joy to behold: "Cleanly, swiftly, scientifically, the olive-green uniforms darted hither and thither . . . opening up every corner to the bright light of science . . . so swiftly that it was like watching a huge machine, well oiled and efficacious, performing a marvelous task with perfect show of ease."[71]

The U. S. Public Health and Marine Hospital Service represented a national orientation that was slowly but surely taking precedence over local bases of power and prestige. Commercial and transportation interests of regional or national scope advocated and supported federal services that facilitated interstate trade and travel by eliminating the diversity and disruption of local regulations. Capitalists and federal health officers could readily agree that centralization and uniformity served as rational means to achieve the expressed goals of efficiency and economy. Surgeon White, in taking control of the New Orleans campaign, moved quickly to reorganize his officers and work force in a bureaucratic, hierarchical system. Telephone communication was utilized for more effective coordination, and officers in charge of ward subdivisions were directed to report by phone each hour to central headquarters. White issued general orders to his subordinates, notices to the New Orleans press, and circular letters to the medical profession of the city. He promulgated rules and regulations outlining with great specificity what was to be done, in what manner, and by whom.[72]

Printed instructions were provided to foremen of work gangs spelling out in fine detail the step-by-step procedures to be followed in fumigation and inspection. White's directions also emphasized discipline, sobriety, and steady work. He assigned the foremen of the screening and fumigation gangs chief responsibility for discipline of workmen. Drinking on the job and loafing were designated as grounds for "instant dismissal." Each gang was required to have one member who could speak Italian and serve as interpreter, but the foreman would be the only official spokesman in talking with householders, and he was instructed not to let others "butt" in. Discipline of self and others was being taught by the rulebook. Directly or indirectly, the instructions stressed the need to depersonalize activities, to separate self from the job, to control feelings, to perform as a cool rational functionary and not in a reactive, emotional manner. For example, in concluding one lengthy set of instructions to foremen of fumigation gangs, Dr. White directed: "Foremen must remember that they are invading the property of homes and disturbing the comfort of individuals. They must expect tongue lashings and other abuse, as part of their day's work for which they are being paid. They must keep their temper, try to make friends with these people, and *do the work assigned them.*"[73]

Previously, during the 1897 epidemic in New Orleans, the Louisiana State Board of Health had instructed its commissioned sanitary officers to "Be polite and positive" in performing their duties and to keep accurate records of inspections and other work. In 1905 Dr. White prepared and provided various blank forms to be used by workers engaged in sanitary inspection and other activities. The use of these forms allowed for more consistent and accurate record-keeping and ease of cumulative reporting, as well as facilitating uniformity and efficiency in the process. More and more value was being assigned to precision in measurement, quantification of data wherever possible. Reports included the numbers for virtually everything that could be counted, cases and deaths from the fever, miles of gutters salted, pounds of salt or sulphur used, gallons of oil poured in cisterns and privies.[74]

Mass communication techniques played a prominent role in propagandizing the mosquito doctrine and measures designed to curb the epidemic. Newspapers cooperated fully with local, state, and federal health officials in providing extensive press coverage to educate and to mobilize the populace in the anti-mosquito crusade. Posters displayed on billboards throughout the city and widely distributed official circulars and pamphlets also carried authoritative messages to the public. Lapel buttons, which served to advertise the cause and encourage participation, gave cooperative citizens the chance to boast that they were doing their part and to remind others to join them. Public lectures, complete with visual aids (the *sine qua non* of the modern scientific seminar), brought out hundreds of persons almost nightly to be entertained and instructed by Dr. Kohnke's lantern slides illustrating the life-cycle of the *stegomyia* and the means for its eradication. Clergymen preached the message to their congregations.

Physicians delivered lectures to workers in factories and to children in schoolrooms. Health officials and the local medical profession recognized that only through a vigorous program of mass education could popular support be obtained for the precise and systematic effort needed to contain the epidemic. Active public participation was desirable, but widespread public acceptance, or at least non-resistance, was absolutely necessary for official measures to work at all.

The administrative strategy of the 1905 campaign and the language used in journalism and official reports reveal the emerging outlines of structures, processes, and values that would soon be taken for granted as the dominant and indeed the defining features of modern society. The successful drive against yellow fever in 1905 demonstrated, and further contributed to, the growing power and influence of modern scientific medicine, bureaucratic management, and mass communication.

After 1905

The campaign of 1905 settled once and for all the widespread doubts about the role of the *Aedes aegypti* and transformed the mosquito theory into the mosquito doctrine. The 1905 report of the Charity Hospital administrators stated that the experience with fever patients had "confirmed in every respect, the soundness of the dogma of the mosquito being the sole transitory agent in propagating yellow fever." In handling about a hundred cases of yellow fever during the epidemic, hospital authorities had been extremely careful to use mosquito bars and to screen the fever wards. Not one case developed amony physicians, nurses, students, Sisters of Charity, or other patients in the hospital.[75]

At least one prominent New Orleans physician continued to oppose what he called "The Mosquito Craze." Dr. Charles A. Faget wrote a lengthy article for the *New Orleans Medical and Surgical Journal* in 1906, expressing his skepticism with regard to the mosquito theory and upholding the nineteenth-century view of the fever's transmission by fomites. He recommended that articles of clothing and certain kinds of merchandise still be watched very carefully and disinfected as in previous years. Although admitting the possibility of mosquito transmission, he considered it the exceptional or experimental case and not the normal avenue by which the disease was spread. Dr. Faget said he knew of many cases that could not be explained by the mosquito and other cases where mosquitoes had been present but the fever failed to spread. He considered the compulsory screening procedure, fumigations and refumigations, and hasty removal of patients to crowded hospitals not only annoying but actually dangerous to the lives of the sick. "Such practices," he declared, "remind one of the bear who, wishing to deliver his sleeping master of an obnoxious 'mosquito,' crushed his head with a huge rock."[76] By this time, however, Dr. Faget's views represented the exception and not the rule.

Having failed to prevent the entry of yellow fever into the state, Dr. Souchon and the other members of the Louisiana State Board of Health completed their report for 1905 and resigned as a group, following the precedent set in 1897.[77] Early in 1906, after the first meeting of the newly-appointed state board, Dr. Clifford H. Irion, its president, announced the board's plan for a statewide educational campaign. At a conference held in Alexandria in February, the board brought together some two hundred persons representing a variety of public and private interests, more or less united in a common desire for the best health protection with the least inconvenience to commerce. Attending this health conference were state legislators, local health officials, and representatives of transportation interests, commercial and agricultural organizations (such as the Merchants and Manufacturers Association of New Orleans, Louisiana Sugar Planters, and Southern Cotton Growers), and other important associations "including those composed of intelligent and public spirited women" (a reference to the Federation of Women's Clubs).[78]

The delegates considered the lessons of 1905 and passed resolutions recommending state and local health measures to bring law into line with the new knowledge made available by science. After this conference, many town governments sponsored educational sessions to teach the new doctrine and the correct procedures for eliminating the cistern mosquito and the disease it transmitted. The state board also arranged more than one hundred educational institutes in areas infected by yellow fever the previous year. At these programs, the mosquito doctrine was presented in a series of illustrated lectures in English, French, German, and Italian. These "popular health conferences" resulted in the widespread fumigation of houses and the passage of compulsory screening ordinances in many Louisiana towns.[79]

The new state board was determined not to let yellow fever get a head start in 1906 as it had done in the past while officials argued about their diagnostic uncertainties and waited for an autopsy to remove all doubt. The old rule had been a negative presumption: consider all suspicious cases every possible malady but yellow fever, until someone dies and the disease is confirmed by autopsy—if or when one is finally permitted. Meanwhile the fever could be spreading beyond control. The new rule, developed from the experience of 1905, was one of positive presumption: consider yellow fever a possibility in every case of disease until certain that it is not; and if in doubt, proceed with screening and fumigation as if the case were yellow fever.

Several "suspicious" cases were reported to the board in the summer of 1906. As each case was being investigated and carefully monitored, the state board president kept the health officials in Alabama, Mississippi, and Texas fully informed of the situation. All precautions were taken *as if* the cases were actually yellow fever. Only one suspicious case was confirmed as yellow fever by the board's experts, a case reported on August 17 by the local health officer of New Iberia. Two "fever experts" from New Orleans, Drs. Charles Chassaignac and P. E. Archinard, at the request of the state board, went to New Iberia to examine the patient, a fourteen-year-old mulatto boy named Guildmaire Mouton. After carefully checking the patient on two different occasions, the New Orleans experts and the local physicians agreed on August 19 that it was indeed a case of yellow fever, and notified the state board immediately.

President Irion telegraphed other southern state health officers and the surgeon-general of the U. S. Public Health and Marine Hospital Service, informing them that he would deal promptly and carefully with the situation in New Iberia. No quarantines were declared. The Louisiana board did prohibit the Southern Pacific Railway from selling tickets out of New Iberia, and trains were not permitted to stop there except for water. Dr. Irion went to the town, taking with him "expert fumigators," supplies, and equipment in a special car that the train dropped off in New Iberia. For the next three weeks, the experts conducted a thorough campaign of fumigating and screening throughout the town. The patient recovered and no other cases developed. The board was never able to determine the source of infection.[80]

Perhaps an infected *Aedes aegypti* had survived the winter and enjoyed an unusually long life, but this hypothesis seems unlikely. The disease might not have been yellow fever at all since other ailments can present strikingly similar symptoms. Young Mouton could have had typhoid fever (prevalent in New Iberia at that time), malaria, influenza, dengue, or hepatitis.[81] In 1914, Dr. Henry R. Carter, one of the nation's leading "yellow fever experts," commented on the difficulties of diagnosis: "Well, I have seen typhoid fever mistaken for it, but that was not necessary. I have seen it mistaken for sunstroke. But you may, I think, legitimately mistake it for malarial fever, dengue, influenza, and measles." In any case, he advised, "you must regard every sick person as having yellow fever until the contrary is proved."[82]

Under the circumstances in 1906, it would not be surprising if all the physicians involved decided to play it safe in calling the New Iberia case yellow fever since it presented so many of the right symptoms. Only an autopsy could verify the diagnosis, but the patient did not die. Whatever the explanation for that case, the state was otherwise clear of yellow fever in 1906, and since that time has continued to enjoy freedom from its traditional summer scourge. Louisiana's last yellow fever epidemic, in 1905, was also the last to occur within the United States.

Directly and indirectly, the epidemic of 1905 produced a number of significant results. According to Dr. Rudolph Matas, the victorious crusade brought a renewed confidence in the future of New Orleans and the entire American Gulf Coast by demonstrating that the disease could be eradicated. "It put a new spirit and a new faith in a once apathetic plague stricken, discouraged population," he said. The episode also shocked the community into an awareness of the obsolete methods of sanitation, or rather *"insanitation,"* which, according to Dr. Matas, "had long ceased to be fit even for a colonial regime." Cisterns, open gutters, unpaved streets, and other "perpetual culture media" for mosquitoes had to go.[83]

Under the impetus of the yellow fever outbreaks in the late 1890s, local officials initiated arrangements for the construction of city-owned systems of drainage, sewerage, and water supply. The drainage system was in partial operation by the turn of the century; work had begun on the sewerage system in 1903, and on the water system in 1905. The 1905 yellow fever epidemic provided the necessary pressure to bring about the completion of drainage, sewerage, and water supply systems, all of which were in operation by 1909. One New Orleans historian called the installation of these systems "the most significant incident" in the city's history during the first quarter of the twentieth century. After 1905, cisterns were inspected annually to see that they were oiled and screened properly—and after the completion of the sewerage and water systems, all cisterns in the city were ordered removed. Local mosquito control programs, in New Orleans and elsewhere, became more systematic as an aspect of health protection.[84]

Despite the protests of conservative newspaper editors and states-righters, objections from the state health board, and opposition from some New Orleans commercial interests, the federal role in maritime quarantine was expanded by Congress in 1906. The federal government purchased Louisiana's quarantine facilities, and in the spring of 1907 the U. S. Public Health Service took control of the Mississippi River Quarantine and the state's other maritime stations. The appointment of the popular Dr. Joseph H. White as quarantine director and the retention of well-known state quarantine officers in the service of the federal agency were first-rate public-relations maneuvers, effectively silencing the voices that had opposed turning over quarantine authority to "strangers."[85] New Orleans remained anxious for a number of years after 1905, expecting the reappearance of Yellow Jack. Some worried that federal quarantine regulations might not provide adequate protection against the disease. The state board kept a close watch on federal policies and in 1910 requested that the practice of examining passengers from suspected ports be restored when the federal officials had ceased to consider it necessary.[86]

Although an occasional case appeared at various quarantine stations, no more epidemics developed in the United States after 1905. Yellow fever has been kept in exile by national health officials through the careful supervision of international travel to and from yellow fever zones that still exist in Latin America and Africa. Such public health safeguards are now taken for granted, and most citizens are unaware of the dangers beyond the confines of protective barriers.

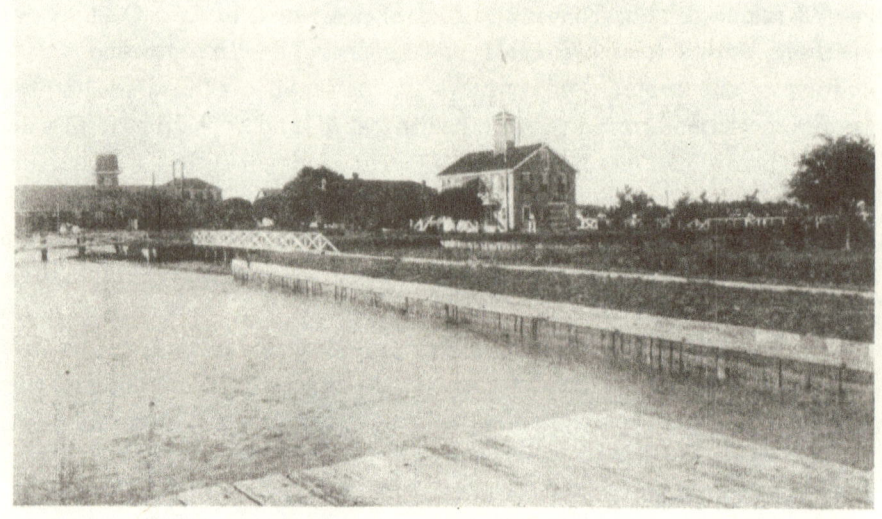

General View of the Quarantine Station.
Courtesy the Historic New Orleans Collection, Museum/Research Center, Acc. No. 1974.25.11.181 (detail).

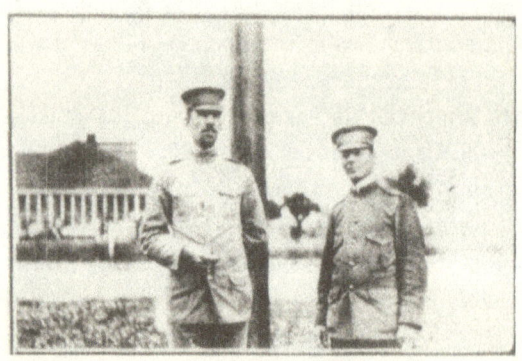

Dr. R. H. von Ezdorf (left), who was in charge of the quarantine station, and his assistant, Dr. de Valin. Courtesy the Historic New Orleans Collection, Museum/Research Center, Acc. No. 1974.25.11.181 (detail).

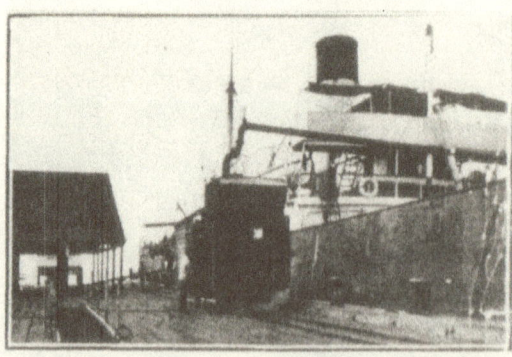

Fumigating an ocean liner with sulphur. Courtesy the Historic New Orleans Collection, Museum/Research Center, Acc. No. 1974.25.11.181 (detail).

The Last Epidemic, 1905

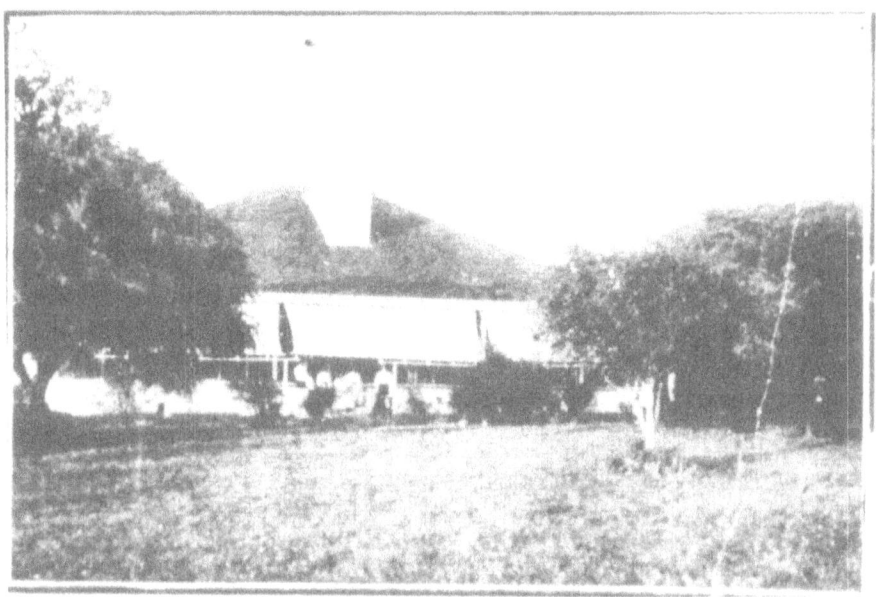

Cozy home of the resident physician.
Courtesy the Historic New Orleans Collection, Museum/Research Center, Acc. No. 1974.25.11.181 (detail).

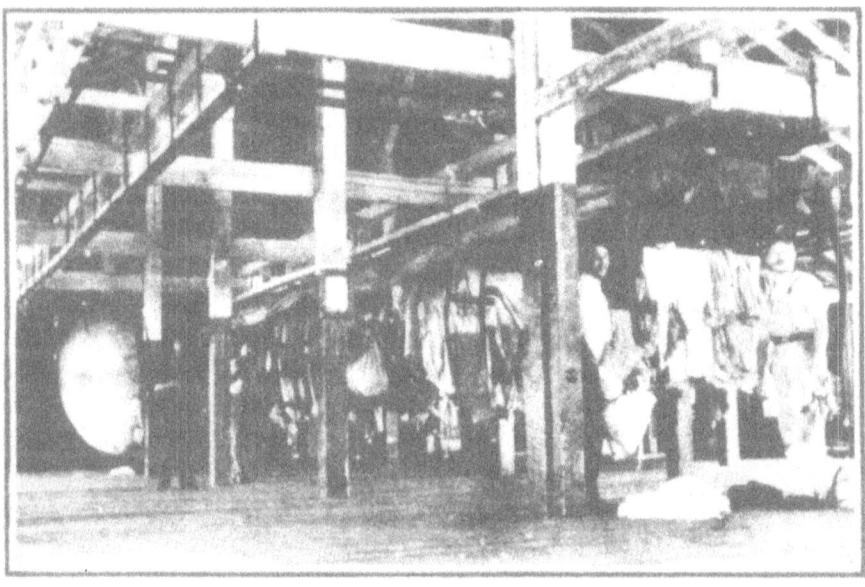

Disinfecting bedding and clothes.
Courtesy the Historic New Orleans Collection, Museum/Research Center, Acc. No. 1974.25.11.181 (detail).

X

THEORY AND CONTROVERSY: ORIGIN, CAUSATION, AND TRANSMISSION OF YELLOW FEVER

For more than a century the mystery surrounding yellow fever's origin, causes, and mode of transmission plagued every medical philosopher who attempted to formulate an explanation. The sudden appearance of the disease in a community, its irregular spread, revolting symptoms, and fatal effects created a terrifying situation that demanded explanation. Yet in terms of the epidemiological concepts available in the eighteenth and nineteenth centuries, an adequate interpretation proved impossible. Transmitted by the yet-unsuspected mosquito, yellow fever exhibited an enigmatic quality beyond the grasp of the theorists.

Theorists abounded, nevertheless, and each contender chose his weapons and dogmatically took up combat with those defending different positions. The expression of different viewpoints could provoke intense personal antipathy. On one occasion, in Jamaica, two doctors terminated their debate on the nature of yellow fever with a duel in which both men were killed.[1] Most of the battles, however, were waged by means of scathing book reviews and rejoinders, journal articles demolishing previous articles, and letters to editors. Until the late nineteenth century, the dominant style of medical writing was personal, literary, philosophical, contentious, wordy, often sarcastic and witty. The literature on the subject of yellow fever increased to a tremendous volume.

Contagion, Miasmata, and Epidemic Constitution

Debated, modified, and amplified into countless variations by determined yellow fever philosophers, epidemiological concepts until the mid-nineteenth century were scarcely different from those employed by ancient Greeks and Romans. For centuries, three fundamental ideas had been used to explain epidemic disease: contagion, local miasmatic influences, and atmospheric conditions. Some diseases, highly communicable through direct contact or association with the sick, were readily recognized as contagious, although the nature of the disease-producing "seeds" transmitted from one person to another was not understood. Other epidemic maladies, more difficult to explain, seemed to require some unknown intermediary influences to account for their mysterious appearance and erratic spread.

Observing the spread of epidemics from one locality to another, laymen considered almost all diseases portable and "catching." Physicians, however, knowing in greater detail the erratic progression of certain diseases, recognized that the theory of contagion as then formulated could not account for all the facts. Contagion was conceived by medical philosophers to be the direct transmission of some chemical or physical substance from a diseased person to the next victim by means of personal contact, or by exposure to the infected exhalations, excretions, clothing, or bedding of the patient. Some diseases clearly and invariably exhibited this tendency to spread by direct contact. But physicians knew that some maladies did not operate in this manner. Cases often developed without any exposure to prior cases, and close contact with a patient often failed to produce disease in the exposed person. Many epidemics simply could not be explained by the narrow concept of direct transmission in the days before the role of pathogenic microorganisms, human and animal carriers, and insect vectors was understood. As one twentieth-century medical historian has pointed out, "We cannot dismiss the resistance of the medical profession to the doctrine of contagion as merely an evidence of hidebound conservatism. There were sound reasons for this attitude."[2]

Epidemics that could not be adequately accounted for by the theory of contagion were usually explained by two other plausible concepts. These concepts, formulated in the second century A. D. by Galen, a Graeco-Roman physician, dominated medical thinking until the refinement and validation of germ theory by Louis Pasteur, Robert Koch, and other laboratory researchers in the late nineteenth century. Although recognizing certain maladies as communicable from one person to another, Galen explained widespread epidemics in terms of local "miasms" and the condition of the atmosphere. Miasms or miasmata included pestilential emanations or foul-smelling effluvia arising from decaying animal and vegetable matter, swamps, stagnant water, accumulations of excrement, and filthy living conditions in general. Presumably, such noxious gases polluted the air, and when inhaled or otherwise absorbed into the system they could produce disease.

Epidemic constitution of the atmosphere, a somewhat broader and even more elusive concept, consisted of an atmospheric condition produced in part by miasms, but also influenced by weather, especially excessive heat and dampness. Sometimes astronomical influences such as comets and meteors were believed to play a part in creating an appropriate atmospheric medium for the widespread occurrence of disease. Since local filth did not *always* cause epidemics, some conditional element in the atmosphere that worked in conjunction with miasmatic poisons had to be postulated.

In addition to local effluvia and an atmosphere influenced by climatic and other large forces, another factor had to be included in the cluster of epidemiological influences—individual predisposition, to explain why the external causes in a given area affected some but not all persons. Within a contaminated atmosphere, those persons accustomed to a sedentary, intemperate way of life and suffering a "general obstruction of the pores" would be more likely to inhale and harbor the seeds of disease than would the active, moderate, healthy individual. For centuries these epidemiological constructions persisted as physicians applied the vague but plausible explanations to various epidemic experiences, modifying the component elements to fit the situation at hand.

Late Eighteenth-Century Explanations

The severe yellow fever attacks along the Atlantic Coast of North America in the late eighteenth century, and particularly the Philadelphia epidemic in 1793, stimulated a new wave of theorizing. In the 1790s two important American epidemiological thinkers, Benjamin Rush and Noah Webster, articulated the pattern of explanation for yellow fever that persisted in American medical thought for almost seven decades. Dr.

Rush, one of the most influential physicians of his time, published extensively and taught at the Medical College of Philadelphia. His ideas were accepted as gospel and his "heroic" therapeutic methods carried to even greater extremes by two or three generations of American practitioners. In an age before professionalization and specialization, when most medical literature was as comprehensible to the general scholar as to the "trained" physician, Noah Webster, famed Connecticut journalist and lexicographer, turned his attention to epidemiology and in 1799 published a two-volume *History of Epidemic and Pestilential Diseases*, tracing the development of epidemiological concepts and presenting the dominant views by the late eighteenth century.

Both Rush and Webster first toyed with the idea that contagion (as well as local miasms) might have some influence in the spread of yellow fever, but both eventually came to reject contagion altogether. They also denied that the disease was imported, therefore opposing quarantine measures as inappropriate and useless. Both concluded that yellow fever was a product of local miasms generated by decaying animal and vegetable matter and influenced by heat and moisture; hence, they advocated sanitary measures for the removal of local causes.

Both believed in the influence of the epidemic constitution of the atmosphere, but Webster gave it more emphasis than Rush. Webster considered the pestilential condition of the atmosphere to be a primary force in epidemics, spreading over many parts of the world at one time, interacting with epizootics (animal epidemics), earthquakes, volcanic action, and comets. While Rush noted the presence of mosquitoes in large numbers, the abundance of dead cats, and the occurrence of a meteor as signs of an essentially unhealthy atmosphere, he gave more attention to the influence of *local* miasms in the production of yellow fever. He also believed that individual "predisposing" and "exciting" causes, such as fatigue, intemperance, fear, and grief, facilitated the development of the disease.[3]

In the writings of Rush and Webster one finds all the elements that would be juggled into various patterns during much of the nineteenth century as medical theorists tried to account for the conditions producing yellow fever (and other) epidemics. The "contagionists," finding more support among laymen than physicians, ordinarily favored quarantine barriers to halt the importation of disease. "Local causationists" opposed quarantine and argued for sanitary measures to eliminate the indigenous filth they considered the source of pestilential miasms.

During the 1790s when Rush and Webster were promulgating their theories, New Orleans experienced its first clearly identified yellow fever epidemic. According to a contemporary, Joseph X. Pontalba, the people of New Orleans and many of the physicians identified the epidemic of 1796 as the same yellow fever that Philadelphia had experienced. Many also believed the pestilence had been brought into New Orleans by the Americans. On the other hand, Pontalba himself, as well as Attorney general Don Gabriel Fonvergne, blamed local noxious effluvia for contaminating the atmosphere and producing the epidemic.[4] As yellow fever continued to appear almost annually in New Orleans after 1796, the doctrine of local miasms gradually took precedence over importation in explaining an outbreak of the disease. Published accounts by travelers in the early 1800s invariably included descriptive passages about the pestilence for which New Orleans was becoming notorious. Almost without exception, commentators attributed yellow fever to morbific effluvia in the atmosphere, emanating from filth and acted upon by the excessive heat of the climate. Most writers (reflecting the prevailing medical view) emphatically denied that the disease was personally contagious.[5]

Local Causes and Atmospheric Influences

Although the theory of local causation had become the dominant view, many fine points were still open to question, and physicians and laymen continued to debate the issue throughout the country whenever yellow fever appeared. The *Medical Repository*, published in New York in the late eighteenth and early nineteenth centuries, filled its pages with articles, reviews, and notices concerning yellow fever visitations in various American port cities. Articles dealt with the recurring controversies about yellow fever's contagious or non-contagious nature; its imported or local origin; its prevention by quarantine or sanitation—all questions that remained unresolved for most of the nineteenth century. While a few medical writers continued to support the doctrine of contagion, most early nineteenth-century physicians cast their vote for miasmatic influences.[6]

As American medical thought became increasingly involved in elaborating the patterns of local and atmospheric influences believed to produce yellow fever epidemics, an English physician, Colin Chisholm, published a work in 1809 to correct "the pernicious doctrine" so popular among American physicians. Arguing strongly against local causation by miasmata, heat, moisture, and putrefaction, Chisholm considered the disease personally contagious and capable of being spread through clothing or other fomites. He also dismissed the mysterious "epidemic constitution of the atmosphere" along with the alleged connection of disease with eclipses, comets, volcanoes, and earthquakes as mere superstitions, coincidental factors but not causal forces.[7]

Nevertheless, the "pernicious doctrine" of local causation continued to find favor among American physicians, especially in New Orleans where the annual appearance of the fever from 1817 onward provided ample grist for the theory mill. During the epidemic of 1817, a New Orleans newspaper published an article entitled "The Prevailing Fever" signed by "Philanthropy." Although a citizen with "no pretentions to medical knowledge" except from practical observation, the writer offered his conclusions to the public. He was convinced that the pestilence was not contagious. Common to the southern states, it varied in malignancy because of variations in soil, climate, and individual predisposing causes. Despite its different degrees of virulence, the writer believed this "inflammatory bilious fever," wherever it occurred, was caused by "miasmal exhalations produced by the ardent rays of a vertical sun, striking against the earth's surface, and operating on putrescent vegetable matter."[8]

Dr. Jabez Heustis, practitioner in New Orleans, summarized his views of yellow fever in 1817, delineating three types of causes. The *remote cause* consisted of "marsh miasmata"; the *predisposing cause*, the constitution of an individual not accustomed to the climate; the *exciting cause*, a state of intoxication or exposure, perhaps to excessive heat or rain. Sometimes miasmata alone might be potent enough to produce a serious attack, he believed, even without the other influences. A confirmed non-contagionist, Heustis stated that he had never seen a case of yellow fever transmitted from one individual to another.[9]

Drs. Gros and Gérardin in a report on the New Orleans epidemic of 1817 prepared for *La Société Médicale* (the organization of French-speaking physicians in the city) concluded that the disease resulted from the "peculiar topography" of New Orleans, the abundant rains and excessive heat of that summer, and the recent influx of numerous strangers.

Although the disease had not been contagious, they believed that under different circumstances it might assume the power of contagion. Two years later, a committee appointed by *La Société Médicale* to investigate the epidemic of 1819 attributed the fever to the blistering heat of July, August, and September, the frequent rains of summer, and stagnant water in the swamps. The report described yellow fever as neither contagious nor imported, but an indigenous product of spontaneous origin.[10]

In 1820 the Physico-Medical Society of New Orleans, the association of American physicians, appointed a committee to investigate and report on the yellow fever outbreak of that year. Avoiding any extended discussion of the controversy over contagion, the committee, although noting that the earliest and latest cases had appeared on board ships at the wharves, concluded that the unsanitary condition of the vessels together with the accumulated filth of the city played some part in causing the pestilence.[11]

The published works of other New Orleans physicians also reflected the increasingly firm medical opinion in favor of local causes. Dr. Jean Louis Chabert, physician from France who practiced medicine for a time in New Orleans, published his thoughts on yellow fever in 1821, declaring that the disease was caused by noxious miasms intensified by heat and humidity, not by a specific contagious substance transmitted from person to person. Dr. Pierre F. Thomas, after observing yellow fever in New Orleans in 1822, also attributed the pestilence to "*les miasmes délétères*" emanating from the putrefaction of vegetable and animal matter and stagnant waters. Thomas saw no need to demonstrate the proposition of non-contagion, an obvious truth, he said, almost universally accepted by physicians who had observed several epidemics.[12]

Contagionists and Quarantine

The non-contagious nature of yellow fever was by no means so clear to non-medical observers of New Orleans epidemics. In his address to the Louisiana legislature in January, 1818, Governor Jacques Villeré, a determined "contagionist," urged the passage of quarantine laws to establish safeguards against the pestilence. The governor was not alone in his contagionist views; the Louisiana legislature in March, 1818, provided for the establishment of a quarantine station near the mouth of the Mississippi River and a board of health to administer the regulations. The appearance of yellow fever that summer seemed to discredit the efficacy of quarantine, and with it the doctrine of contagion. The following March, 1819, the quarantine act was repealed. Shortly thereafter, in the summer and autumn of 1819, New Orleans experienced another dreadful epidemic, worse than any previous outbreak. The scourge struck again the following summer. In November, 1820, Governor Villeré urged the legislature to pass new quarantine measures. Despite the judgment of the New Orleans medical profession, the governor still considered the disease both imported and contagious, not an indigenous product.

Governor Thomas Bolling Robertson, Villeré's successor, in his inaugural message in December, 1820, also recommended another trial of quarantine to prevent the importation of yellow fever. In February, 1821, the legislature again passed an act establishing a quarantine station near the mouth of the Mississippi River and providing a board of health for New Orleans. When that summer and autumn passed with only a few cases of yellow fever, the contagionists claimed credit for their side. When the following summer and fall, 1822, brought the most devastating epidemic yet to occur, the local causationists hastened to point out the futility of quarantine against an indigenous disease.[13]

After the epidemic of 1822, Governor Robertson was ready to admit that the effort to legislate against the fever had been in vain. "It is an idle waste of time for me to inquire into the causes, origin and nature of this dreadful malady," he declared. "The State resorted to quarantine, under the expectation that it would add to the chances of escape from this dreadful visitation. If this hope be fallacious, . . . then should it be abandoned, and our commerce relieved from the expense and inconvenience which it occasions." The board of health continued to express faith in the potential value of quarantine, but failed to persuade the dominant commercial and medical interests of the city. On January 23, 1823, a large meeting of New Orleans citizens resolved that the quarantine regulations, proved useless by the late epidemic, were "oppressive and injurious to the commerce of this city," and asked the legislature to repeal the act of 1821. The House Committee on Quarantine Laws admitted that the measures had not yet been effective in screening out the disease, but recommended that quarantine be continued in force "because it had not been tried sufficiently long, and because other States had similar regulations." New Orleans was fairly healthy in 1823, but in 1824 a sufficient number of yellow fever cases and deaths occurred to give weight to the argument that quarantine was more a hindrance to commerce than to disease. In February, 1825, the Louisiana legislature abolished its second experiment with quarantine barriers, and not until 1855 did the state again provide for such restrictions.[14]

The severe epidemics of the 1840s stimulated a renewed clash of opinions. The establishment in 1844 of the *New Orleans Medical Journal*, the first successful medical periodical in Louisiana and the South, encouraged the philosophical jousting by providing a ready medium of expression for the contenders. The first two issues of the journal contained at least six lengthy articles on yellow fever. In the second issue the editor expressed the hope that "we shall not fatigue our readers with the subject of Yellow Fever; [but] it is the *great disease* of our City and region, and in as much as very discordant opinions in relation to it seem to prevail, we think it deserves a patient, and thorough investigation."[15]

In the July, 1844, issue of the new journal, Dr. P. H. Lewis of Mobile reviewed two papers that had been read before the Mobile Medical Society in June, both supporting the contagious nature and foreign origin of yellow fever. The ideas presented in the papers indicated the persistent strength of contagionism among some medical thinkers; the tone of Dr. Lewis's critical reviews and the response from one of his targets reveal the extremely personal nature of nineteenth-century medical controversies.

In one of the papers, Dr. J. W. Monette of Washington, Mississippi, declared that yellow fever was indigenous to the West Indies, but not to New Orleans or Mobile where it only occurred when imported. According to Dr. Monette, the infection was carried from place to place in certain porous goods, blankets, and feather beds, and was rendered more virulent by the heated atmosphere within the holds of vessels transporting the goods. Point by point, Dr. Lewis disagreed with Monette, frequently attacking his argument with ridicule. Rejecting the influence of contagion altogether, Lewis cited many instances of close contact with fever patients that failed to produce new cases of the disease.[16] Dr. Lewis also reviewed a paper on yellow fever "disproving its Domestic Origin, and demonstrating its Transmissibility" by Dr. W. M. Carpenter, professor in the Medical College of Louisiana in New Orleans. Carpenter believed yellow fever to have been imported originally to the West Indies from Africa, while Monette believed the disease indigenous to the West Indies. Otherwise the papers reached similar conclusions by similar paths of argument. The arrogant Dr. Lewis of Mobile expressed his regret "that the labour and talent employed on these works should have been so misdirected."[17]

Carpenter apparently ignored the review, but Monette responded in the October issue of the *New Orleans Medical Journal*. He protested that "no display of wit or of ridicule" could ever substitute for "enlightened research . . . in illuminating the path of truth." Correcting Lewis's misinterpretations of his paper, Monette said he had not proposed the "unconditional contagious nature of yellow fever" nor other extreme views attributed to him by the reviewer. The Mississippi doctor rested his case with the medical profession at large, "believing that the intelligent and discriminating will award to me such judgment as is right and proper."[18]

The Dominant Miasmatic View with Variations

Even if one accepted the orthodox miasmatic theory, there were countless ways to arrange the various explanatory elements into different combinations, proliferating theories and provoking further disagreement. In 1843 Dr. P. A. Lambert read an essay on yellow fever in French before the Louisiana Medico-Chirurgical Society, offering a slightly different formulation of the traditional miasmatic view: In early summer, under the influence of the burning sun, stagnant waters around New Orleans evaporated, and the miasmatic particles ascended into the higher regions of the atmosphere. Later in the form of rain they scattered disease over many regions. Lambert pointed out that the coming of frost terminated a yellow fever epidemic by condensing the deadly particles. "It is impossible," he admitted, "in the present state of science, to determine the nature of these miasms, and to say what are the material causes and conditions of their development." Their existence was known only by their effects; otherwise, nothing was clear. Variations in the quantity of miasms and the influence of meteorological conditions probably accounted for the different degrees of yellow fever's virulence. With few exceptions, he believed the infection was acquired through "pulmonary absorption." In addition to miasms arising from putrefaction, Dr. Lambert postulated another miasm expelled by the yellow fever patient in his excretions and his breath: "This being premised, we can understand how Yellow Fever may be communicated to unacclimated persons, by means of the miasm which is exhaled from a large number of persons, congregated in small and badly ventilated apartments."[19]

In 1847, Dr. John Harrison, professor of physiology and pathology at the Medical College of Louisiana, published his "Speculations on the Cause of Yellow Fever," advancing his own particular construction of local causation. In a lengthy demonstration he arrived at this conclusion: under certain meteorological conditions, from the accumulated filth of large cities (mainly the animal matters of urine and feces), a "poison" is generated, "which, either in the form of a volatile oil, or other organic matter, held in solution by ammonia, floats in the atmosphere; is inhaled during respiratory movements; is taken into the circulation and poisons the system." For prevention of yellow fever, he suggested the removal of filth from streets, gutters, private yards and lots, the emptying of privies at least once every three months, the paving of streets, and the construction of an effective system of drainage and waterworks.[20] Dr. Harrison cited many specific cases as evidence and quoted liberally from "authorities." Like some latter-day scholastic, he lined up the possible answers to the questions at issue and posed objections that destroyed each proposition in turn except one. Then he set forth the objections to that proposition and answered them one by one, leaving the victorious principle firmly established as sound doctrine.

When the widespread epidemic of 1847 prompted further speculations on yellow fever, the editor of the *New Orleans Medical and Surgical Journal* commented that it might seem useless to write anything more on the subject. "Medical are very much like religious controversies: in either case, when men have formed and expressed opinions, they seem to shut their eyes against all farther light, and hold on to them with like pertinacity." Nevertheless, the editor felt it necessary to pass along all observations with the hope that someone eventually might be able to analyze the information, "winnow the grain from the chaff, and establish the truth by facts and logic." The epidemic of 1847 had provided many interesting facts that the editor expected "would give rise to deductions which would probably vary according to the diversity of intellect by which they were examined."[21] With so many unknown variables, every man was his own yellow fever philosopher.

In 1852 Dr. J. C. Massie of Houston, Texas, outlined his observations and deductions regarding the "circumstances which conspire . . . to produce a pestilence." Among those circumstances he listed irregular weather and local impurities, including putrefying animal and vegetable matter. Although an anti-contagionist, Massie believed that a filthy vessel might convey a disease from one place to another, and in a filthy area the infection might somehow "find an affinity in the atmosphere" and "act as a spark to ignite the whole material." Massie was one of the medical thinkers who had decided that yellow fever, although not personally contagious, might be carried from place to place—that the characteristics of contagion and transportability need not be inseparable. He denounced the doctrine of contagion as a product of the "Romish Church." According to Dr. Massie, in 1545 when Pope Paul III wanted to remove the Council of Trent to Bologna, he seized upon the prevailing plague at Trent as a means to his own ends, proclaimed the disease contagious, and persuaded some physicians to support this judgment. Thus by authority of the Church, said Massie, the belief in contagion had been established and sustained through the ages. He was certain that at least nine-tenths of the medical profession agreed that scientific investigation failed to confirm the doctrine of contagion in epidemic fevers.[22]

Explaining the Great Epidemics of the 1850s

A large majority of the medical profession would have agreed with Massie in 1852 on the non-contagious nature of yellow fever. But the Great Epidemics of the 1850s attracted a number of supporters, including some physicians as well as many lay observers, to the contagionist camp, when the extraordinary virulence and widespread extent of those epidemics provoked a new outburst of theorizing. Other medical philosophers, however, from their experience in the 1850s accumulated even more evidence to bolster their firm faith in the powers of miasmata. Dr. Erasmus Darwin Fenner of New Orleans, for many years a staunch exponent of local causation, relied on the traditional *combination* of filth and the "peculiar constitution of the atmosphere" to explain the epidemic of 1853, unprecedented in its widespread devastation of the city, the state, and the Gulf Coast area. To account for the spread of the fever in 1853 to many places never affected before, Fenner believed the "epidemic constitution" covered a more extensive region than ever before. Wherever local causes were also present within the boundaries of this peculiar atmosphere, the two influences combined to generate the disease. Fenner would not say that yellow fever was *never* communicated from one person to another. Although he himself had never seen a case caused by contagion, reliable testimony indicated that such rare cases had occurred. Nevertheless, the majority of the profession agreed that yellow fever seldom, if ever, was spread by infected ships, goods, or persons. Thus he dismissed the doctrine of contagion.[23]

At the close of the epidemic of 1853, the New Orleans City Council created a sanitary commission to investigate the facts of the Great Epidemic. In his portion of the final report, Dr. Edward H. Barton, chairman of the commission, concluded that yellow fever, although not a contagious disease, was communicable within a foul atmosphere. That is, the disease could be propagated by an individual or a vessel only in an atmosphere favorable to its spread. Sporadic cases of fever might be produced by miasms arising from filth, but the meteorological elements, the unusual constitution of the atmosphere, also had to be present for the production of a full scale epidemic. Like Fenner, Barton believed that the conjunctive action of both influences, local filth and special atmospheric conditions, was required for the production of a widespread epidemic. Heat and moisture constituted the two most important elements in the climatic influence; "malaria" (literally bad air) or miasmata included all impurities of the air resulting from filth and decomposition, such as street and kitchen offal, drainage from sugar and molasses barrels,[24] the refuse of stables, slaughterhouses, soap and tallow factories, privies, cemeteries, swamps, hospitals, and crowded tenements. Whatever factors contaminated air, food, and water, Barton listed among the local or terrene causes.[25]

Further, to explain the spread of yellow fever over a large portion of the South in 1853, Dr. Barton postulated that some "vast influences" or "apparent irregularity" had developed within the ordinary state of the atmosphere "that was at war with its being." He described the epidemic constitution as a combination of terrene and meteorological constituents arranged in some manner different from the normal condition. "We have no proof of anything *specific*," he said, "behind this combination, and this is *two-fold*, the meteorological part probably forming the predisponent is innocuous without the other . . . [and] the second is the local circumstances and influence—the true localising or fixing power."[26]

The "false fact" of contagion had arisen, Barton explained, when a case of fever transported into an impure atmosphere was followed by other cases. Within a pure atmosphere, however, no other cases would have developed. The defining characteristic of *true contagion* was its independence of climate, season, place, or atmosphere—its action under all circumstances. Barton considered the concept of contingent contagion a "medical misnomer." To say that yellow fever might become contagious under certain contingencies was only to say that it might be propagated in an impure atmosphere by the impure air introduced by persons, ships, clothing, or other materials or containers. Independent circumstances then accounted for the "seemingly contagious quality."[27] Thus Dr. Barton had separated the two concepts ordinarily linked together—contagion and transportability. One could admit that the "spark" of yellow fever might be brought into a community from the outside, by a person or other mode of conveyance, and still argue that local sources of filth provided the explosive material without which the spark had no effect. Even so, Barton continued to insist that the epidemic of 1853 had originated in New Orleans, vehemently rejecting the idea of foreign importation.

In summary, Dr. Barton declared that his facts and logic had demonstrated four postulates as clear truths: (1) that a close combination of meteorological and terrene conditions was absolutely necessary to the origin and transmission of yellow fever, (2) that all the terrene conditions might be removed by human effort, (3) that such cleanliness would render the atmospheric element innocuous, and (4) that the "irresistible corollary" followed that "yellow fever is an evil, remediable and extinguishable by human agency." He hoped that a great sanitary reform movement might be instituted throughout the South. The idea that the course of epidemic disease could not be altered Barton considered positively un-American and entirely out of step with the progressive spirit of the age. Sanitary measures, in his scheme, would eliminate the local terrene influences and thereby banish once and for all the scourge of yellow fever.[28]

Regardless of what Fenner, Barton, and many others might have thought about the causative powers of filth, one New Orleans physician during the epidemic of 1853 advanced an astonishing theory on the negative influence of filth. Dr. J. S. McFarlane, New Orleans practitioner for some thirty years, addressed a letter to Mayor A. D. Crossman, published in the New Orleans *Daily Delta* on July 28, 1853, during the raging epidemic. Noting that many medical men saw filth as the source of yellow fever, McFarlane announced "that so far from believing that the filth, offal and impurities around and about us have anything to do with the formation of what physicians designate an epidemic constitution of the atmosphere, I believe that these very impurities ... to a certain extent ... are calculated to retard its formation."[29] In a tirade denouncing the doctor's extraordinary notion, the editor of the New Orleans *Crescent* remarked that if filth were a protective influence, New Orleans would undoubtedly be the healthiest city in the world. On another occasion, that editor also suggested that the citizenry be supplied with nose-bags containing the noxious vapors so highly praised as a yellow fever preventive by Dr. McFarlane.[30]

To defend himself against the denunciations, both lay and professional, McFarlane attempted to make his theory more explicit and intelligible in an article in *DeBow's Review* in May, 1854. He hypothesized that the pestilential atmosphere conducive to the production of intermittent, remittent, swamp, and congestive fevers served to counteract the development of a yellow fever atmosphere. As evidence, he pointed out that some parts of the swamps behind New Orleans, into which the city's filth flowed, had been cleared of trees, partly drained, and bared to the burning heat of the sun for several years prior to 1853. The fumes from filth exposed to the sun produced various forms of fever during those years, but almost no yellow fever appeared. In contrast, during the summer of 1853, frequent rains and the interruption of the draining machines left the filthy swamp covered with water, preventing the exhalations. Intermittent and remittent fevers then disappeared, and "yellow fever established his dread empire over our devoted city." McFarlane wondered "what extravagance could there be in describing the foul drainage and percolations, vegetable and animal, of the city of New-Orleans, when combined with the perishable deposit of the swamp . . . and declaring it as my opinion, that to a certain extent we *might* be protected from yellow fever by an atmosphere teeming with their exhalations?" After his thoroughly complicated explanation, he restated his firm opinion that miasmata from filth and swamps, when exposed to the burning sun, created an atmosphere productive of other fevers (malarial, bilious, and so on), but basically antagonistic to yellow fever.[31]

In a pamphlet published in 1853, Dr. McFarlane expressed the view that nothing so far was known with any certainty regarding yellow fever: "We are . . . as yet not even at the threshold of science." He than proceeded to summarize his own "opinions," as he called them, with force and vigor and an acid pen. Believing yellow fever neither contagious nor produced by filth or decomposing matter, he considered quarantine as well as drainage and sanitation futile efforts to control the disease. McFarlane predicted that yellow fever would eventually wear itself out in New Orleans and disappear, even as it had done in many other places.[32]

Microscopic Organisms

At least one physician in antebellum New Orleans more closely resembled a modern scientist in his approach to yellow fever. Dr. John L. Riddell, a member of the Sanitary Commission of 1853, had arrived at conclusions different from those of Dr. Barton, although he agreed that yellow fever had not been personally contagious. Professor of chemistry at the Medical College of Louisiana, Riddell was more a laboratory scientist than a traditional medical philosopher. Not satisfied with the intangible properties of the epidemic constitution, he attempted to delve more deeply into material entities that could be observed and quantified, asking new questions and seeking an approach beyond mere logic. Previously Riddell had devised experiments to measure the amount of "organized matter" in the atmosphere while yellow fever was prevailing in New Orleans. His investigations revealed "myriads of microscopic motes" in the air and convinced him that the atmosphere contained countless other forms of organic life so minute as to elude observation even with the aid of the microscope. Furthermore, he suggested that the "living motes" in some manner produced the "miasmatic maladies."[33] His interest in microscopic and ultra-microscopic organisms involved Riddell in the kind of laboratory research that would eventually lead others to the germ theory. Ever since the early microscopes had opened a view of the world of tiny living creatures in the seventeenth century, various speculations had been offered relating microorganisms and disease, but the "animalcules" revealed by the primitive instruments seemed harmless enough, and no persuasive demonstration of causal connection could yet be made.

In his conclusions regarding the epidemic of 1853, Riddell attributed its infectious communicability to "poisonous matter (doubtless of some living organism) maturing its germs or spores . . . surrounded by confined or impure air; which germs became diffused in the impure atmosphere." Among the various conditions favorable to the development of the infection, he included emanations from putrefying matter, consisting of gaseous, liquid, and solid particles ("the pablum . . . of cryptogamic growths"), and the "presence of the specific organism whose perfected spores constitute the material cause of yellow fever."[34] Although Riddell seemed to accept the role of impure air as the fertile field in which the disease could spread, the resemblance to Barton's local miasmatic elements is largely superficial. Riddell's laboratory work suggested to him that a specific microorganism, plant rather than animalcule, might be the vital principle in the production of yellow fever. In calling attention to minute cryptogamia (plant life that propagates by spores) and in referring to a "specific organism" as yellow fever's "material cause," Riddell had moved beyond his colleagues who were still constructing an abstract world of intangible compound essences of miasmata, theoretical constitutions of the atmosphere, and general principles of causation for a general class of fevers, the nature of which remained obscure.

Challenges to Prevailing Theories

Another New Orleans physician writing in the 1850s, Dr. Morton Dowler assumed a negativistic, fatalistic position, dismissing all the various theories proposed over the years. Dowler declared that he was no defender of filth, but the erratic spread of yellow fever seemed to him powerful evidence against the filth theory, since the disease exhibited no "special predilection" for locations characterized by excessive heat, moisture, or animal and vegetable putrefaction. "The ship-hold and gutter-philosophers desire to claim sway," he said, "and in their crusade against filth, on the yellow fever basis, go for expending millions of the public money, and devouring the commerce of New Orleans." He was referring to the increasing demand in some quarters for sanitation and quarantine regulations, both expensive propositions. Dowler also rejected Riddell's cryptogamic theory which he thought had been deduced primarily from the filth premise.[35]

On another occasion, Dowler again dismissed all the theories thus far advanced, declaring that "Whoever discovers the objective or external cause of yellow fever, must look beyond the crude dealings in gases, animalculae, cryptogamia, quarantine, filth, and meteorology which are now being exhibited before the world." Such a discovery would require that "new laws . . . be investigated and new problems solved," by which time a "higher scientific era" would have begun. Although few physicians would deny that almost nothing was known about the causation of yellow fever, Dowler pointed out that almost all medical works on the subject presented a fine array of causes. "The writers cautiously make out these by giving a little 'meteorology,' a little 'medical topography,' a little 'geology,' a little 'putrefaction and exhalation,' together with a very circumspect reference to the organic, microzoic, cryptogamic, electric, calorific, gaseous, and filth theories, and so forth." In this fashion a "very specious appearance" of knowledge and impartiality could be created, despite the lack of any positive knowledge whatsoever. "It does not comport with the dignity of authorship or professorship," Dowler explained, "to say, 'I don't know.' It must be said gradually, and with the appearance of knowing everything."[36]

Although rejecting all theories as well as the proposals for sanitation and quarantine, Dowler insisted that he was not painting a hopeless picture for New Orleans. On the contrary, he proposed in 1855 a "doctrine of hope" for the eventual spontaneous cessation of yellow fever, not unlike McFarlane's suggestion in 1853. When the population became stabilized and acclimated by fever attacks, when European immigration slowed and finally ceased, he believed the disease, lacking new victims, would disappear of its own accord. Widespread epidemics as in 1853 would also immunize many persons throughout the country who might later move to New Orleans. Observing that yellow fever had been "emphatically a German and Irish disease," Dowler believed a halt to immigration would remove one source of the fever's fuel. The "unfeasible expedients" of sanitary reformism would bring nothing but "disappointment and heavy taxation," he maintained, but if allowed to run its course, ultimately the disease would burn itself out.[37]

Dowler was not altogether wrong. Disrupted by the Civil War, foreign immigration to New Orleans was a mere trickle in the postbellum era compared to the numbers before the war. The city's altered demographic pattern was probably one of the conditions contributing to the decline of yellow fever in the late nineteenth century. Dowler's fatalistic, laissez-faire policy toward the pestilence, however, found little favor in the 1850s among those reformers who refused to believe that the situation could not be remedied by human effort.

Some physicians, although supporting sanitary reform, agreed with McFarlane and Dowler that filth alone could not account for the development of yellow fever.[38] Even Louisiana's recently created state board of health, in its report for 1857, took the position that filthy conditions were apparently not sufficient to generate yellow fever: "If refuse organic matter in any of its forms . . . [had] any agency in the production of yellow fever, its attributes were fairly put to the proof this past summer on a scale of grandeur that would be shocking to the eyes of one accustomed to the filth of Constantinople or Cairo." For weeks the streets had remained uncleaned, while two of the city's largest hotels poured the refuse from their privies into one of the main streets. The refuse from Charity Hospital supplemented "the stifling current." Although gutters and canals were "seething and bubbling with their putrid waters," the yellow fever cases that appeared in New Orleans, with few exceptions, remained in an unusually clean portion of the city. "If infectiousness were a property resulting from filth and putrescent organic matter," the board of health contended, "the whole city was a laboratory for its generation, unsurpassed in magnitude and extent . . . ." Yet the yellow fever of 1857 did not assume epidemic form.[39]

While the filth theory was debated *pro* and *con*, the questions of yellow fever's portability and its local or foreign origin also engaged the attention of theorists, especially after the widespread epidemic of 1853. In the report of the Sanitary Commission of 1853, Dr. Barton denied the allegation of foreign importation. That proposition, he said, was prompted by "a patriotic, but mistaken impulse, which is pretty universal, as well among savages, as those more civilized, viz: *never to acknowledge the paternity of a pestilence!*" He felt certain that the epidemic fever had originated in New Orleans.[40] Dr. Riddell, on the other hand, while admitting that the disease might sometimes originate locally, believed the seeds of the 1853 epidemic had been introduced to the city from Latin America and spread from New Orleans to other towns and plantations throughout the South. Hence, Riddell advocated quarantine measures to detain and to fumigate filthy persons, clothing, and ships, as well as all goods from the West Indies, Mexico, and South America.[41]

Transportability, Contagion, and the Animalcular Hypothesis

Another southern physician stimulated by the epidemic of 1853 to reexamine the issue of yellow fever's transportability and the highly controversial doctrine of contagion was Dr. Josiah C. Nott of Mobile, Alabama. The extraordinary spread of the pestilence in 1853 reopened the "long neglected idea of contagion," which Nott, along with the majority of the medical profession, had considered obsolete. Believing the spread of yellow fever too irregular to be explained by gaseous substances in the atmosphere, Nott saw the need to search for a more plausible explanation. He was beginning to think that the cause of yellow fever "exists in an organic form and possesses the power of propagation and progression by organic laws." Attempting to distinguish between two issues so often confused—transportability and contagion, he argued that a disease need not be communicable from one person to another like smallpox for its germ to be transported from place to place in vessels or baggage. Earlier epidemics had provided evidence against contagion, but the conflicting facts of 1853 left Dr. Nott in a state of indecision. He was inclined to believe the disease contagious, and he considered transportability even more certain as the fever had clearly traveled along the coast and rivers, striking those towns frequented by ships, boats, and railroad trains.[42]

Several years earlier Nott had published an article advancing the animalcular hypothesis as a better explanation of the "erratic habits" of yellow fever than any other theory yet offered, although many objections could be raised against this proposition. One critic had pointed out that none of the known animalculae (microscopic animal life) was poisonous; indeed, he had swallowed water on numerous occasions containing minute animal life without the least effect. Nott responded that one might also swallow viper's poison without perceptible effect. He was well aware that the precise manner, direct or indirect, of transmitting the poison of animalculae to persons had not yet been ascertained. Coming closer to solving the puzzle than any other antebellum medical thinker, Nott suggested that insects, the mosquito among others, might be involved in the transmission of disease.[43] In attempting to depart from traditional paths that had led nowhere, and for postulating something other than the customary miasms, Nott of Mobile and Riddell of New Orleans both deserve special recognition.

The epidemic of 1853 led Dr. T. A. Cooke of Washington, Louisiana, to believe in the transportability of yellow fever as well as the animalcular theory. Although rejecting the doctrine of personal contagion, he did seem to allow for contagion under certain conditions. Having no doubt that the disease had been transmitted from New Orleans to other places in 1853, Cooke believed that the "morbific cause" had been conveyed by effluvia from sick persons as well as by fomites. In his formulation, fomites carried the "cause" itself, which if accumulated in a sufficient quantity would produce the disease in all persons "predisposed" to it. On the other hand, emanations from the sick were harmless unless the surrounding atmosphere was suitable for the propagation of disease germs coming from the patient's body. Dr. Barton of the Sanitary Commission had also allowed for this contingency which he called "false contagion." Unlike Barton,

Cooke believed in yellow fever's foreign origin and importation to New Orleans, and its direct transmission from there to other communities: "The facts in proof of the importation of the disease through the medium of such persons, and of merchandize, are as numerous as the leaves on the trees, at least in the opinion of most country people destitute of prejudice, or a taste for metaphysical disquisitions." Along with many other "country people," Dr. Cooke strongly favored quarantine measures to prevent the future importation of yellow fever.[44]

As links in the chain of causation, Cooke noted the summer heat, an extraordinary condition of the atmosphere, and a crowded population, as conditions favorable to the action of the *imported* morbific influence. He expressed serious doubts, however, about this traditional litany of causes, having observed that emanations from filth, organic or inorganic poisons, and meteorological conditions—alone or combined into any possible arrangement—always encountered contradictions and therefore failed to provide an adequate explanation for yellow fever epidemics. Referring to the animalcular theory proposed several years before by Dr. Josiah Nott, this insightful small-town practitioner announced that he had "long been inclined to the opinion that the time is fast approaching, when most febrile diseases will be attributed, and justly, to a similar cause—to an animalcular origin." Cooke recognized, however, that the yellow fever poison was essentially different in its action from that of contagion, which produced disease by direct personal contact, without regard to zone, climate, season, or other influences. Somehow yellow fever was different; this he knew, but exactly in what manner it operated he could not say.[45]

During the 1850s more and more people came to believe the disease transportable, first from Latin America to New Orleans, then from the Crescent City inland along river and rail or along the coast. Many laymen, especially in the interior, after the epidemics of the 1850s considered yellow fever both portable and contagious. Many physicians also came to accept the idea of transportability through infected goods or baggage (fomites), but most continued to reject the doctrine of personal contagion. There was simply too much evidence to the contrary. Contagious diseases such as smallpox and measles followed certain discernible laws; yellow fever did not. Sometimes cases *appeared* to result from contact with a patient, but far too often no traceable connection between cases could be found. To account for these anomalies, the concept of

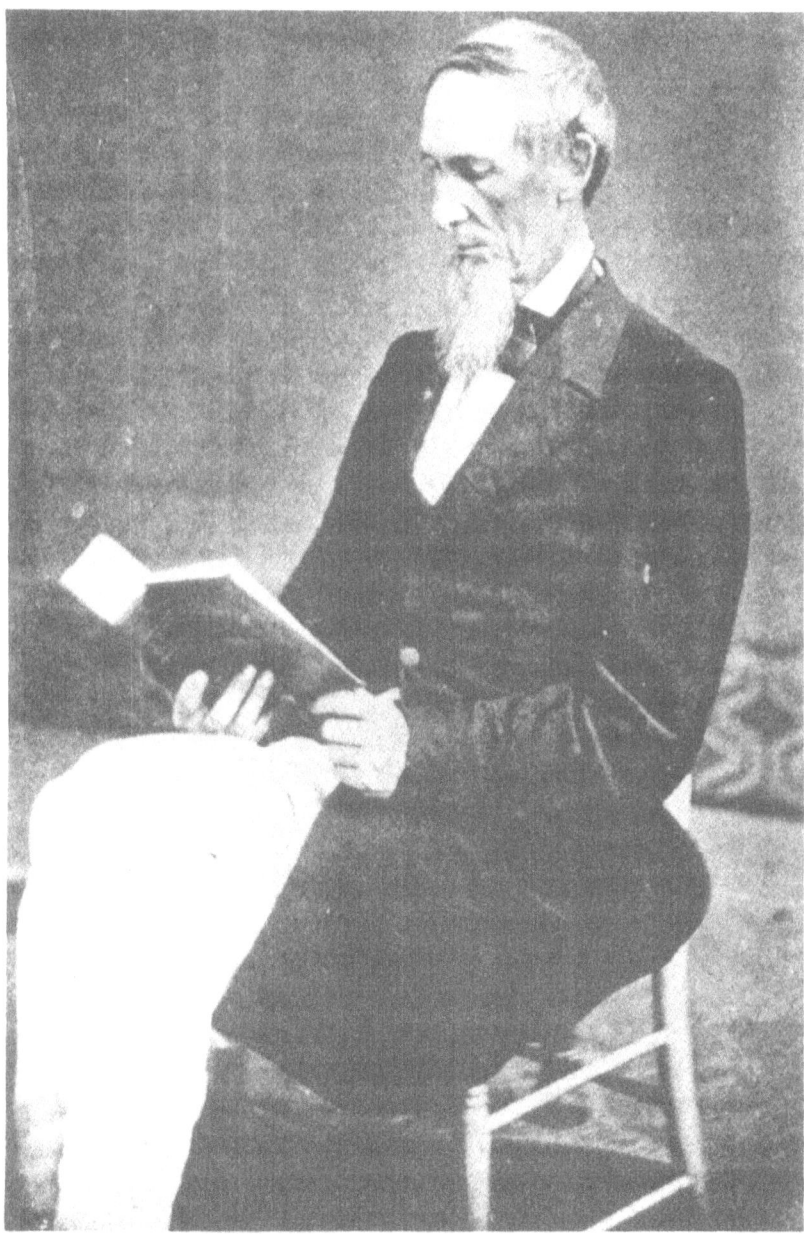

Josiah C. Nott (1804-1873)
Nott of Mobile challenged traditional views and offered new hypotheses. Nott suggested that yellow fever might be transmitted by an insect such as the mosquito.
Courtesy Rudolph Matas Library, Tulane University Medical Center.

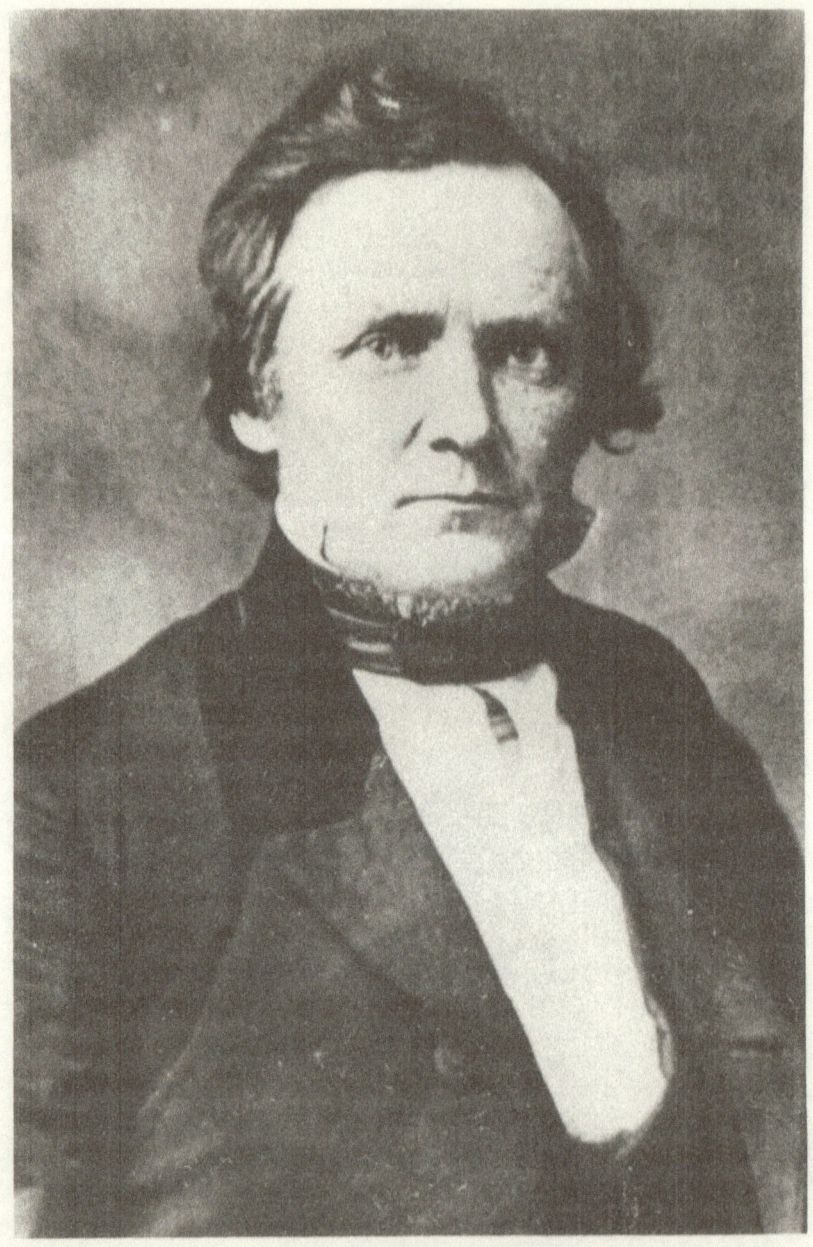

John L. Riddell (1807-1865)
Riddell, professor of Chemistry at the Medical College of Louisiana, also challenged traditional views and offered new hypotheses. Riddell was interested in microorganisms as the possible cause of yellow fever. Courtesy Rudolph Matas Library, Tulane University Medical Center.

Origin, Causation, and Transmission 229

"contingent contagion" was advanced, but few considered this a satisfactory explanation.

The opponents of contagion, and they were numerous, had accumulated ample evidence to cite against that position. Over the years various physicians had experimented with the saliva, perspiration, and even the black vomit of yellow fever patients. They had swallowed, inhaled, and inoculated themselves with those materials and yet experienced no ill effects. According to one source, a physician in Philadelphia in the early nineteenth century fed "black vomit" from yellow fever patients to dogs and cats for several weeks, inoculated the animals and himself with it many times, rubbed the matter into his eyes, drank a large amount in diluted and in pure form—all without harmful result. On one occasion, a surgeon in the British Army "swallowed a wine-glass full of fresh black vomit and felt no more effect from it than if so much water had been taken into the stomach. It did not impair his appetite for dinner."[46]

In further experimentation, physicians had slept in beds where yellow fever victims had recently died and also had worn the victims' supposedly infected clothing without contracting the fever.[47] Theodore Clapp, Unitarian minister in New Orleans, told of a man who had slept in the same bed with a friend dying of yellow fever during the epidemic of 1822. This man had been "absolutely inundated by a copious discharge of the vomito." Even after his friend's death, he continued to occupy the same room and enjoyed the best of health. Dr. Clapp said he knew of many similar cases.[48]

In 1855, in the midst of the escalating controversy over contagion, René La Roche of the College of Physicians of Philadelphia, published a 1,400-page, two-volume compendium of observation, theory, and argument, demonstrating among other things that there was far more to be said against contagion than in its favor. His forty-five page bibliography, listing approximately one thousand items, shows the great volume of writing on yellow fever by the mid-nineteenth century. Volume One included a historical sketch of yellow fever and a full discussion of its symptoms, pathology, complications, diagnosis, prognosis, incubation, and other medical aspects. Volume Two dealt with acclimation, second attacks, predisposing factors, facts and arguments for and against contagion, contingent contagion, nature of the poison, treatment, and related problems.[49]

In one sense, La Roche's treatise represents a *Summa* of yellow fever philosophy by the middle of the nineteenth century. Yet it was by no means a synthesis as the author made no attempt to reconcile the conflicts. He devoted almost ten times more pages to the facts and arguments opposing contagion than to those supporting it, commenting that prevailing medical sentiment favored non-contagion and indicating his own inclination in that direction. Otherwise, his encyclopedic coverage offers mainly a detailed description of the conflicting evidence and theoretical debates on the subject of yellow fever.

Reviewing the work of La Roche for the *New Orleans Medical and Surgical Journal* in January, 1856, Dr. Bennet Dowler remarked that almost one-fourth of the "huge volumes" had been devoted to the contagion question, but even this "massive logic though wrought out with the patience of Job, will not convert the contagionists against their will."[50] According to Dr. William Holcombe, homeopathic practitioner in New Orleans, La Roche had simply paraded forth the arguments for all theories and all sides of the issues and then assumed a "negative, conservative, indefinite amalgam of opinion"—or no opinion at all. "There is nothing positive and definite," said Holcombe, "in all this pile of literary lumber; not one proposition which others have not scouted, not one affirmation which many others have not denied."[51]

Although he provided a gigantic reference work on yellow fever, La Roche settled no issue, ended no argument. His volumes appeared at the time when yellow fever theories were being debated more furiously than ever. Old concepts were beginning to break down under the mass of conflicting and anomalous evidence accumulated during the widespread epidemics of the 1850s. Local causation came under severe attack from many quarters, and traditional views underwent gradual modification. Laymen, together with a small portion of the medical profession, began to advocate quarantine as well as sanitary measures to fight the disease. Even if yellow fever might not be contagious in the medically defined sense of the term, a person suffering from the disease was obviously associated in some way with the spread of the fever to other persons and places.

Revival of Quarantine

In 1855, for the first time in thirty years, the Louisiana legislature again passed an act providing for quarantine and at the same time establishing the Louisiana State Board of Health, the first permanent state health agency in the country.[52] In its report for 1856 the new board of health suggested that neither atmospheric nor terrene influences operating alone or combined were sufficient to produce yellow fever, although they might serve as contributing elements in the development of an epidemic. The great volume of evidence and testimony collected since 1853 indicated "that a material virus, originating in the body of the sick man, is also a potential means and perhaps the most so, under favorable circumstances, of all the others." But local variations in pollution and climate must also be essential, the board concluded, since the "morbific poison" from the patient's body, whether as exhalations into the air or transferred to fomites, did not always and invariably transmit the disease to susceptible individuals on exposure.[53]

Addressing the same problem in its 1857 report, the Louisiana State Board of Health stated that prevailing opinion prior to 1853 had considered yellow fever non-contagious. But the experience of the great epidemics of 1853, 1854, and 1855 necessitated a revision in judgment: "The common sense of the people, unskilled in the refinements of scientific hypotheses, solved the problem, by a process quite as logical as, and certainly far more practical than the conjectures of the learned." A yellow fever patient was in some unknown manner a source of disease. If not directly contagious, yellow fever was clearly infectious, communicable, and portable. Hence, came the general sentiment in favor of quarantine. "The policy [of quarantine] was then inaugurated," according to the board, "not in obedience to the judgment of the medical community, but in spite of it."[54]

Many Questions, Few Answers

Although most physicians continued to deny that yellow fever could be personally contagious (and with good reason), many began to question other traditional concepts. Several French Louisiana practitioners, writing after the epidemics of the 1850s, enumerated the usual contributing influences—miasmatic poison, filth, heat, humidity, and predisposing causes—but went on to admit that essentially nothing was known of yellow fever's etiology. More clearly than ever before, they realized that something basic was lacking in all previous explanations.[55]

One French Louisiana physician, Dr. D. Durac, raised an important question: exactly what is a miasm? Although the majority of medical writers had long agreed that yellow fever resulted from miasmatic influences, Durac pointed out that science had not yet found any means for analyzing that mysterious something called a miasm. Perhaps the active principle in miasmatic poison might be animalcules, he suggested, such as the ones black vomit exhibited under microscopic observation. Like John Riddell, Durac insisted that miasmata required further analysis, claiming that absolutely nothing had been settled about the disease.[56]

Disturbed by the theoretical conflicts since the 1840s, Dr. Bennet Dowler had tried to keep open to further investigation a path rapidly becoming cluttered with dogmatic abstractions. Dowler charactrized the "alleged causes" of yellow fever as completely inadequate in spite of, or because of, the "hundreds of inconclusive and contradictory volumes, filled with special pleadings, diluted logic, theoretical biases, and irrelevant facts." This doctor believed it was "better to acknowledge ignorance than to advocate an error."[57] Medical philosophers, in Dowler's judgment, generally assumed a cause without ample proof. When the effect appeared without that cause, they subtly substituted some closely related influence. When their cause existed without the appropriate effect, they assumed a counteracting contingency. Dowler compared this kind of sophistry to the story of a Frenchman who, having observed that an Englishman recovered from an illness after eating a red herring, fed one to a fellow Frenchman with the same malady. When the patient died, the would-be empiricist concluded that a red herring would cure an Englishman of a fever, but the same treatment would kill a Frenchman.[58]

Dowler considered the epidemic constitution of the atmosphere a useless assumption except as "a cloak to ignorance" and declared that it "might as well be called an epidemic deception."[59] The state board of health in 1858 struck another blow against the concept of the epidemic constitution. According to the board, sufficient evidence existed to demonstrate that yellow fever patients served as one means of diffusing and propagating the poison of the disease. Although many cases occurred without a traceable connection to sick persons or fomites, the "traditional and hackneyed solution" so long employed to account for yellow fever's irregularities—epidemic constitution of the atmosphere—was now considered a completely inadequate explanation. The board declared that "the assigning of an unknown cause ... [was not] a whit more rational and satisfactory, than an unqualified denial of any causation whatever for the event."[60]

Origin, Causation, and Transmission 233

And so the disagreement and uncertainty continued. Enforcement of extraordinary quarantine and sanitary regulations in federally-occupied New Orleans during the Civil War, based on General Butler's synthesis of yellow fever theories (effluvia from decomposition plus an imported "seed"), was accompanied by a period of freedom from the disease. This phenomenon provided compelling evidence to some that yellow fever was an imported disease and could be screened out by strict quarantine—and to others that the scourge was indigenous but could be prevented by thoroughgoing sanitary measures. Still nothing was settled.[61]

XI

THEORY AND CONTROVERSY: SUSCEPTIBILITY, ACCLIMATION, AND IMMUNITY

As if the questions surrounding yellow fever's nature, causation, and transmission were not enough to confound the truth-seekers, several other issues arose concerning the seemingly unpredictable disease. Why did certain groups seem more susceptible to yellow fever than others? Did "acclimation," that is, becoming accustomed to the southern climate, carry with it immunity to the "Saffron Scourge"? Or could immunity be acquired only by living through an attack of the disease? What roles did age, race, sex, nationality, economic class, or "mode of living" play in determining degrees of susceptibility or resistance? An examination of these questions and the various answers offered during more than a century of yellow fever epidemics in Louisiana reveals a close relationship between medical theories and social attitudes.

Strangers' Disease

Beginning with New Orleans' first major epidemic, yellow fever exhibited an apparent preference for newcomers to the area. Both Pontalba in 1796 and Governor Claiborne in the early nineteenth century had commented on the vulnerability of newcomers to the fever. The medical tradition linking climate and disease gave rise to the belief that the "unacclimated stranger" was more susceptible to yellow fever than the native simply because he was not yet adapted to the subtropical heat and humidity of the region, hence not yet resistant to maladies associated with that climate.

According to Berquin-Duvallon, French traveler in Louisiana in 1802, different degrees of adaptation to the hot climate and different habits of eating and drinking explained why yellow fever proved so fatal to the Americans in New Orleans and left the French and Spanish inhabitants virtually untouched. He reasoned that Americans, coming from a colder region, had their veins "copiously" filled with blood and suffered greatly from the intense heat, which made them more "susceptible of inflammation and corruption." Making matters worse in the judgment of this moderate Frenchman, the intemperate American "revels on succulent meats, and spices, and has often the bottle or glass to his mouth."[1]

After the purchase of Louisiana in 1803, the American population of New Orleans increased in number year by year, both permanent residents and the so-called "floating population" of transients. As yellow fever became an annual visitor and occasionally a city-wide epidemic, the recently arrived Americans from the upper Mississippi Valley and the northeastern states continued to furnish most of the victims. In 1817 Dr. Jabez Heustis, as others before him, noticed that yellow fever appeared more often among Americans in the city than among the French creoles. To account for the fever's peculiar selectivity, Heustis emphasized the difference in national attitudes toward temperance and sobriety. While the French drank wine, Americans consumed great quantities of distilled spirits on the false assumption, he said, that hard liquor would "preserve them against the fogs, damps, and sickly vapours of the climate." Dr. Heustis also believed that American susceptibility to the fever was related to their excessive use of animal food, especially when it was likely to be in a partially spoiled condition.[2]

As New Orleans grew rapidly in the antebellum decades, from 10,000 in 1803 to almost 170,000 in 1860, yellow fever continued to exhibit an obvious preference for those persons, whether American or European, who had recently come to the city. By the 1840s and 1850s the disease was most visible among Irish and German immigrants and newcomers from the northern states, the most numerous groups among the laboring poor. Between 1820 and 1860 the port of New Orleans received more than one-half million immigrants, many moving on to other destinations, but many remaining in the city, swelling the ranks of the living and the dead. By 1850 approximately 80 percent of New Orleans' population was white; almost half the white population was foreign-born; and 20 percent of the white population had come from Ireland. In the epidemic of 1853, Irish and German immigrants accounted for 75 percent of the yellow fever mortality among victims whose place of birth was recorded. Information on nativity was available for about half of the yellow fever deaths reported.[3]

Yellow fever was often called the "Strangers' Disease" or the "acclimating fever," and the term "acclimation" itself acquired a somewhat ambiguous meaning, suggesting not only adaptation to the climate but the possession of immunity to yellow fever as well. Summarizing current opinion in the 1840s on acclimation and immunity, Dr. John Harrison, professor of physiology and pathology in the Medical College of Louisiana, asserted that the disease attacked "only strangers, those born in the city being perfectly exempt from the disease, though it is still a question whether they do not pass through it in infancy." Yellow fever in children, as well as in blacks, was usually mild and rarely fatal. Persons moving to New Orleans from other southern or Latin American localities where yellow fever was common seemed to enjoy immunity although not having experienced a recognized attack of the disease. Other newcomers to the city who lived through one of its *violent* epidemics without contracting the fever were also considered "fully acclimated." But, as Harrison cautioned, passing through a *mild* epidemic without being affected provided no guarantee of immunity. Those who actually survived a case of the fever were said to be definitely acclimated and immune to future attack. According to Harrison, even that immunity was not absolute because second attacks, although rare, had been known to occur.[4]

Other nineteenth-century physicians also referred to occasional "second attacks" they had encountered. Dr. Erasmus Darwin Fenner claimed that many persons had experienced yellow fever a second time during the epidemic of 1847. He suggested that mild first attacks did not provide the same degree of future protection as severe cases. Fenner and others also believed that immunity was lost by lengthy exposure to a cold climate—that is, by living for some years outside the areas where yellow fever often prevailed.[5]

One attack of yellow fever confers lasting immunity to the survivor, and second attacks are highly improbable. In such cases as Fenner observed, the diagnosis of either the first or the second illness was almost certainly mistaken—possibly dengue, influenza, malaria, or typhoid fever, diseases that have sometimes been confused with yellow fever because of similarities in superficial symptoms. The medical opinion that immunity could be lost through extended residence in a colder region is consistent with the theory of acclimation, but the empirical basis is uncertain. It had probably been observed on more than one occasion that a native or long-term resident of New Orleans, presumed to be acclimated and immune to yellow fever (but never actually having experienced the disease), returned to the city after a long absence and found himself susceptible to the fever after all. To explain such cases without weakening the theory of creole immunity or gradual acclimation, it was necessary to declare that immunity was lost through de-acclimation rather than admitting that none had existed in the first place.

Strangers from the North or from Europe might reasonably fear for their lives in New Orleans until "acclimated" directly by the disease, or gradually through five or six years of continuous residence—or so it was believed during much of the nineteenth century. Dr. Bennet Dowler, one of New Orleans' yellow fever experts and leading medical journalists, stated in 1850 that "Long urban residence (with or without having had yellow fever), is, in a sanitary sense, an equivalent to nativity, . . . a kind of naturalization, or rather creolization. . . ."[6]

Characterizing the confident, self-assured "acclimated man" in the midst of the dreadful epidemic of 1853, the New Orleans *Weekly Delta* declared: "You can tell this man the moment you see him. He walks along the street with a tremendously bold swagger." To the acclimated, yellow fever was a "mere nothing"; in fact, it was "rather a pleasure to have it than not, it results in such a splendid appetite *when* you get over it."[7] The confidence that came from a sense of immunity helps to explain the tendency of many New Orleanians to discount the severity of epidemics and to insist that their native or adopted city was not really so unhealthy after all.

Physicians and laity alike sometimes exaggerated the benefits of "acclimation." In July, 1853, one diarist wrote that although New Orleans had many cases of yellow fever, "it only requires gentle medicines and good care, when taken in time to insure recovery, and then the system is invigorated by it and the health is usually better after than before."[8] A member of the Howard Association declared that a yellow fever patient who survived the disease thereafter enjoyed "immunity not only from all fevers, but from the rheumatisms and complaints generally of the nervous system." Believing this principle confirmed by his years of observation, this acclimated New Orleanian comforted a sick friend with the thought that "a successful issue was a safeguard against all other ills indigenous to a southern latitude."[9] Dr. Edward Hall Barton, and others, had also concluded that this "ordeal by disease," although severe, provided the key to a safe and secure southern residence.[10] Unfortunately, more than 8,000 persons in the New Orleans epidemic of 1853—and thousands more in other years and other southern towns—did not survive to enjoy the benefits of security, good health, and an invigorated system. And many more survived yellow fever only to fall prey to some other malady among the "fevers and fluxes" so common throughout the South.

Persons coming to the Crescent City to live must have felt some anxiety about the "acclimating fever," at the same time hoping they might have an attack, recover, and settle the matter of "creolization" once and for all. Isaac H. Charles, a youth who had recently moved to New Orleans, wrote his Philadelphia cousin in September, 1847, "It is with great pleasure that I am able to tell you with certainty, that both [brother] Dick & I are *acclimated*." The epidemic had been severe that summer, and "I knew that we were running some risk by remaining here during the sickly season, but as we expect to reside here altogether, it was much better to get through with it at once. . . ." They had not been extremely frightened for their lives, he said, since yellow fever when treated in time was not as deadly as many believed. Already weakened by a previous attack of "the Chills & Fever" (malaria), brother Dick had "a very bad time of it," but Isaac had an attack "just sufficient to answer all purposes of Acclimation," and he boasted, "I feel strong as ever."[11]

This letter apparently provoked a sharp response from the Philadelphia cousin on the subject of New Orleans' pestilential reputation, for the recently "creolized" young New Orleanian felt it necessary in his next letter to defend his adopted city with as much patriotism as any native. "As for our Fevers Ned, I must beg of you to speak of them in a more respectful manner. You seem to place your 'City of Brotherly love,' against or rather before, our beloved 'Crescent,' as regards health—But there I think you are wrong." (Actually, the Philadelphian was right; New Orleans suffered an annual mortality two and sometimes three times the death rate in the City of Brotherly Love.) In defending New Orleans, Isaac Charles set forth the usual argument based on local tradition and wishful thinking rather than vital data and comparative analysis. He had learned his lesson well, and quickly. He had become intellectually as well as physically acclimated. From 1842 to 1847, only one yellow fever epidemic had occurred, and New Orleans' total mortality for that six-year period, he conjectured, was probably no greater than that in Philadelphia during the same time. As a rule, New Orleans suffered a sickly season only about once every six or seven years—"And besides—the Yellow Fever is not so terrible a disease after all."[12]

At this point in his letter, young Charles introduced another line of defense which recurs throughout the nineteenth century, an appeal to upper- or middle-class consciousness and nativist elitism. He admitted that the disease carried off large numbers of persons, "but by far the greater part of the victims are the Irish & the Dutch [probably German], who have just arrived from a country where the Climate is totally different to ours—And if you could accompany me thro' parts of this place, & see the miserable, filthy, loathsome manner in which the lower orders live, you would not be at all surprised, that when a fever once broke out, that it should spread & become as malignant as it does here."[13]

At least a few New Orleanians seem to have viewed epidemics as providential instruments for keeping down the number of undesirables in the population. According to Charles Gayarré, a nineteenth-century Louisiana historian, some French creole inhabitants in the early 1800s even "felt friendly to the scourge" as a means of slowing down "the tide of immigration which, otherwise, would have speedily rolled its waves over the old population, and swept away all those landmarks in legislation, customs, language and social habits to which they were fondly attached."[14] In discussing the pressing need for sanitary reform in 1845, the editor of the *New Orleans Medical and Surgical Journal* took issue with "some narrow-minded and selfish individuals, [who believe] that our city is already *too healthy*, and that nothing but frequent and severe epidemics can keep off the million who are eager to come here, and who, they say, would divide and fritter away the business of the place until it would be worth nothing to any one." He doubted that such opinions would be held by "the liberal and philanthropic members of the medical profession, nor, we trust of our enlightened councilmen." On the contrary, he argued that business and prosperity would grow with an increasing population.[15]

Those who welcomed periodic epidemics to sweep away a portion of the strangers and lower classes probably constituted a small minority in New Orleans. But in decades to come, some physicians and journalists began to doubt that population growth alone always meant greater prosperity. As the epidemic of 1855 was coming to a close, Dr. Bennet Dowler declared that the present population of the city consisted almost entirely of persons now immune to yellow fever—the natives, the acclimated, and the recent survivors, "being, by the way, sufficiently numerous to conduct all its business." The deluge of poor immigrants to New Orleans "where manufactories scarcely exist" did not contribute to prosperity but seemed to intensify the problems of pauperism and pestilence. "A redundant population, without employment, tends to increase crime, sickness and misery," wrote Dowler.[16]

In a similar vein, at the end of the epidemic of 1867, the *Picayune* warned strangers not to come to New Orleans seeking their fortunes and believing that yellow fever had killed off the labor force and created grand opportunities. Recalling the situation after the pestilence of 1853 when hundreds streamed into the city with the mistaken notion that depopulation had driven up wages and salaries, the *Picayune* announced that "Our population now is more than sufficient to transact all the business which we can reasonably look for."[17]

In 1853 Dr. Samuel Cartwright had proposed that New Orleans develop "handicraft employments and fancy trades" to provide suitable work for all the male and female immigrants who came to the city. Such industries and shops, he believed, would benefit New Orleans as well as the newcomers, and by eliminating the need for whites to engage in "drudgery work" in the semitropical heat, they would also prevent yellow fever.[18] Reflecting a less positive approach as well as a defensive xenophobia not uncommon in the 1850s, another New Orleans physician, Dr. J. S. McFarlane, considered the "floating population" of strangers responsible for the city's bad reputation as a center of disease and immorality. "Every evil with which we have to contend," he complained, "is introduced by strangers . . . who periodically visit this city." After the devastating plague of 1853, McFarlane felt it was high time that New Orleanians "fix the charge of vice and insalubrity where it properly belongs—on those who, coming temporarily among us . . . indulge . . . in every evil propensity and passion, until they are overtaken by those retributive diseases . . . ordained as the punishment of vice and immorality."[19]

In the absence of a significant manufacturing sector, New Orleans had a limited range of job opportunities as well as serious seasonal underemployment. Its commercial economy based on agricultural products made the Crescent City a "six-months-a-year town." The business season began in late October or early November as the harvest of the hinterlands was shipped to the city. By April and May trade slacked off, and by July the business season was virtually over until the following November. The slow season (May through October) coincided with the sickly season when many prosperous New Orleanians left town for healthier and more comfortable locations elsewhere.[20]

After visiting New Orleans in 1835, Harriet Martineau remarked that some residents denied the insalubrity of the city as vigorously as others denied its immorality. In her view, no place could claim to be healthy where the residents had to leave for several months each year "on pain of death." Drainage and paving were then being considered as a means "to render the city habitable all year round," an objective that she hoped might be achieved because "the perpetual shifting about which they are subjected to by the dread of the fever is a serious evil to sober families of an industrious turn."[21]

Ironically, the "permanent residents" who left home each summer were just as much a part of the so-called "floating population" as the business agents who arrived during the months of trading activity and took up residence in hotels or boarding houses, leaving their families safely at home elsewhere and rejoining them during summer and early fall. Sailors, river boatmen, transients of every sort, gamblers, prostitutes, visiting planters with their families, and various other legitimate and illegitimate occupational groups swelled the population during the busy season and departed at its conclusion. This much-maligned "floating population" was rarely even on the scene during the sickly summer season. Thousands of immigrants did indeed pass through antebellum New Orleans, especially in the 1840s and 1850s, arriving at port and moving on for points north or west. The poor foreigners who remained in the city, however, were less likely to "float" in and out each year than the well-to-do "permanent residents." While many newly arrived strangers found a resting place in the cemeteries of New Orleans, the foreign-born survivors of yellow fever epidemics were perhaps the most permanent residents of the city, the truly acclimated, though hardly protected against other ills to which many would later fall victim. Immigration to New Orleans declined greatly in the post-Civil-War years, and the proportion of foreign-born persons in the population dropped to about 10 percent by 1900; in

1850, however, the foreign-born constituted a majority of New Orleans' white population and about 40 percent of the total.[22]

The Lower Orders

Almost all commentators on the subject associated the origin and prevalence of yellow fever and its worst effects with the unsanitary living habits of the lower orders of society, who were usually but not exclusively of foreign background. Even when the disease leaped across socioeconomic boundaries and attacked members of all classes, the chances for recovery seemed to increase in proportion to one's status. In 1839 the New Orleans *Bee* reported that the epidemic had affected mainly "the laboring classes and strangers," while the "better classes" suffered negligible losses. During the 1847 epidemic a merchant commented that yellow fever "attacks indiscriminately but proves fatal to but few except the dissipated and filthy—nine tenths of the funerals that have been seen by the writer within a fortnight were *Irish*. These die as a matter of course."[23]

In a superior tone reflecting his social class, Dr. Erasmus Darwin Fenner declared in 1848 that "No one aware of the stupid imprudence of the labouring classes can be surprised at the mortality amongst them. They receive high wages for their labour, and having no idea of economy, it too often causes their ruin."[24] After a limited outbreak of yellow fever in 1849, the *New Orleans Medical and Surgical Journal* reported that the disease had been "confined almost exclusively to the laboring and lower class of the community." Few in the upper "walks of life" who attended to the usual "hygienic precautions" experienced an attack. Did the difference in living habits account for "this preference of the disease for a particular class of persons"? The editor's answer was yes; if the social and moral conditions of the lower class could be "ameliorated and raised to a level with the better class of our citizens, the yellow fever would seldom visit our city."[25]

During more than a hundred years of epidemics, New Orleans analysts of such matters always focused attention on the "habits and modes of living" and even the temperament of Yellow Jack's targeted groups. Emotions such as melancholy or intense fear could serve as predisposing or exciting causes of the fever, according to early theorists. Frightened strangers could therefore bring the disease upon themselves. As late as 1905 one physician attributed the extremely low death rate among blacks to their "fatalistic attitude," their lack of fear or worry.[26]

Intemperance and "imprudence" in the consumption of food and drink were standard judgments applied to the fever victims of whatever nationality or class, although the specific features of their dietary indiscretions varied with each group under analysis. In the early nineteenth century when American newcomers, in contrast to French and Spanish creoles, bore the brunt of the fever, their indulgence in distilled spirits and consumption of too much meat became part of the explanation for their susceptibility. In 1853, Irish and German immigrants and other working-class victims of the pestilence were said to "gorge themselves with fat bacon and corn bread . . . and eat imprudently of fruit." And many, of course, were judged guilty of dissipation through alcoholic intemperance.[27]

Physicians and journalists charged that immigrants and others among the laboring poor brought on the disease by their ignorance, recklessness, and refusal to alter their dietary habits to conform to the hot climate or to cope with the rigors of a serious illness. Eating "green unwholesome fruit" or "immature and pernicious fruit" was often singled out as the exciting cause of a yellow fever attack. During the final epidemic in 1905, the Italian immigrants received special criticism for their resistance to "modern medical treatment." In their case, according to the newspapers, the macaroni and bananas that Italians insisted on consuming throughout the illness contributed to the high death rate among them. It was also said that they refused to seek medical assistance, and when it was available they rejected everything offered for their benefit; in short, they were guilty of classic noncompliance.[28]

Heavy consumption of alcohol as well as hard-to-digest foods might have compounded the damaging effects of yellow fever on the liver, kidneys, and stomach, thereby reducing the chances for survival. Whether the consumption of hard liquor or certain foods would render one more likely to contract the disease in the first place is debatable. Dietary factors and the state of health associated with good nutrition, however, may actually serve to strengthen resistance. Likewise, the lack of an adequate, well-balanced diet, usually associated with poverty, together with the excessive use of alcohol could have diminished the capacity to resist yellow fever as well as other maladies.[29]

Aside from their food and drink, other aspects of lifestyle believed to predispose the lower classes to yellow fever included the circumstances of their work and the conditions of their housing, matters about which they had little choice. Medical journals and newspapers repeatedly pointed out that the laboring classes "live in the filthiest hovels imaginable" and that "they congregate in damp and unwholesome places," as if they deliberately sought out such places to reside. Workers also toiled, it seems, in sun and rain, exposing themselves to the noontime heat and the afternoon dampness, circumstances believed by some to serve as predisposing causes of yellow fever. The *Picayune* in 1839 advised the strangers in New Orleans to protect themselves against yellow fever by "regular living," cleanliness, moderation, and avoidance of exposure to the mid-day sun. Not all of the strangers could afford the advice.[30]

Dr. A. F. Axson, describing the terrible yellow fever mortality among "our poor and foreign population" in August, 1853, argued for preventive measures in the future: "We must learn to interpose in their behalf for our own safety and welfare." In another editorial in the *New Orleans Monthly Medical Register* in September, he again urged that attention be given to sanitary reform. In view of the poverty and ignorance of the immigrant population, Axson called for the enactment of regulatory measures to deal with their "disorganized condition and mischievous habits" that served to intensify disease and facilitate its spread. "We must therefore look to their domestic relations, we must subject their social irregularities to control and discipline, if we wish to do them good service, and to exempt ourselves from the destroying ravages of a cruel pestilence." Those people had to be taught good sanitary habits and the importance of a "well-ordered, salubrious home."[31]

In 1870 Dr. Samuel M. Bemis, a New Orleans professor of medicine, also made the case for "sanitary science" and social control. Because the behavior of some persons posed a threat to the health of the whole community, Bemis advocated compulsory enforcement of a strict sanitary code, "although involving inconvenience, expense and some sacrifice of individual liberty."[32] Most New Orleanians with power and influence were not yet sufficiently worried for their own safety or their city's image. Nor were they yet convinced that health legislation could produce benefits worthy of the inconvenience and the expense.

As yellow fever almost always made its first appearance in the dilapidated tenements and boarding houses near the waterfront (after its introduction in the shipping from Central America or the Caribbean), it seemed logical to relate the disease to the unhygienic living conditions of the lower classes in those run-down districts. Sometimes the pestilence spread to the homes of the well-to-do, but the fever seemed less severe among the upper strata of society—or so it was perceived, probably because the scourge struck only here and there where the numbers of nonimmunes were not so concentrated. Perhaps the patients with more resources also had more physical resistance to the disease. In seeking immediate medical attention the affluent probably also obtained the best possible nursing care, while the laboring poor, especially single men, were more likely to die unattended.

The Myth of Creole Immunity

In the postbellum era when New Orleans enjoyed a number of years of complete exemption from yellow fever, the disease began to strike more visibly among the natives of the city—including French and Spanish creoles, by then almost the only white New Orleanians who still referred to themselves as *creole* (and who by deliberate design and organized effort now claimed for themselves alone the label which in previous decades had signified all those born in New Orleans of whatever race or national origin).[33] Having missed the opportunity to acquire immunity through an inapparent case in childhood, the native-born found themselves quite as susceptible to the fever as the recently arrived immigrant. The virulent outbreak in 1878, occurring eleven years after the last major epidemic in 1867, claimed many victims among the affluent, especially their small children, and led to a crisis of confidence and another turning point in the attitudes of many upper- and middle-class New Orleanians regarding the health of their city.[34]

That persons born in New Orleans exhibited an apparent immunity to yellow fever had long been a clearly observed and well-noted fact; why they did so was a matter for speculation and debate. In the 1850s and 1860s the question of creole immunity became a heated issue among the physicians of New Orleans. Before the epidemic of 1853 a large majority of the New Orleans medical profession believed that persons born in the city and gradually acclimated to local meteorological influences were not susceptible to yellow fever. A few medical dissenters contended that creole children did experience the disease, but in cases so mild as to escape diagnosis. During the epidemic of 1858 the editor of the *New Orleans*

Medical News and Hospital Gazette declared creole immunity a fallacious notion that should have been set aside after the numerous yellow fever cases and deaths among native New Orleanians in 1853. Some physicians had raised the issue as early as 1847, when they saw a number of unmistakable cases in creole children. But the doctrine was still widely accepted in 1858, the editor complained, and although creole children were dying daily of fever exhibiting yellowness, black vomit, and other obvious symptoms, the current illness among those children was labeled "pernicious fever" because of the firm belief that the native-born possessed immunity to the disease.³⁵

This controversial malady of creole children in 1858 set off a lively discussion among New Orleans physicians, with Dr. Jean Charles Faget and Dr. Charles Deléry representing the two opposing views. Faget insisted that both creoles and blacks enjoyed immunity to yellow fever and that the disease they experienced, incorrectly diagnosed by some as yellow fever, was actually "fièvre paludéene" ("swamp fever," or malaria). Deléry, on the other hand, argued that neither creoles nor blacks were *ipso facto* exempt from the disease. The discussion grew more and more heated in tone, with physicians throughout the city joining one side or the other and writing spirited articles in medical journals and newspapers. Eventually, the personal element in the debate between the leading contenders became so intense that Dr. Deléry challenged Dr. Faget to a duel. Declaring himself a Christian, Faget refused to accept the challenge.³⁶

After the epidemic of 1867, the first severe outbreak since 1858, Dr. Deléry wrote a book designed to refute the belief in creole immunity. His opposition to the traditional view had been reinforced by further observations in 1867. The tradition had started, he said, when strangers had borne the chief burden of the pestilence while attacks among the native-born were rare. In time it was assumed that creoles must be immune. Hence, whenever a disease resembling yellow fever occurred in creole children, the doctors called it malignant, putrid, or ataxic fever—anything but yellow fever. The tradition had long been sustained by a powerful prejudice associated with the privileged status of old creole families. Although he realized it was no easy task to destroy a belief cherished by the privileged, Deléry outlined his arguments, described numerous cases, and once again concluded that, contrary to popular opinion, yellow fever did occur among creole children.³⁷

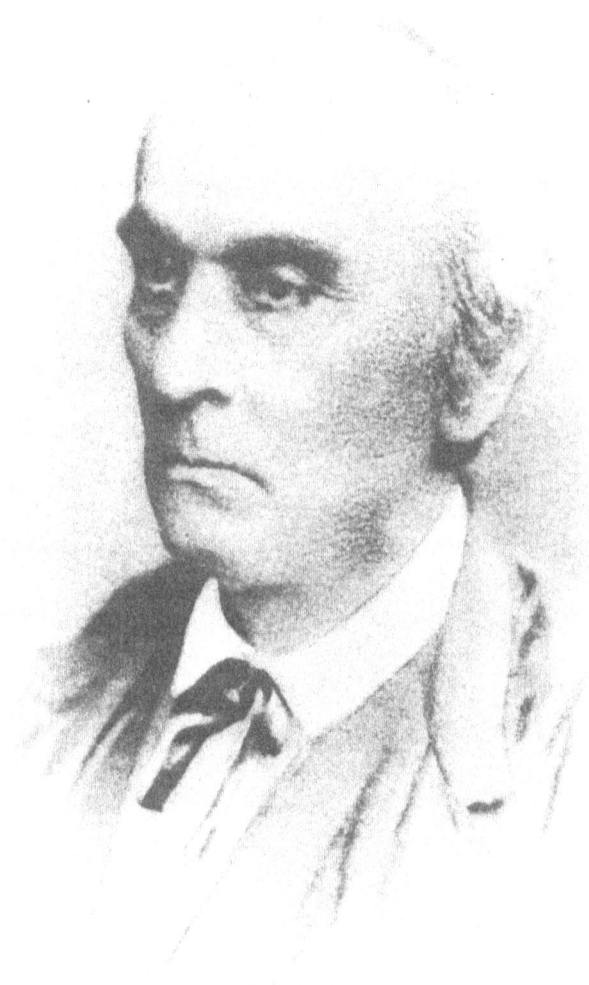

Charles Deléry (1815-1878)
By careful studies during a succession of epidemics, Deléry challenged the "myth of creole immunity," a matter on which he and Faget had a serious disagreement.
Courtesy Rudolph Matas Library, Tulane University Medical Center.

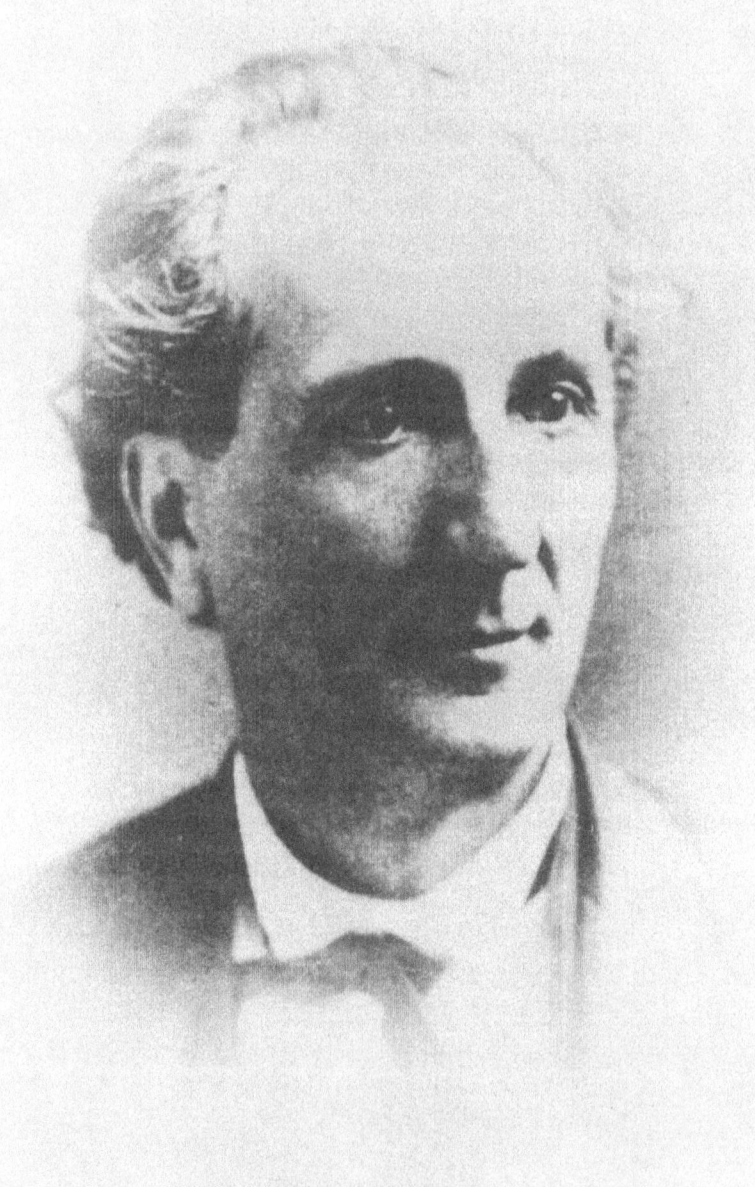

Jean-Charles Faget (1818-1884)
Faget's careful observation and measurement of the relationship between pulse rate and temperature in yellow fever cases gave rise to "Faget's sign" which he formulated in the 1870s, still useful in differential diagnosis. Courtesy Rudolph Matas Library, Tulane University Medical Center.

By 1880 the New Orleans medical profession generally accepted this judgment, except for two of the leading French creole physicians, Drs. Jean Charles Faget and Armand Mercier, who held fast to the old belief. Writing in the *New Orleans Medical and Surgical Journal*, Dr. Stanford Chaillé explained the change in medical opinion. Until 1858 New Orleans had suffered "almost biennial epidemics." Since that time only two serious outbreaks had occurred—in 1867 and 1878. "The longer the intervals between epidemics, the larger necessarily must be the number of those who have failed to acquire immunity, and the more glaring becomes their liability to the disease." Wherever the fever was an unusual occurrence, natives seemed as vulnerable to attack as anyone else; where the disease made frequent appearances, creole adults seemed generally immune—obviously because of mild attacks in childhood. With evidence from Cuba as well as New Orleans, Chaillé destroyed once and for all the old notion that becoming accustomed to the climate conferred any degree of immunity. He considered it "an abuse of language" to refer to yellow fever *immunity* as *acclimation* when the terms signified two entirely different processes.[38]

The Myth of New Orleans' Salubrity

Closely associated with the muddled concepts of acclimation, creole immunity, and the "floating population" was the belief in New Orleans' status as a healthy city relative to all others, despite its occasional epidemics. In the absence of accurate records, quantitative judgments were based on estimates that left considerable room for maneuver. Especially in the early decades of the nineteenth century, journalists, travelers, and other commentators often mentioned the impossibility of obtaining accurate and complete information on the city's mortality. Despite the lack of reliable records, the city directories, newspapers, and periodicals repeatedly insisted that the mortality of New Orleans was no greater than that of any large city anywhere in the world.[39]

From time to time the various temporary boards of health collected the burial lists from the city's cemeteries and published a report of the death count, but even then almost everyone acknowledged the problem of "imperfect data." Sextons of cemeteries were expected to keep registers of burials recording the details from each death certificate, required as a condition of interment. State legislation in 1848 establishing a new health board for New Orleans also provided that sextons could be fined for failure to supply detailed reports of all interments to the board. Enforcement was lax, however, and record-keeping remained haphazard and incomplete. Many burials recorded by the sextons were performed without the required certificates, and specific information (especially on nativity and age) needed for thorough statistical analysis was not consistently available.[40]

Dr. J. C. Simonds in the late 1840s decided to seek out the data to determine how the annual mortality of New Orleans compared with that of other cities. While attending a meeting of the American Medical Association in Boston, he had discovered that New Orleans was considered one of the unhealthiest cities in the country. He was also well aware that New Orleanians, on the contrary, believed their city one of the healthiest in the Union. Although Simonds had started with the idea of proving the city's claim through data analysis, he soon discovered that the "theory of the salubrity of New Orleans" would not hold up under careful scrutiny, even with the incomplete records that left many deaths unreported. The only way to prove New Orleans among the healthiest cities in the country, he said, was to "Throw out of the estimate of deaths those not native; if cholera, or yellow fever, or any other disease, cause many deaths, deduct these also from the calculation; but in comparing the remaining deaths with the population, do not even admit the correctness of the census, but add from twenty to fifty thousand for errors and floating population."[41] This procedure is essentially what boards of health, journalists, and other medical and lay spokesmen for local interests had been doing for some years, and would contine to do for many more.

Dr. Stanford E. Chaillé, writing in a New Orleans medical journal some twenty years later, in 1870, found it necessary to justify the study of vital statistics, to explain the benefits of statistical knowledge, and to outline in an elementary fashion for his medical readers some of the basic principles and common sources of error in comparing the health status of different locations. Carefully compiling his data from official records and reports, Chaillé argued that his calculations and tables proved beyond doubt

> . . . that New Orleans has been an unhealthy city not only during her epidemics, but also when free from them; not only extremely unhealthy from May to November, but also fails to attain the standard of a healthy death rate from November to May; not only unhealthy for foreigners, but

also for natives; not only for the whites, but also for the blacks; and not only for youthful manhood, but also for infancy alas! and for old age.

Only the "credulous inhabitants" of New Orleans believed it to be a healthy city.[42]

In the 1849 report of the New Orleans Board of Health, Dr. Edward H. Barton had admitted that the Crescent City suffered a mortality greater than any other city in the country, "mainly attributable to removable causes." According to his calculations, after subtracting the deaths from cholera and from causes other than diseases, the city's death rate for 1849 was almost six percent. He hastened to add, however, that a large number of deaths came from the "mass of floating population, not enumerated in the census," and not consistently recorded as such in the burial certificates as requested by the board. Even so, Barton believed the death toll was twice what it should be, and he strongly recommended the construction of drainage and sewerage systems and sanitary reform in general. "The removable causes of disease which afflict mainly the laboring population, hover like avenging angels over the heads of those in more elevated circumstances . . . ," he warned. *DeBow's Review* in an 1850 editorial referred to the convincing research of both Dr. Barton and Dr. Simonds and admitted that "We have been the last to yield assent to the proposition that New Orleans is an unhealthy city. . . . The facts are, however, against us."[43]

Although the 1849 report had offered many pages of data on the deaths among various categories of population in New Orleans (the first such effort at detailed tabulation of the city's mortality records), Dr. Simonds found much to criticize in its unwieldy organization, self-serving estimates and assumptions, statistical naivete, and numerous typographical errors and mathematical discrepancies. "If a board of health desired to mystify the facts and conceal the truth furnished by tables of mortality," he said, "it should carefully copy the example given in the tables accompanying the late report of our Board." Simonds pointed out the difficulties in trying to interpret the tables when the causes of death were presented in alphabetical order, an illogical arrangement that brought together dissimilar diseases and separated related ones. The problem was made worse by the lack of a standard nomenclature, as the tables simply listed the various causes of death recorded on the death certificates, many of which were provided by non-medical persons.[44]

Simonds also complained that the failure to organize and digest the details in the tables served only to "obscure the truth." The tables provided statements about some 244 diseases (including many synonyms for the same disease), occurring or not occurring among eight categories of persons (defined as adult or child and by race and sex), during each of the twelve months, making a total of more than 25,000 assertions, of which perhaps ninety percent were negative. For example, in September,

    Of *Jaundice* there died *no* white male adult.
       "   "   *no*   "   "   child.
       "   "   *no*   "   female adult.
       "   "   *no*   "   "   child.

And so on for each month, the number of deaths from each disease, under all its variant labels, was listed for male and female, black and white, adult and child, even when the number was zero. Yet nowhere in the report could one find, without "laborious calculation," the total deaths in a given month, the total number from a particular disease, the total mortality of children, or females, or blacks, and other matters of interest and importance. Simonds was exasperated with the board of health for presenting such valuable data in a form that could only "perplex and mislead those who may have occasion to refer to them." He also criticized the report for drawing erroneous conclusions from the data and failing to consider the population actually at risk in any given calculation. No effort was made to deal with age-specific rates or other population variables. In fact, the report did not even state the age used to draw the line between childhood and adulthood in the tables.[45]

The New Orleans board used the average age at death to show "expectation of life" without due regard for the age distribution of the population. Since New Orleans had a higher average age at death than "the northern cities," the report concluded that New Orleans was "much more favorable to infantile life," without taking into account the large proportion of New Orleans' population between twenty and forty years of age. The report also tried to show New Orleans in a favorable light by using the proportion of the total mortality caused by a particular disease as a basis of comparison between cities. Thus the board made it appear that New Orleans suffered less from lung disease "than any large city in this hemisphere" by its finding that tuberculosis caused a smaller proportion of the total mortality in New Orleans than it did in Philadelphia, New York, or Boston.[46] When the figures are expressed in terms of deaths per thousand population, New Orleans actually had a higher death rate from "consumption" than the northern cities. Tuberculosis claimed a smaller percentage of the total in New Orleans only because yellow fever and other diseases contributed so heavily to an annual mortality greatly exceeding that of other cities relative to population.

In an article published in the *Edinburgh Medical and Surgical Journal* in 1851, Dr. James Stark, a British physician, analyzed the 1849 report on New Orleans. Prior to its publication, he said, "we knew almost nothing of the mortality prevailing among the inhabitants of the southern cities of the American Union." Stark pointed out most of the same statistical flaws in the report that Simonds had noted, as well as certain "laughable peculiarities" and "curious anomalies" in the table of diseases, which made him "fear that pathological knowledge in that far-famed commercial capital is not in such a satisfactory state as it ought to be." The death rate of New Orleans he found to be about twice that of Philadelphia and three times that of Boston. Using figures derived from the report, Stark also concluded that New Orleans was a healthy place for blacks, but "preeminently unhealthy" for the white population.[47] During the antebellum years, with yellow fever a principal cause of mortality, the overall death rate of whites in the city at times greatly exceeded that of blacks.

Black Resistance

Black resistance to the scourge always perplexed and intrigued the medical profession. The contrast between yellow fever's effects in white and black populations was so great during the first half of the nineteenth century that many physicians considered blacks completely immune. From time to time some blacks did contract observable cases of the fever, but its effects were seldom severe. In his account of the epidemic of 1853 Dr. Erasmus Darwin Fenner stated: "It is a well established fact that there is some thing in the negro constitution which affords him protection against the worst effects of Yellow Fever; but what it is I am unable to say." Blacks came down with yellow fever as readily as whites in 1853, but few died of the disease. Fenner had observed that "the least mixture of the *white race* with the *black* seems to increase the liability of the latter to the dangers of Yellow Fever; and the danger is in proportion to the amount of white blood in the mixture."[48]

Dr. Samuel A. Cartwright, advocate of a specialized medical practice for the "peculiar" Negro constitution, advanced a timely theory in 1853 regarding yellow fever and race. Classifying yellow fever as a form of tropical typhus, Cartwright contended that the disease resulted from the violation of nature's laws:

> Nature scorns to see the aristocracy of the white skin—the only kind known to American institutions—reduced to drudgery work under a Southern sun, and, has issued her fiat, that here at least, whether of Celtic or Teutonic origin they shall not be hewers of wood or drawers of water, or wallow in the sloughs of intemperance, under pain of three fourths of their number being cut off.

Furthermore, he insisted, "Until this immutable law which has made the white race rulers . . . be properly respected, the deaths arising from its violation will continue to swell the bills of mortality, and to lead the world into the error that New Orleans is a most sickly location." Who were the prime sufferers from yellow fever? Northern emigrants, said Cartwright, who fell prey to an artificial complaint of their own creation. They produced the disease by their intemperate living habits and their "drudgery labor" in the hot summer sun. According to Dr. Cartwright, yellow fever in New Orleans occurred almost exclusively among those "unacclimated persons who attempt to jostle the negro from his stool, and to take from him those outdoor, laborious employments in the sun, wisely given to him as a precious inheritance to lift him up from brutish barbarism upon the platform of civilization, by forcing him to expand his lungs and oxygenate his blood."[49]

Although the epidemic of 1853 affected more blacks than ever before, Dr. Cartwright continued to support his race theory. Yellow fever fatalities that year among New Orleans blacks, in his judgment, resulted more from panic than from the disease itself. "A negro never dies with it in any locality, when treated with regard to his ethnical peculiarities; . . . even under mal-practice," he said, "death is the exception—and recovery the rule."[50]

Dr. Morton Dowler ridiculed Cartwright's view of a special methodology for the treatment of blacks. During the epidemic in 1854, Dowler had dealt with five cases of yellow fever among blacks. "I treated them without reference either to free-soilism or the ultraism of . . . Dr. Cartwright, who, whatever he may expect from the laity, cannot expect any medical man, be he fire-eater, unionist or abolitionist, to swallow his paradoxes with regard to negroes." Dowler described the case of a black woman whom he had treated "on the same principles I would have treated a golden-haired daughter of Japhet," and she had responded well and exhibited no ill effects from "white folks' diet" or the other usual treatment for Caucasians.[51]

When in the epidemic of 1867 yellow fever affected a large number of blacks, the *New Orleans Medical and Surgical Journal* cited that phenomenon as an unusual feature of the epidemic, "following the solitary precedent of 1853." Mixing a bit of Reconstruction politics with pathology, the editor commented, "We infer that this is one of the *civil rights* conferred on that fortunate class by the late enlightened Congress, of which they are already availing themselves."[52] Other southern communities in the postwar era also noticed a remarkable increase in yellow fever cases among blacks when freedmen moved from plantation to town and encountered the virus for the first time. In the widespread epidemic of 1878, thousands of blacks in New Orleans, Memphis, and other towns along southern waterways came down with yellow fever. The contrast between the races in case fatality rates, however, continued to show an unmistakable black resistance to the worst effects of the disease. Ninety percent or more of black cases survived. In some communities the white case fatality rate was as high as 70 percent.[53]

In the crusade against the yellow fever mosquito during New Orleans' final epidemic in 1905, when white health officials needed to enlist blacks in the city-wide effort, the lectures and appeals in black churches suggested that all persons were equally vulnerable regardless of race. And whatever they might have believed about their resistance to the fever, black ministers and other professionals participated in mobilizing black New Orleanians for the war against Yellow Jack.[54]

According to Dr. Charles Chassaignac, dean of the New Orleans Polyclinic and editor of the *New Orleans Medical and Surgical Journal*, the experience of 1905 clearly demonstrated that blacks were just as susceptible to yellow fever as whites but less likely to die from it. Mortality statistics from the areas around Tallulah, Louisiana, supported his conclusion: among ninety white cases, eighteen died; of 950 black cases, only five died. Patterson and vicinity reported about 500 white cases with fifty-one deaths, and 200 black cases with only one death. In New Orleans, blacks accounted for less than one-half of one percent of the total yellow fever mortality, while constituting more than 25 percent of the population. Attempting to account for the racial difference, Dr. Chassaignac admitted the possibility of a greater black resistance to the yellow fever poison after it entered the system, but he was more inclined to think that "the Negro" actually received a lesser dose of the infection in the first place because he was bitten less by the mosquito. "This may be due to his tougher skin," the doctor speculated, "or to the strong musky smell coming from his surface which may keep the mosquitoes away in a way analogous to that of pennyroyal and other strong scents which are used with that end in view."[55]

Although the specific genetic basis for black resistance to yellow fever remains uncertain, twentieth-century historical and epidemiological studies have suggested that the phenomenon is not surprising if one accepts Africa as yellow fever's place of origin. A population exposed to a killer disease over countless generations would either die off or develop some defenses against the effects of the virus through natural selection. Persons of African ancestry, in striking contrast to whites, historically have exhibited some innate resistance to the lethal effects of yellow fever—not absolute immunity but some defensive mechanism that enhances survival.[56]

Female Resistance?

Because of the remarkable preponderance of males among yellow fever victims, some physicians suggested that females also possessed an inherent resistance to the disease. Others devised an explanation based on the circumstances of the sexes in their daily lives. While women were confined largely to their households, men had greater exposure to the harsh elements of the weather and more opportunities for encountering yellow fever as they moved about the city and came in contact with a variety of persons and places. It was also postulated that men might be more vulnerable to the fever because they were generally more reckless and intemperate in their habits than women. Dr. Edward H. Barton stated that females constituted only one-seventh of yellow fever deaths in New Orleans during an eight-year period in the 1840s. He considered this statistical fact an argument in favor of temperance since women, unlike men, were "proverbially temperate everywhere."[57]

In the 1850s Dr. Elisha Bartlett in his volume on the fevers of the United States also observed that yellow fever epidemics always seemed to destroy more males than females. Because more males than females were always exposed to the disease, Bartlett was not yet persuaded that females enjoyed any special resistance. Most fatalities occurred among the immigrant populations in the southern yellow fever cities, and among immigrants men always greatly outnumbered women. While the number of male victims in port cities exceeded female fatalities, in several large inland towns with fewer strangers Dr. Bartlett at times had found females outnumbering males in the death toll from yellow fever. He did not reject the possibility that women might be less susceptible to the fever; he only wanted to show that the male population *at risk* was generally much more numerous than the female and to explain that absolute mortality figures alone could not warrant such a conclusion without further investigation.[58]

In his report as a district sanitary inspector in New Orleans in 1878, Dr. Joseph Holt pointed out that male fatalities greatly outnumbered female, "a curious fact" that could not be explained in terms of population composition since his district actually had more resident females than males. In 1880 Dr. Stanford Chaillé argued that what seemed to be a lesser degree of female susceptibility or a greater degree of resistance might best be explained by the circumstances of exposure.[59]

Sex-specific case fatality rates were seldom available, partly because of the lack of systematic reporting of cases, partly because mild cases were diagnosed or labeled as some other kind of fever or escaped attention altogether, and partly because the subject of sex-linked resistance probably attracted less interest than that of race differentials in morbidity and mortality. Specific information as to age, sex, race, ethnicity, and place of birth was hard enough for nineteenth-century statisticians to obtain for even a fraction of the deaths; for information on cases, estimates of numbers alone had to suffice. Hence, the question of female resistance to the disease remains open. There is some evidence, however, that females may actually possess a "superior immunocompetence."

Two medical researchers in 1979 summarized a "substantial" body of data supporting "the concept that X-linked immunoregulatory genes" play a major role in the "immunological superiority" of females. In their words, "Females have . . . superior ability to form antibodies to infectious agents, and experience a lower incidence of viral and bacterial infectious diseases." Although their work did not refer specifically to yellow fever, their findings are applicable, as they suggest a genetic basis for female "resistance to many disorders that are prevented or modified by immune responses."[60]

Privilege, Prejudice, and Theory

From one epidemic to another, yellow fever always evidenced considerable variation in the scope and intensity of its effects. Some strains of the virus may be more virulent than others. The number and density of human and mosquito populations as well as transportation technology are important determinants in the spread of the disease. Environmental, circumstantial, and demographic influences can account for much of the apparent group or individual susceptibility, with the exception of black resistance which does appear to have a genetic component, and possibly that of females as well. The connection between lower class whites, especially immigrants, and the prevalence of yellow fever had a real basis. The slum areas were located near the waterfront, and the laboring classes who worked on the docks usually contracted the first cases of yellow fever after its arrival on vessels from Latin America. When the disease gradually spread beyond its original focus of infection, the well-to-do of New Orleans, if not immune by prior attack, could be quite as susceptible when bitten by an infected mosquito as the lowest person on the socioeconomic scale.

At times, however, the antebellum pattern of yellow fever activity did indeed serve to reinforce the identity and cohesiveness of creoles as a privileged immune class. It seemed to support the superiority of the "better element" of New Orleans as well as the nativist prejudice against immigrants. The perceived patterns of the disease and its apparent selectivity of certain groups provided material for the medical proslavery argument (and the opposing position as well), the temperance movement, and the drive for middle-class order, regularity, prudence, and discipline. In the absence of a clearly demonstrable scientific explanation for the transmission of the disease, judgments related to social privilege and prejudice filled the vacuum. Medical theories reflected social attitudes, and each reinforced the other.

The widespread acceptance of germ theory in the 1870s and 1880s provided a different framework for theorists, but one that still related disease to filth and the lower orders of society. Pathogenic microbes replaced noxious effluvia, and germ-laden fomites (clothing, bedding, materials believed capable of absorbing and transmitting infection) were added to contaminated air, water, and soil as possible sources of disease. Much uncertainty remained regarding the precise means by which yellow

Susceptibility, Acclimation, and Immunity

fever could be transmitted from person to person and place to place. After 1878 yellow fever did not recur in epidemic form until the late 1890s, by which time the scourge was uncommon enough to cause great consternation. Fortunately for the large number of nonimmunes in the city, the disease appeared as a pale reflection of its earlier form.

By the 1880s the myth of creole immunity and the related theory of acclimation (or "creolization") had finally been laid to rest. The theory of black immunity had been refined to the more accurate concept of black resistance. During the outbreak of 1897 and the final epidemic of 1905, Italian immigrants became the new foreign scapegoats. The laboring poor in general were still considered more vulnerable to attack and less likely to recover than the better classes, probably an accurate observation since health status and standard of living are not unrelated.

Most New Orleanians by the end of the nineteenth century probably recognized that their city was not among the most salubrious, although some still argued its merits relative to the health of other American cities. Businessmen had become more concerned about the city's poor health reputation as an obstacle to population growth, capital investment, and commercial prosperity. Some medical theories had changed; some controversies had been settled; but other puzzles remained—soon to be solved by "the mosquito doctrine" which made possible the liberation of New Orleans and the South from the annual threat of yellow fever.

XII

THEORY AND CONTROVERSY: SPECIFICITY, GERMS, AND MOSQUITOES

The last third of the nineteenth century witnessed the articulation of germ theory, the development of laboratory techniques, and the bacteriological revolution that transformed the field of medicine. With a turn of the mental kaleidoscope the world of infectious diseases was redesigned and opened to new ways of exploration. The traditional historical, narrative, macroscopic investigation of disease had recounted observations of individual constitutions, environmental conditions, and all possible influences in constructing plausible explanations of epidemics. This approach would gradually give way to the new reductionist, microscopic, laboratory-centered, experimental, and statistical investigation of specific disease entities presumed to have specific causative microorganisms and specific modes of transmission.

The new ways of seeking etiological and epidemiological "truths" required conversion to the new faith, the acquisition of skills in experimental design and operational techniques, and adequate institutional resources for specialized equipment and supplies. Any astute medical practitioner could participate in writing the old natural history; the new science was not open to amateurs, but it soon won their faith in its "mysteries" because of its impressive achievements in the late nineteenth century.

In pursuing new paths and defining standards for experimental proof, scientists narrowed the arena for disagreement while increasing the technical complexity, but the necessity for judgment of skills and interpretation of results became more important than ever. Professional power and prestige were associated with the discovery of new truths. Such knowledge could have practical results in controlling disease, thereby saving great sums of public and private money as well as lives. Aside from the technical difficulties of evaluating, interpreting, or replicating research, scientists' initial judgments about the credibility of others' work, and their decisions about which questions and whose claims warranted attention, were sometimes influenced by ambition, jealousy, and pride; personal, institutional, or national rivalries; and the political and economic context in which they functioned.

Yellow fever with its submicroscopic virus and its specific timetable for transmission by one type of mosquito provided a more complicated puzzle to solve than many other major infections with more readily identifiable causative microbes and more obvious means of transmission. While Dr. Carlos Finlay correctly identified the mosquito vector of yellow fever as early as 1881, the work of this Cuban physician was virtually ignored by American and European researchers who were then preoccupied with the elusive yellow fever germ. As years went by some medical investigators came to believe (correctly, as it turned out) that yellow fever's cause was a submicroscopic entity not to be isolated by the instruments and techniques then available, and interest shifted toward investigating the means by which the causative agent spread from one case to the next. British and European work in the 1890s pinpointing a mosquito as the vector of malaria was one of the influences prompting Walter Reed and his colleagues in 1900 to add Finlay's hypothesis to their list of items to investigate in Cuba. The threat posed by yellow fever to the American troops in Cuba since the Spanish-American War (and to American expansionist interests in the Caribbean) provided both the stimulus and the opportunity for a major research effort sponsored by the U. S. Army. Finlay's theory was finally worth investigating. With the power and resources of the U. S. Army Medical Corps behind them, with Finlay's cooperation, and with new epidemiological information on the timing of yellow fever's progression from case to case, the Reed Commission was soon able to demonstrate that Finlay's mosquitoes were indeed the transmitters of yellow fever.

Competing Theories

In an 1870 publication Dr. Stanford E. Chaillé, professor of physiology and pathological anatomy at the University of Louisiana (later Tulane), remarked that scientific boundaries had to be greatly expanded "before the wearisome discussions of doctors can confer any substantial benefits on the public." Summarizing the yellow fever theories then competing for ascendancy, Chaillé listed three basic positions and a fourth representing the various possible combinations: (1) Yellow fever is both contagious and portable, spread by persons as well as fomites (clothing, baggage, and other materials by which germs were presumably conveyed from one place to another). (2) Yellow fever is portable but not contagious, spread by fomites but not by persons. (3) Yellow fever is neither portable nor contagious, transmitted by neither persons nor fomites, but the poison is sometimes present in certain localities where it affects those susceptible to its action. (4) Yellow fever may be produced by two different poisons, or by one poison producing variable results, depending on individual or atmospheric conditions; therefore, at various times, the disease may be contagious or portable or both or neither. Some physicians believed that an imported poison caused *epidemic* yellow fever and that a poison of local origin produced *sporadic* cases of the disease.[1]

Throughout the rest of the nineteenth century the subject of yellow fever continued to generate controversy, but several significant modifications occurred. As yellow fever spread throughout the South and the Mississippi Valley in 1878, the experience of inland communities along rivers and railroad lines left little remaining doubt about the portability of the disease. The infectious agent was now generally conceived to be a living microorganism (not yet identified), which could propagate itself, adhere to clothing, bedding, baggage, and other cargo, and be transported by these fomites and by infected persons as well. As least in some places in 1878, the effectiveness of a strict quarantine barrier had been clearly demonstrated.[2]

When four years during the 1880s and the first seven years of the 1890s went by without the appearance of yellow fever in New Orleans, it became harder to believe that the disease was in any sense indigenous. Proponents of quarantine claimed that the improved system of the Louisiana State Board of Health, which emphasized disinfection of ships and cargo, had protected the city and the region from the pestilence.[3] Various fumigants and disinfectants from the 1860s on became a standard weapon used by public health authorities as a shotgun in the dark against all infectious "poisons" or germs whether known or merely assumed, used to fight the invisible enemy believed to be lurking in the holds of ships, in cargo and baggage, in apartments and neighborhoods where disease had occurred, along streets and alleys, in gutters and privies. (Fumigation with burning sulphur would have killed mosquitoes in closed apartments and the holds of ships.)

In antebellum days health officials exploded gunpowder and burned tar in the streets with the hope of neutralizing "noxious effluvia" or counteracting the "epidemic constitution of the atmosphere"; after the war they generously applied carbolic acid, sulphur fumes, and other chemical compounds wherever the "germs" or "seeds" of disease were believed to be—again a matter of preventive practice determined by theory. Although the puzzles of yellow fever's etiology and epidemiology were yet to be solved, germ theory at least provided a map with more promise than miasmatic influences and epidemic constitutions, vague concepts that soon disappeared from medical discourse as their proponents were converted to the new beliefs, or eventually died off.

Germ theory (linked with methodological principles, technical precision, and refined instrumentation) emerged from the laboratories of Louis Pasteur, Robert Koch, and other European researchers. It was no less than a scientific revolution, a "paradigm shift." The introduction of this new explanatory framework found general acceptance within a large community of investigators and practitioners because it answered so many of their questions of greatest immediate concern, while other issues (chronic diseases) for a time faded into the background. Adoption of a new paradigm transforms the way the world is seen, gives meaning to "facts" previously overlooked, resolves the accumulation of anomalies not accounted for by old schemes, and points the way to further exploration, testing, and refinement of theory.[4] Once researchers have a "map" of sorts and know what they are looking for, they are more likely to find it. During the 1880s and 1890s skilled researchers in the new bacteriology (almost entirely European) isolated the specific microorganisms causing more than twenty major infectious diseases. By the 1890s it became clear that in some diseases the causative agents were too small to be seen with the microscopes then available. Known only by their disease-producing effects through inoculation, these entities were called filterable viruses because they could pass through filters that held bacteria.[5]

Although the new field of bacteriology led researchers and many practitioners to abandon traditional miasmatic concepts, the basic question of how persons contracted "yellow fever germs" remained a mystery as did the yellow fever germ itself, despite the efforts of researchers. The doctrine of direct personal contagion still had more medical opponents than advocates, but few after 1878 would challenge the belief that yellow fever was spread by fomites. Although the connection between any given case of fever and the source of the infection was not always clearly discernible, fomites provided the most plausible answer until the discovery of the mosquito vector in 1900.

Writing in 1880, Dr. Chaillé pointed out that the "poisons" of cholera, typhoid fever, and yellow fever were alike in being portable but not contagious, "being characterized apparently by the peculiarity that, while they come from a sick person, they yet require outside of the body, favorable conditions for further change or development, before acquiring any infective poisonous power."[6] He was correct in his observation. These diseases are not directly contagious but require a link or intermediary from one case to the next: the transmission of cholera and typhoid germs by food or water contaminated by germ-laden fecal matter from a sick person or a healthy carrier, and the transmission of the yellow fever virus from one host to the next through the bite of the *Aedes aegypti* mosquito. Within a few years after Chaillé's publication, the microbes causing typhoid fever and cholera were both isolated and their modes of transmission clarified. Yellow fever remained an enigma for years to come (despite Finlay's efforts), with its specific insect vector and precise timetable for the acquisition and transfer of the causative agent—a filterable virus, known only by its effects until the development of electron microscopy.

In a brief article on "Extra-Microscopic Organisms" also published in 1880, Chaillé stated that he had long favored germ theory as an explanation for yellow fever. Those opposing the theory with regard to yellow fever demanded that the specific germ be demonstrated with the microscope. But, according to Chaillé, there were reasons to believe in the existence of organisms so small that not even the most powerful microscope could reveal them. He thought such a belief "just as logical as the universal belief in extra-microscopic atoms and molecules."[7]

Specificity of Fevers

In addition to the age-old controversies about causation and transmission, now being transformed by germ theory, another closely related issue that had confounded medical philosophers until the 1870s concerned the very nature of yellow fever: was it a disease *sui generis* or was it simply one among a class of interrelated fevers? For centuries physicians had dealt with illness mainly in terms of superficial symptoms, viewing disease as a disordered condition manifested by a human body, a pathological response to environmental influences and inherited constitution. Diseases were not objectified as distinct entities, each with its own specific cause. Some ailments did indeed exhibit marked characteristics that made them easy to recognize and label, such as smallpox, bubonic plague, and venereal disease. Maladies not so readily differentiated included those producing high fever together with respiratory, intestinal, or nervous disorder, but without distinctive skin eruptions or other consistent features to set them apart from each other.

Dr. Benjamin Rush, the widely known American physician of the late eighteenth and early nineteenth centuries, opposed the European trend away from the unity of fevers, believing that the multiplication of diseases was "as repugnant to truth in medicine, as polytheism is to truth in religion." The physician who considers every different bodily disorder as a distinct disease, said Rush, is like "the Indian or African savage, who considers water, dew, ice, frost, and snow, as different essences; while the physician who considers the morbid affections of every part of the body (however diversified . . .) as derived from one cause, resembles the philosopher, who considers dew, ice, frost, and snow, as different modifications of water." To Dr. Rush, yellow fever was simply the most malignant form in the hierarchy of fevers believed to be produced by miasmata (noxious fumes from filth and decay). His lexicographer-epidemiologist contemporary, Noah Webster, also concluded that yellow fever was nothing more than a high grade of bilious fever.[8]

This view of yellow fever as the most malignant degree of a disease that assumed many interchangeable forms prevailed as the majority opinion throughout the first half of the nineteenth century. In 1817, Dr. Jabez Heustis described the saffron scourge of New Orleans as a "more aggravated degree of intermitting and remitting fever, . . . the grand climax of malignity, analogous in its origin and nature [to the other forms], and standing at the top of the same scale." All such fevers, he declared, were modifications of the same basic disease, differing only in strength. Furthermore, the forms were interchangeable; one type could develop into another or assume the prevalent form during an epidemic. Any observer who had ever witnessed this phenomenon and yet doubted the identity of fevers, said Heustis, "must be a skeptic in physics, and a disbeliever in the demonstrative evidence of his own senses."[9]

A few medical writers as early as the 1840s suggested that yellow fever was a specific entity, separate and distinct from all other fevers.[10] Most physicians, however, continued to believe that during an epidemic all forms of fever tended to merge into the most malignant grade, assuming the form of yellow fever.[11] In 1844 Dr. P. A. Lambert of New Orleans tried to classify the forms of epidemics as well as the types of yellow fever. In his construction, the epidemic forms included inflammatory, bilious, bilious inflammatory, mucous, putrid, and nervous, depending on the dominant symptoms characterizing the epidemic disease. As types of yellow fever, he included remittent, intermittent, and continued, categories based on the pattern of fever exhibited by an individual. Lambert said he did not intend to devise "an algebraic formula" for the application of his theory of types because variations were far too subtle to allow for such precision.[12]

According to Dr. Erasmus Darwin Fenner, one of the leading defenders of the doctrine of interrelated fevers, "the terms of *bilious remittent, yellow* and *typhus*, applied to the fevers seen in New Orleans, in the months of August and September, more properly designated *certain conditions of the system* produced by *a common cause*, or rather, certain stages of some general disease, than they do the existence of *diseases altogether separate and distinct* . . . ." He claimed that he had witnessed all the various types of fever exhibited in one individual during one illness.[13]

Although accepting the unity of fevers, Fenner disagreed with Rush and others who classified yellow fever as the highest grade of bilious fever. His experience convinced him that ordinary bilious fever at times could be more malignant than yellow fever without exhibiting the hemorrhagic tendency. To attribute the varied forms of fever to modifications of one basic cause was, in his judgment, "*certainly a more rational supposition than to attribute the various types of concomitant fever to the simultaneous action of separate distinct and specific causes.*"[14] Addressing himself to those who considered yellow fever a distinct disease, Fenner asked, "If you maintain that one of these types (yellow fever) is a disease *sui generis*, why not contend for the same in respect to intermittent, typhus, typhoid, remittent, bilious, congestive, malignant, pernicious, ephemeral, continued, gastric and solar fever. . . ?"[15] (Why not, indeed? From that list of fever "types," at least three in addition to yellow fever would survive as distinct diseases with specific causes and not merely descriptive labels: intermittent fever or malaria, typhus, and typhoid fever.)

Dr. Edward H. Barton, in the Sanitary Commission Report on the epidemic of 1853, stated that bilious, intermittent, and yellow fevers had been observed to "run into each other." As Barton and others perceived it, many cases began with the symptoms of intermittent or remittent fever but ultimately turned into yellow fever, terminating in black vomit and hemorrhagic activity; other cases initially exhibited signs of yellow fever but concluded favorably as the intermittent type. Barton attributed this convertibility of fevers to variable concentrations of the same cause and differences in individual susceptibility.[16] The perception of blending or overlapping diseases can perhaps be explained by the similarity of readily observable symptoms in yellow fever, malaria, and several other maladies, as well as the diversity of symptom patterns manifested in different cases of the same disease. It is also possible that some persons were suffering from more than one disease. Given the diagnostic framework in which "miasmatic fevers" were seen as a single category of disorders with variations in dominant symptoms and degrees of severity, it is not surprising that physicians interpreted their observations as blending symptoms and convertibility from one form of fever to another.

Although still in the minority, by the 1850s a few more physicians were beginning to view yellow fever as a specific entity, distinct from other fevers. Dr. A. J. F. Cartier, for example, called attention to what he considered fundamental differences between yellow fever and the intermittent fevers: Yellow fever conferred lasting immunity after one attack; the others did not. Although it might appear that diseases sometimes intermingled, yellow fever always disappeared as winter approached, while other fevers were not so clearly affected by the season. Yellow fever exhibited a different pattern of chills and fever, a continued type rather than intermittent. To Cartier, yellow fever was distinguished from all others by its own essential characteristics: yellowness, passive hemorrhage, and black vomit, symptoms not occurring together in any other known fever.[17]

Drs. T. A. Cooke of Washington, Louisiana; W. J. Tuck of Memphis; James Jones of New Orleans; and others also argued in the 1850s that yellow fever was a specific disease with a specific cause.[18] Cooke maintained that "the time is now approaching when many diseases now assembled into one group or family, considered mere modifications of a type, having a presumed identity of causes and similarity if not identity of nature, will take separate and distinct places in nosology."[19] In foreseeing the ultimate breakdown of symptom-complexes into distinct diseases, each with its own cause, Dr. Cooke was approaching the principle of specificity, which in alliance with germ theory in the late nineteenth century would provide a new foundation for medical science and public health practice.

From the mid-nineteenth century onward, the investigation of yellow fever became more "scientific," methodical, quantitative, reductionist, technical, and concrete; less philosophical, argumentative, "rational," speculative, and abstract. Instead of relying on traditional concepts and deductive structures, some medical thinkers, in Louisiana as elsewhere, began to delve into the particulars in the laboratory, employing methods first utilized on a large scale by French clinician-pathologists in the hospitals of Paris in the 1820s and 1830s.[20] Dr. Joseph Jones, for example, after returning to New Orleans from Europe in 1870, began a study of the yellow fever cases in his wards in Charity Hospital, undertaking a number of painstaking postmortem examinations. With the microscope, he made intensive studies of the blood, black vomit, urine, heart, brain, lungs, liver, spleen, and kidneys of the patients who died. He filled a research notebook with close descriptions of the cases, their symptoms, urinalyses, and comparative results of autopsies, including drawings of the various organ tissues under microscopic view.[21]

Jones believed that systematic, analytical laboratory research was necessary to extend the boundaries of knowledge relating to "this terrible scourge of tropical and sub-tropical America." Not until crude observations and hasty generalizations had been replaced by careful, accurate, quantitative, and comparative analysis, he said, could yellow fever's effects on the various organs of the body be understood.[22] His study of specific pathological features led him to conclude that yellow fever "differs essentially from the different forms of Malarial fever. . . ."[23] The confusion of fevers resulted mainly from the similarity of superficial symptoms. Probing beneath the surface disclosed fundamental differences in the effects of similar diseases on the organs and fluids of the body. The correlation of closely observed symptoms in living patients with postmortem studies of the same patients provided a firm basis for the concept of specificity and a better means of differentiating one disease from another.

Another Louisiana physician, Jean Charles Faget, investigated the specific action of yellow fever in relation to the patient's pulse and temperature. In the 1870s he delineated the phenomenon that came to be known as "Faget's sign," still cited in modern medical works as a clear indication of yellow fever, useful in differential diagnosis.[24] In the New Orleans epidemic of 1870 and the Memphis epidemic of 1873, Dr. Faget (with the aid of several colleagues) studied the action of the pulse and temperature in numerous cases and observed that the pulse rate did not increase with the rising temperature, as in other fevers. Instead, after an initial rapid ascent, the pulse gradually declined as the temperature went up. Faget declared this pattern to be one of the best ways to detect yellow fever in its early stages. He also contended that this peculiar sign demonstrated the specific nature of yellow fever, distinct from all other diseases, its "essential principle" being the effect on the heart.[25]

As early as the 1850s, Faget and at least two other French-trained physicians had independently noticed and commented on the declining pulse with rising fever as a peculiarity of yellow fever.[26] Their observations received little attention at the time. In the United States, measuring body temperature was not a common practice in clinical medicine until some years after the Civil War. When Dr. Just Touatre came to New Orleans in 1865, he brought a clinical thermometer with him. Years later he claimed to have been "the first in New Orleans to have used it for the study of the march of temperature in yellow fever during the epidemics of 1866, 1867, and the following ones." He also claimed to have been "one of the first to note the divergence between the pulse and temperature in yellow fever." But he agreed that Dr. Faget deserved full credit for establishing "the magnificent law which bears his name."[27]

While others had noticed the unexpected decline in pulse rate, until Faget's work in the 1870s, no one had systematically and repeatedly measured and recorded patient temperatures and pulse rates. Using a thermometer and a watch with a second hand, Faget charted the relationship between the progression of the two measures, described the results, and formulated a clear principle, a means of distinguishing yellow fever from malarial fevers. His work marked an advance in technical precision with the use of instruments and made a lasting contribution to theory and practice, offering persuasive evidence in support of yellow fever's specificity as well as a useful diagnostic rule.

In 1878 the members of the Orleans Parish Medical Society took a vote on several long disputed questions about yellow fever. Although no unanimity existed on any single position, the majority did agree that yellow fever was a specific disease caused by a microorganism and therefore not interchangeable with any other fevers.[28] As the germ theory steadily gained more adherents, the doctrine of specificity would replace the monistic theory of fevers. Nevertheless, there were always some who resisted conversion. In an address before the New Orleans Academy of Sciences in December, 1879, Dr. U. R. Milner paraded forth all the traditional conceptions of yellow fever's nature, causation, and transmission. Neither imported nor contagious, the fever was indigenous to the area, he insisted, and spread by "infectious gases" generated from animal and vegetable effluvia. Dr. Milner also persisted in believing that "The true yellow fever is the topmost grade in a regular ascension from the simplest intermittent. . . ."[29]

Germ Theory

The Louisiana State Board of Health did not officially "accept" the germ theory in explaining yellow fever until 1877.[30] Its annual reports, however, had included some earlier discussion of the hypothesis, and at least some of the board's members and inspectors had already been converted to the new faith in pathogenic microorganisms. The 1871 report had referred to a general belief among the medical profession that yellow fever was spread by "minute germs or spores" present in the air of a patient's rooms or adhering to clothing, bedding, carpets, or furniture. Many doctors, however, were still concerned about noxious effluvia. Admitting that the use of disinfectants was "empirical" and theories about their "mode of action" still open to question, the board argued that experience thus far justified the continued use of sulphurous acid gas and carbolic acid as a means of limiting the spread of yellow fever.[31]

In its report for 1878, the year of the worst epidemic of the postbellum years, the state board cautiously explained that disinfection was based on "the hypothesis that the *materies morbi* of yellow fever consists of living germs, probably animalcular." The germs were assumed to be "wingless animalcula," likely to travel on or near the ground. The *New Orleans Medical and Surgical Journal* in 1878 also stated in an editorial that "The more one studies the mode of progress of the yellow fever poison in epidemic visitations, the more likely he is to adopt the belief that it creeps along the surface of solid substances—probably by gradual growth and accretion." This hypothesis would explain "its steady, deliberate progress whether along with, or against atmospheric currents." It would also explain why yellow fever was "rarely communicable, except within the fatal circle of an infected locality."[32]

In the 1850s and 1860s, Louis Pasteur, a French chemist, with a series of remarkable laboratory experiments had clearly demonstrated that fermentation, putrefaction, and certain kinds of infection were all dependent on living, propagating microorganisms, present in the air but not the product of spontaneous generation, a doctrine which had persisted since ancient times. Proponents of spontaneous generation had previously argued that microbes were a *result* of the processes of decomposition and infection rather than a *cause*. Their position was less tenable after Pasteur's demonstration that microscopic life did not appear in fermentable liquid when it was sterilized by heat and protected against contamination by germs or spores in the air.

In the 1870s Pasteur and Robert Koch, a German physician and laboratory scientist, independently investigated anthrax, and other diseases of animals and humans, and in the process established the new field of bacteriology. Koch set the standards for identifying the causative agent in a disease ("Koch's Postulates"). It was necessary to isolate specific microorganisms from diseased tissue, grow them in a pure culture, use them to produce the disease by inoculating experimental animals, and recover the same kind of microbes from the diseased animals. Koch also introduced the use of solid media for cultures, developed staining techniques for microscopic specimens, and made other technical innovations that established the foundations for this new experimental science with so much promise for the medical field. Pasteur had broken new ground with his earlier work on the role of microbes in the making of wine and beer, the souring of milk, the putrefaction of food, and diseases of silkworms. In the 1850s, from his earliest work on fermentation, he had suggested that germs probably played a role in human diseases as well. In the 1870s he studied anthrax, confirming and extending the work of Koch and going on to develop the conceptual and experimental basis of immunology, first with a vaccine for anthrax, then for chicken cholera, and later for rabies. Using the concepts and techniques pioneered by Pasteur and Koch, bacteriologists in the 1880s and 1890s succeeded in identifying the microscopic agents responsible for most of the major infectious diseases of humankind.[33]

During these years only a few American scientists with European training were actively engaged in the laboratory search for the specific microbes that caused specific diseases—mostly young microbiologists in the Army Medical Department, the Department of Agriculture, and Johns Hopkins Medical School.[34] But many physicians and public health authorities seem to have accepted the theory in its broad outlines rather quickly, even before the impressive number of European discoveries in the 1880s, judging from official reports and articles in medical journals. Medical practitioners writing for medical periodicals still dealt mainly with clinical observations and the natural history of epidemics, still speculating and attempting to construct plausible accounts of "what happened." But now they had a new "belief," a doctrine with far greater explanatory power than miasmatic poison ever had, and a firm faith that in time the specific "contagium vivum" would be identified. In the meantime, disinfection made more sense than ever before.

Louisiana physicians continued to write many articles on yellow fever for the *New Orleans Medical and Surgical Journal* in the 1870s, and most subscribed to some version of the germ theory. Dr. S. S. Herrick, writing in 1875 on the past six years of New Orleans' experience with its peculiar disease, stated that "the *materies morbi* of yellow fever, not having been brought within range of our outward senses, has still to be studied solely by its effects. Accumulated observation of its mode of action tends to the belief that it exists in living germs, propagated rather without than within the human body." As evidence for this conclusion, he cited the apparent spread of the disease by infected materials, or fomites, but not directly by sick persons; the slow development of the disease from the original location; and the utility of disinfectants in limiting its spread.[35]

In 1879 the *New Orleans Medical and Surgical Journal* praised the work of the state board and the Citizens Auxiliary Sanitary Association in cleaning up the city. Although yellow fever was not a "dirt disease" like cholera, the editors pointed out, no one really knew how much influence filth might have in promoting the growth of the yellow fever germ. It had long been assumed that the germs adhered to surfaces when infecting a given area; hence, they argued, cleaning and scrubbing could be considered a "rational mode."[36]

Dr. John Shaw Billings, U. S. Army Medical Department, one of the leading figures in American medicine and public health, active in the American Medical Association and the American Public Health Association, and member of the National Board of Health, wrote an essay on yellow fever in 1880 for the *International Review*. He denied that yellow fever ever developed spontaneously from filth, moisture, heat, or whatever. Its cause, he said, may be a microorganism or the product of a living microbe, some entity with the capacity to reproduce itself outside the bodies of sick persons. According to Billings, "The great mass of the people agree with the old farmer that 'yellow fever can't go anywhere unless yer tote it.'"[37]

One of New Orleans' leading pathologists and microscopists, Dr. Henry D. Schmidt, would never be converted to the new doctrine; knowing more than the average practitioner, he was not so willing to accept the theory on faith. In an 1880 publication he summarized the current competing theories of infectious diseases: (1) the "gaseous" theory was concerned with the old miasmatic poison, a gaseous or molecular substance believed to emanate from decaying animal or vegetable matter or from the soil in certain areas; (2) the "glandular" theory postulated a poison produced by specific pathological changes in blood and tissues, caused by the absorption of this poison from a previous case into a person's system, which then gave rise to secretions with the poison's specific properties; and (3) the "contagium vivum" or germ theory dealt with certain minute organisms, believed to enter the body through the lungs, digestive tract, or wounds, and once in the blood, producing the symptoms of disease. Schmidt maintained that no positive proof yet existed for any of these theories with regard to yellow fever. The germ theory, he said, was especially popular with a considerable number of physicians, being more recently advanced. But he had found no satisfactory proof with his microscope that organisms in the blood or tissues were the cause of yellow fever. Schmidt supported the "glandular" theory that the diseased body itself produced the yellow fever poison, the result of "a modified or vitiated secretion," which emanated from the patient as minute protein-particles in vapor from the skin and lungs. Once introduced by inhalation or ingestion into the next subject, the yellow fever poison transferred its noxious powers to the patient's natural secretions. Schmidt also believed these hypothetical particles might stick to clothing, bedding, and walls.[38]

Mistaken Identities

The yellow fever germ continued to elude the microscopists who tried to track it down, but unlike Schmidt, other researchers did not reject germ theory on that account. Dr. George M. Sternberg, Surgeon, U. S. Army Medical Department, and pioneer American bacteriologist, went to Havana in 1879 as a member of the Yellow Fever Commission appointed by Congress to investigate the disease. His task was to study the yellow fever poison: was it a gas, a germ, or a vapor from the body? In a paper presented to the Louisiana State Medical Society in 1880, Sternberg offered the results of his Havana research: "there is no gross and conspicuous germ or organism, . . . either in the blood of yellow fever patients or in the air of infected localities, which by its peculiar appearance or abundant presence might arrest the attention of a microscopist and cause suspicion that it is the veritable germ of yellow fever." Nevertheless, Sternberg was willing to assume the existence of "microbes infinitely smaller" with "natures and properties" yet unknown, and he strongly believed that Americans should be investigating this subject as the English, French, and others were doing.[39] In 1881 the *New Orleans Medical and Surgical Journal* published a summary of the conclusions of the Havana Yellow Fever Commission, which had been chaired by Dr. Stanford E. Chaillé of New Orleans. Although not able to isolate the microbe, the investigators believed the yellow fever poison to be a living organism, capable of spreading and multiplying, but never the product of spontaneous generation.[40]

By the 1880s a large majority of the medical profession considered yellow fever an infectious disease caused by a specific "poison," the identity of which was still in doubt despite the claims of several would-be discoverers.[41] Various pathogenic microbes were "discovered" and identified as causative agent in an impressive number of major diseases during the 1880s and 1890s as the new paradigm was applied in the laboratory. The hunt was on, and the yellow fever germ was considered prime quarry. Several researchers claimed to have captured it, but each time other bacteriologists were unable to replicate the results and found flaws in the techniques or interpretations of the claimants.

Medical journals gave much attention to these controversies, which centered not on any disagreement with germ theory or the proper methods for proving one's case, but on matters of skill in performing the required techniques and judgment in interpreting the results. Applying "Koch's postulates" and obtaining consistent and unequivocal results was not as simple a process as it might appear to the uninitiated. Different researchers had different interpretations of the microscopic evidence. It was necessary to distinguish the specific causative microbe from the common bacteria present in the body, from a secondary infection of the weakened body, from a contaminant accidentally introduced into the blood sample, from the microorganisms of a decaying cadaver, and from the microscopic "debris" in diseased blood and tissues that could be mistaken for microbes.

Once isolated and cultured, the suspected microbe, when inoculated into an experimental animal, was expected to produce yellow fever. Interpreting symptoms in animals proved even more difficult than in humans. Yellow fever was never easy to diagnose, even during epidemics, since few cases exhibited all the "typical" symptoms, many mild cases exhibited none at all, and other infections can produce similar effects. Deciding whether "true" yellow fever rather than some other infection had been produced in an experimental animal (or person) was no simple matter. The search for the germ required access to yellow fever cases (living and dead) whose blood and tissues could be subjected to microscopic study. Between the outbreaks of 1879 and 1897, yellow fever was a scarce item in the United States. Hence, most of the research, whether by American, European, or Latin American scientists, had to take place where the disease was a common phenomenon—Cuba, Mexico, Brazil.[42]

The first two contenders for the honor of having found the germ of yellow fever came from the Latin American medical community, each publishing a lengthy account of his research claims in 1885 in the French language. Dr. Domingos Freire of Rio de Janeiro in a 650-page work entitled *La Doctrine Microbienne de la Fièvre Jaune* described his discovery of the yellow fever microbe, *cryptococcus xanthogenicus*, and his success in producing a preventive vaccine. Dr. Manuel Carmona y Valle of Mexico in a 300-page book nominated his yellow fever germ, *peronospora lutea*, and also claimed to have developed a preventive inoculation. The *New Orleans Medical and Surgical Journal* devoted an enormous amount of critical attention to these claims and to the proposal being considered by Congress in 1886 that a commission of American medical experts be sent to

Brazil and Mexico to evaluate the claims. The prospect of a protective vaccine against yellow fever had excited both physicians and laity and prompted Congressional interest in pursuing the matter. In a series of lengthy, acerbic critiques, however, the New Orleans medical editors insisted that there was nothing worth investigating further in the works of either claimant and strongly objected to the proposed commission as a waste of time and money.[43] Their negative judgment of both claims would eventually be confirmed by other laboratory investigators. Neither germ was yellow fever's cause; no protective vaccine had been found.

From their first review of Freire's book, the journal's editors pointed to many discrepancies in his work. They considered it imprecise, inexact, filled with hasty conclusions, and based on an inadequate number of experiments. Freire claimed to have found the microorganism in the blood of yellow fever cases with a microscope less than half as powerful as those used by the U. S. Yellow Fever Commission in Havana in 1879, which had *not* revealed this microbe in blood from undisputed cases of the disease. The editors found his research totally unconvincing, and in another issue a few months later, referred to Freire's germ as "Xanthogenic cryptocockeye."[44] Still another editorial declared Freire's claims "no less absurd" than that of two doctors in 1864 who supposedly had found that inoculation with "natural dew" would provide protection against yellow fever; or the alleged discovery by a Dr. Humboldt in 1853 that yellow fever could be prevented by vaccination with the venom of a certain Mexican snake.[45]

Nor did these New Orleans medical editors have any more confidence in Carmona y Valle, whose work they found "altogether opposed to sound logic and accurate observation." Although expressing support for the germ theory as the most plausible yet offered and hoping that a protective inoculation would eventually be developed, the editors stressed the necessity for caution and care in evaluating research claims. They noted that Carmona had dealt with only three or four actual cases of yellow fever, having had to rely on specimens sent from some distance, or on the observations of others. Careless handling could easily have introduced extraneous microbes into the materials. Although Carmona said his germ could be readily observed in all the organs and fluids of yellow fever victims, the editors in their own investigations had been unable to find it anywhere. A pathologist at Charity Hospital who examined a thousand preparations found a *peronospore* in only one liver-section, which he judged to be a fungus introduced inadvertently into the specimen. As proof of the protective power of his vaccine, Carmona described how he had inoculated more than a hundred persons who went from Mexico to New Orleans for the World's Exposition in 1884 and 1885 and not a single one contracted the disease. The *New Orleans Medical and Surgical Journal* pointed out that for months before and after the fair, not one case of yellow fever had appeared in New Orleans. Even if the infection had been present in the city, how, the editors asked, without the vaccine, did thousands of other visitors as well as New Orleans' resident population avoid the pestilence?[46]

Having read (in French) the 950 pages constituting the complete works of both men, the New Orleans medical editors declared them "utterly devoid of all scientific value" and considered it ridiculous to spend money to investigate further. They did suggest that one "competent bacteriologist" such as Dr. George Sternberg, already in government service as an army surgeon, might be sent to settle the questions at no additional cost. He could look for the germ again as he had done in Havana in 1879, and he should be allowed to stay "until he had satisfied himself either that he had discovered the pathogenic microbe and a method of protective vaccination, or that these were not to be discovered by any of the means and methods at present known to science."[47]

Congress finally decided against creating a commission, and Sternberg was given the assignment in 1887—much to the delight of the New Orleans editors. After a sojourn in Brazil and Mexico, in 1888 Sternberg successfully demolished the claims of both Freire and Carmona y Valle. He continued his research in Havana in 1888-89, and while he did not achieve a positive identification of the yellow fever germ, Sternberg did demonstrate that most of the microorganisms he encountered in culture experiments, as well as those "discovered" by other researchers, were *not* the cause of yellow fever. This was "negative research" that failed to elicit public enthusiasm, but it was necessary and valuable work. One microbe isolated from the intestines, which Sternberg called *bacillus x*, met some of the conditions, but the results of animal experiments were inconclusive. Still he believed that this particular germ might be worth further investigation.[48]

After Sternberg's exhaustive studies, some measure of caution prevailed and not until 1897 was the discovery of the yellow fever microbe again proclaimed, this time by a well-trained, highly respected European microbiologist, Professor Guiseppe Sanarelli of the University of Bologna, who had been studying yellow fever in Montevideo, Uruguay. He reported his discovery of the causative agent, which he called *bacillus icteroides*, in the prestigious *Annales de l'Institut de Pasteur* published in Paris. This claim was more readily acceptable on faith by the medical profession than previous assertions largely because of the source and setting, Sanarelli's reputation and the prestige of the Pasteur Institute. But the discovery was still open to dispute among laboratory scientists for many reasons having to do with the complexity of the research, the difficulties in reproducing (and interpreting) results, and the potential for diagnostic disagreement in deciding whether the disease had actually been produced in experimental animals. Sternberg expressed doubts almost immediately, although he suggested that *bacillus icteroides* might be the same as his own *bacillus x*. He was now Surgeon-General of the Army, and he proceeded to assign some of his research men—Walter Reed, James Carroll, and Aristides Agramonte—to investigate the claims of Sanarelli. They found that Sanarelli's germ and the *bacillus x* were two entirely different microbes, and they all raised serious questions about the validity of Sanarelli's work.[49]

Other bacteriologists arrived at different conclusions. Drs. Paul E. and John J. Archinard of New Orleans, both bacteriologists employed by the Louisiana State Board of Health, claimed that they successfully isolated the *bacillus icteroides* in thirty-two of thirty-nine yellow fever cases, a higher percentage than Sanarelli himself had been able to achieve. By Koch's standards, however, *the* causative agent should have been present and recoverable in *every* case. Dr. Walter Wyman, Supervising Surgeon-General of the U. S. Marine Hospital Service, sent two of his officers, Drs. Eugene Wasdin and H. D. Geddings, from New Orleans to Havana to continue their yellow fever studies and to evaluate Sanarelli's findings. Their research, published in 1899, seemed to confirm Sanarelli's *bacillus icteroides* as the cause of yellow fever and to deny any role to Sternberg's *bacillus x*, which they found in the intestinal tract of healthy animals and humans and in other secretions as well. After reviewing the conflicting positions, the editors of the *New Orleans Medical and Surgical Journal* decided that the "weight of opinion" seemed to be leaning toward Sanarelli, and the "burden of disproof" was assigned to Sternberg and his associates.[50]

Extrensic Incubation Period

The controversy continued, and bitter words passed back and forth between Sanarelli and the Sternberg team. Whichever side was right, no practical results were immediately in view, no dramatic cures or demonstrably effective immunization procedure or new methods to prevent the spread of the disease. Even for those physicians who accepted the Sanarelli microbe as yellow fever's cause, nothing had really changed in practice. Other questions attracted attention; other puzzles remained. Dr. Just Touatre of New Orleans, in his "clinical notes" published in 1898, observed that yellow fever always took a long time to propagate itself after the introduction and appearance of the earliest cases. "The day that we know how and where the germs of Yellow Fever develop outside of the patient," he wrote, "a great advance will have been made in protective sanitation." While accepting Sanarelli's bacillus as the probable cause of yellow fever, Touatre thought it necessary during the next epidemic to search for that microbe in the mud and filth of the streets and gutters "to determine the dens of this terrible enemy." From a study of New Orleans' past thirty-three epidemics, he had concluded that the first imported cases of the disease did not immediately or directly produce the epidemic, but they apparently carried the seeds, probably Sanarelli's bacilli. These germs were believed to emanate from the patient's body, and they seemed to need some appropriate outside medium for propagating before they could produce more cases of the disease. Touatre suggested that the "favorable culture medium" might be the mud in streets and gutters warmed by the sun.[51]

Dr. Henry Rose Carter, U. S. Marine Hospital Service, had also noticed a time lag between the appearance of the first cases in a community and the development of secondary cases, usually from two to three weeks. He had been observing and recording this phenomenon since 1887. In 1898 he had an opportunity to do a precise epidemiological study in two small farm communities in Mississippi, Orwood and Taylor, where he was able to gather information on the chronology of specific contacts between various households and the later appearance of yellow fever cases. He wanted to determine wherever possible the time interval between the arrival of the first case of fever in a house and the development of secondary cases in that house and among persons thereafter exposed to the infected environment. From these studies Carter documented what he called the "extrensic incubation period," the interval between the appearance of an "infecting case" and the capacity of the house environment to convey the infection to a resident or a visitor. Persons visiting the house only in the early days of the patient's illness did not contract the disease, whereas those who were there about two weeks later became ill with yellow fever within a few days. Carter concluded that at least two weeks were required for the germs to develop outside the body of the "infecting case" before exposure to the house environment could produce infection in another person.[52] These observations would prove of great value to Walter Reed and the other members of the U. S. Army Commission in Cuba in 1900 as they began to focus on the mosquito as a possible transmitter of yellow fever. The "extrensic incubation period" provided an indispensable clue to the importance of a time lapse between the mosquito's first biting a yellow fever patient and its ability thereafter to transmit the infection when biting a susceptible subject.

From Insect Hypothesis to Mosquito Doctrine

For more than a hundred years before the Reed commission transformed the "insect hypothesis" into the "mosquito doctrine," medical and lay observers had often commented on the extraordinary numbers of mosquitoes present during yellow fever epidemics, and some had suggested a causal relationship. Dr. Benjamin Rush noticed during an epidemic in Philadelphia in 1797 "that mosquitoes were more numerous during the prevalence of the fever than in 1793." But he had also seen more ants and cockroaches as well. Dr. John Vaughan, writing about the epidemic of 1802 in Wilmington, Delaware, mentioned the "Myriads of mosquitoes" that infested those areas of town where the fever was most virulent.[53]

The report on the New Orleans epidemic of 1819 published by *La Société Médicale* found it noteworthy that both flies and mosquitoes had been much more numerous than in previous years. Benjamin Latrobe recorded in his journal that "This year 1819 is said to have been by far the most remarkable for mosquitoes within the memory of man." Louisiana would be one of the "most delightful" places in the world, he wrote, "were it not for the mosquitoes. I say nothing of the yellow fever, because I believe that this calamity may be moderated, if not entirely eradicated, by a good medical policy. . . ." Latrobe went on to write several pages on the subject of New Orleans' mosquitoes, "so important *a body* of enemies" that they received much attention in conversation, influenced the use of time, and served as a source of discomfort to all, especially from June until frost. He described four kinds of mosquitoes he had seen, one of which was obviously the *Aedes aegypti,* "the legs . . . ringed with white, like the tail of a racoon." Mosquito bars of canvas, linen, silk, gauze, or muslin, covering the bed from the tester to the floor, provided some protection while sleeping. Latrobe also recounted that some of his friends, "lawyers, & other studious men, put up in their offices a kind of safe, or frame covered with gauze, . . . large enough to contain a table & chair, & write till late at night in perfect security." Astutely observing that the common breeding places for most of the house mosquitoes were pitchers, small vessels, and the casks and wells of rainwater, Latrobe believed that the pests would be virtually eliminated once the city had piped water.[54]

In an account of his travels in the 1840s, Sir Charles Lyell, the noted geologist, quoted what a captain of a Mississippi steamer told him about New Orleans mosquitoes: "That they who are acclimatized, suffer no longer from the bites, or scarcely at all, and even the young children of creoles are proof against them. . . ." Others had also informed him that "when people have recovered from the yellow fever, the skin, although in other respects, as sensitive as ever, is no longer affected by a mosquito bite . . . ."[55] According to Dr. Bennet Dowler, in his "Researches into the Natural History of the Mosquito," scientific observers agreed with popular opinion that mosquitoes exhibited "partiality" for the blood of strangers. Whatever the reason, he said, mosquito bites obviously produced more pain and swelling in newcomers than in the native-born. Dowler also quoted a geographer who believed that mosquitoes were nature's warning in areas subject to disease, that they signified "a state of air injurious to health—the prevalence of bilious complaints and the yellow fever." Dowler was also aware that some persons considered any increase of mosquitoes as a "certain prelude" to a yellow fever epidemic, although he disagreed, pointing out that the disease had been known to occur in places where mosquitoes were not common.[56]

Prior to and during the Great Epidemic of 1853, New Orleans newspaper editors repeatedly offered wry comments on the severity of the mosquito problem, worse than ever before.[57] In 1854 yellow fever struck again, and on November 1, one New Orleans resident wrote in his diary that the epidemic showed little signs of abatement; "no indications of cold weather yet, and the mosquitoes are cruel as ever." Inspired by a clever thought, he added that the mosquitoes were "nature's homeopathic 'cuppers and bleeders'—provided to reduce that redundancy of blood which in a hot climate, might take a febrile direction."[58]

In 1848 Dr. Josiah C. Nott of Mobile published an article rejecting the miasmatic doctrine of fevers and suggesting that the cause of yellow fever was some form of insect or animalcular life. The hypothesis of insect life as a cause of disease was not entirely original, he admitted, having been offered by various writers in the past, but Nott proposed to apply the concept specifically to yellow fever. In the hot and humid regions, the prevalent fevers had long been attributed to the rapid decomposition of vegetable and animal matter. Another common feature of such regions, he noted, was a plethora of insect life and "infusoria" (all microscopic animalcula present in fluids and in the air). Nott believed the insect theory could resolve some of the doctrinal conflicts and provide a far better explanation of the natural history of yellow fever than the "gaseous or molecular" emanations had ever been able to do. "It would certainly be quite as philosophical . . . to suppose that some insect or animalcule, hatched in the lowlands, like the mosquito, . . . wings its way to the hill top to fulfil its appointed destiny." The apparent intensity of yellow fever's morbific cause at night might be accounted for, he said, by the habits of certain insects that are most active at night, such as moths, night mosquitoes, and many others.[59]

In another paper on yellow fever, prepared in 1870 for the New York Metropolitan Board of Health, Nott remarked on the possibility "that even insects may exist a million times smaller than any the microscope has yet reached." Although the "slow and steady progression" of yellow fever could not yet be fully explained, he believed that it had to be caused by some kind of living organism—possibly insect or fungi. "Moreover, it is the business of some insects to distribute certain seeds of plants far and wide; to carry the pollen of one plant to another to fructify it; and it may be the duty of others to disseminate diseases," he suggested. In Mobile, New Orleans, and other southern towns that commonly suffered from great swarms of mosquitoes, Nott had often noticed that light-skinned strangers from a colder climate, especially children, were painfully afflicted by the bites of these insects, while native-born children went relatively unscathed; "they seem to become acclimatized against the poison of these insects," he said, "as they do against the poison of yellow fever."[60]

Other observers, such as Dr. Louis Daniel Beauperthuy of Venezuela in the 1850s and Dr. Greensville Dowell of Texas in the 1870s, focused more specifically than Nott on the mosquito as a probable source of yellow fever. All these suggestions, however, remained in the realm of natural history and speculation, until Dr. Carlos Finlay of Cuba in the 1880s began to experiment with mosquitoes and human volunteers in an attempt to transmit the germ of yellow fever, as yet unidentified but generally assumed to exist.[61] Not until experimental proof became the normal procedure for scientific verification of hypothesized relationships was it conceivable that experiments such as Finlay's would be attempted. While he was on the right track, his experimental results were inconsistent and failed to persuade North American and European scientists that the hypothesis was worthy of attention.[62]

Dr. Finlay had begun his investigations in 1879, and in August, 1881, he presented the preliminary results to the Royal Academy of Medical, Physical, and Natural Sciences of Havana. His paper was entitled, "The Mosquito Hypothetically Considered as an Agent in the Transmission of Yellow Fever." Having previously worked on a theory relating alkalinity in the atmosphere to yellow fever epidemics, he concluded that all such theories of atmospheric, miasmatic, climatic, and unsanitary influences were inadequate to explain the anomalies and vagaries of yellow fever. Assuming that a material substance, germs or whatever, had to be transported from one case to the next, Finlay then decided to focus on the intermediary, the agent by which the "pathogenic material" of yellow fever was transmitted. It was necessary to select an organism affected by variations in heat, cold, and altitude in ways similar to yellow fever; some kind of insect seemed probable. Because yellow fever produced major alterations in the blood, it occurred to Finlay that the mosquito might acquire the germs along with its blood meal when biting a yellow fever patient and inject those germs with its "lancet" when biting another person, thus spreading the disease.

After a careful study of the mosquitoes of Cuba, Finlay settled on the *culex* (later known as *stegomyia*, now as *Aedes aegypti*), because it was known to bite several times during its brief lifetime and because its features and habits matched other conditions associated with yellow fever. Using these mosquitoes, Finlay tried to transmit the disease from yellow fever patients to several volunteer subjects and to himself. Of the five experimental cases in his initial report, he described one as "benign" yellow fever, two as "aborted," and two as "light ephemeral." He believed it might take more than one mosquito bite to produce a typical case of the fever.

Cautiously advancing his theory and outlining his experiments, Finlay recognized that more research was required, and he expressed hope that others would join the effort. He believed the evidence supported his theory but knew that "an irrefutable demonstration" would be necessary to win support for such a radically different concept.[63]

Translated from Spanish to English by Dr. Rudolph Matas, Finlay's research report appeared in the *New Orleans Medical and Surgical Journal* only a few months after its original presentation in 1881 to Havana's scientific academy.[64] In 1884 the *Journal* published an extract from another of his papers in English translation, and in 1886, an abstract of his article which had appeared in the *American Journal of Medical Sciences*. Finlay described his continuing experiments with the *culex* mosquito and human subjects, attempting to clarify the transmission process but with inconsistent results. He had applied each mosquito to a yellow fever patient on the third to the sixth day of the illness and two to five days later allowed each one to bite a different volunteer who was believed to be susceptible, not having previously had a recognized attack. A few of these subjects exhibited what Finlay diagnosed as "mild attacks" but not always within the commonly accepted incubation period, and almost half of his subjects displayed no symptoms whatsoever but later seemed immune. Despite the difficulties, Finlay remained convinced that this mosquito was the principal agent of transmission. He knew that the disease failed to spread in locations lacking tropical mosquitoes and that cold temperatures or high altitudes halted mosquito activity as well as the spread of yellow fever. In 1886, the editors of the New Orleans journal commented favorably on Finlay's work as worthy of attention and agreed that "a great deal of plausibility attached to his conclusions. . . ."[65] But, until 1900, no American or European scientist accepted his open invitation to join the research effort or took his work seriously enough to investigate further.

Despite having found the key element in yellow fever's transmission process, Finlay was unable to get clear results because of the crucial importance of *timing* for the mosquito's ability to acquire and to transfer the virus from the sick to the healthy. Only in the first two or three days of illness is the virus sufficiently concentrated in the patient's blood so that a mosquito can ingest it with a blood meal. Finlay had his mosquitoes biting the patients from the third to the sixth day of the fever when most of them could no longer infect the mosquito. The other matter of timing involves the interval of at least ten to fourteen days required before the ingested virus reaches the mosquito's salivary glands, after which time the mosquito is able to inject the virus while taking another blood meal.

Most of Finlay's mosquitoes—including those that might have bitten a patient early enough to acquire the virus—were set upon the healthy subjects within two to five days after biting the sick, long before sufficient time had elapsed for the mosquito to become infective—that is, to have the virus in its saliva. Clinical diagnosis of yellow fever was always problematic. Many true cases manifest no visible symptoms, and some of Finlay's subjects could have been immune from a previous inapparent case. In spite of his equivocal results and lack of recognition, Finlay held firm to his belief and persisted in his work, conducting mosquito inoculations of human subjects more than one hundred times in a twenty-year period, publishing dozens of papers in several different languages. He argued his case again and again without winning any measurable support for his theory, and sometimes he was viewed as "a crank."[66]

His formulation of the original hypothesis, however, was a brilliant achievement based on intense observation, intuition, and reasoning, and he deserves more credit than he has generally received. Unlike his predecessors in the "insect" arena, Finlay conceived of the mosquito as the link between each fever patient and the next case, not as a signal or a byproduct of the atmospheric conditions causing disease, or as a source of the poison like a snake produces venom, or as a carrier of germs acquired from polluted waters. Finlay's theory was essentially different. While his own experiments failed to achieve that "incontrovertible demonstration" he knew to be necessary, in 1900 the U. S. Army Commission in Cuba, with far greater power and resources, applied his theory, working with the *culex* ova supplied by Finlay himself along with copies of all his publications. The American research team quickly obtained experimental results that verified (and clarified) the transmission theory.

Surgeon-General Sternberg had sent this group of medical officers to Cuba in 1900, when the disease was prevalent among the American occupation forces, instructing them to "give special attention to questions having to do with the etiology and prevention of yellow fever." Their first task, as they saw it, was to search again for the Sanarelli germ, widely accepted as the cause of yellow fever, especially since the U. S. Marine Hospital Service report of Wasdin and Geddings in 1899 had confirmed it— or so it seemed. With forty-eight separate cultures from the blood of living patients and from the blood and organs of yellow fever cadavers, examined in more than a hundred preparations in agar plates and tubes of bouillon, not once did the Reed Commission find Sanarelli's *bacillus icteroides*. It must have been a contaminant or a secondary invader in the other experimental demonstrations. Rather than continuing the hunt for the yellow fever germ, the Army researchers then decided, after careful consideration of available data, to study the mode of transmission or propagation of the disease. Testing Finlay's theory was the obvious place to begin.

Walter Reed and his team had developed serious doubts about the power of fomites to convey the disease, as they observed nonimmune hospital attendants failing to contract the disease despite their constant handling of bedding and clothing soiled by patients. The research team decided to try to transmit the disease to susceptible human volunteers (1) by mosquito inoculation, (2) by hypodermic injection of blood from a patient, and (3) by exposure to fomites. As an important consideration in turning to the mosquito theory and for suggesting the necessary time lapse in the transmission process, Reed later credited Dr. Henry R. Carter's work on the "extrensic incubation period," readily applicable to an intermediate host such as the mosquito. Another recent discovery also influenced the commission to give serious attention to Finlay's mosquito; by the late 1890s the investigations of Ronald Ross, a British medical officer in India, and G. P. Grassi, an Italian zoologist, and others as well, had elucidated the role of the *Anopheles* mosquito in the transmission of the parasite that caused malaria, one of the world's major diseases.

After mosquito inoculations produced *two* "well-marked" cases of yellow fever among their first eleven trials with human subjects, the Army research group presented a "preliminary note" to the meeting of the American Public Health Association in October, 1900. By this time, one of their number, Jesse Lazear, had died from yellow fever, having been bitten by an infected mosquito. After the initial results, an experiment station was established, relatively isolated and carefully quarantined from outside contact, and the researchers continued their experiments in Cuba with human subjects, including recent immigrants from Spain (nonimmunes already at risk and attracted by a monetary reward) as well as volunteers from the U. S. troops. The researchers made every effort to ensure that their subjects could not have been exposed to yellow fever outside the confines of the particular experiments—which Finlay, lacking their resources, had not managed to do.

From December, 1900, through early February, 1901, the investigators succeeded in producing yellow fever by mosquito inoculation in ten of thirteen cases attempted. They had discovered that at least ten or twelve days had to elapse after the ingestion of infected blood by the mosquito before it had the power to convey the infection when biting a nonimmune person. They also succeeded in producing yellow fever in nonimmunes by the subcutaneous injection of blood drawn from a patient in the first two days of the disease. The Army researchers found that even when filtered to remove bacteria, blood samples from yellow fever patients retained the infective power when inoculated into another person. Therefore, they set forth the hypothesis that the cause of yellow fever was a "filterable virus" of ultramicroscopic dimensions. Although several more germs were proclaimed as yellow fever's cause within the next two decades, and at least one was a serious contender, the commission's assumption of a submicroscopic entity (a virus) would ultimately be confirmed. Commission members were unable to propagate the disease in a single instance by fomites, although they confined their subjects for an average of twenty-one days to an area screened against mosquitoes and supplied with bedding and garments recently used by yellow fever victims and soiled with excrement and vomitus. The Reed team possessed first-rate experimental skills, but it was Finlay who had provided the theory as well as the targeted mosquito. Knowing where to look saved much time. The initial reports of the commission's work gave Finlay "full credit" for the general theory that their experiments confirmed and refined.[67]

What seemed so clear to the researchers themselves was not entirely convincing in all its particulars to practicing physicians and public health officials. Disinfection had become a standard practice and sometimes seemed effective in limiting the spread of disease. While willing to accept the fact that yellow fever had been experimentally transmitted by the mosquito, most physicians were reluctant to believe that it was the *only* way or even the typical manner by which the disease spread in the world. One Ohio physician wrote: "Does any one imagine, for a single instant, that the destruction of the whole mosquito tribe, that is beyond the realm of human possibility, would result in the disappearance of malaria and yellow fever? For ourselves, we see no science in these experiments, much less common sense." As usual, the editors of the *New Orleans Medical and Surgical Journal* urged caution regarding the acceptance of "newly found truths."[68]

More convincing than the experiments themselves was the practical application of the mosquito doctrine by William C. Gorgas, Army medical officer in charge of sanitation in Havana. In 1901, through a systematic campaign to reduce the mosquito population, Gorgas was able to bring yellow fever under control within a few months in a city long noted as a focus of the disease. He would go to Panama in 1904 to perform the same service, facilitating the American construction of the Canal.[69]

Despite these dramatic results, many were still not entirely persuaded. Although the Louisiana State Board of Health expressed some reservations, New Orleans' health chief, Dr. Quitman Kohnke, accepted the theory immediately and attempted to stir New Orleans to action against the mosquito, but he encountered an uncooperative city council and a resistant public. Overcoming their original misgivings about the claims of the Reed Commission, the editors of the *New Orleans Medical and Surgical Journal*, in 1902, 1903, and 1904, stressed the need for a city ordinance requiring that cisterns be screened and other measures employed to eliminate the yellow fever mosquito. But as long as no cases of yellow fever were present in the city, it was difficult to arouse a public that was largely ignorant of the new theory, or at least indifferent or skeptical, as were some physicians. The *Journal* editors urged the medical profession, through the state and local societies, to take responsibility for educating the public on the role of the mosquito and the importance of ridding the city of these carriers of disease. They also called on the press for assistance in spreading the message.[70]

The president of the Louisiana State Medical Society in his annual address in 1905, prior to the surfacing of the last yellow fever epidemic, discussed the new discovery and declared it the duty of the society's members to "preach the gospel of the mosquito peril and the crusade for his extermination." Doctors and laity, he said, must take up the task and continue until "all unbelievers are converted."[71]

When yellow fever once again struck New Orleans in 1905, the combined efforts of local, state, and national health officials, assisted by journalists, the clergy, and other local leaders, succeeded in mobilizing the New Orleans public for a campaign against the mosquito as a means of halting the epidemic. The successful crusade provided a propaganda victory for scientific medicine and public health practice. Not until yellow fever had been banished from the United States after 1905, and kept out by quarantine and other protective measures based on the mosquito doctrine, was there anything resembling general agreement on the cause and transmission of one of the most controversial diseases in medical history. Other puzzling and threatening facets of this virus and its close relations and their *modus operandi* would continue to arise in years to come, and some remain to this day.[72]

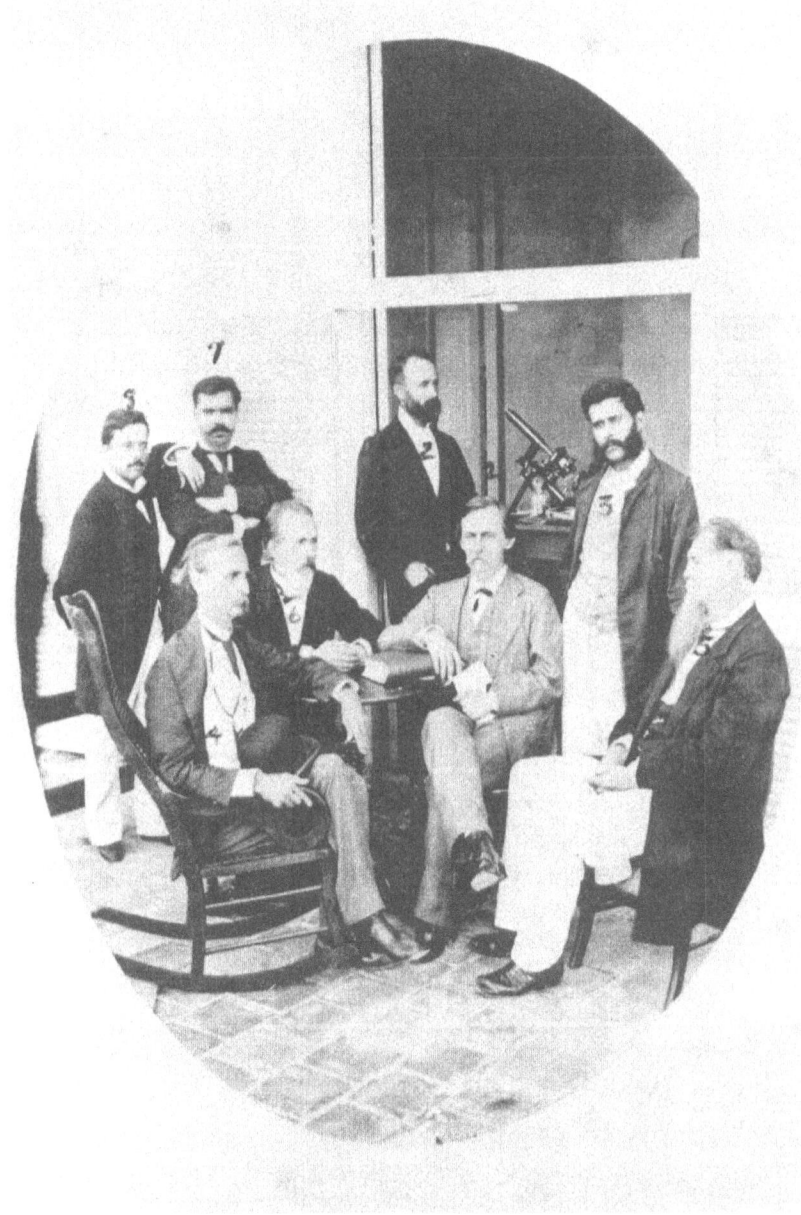

Yellow Fever Researchers
Yellow Fever Commission of the U. S. National Board of Health in Havana, Cuba, August 1879. 1. Stanford E. Chaille, chairman. 2. George M. Sternberg, secretary, bacteriologist. 3. John Guiteras, pathologist. 4. Thomas S. Hardee, sanitary engineer. 5. Daniel M. Burgess, U. S. Sanitary and Quarantine Inspector at Havana. 6. Henry C. Hall, U. S. consul general at Havana. 7. Rudolph Matas, medical clerk. 8. Abraham Morejon, assistant medical clerk. Courtesy Rudolph Matas Library, Tulane University Medical Center.

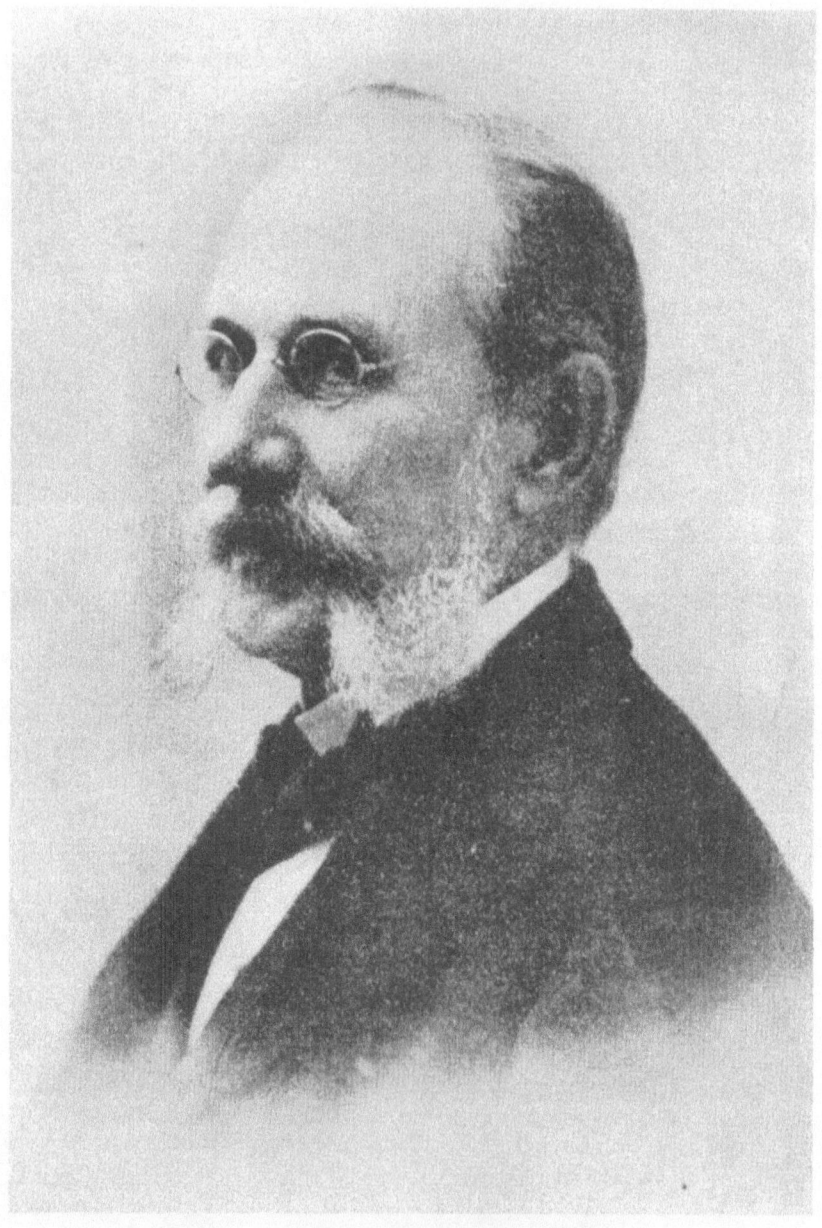

Carlos J. Finlay (1833-1915)
Cuban physician who first theorized that the *Aedes aegypti* mosquito was the transmitter of yellow fever. Courtesy Rudolph Matas Library, Tulane University Medical Center.

Specificity, Germs, and Mosquitoes

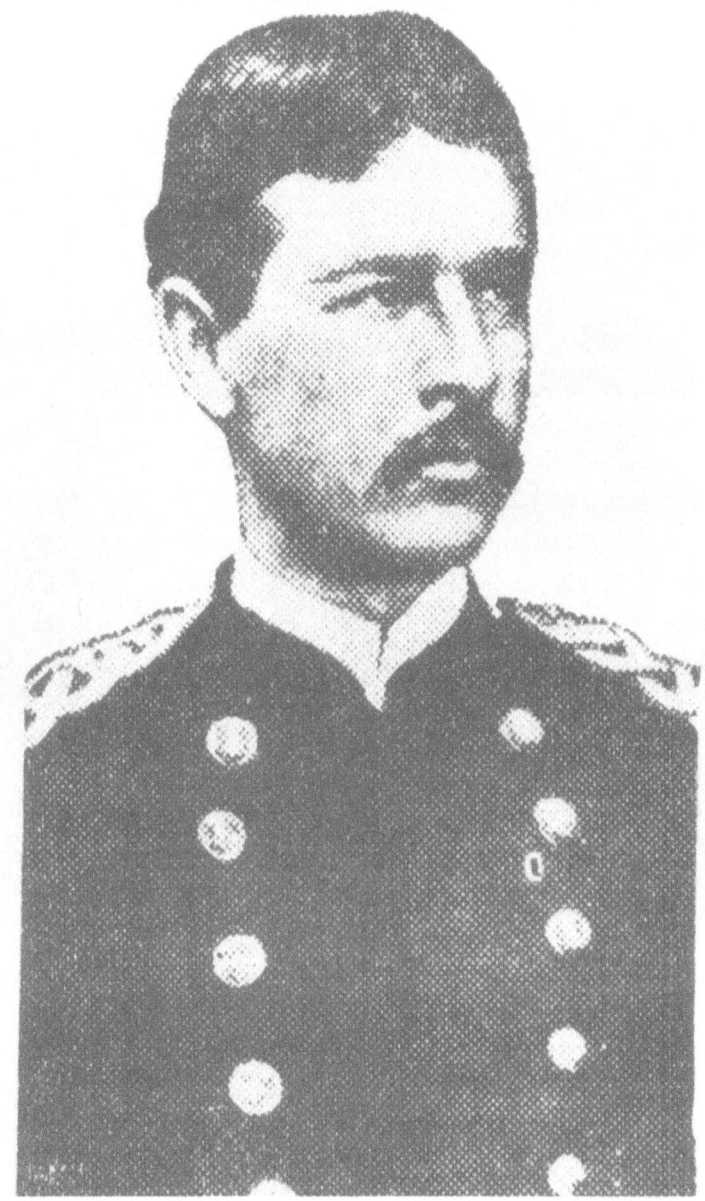

Walter Reed (1851-1902)
Headed the U. S. Army Medical Commission in Cuba that clearly demonstrated the process by which Finlay's mosquitoes served as intermediate host and vector of yellow fever. Courtesy Rudolph Matas Library, Tulane University Medical Center.

XIII

COMPETING MODES OF TREATMENT: A CENTURY OF CONTINUITY AND CHANGE

Treatment of yellow fever varied from epidemic to epidemic, doctor to doctor, and patient to patient, especially in the antebellum years when epidemics were frequent and increasingly virulent. Application of any set of remedies depended on the course of the disease, the experience and judgment of the physician, and the unique characteristics and symptoms of each patient—all highly variable phenomena. General patterns of therapy can be found in contemporary medical literature, but these modes and routines also changed over time as medical theory and practice underwent significant albeit gradual revision during the nineteenth century. Late eighteenth- and early nineteenth-century "rational" therapies, for yellow fever, as well as other disease manifestations, were derived from the speculative theoretical system of Dr. Benjamin Rush and other older medico-philosophical traditions. The continuing failure of these measures influenced many physicians to turn to empirical or experimental weapons against yellow fever, especially in the 1840s and 1850s.[1]

Louisiana's French practitioners from their earliest experiences with yellow fever tended to apply milder remedies than their Anglo-American colleagues, most of whom persisted in believing that yellow fever required aggressive intervention. After the great epidemics of the 1850s, some traditional harsh therapies were gradually abandoned or at least moderated. A mild supportive regimen emphasizing symptomatic treatment and attentive nursing (similar to the French creole tradition) was the course recommended by the most prominent New Orleans physicians during the second half of the nineteenth century.

Despite remarkable advances in medicine, there is still no specific cure for yellow fever; treatment remains symptomatic and supportive, requiring watchful nursing care. The large majority of cases recover whether treated or not and regardless of the kind of treatment. Nothing medicine has to offer will affect the most severe cases, leaving a small proportion in which supportive therapy and good nursing might actually save the patient's life.[2] The most astute southern physicians had reached this conclusion before 1860.

Diversity of Treatments

Antebellum observers often noted the great diversity in physicians' modes of treatment, remarking that some yellow fever patients died and some lived whatever the treatment. For example, in 1845, Dr. John Harrison, professor at the Medical College of Louisiana, said he had once been "called to an Irishman, who had been sick five days, and who had done nothing but drink whiskey the whole time. He was suffering with great irritability of the stomach, but recovered." Harrison also noted that patients sometimes recovered *in spite of* excessive dosing with mercury, *not because of* the treatment. Its advocates argued fallaciously, he said, *post hoc ergo propter hoc*; whenever a patient recovered, as the majority usually did, the treatment employed in that particular case received the credit, whether deserved or not.[3]

William L. Robinson, a member of the New Orleans Howard Association in the 1850s, had ample opportunity to observe all manner of therapeutic approaches. He discovered that "never was a practice devised that has not been marked with some success." Eventually he concluded that the "secret of success" could be found in "the confidence of the patient in his physician, and the hope inspired by a reputation for professional skill. . . ." The Howard Association tried to assign patients a doctor of their own nationality, or at least one able to speak their language. Observing that physicians of Spanish, German, French, Anglo-American, and various other backgrounds prescribed widely differing medications and convalescent diets, Robinson and his fellow Howards "were always as happy as surprised at the results when they proved favorable."[4]

Robinson described an occasion in 1853 in the Howards' Second District Infirmary when a delirious patient shouted a false alarm of fire, causing great confusion as patients ran about in a frenzy trying to escape the building they believed to be in flames. When finally persuaded to settle down and return to their beds, two patients inadvertently switched places. One had been sick only about thirty-six hours; the other was convalescent after nine days of illness. The doctor had ordered different treatments for them based on the stage of the disease and the particular conditions exhibited in each patient, recording the prescriptions not by patient's name but by a number assigned to each cot in the hospital. Each patient thus received the treatment intended for the other that day and for two more days, and both showed steady improvement. The physician finally noticed that he "had been successful by error." Both cases recovered completely, leaving Robinson and others to wonder with amusement if either would have recovered under the original plan of treatment.[5]

During New Orleans' first major yellow fever epidemic in 1796, one observer reported that the doctors generally declared their fever patients to be hopeless cases either "to receive greater credit when any of them pull through, or in order to acquire the reputation of being infallible should these die."[6] In later years, when doctors boasted of the small number of patients they lost, critics suggested that many yellow fever deaths were falsely attributed to other causes, thereby increasing the cure rate.[7]

Therapeutic Foundations

In the generalized monistic pathology shared by most doctors and patients prior to the mid-nineteenth century, disease was viewed as a disorder of the entire system, a manifestation of disequilibrium occurring when the blood or other body fluids (or "humors") were corrupted by some morbific matter of uncertain origin, or when an imbalance resulted from an excess of tension or "irritability" in the nervous or vascular system, or from influences causing general weakness or debility.

According to accepted theory, age, sex, race, nativity, occupation, "mode of living," temperament, physique, and a multitude of other particular features, as well as local environmental conditions, influenced the specific manifestation of disease in a person; hence, a course of treatment had to be carefully tailored to the individual patient. Dr. John Harrison's statement in the 1840s on the importance of individualized therapeutics expressed the prevailing view of the medical profession for much of the nineteenth century:

> As to the details of the treatment, they must be left to the judgment of the physician. Any specific treatment is just as absurd in yellow fever, as in any other disease. The physician is not called in to treat an abstraction, but a sick man. The treatment must be varied accordingly to the peculiarities of the cases. Remedies, beneficial in one case, may be most injurious in another; and success in practice will depend, in a great degree, upon the sagacity and acquirements of the physicians.[8]

Therapeutic measures were designed to counteract the underlying condition, to help the body regain its natural equilibrium, and to relieve pain and discomfort. Bleeding, purging, vomiting, sweating, blistering, and the use of anodynes and stimulants all "worked" in terms of the therapeutic systems of the day; that is, they produced a predictable, visible physiological result.

Depletion therapy presumably cleaned out the system and drained off the morbific poisons through general or local bleeding, vigorous purging of the bowels, and vomiting induced by emetics. Poultices made of irritating substances and placed over the stomach to halt vomiting produced a "counterirritation" in the form of a blister. Painful blisters, often infected and filling with pus, seemed to be drawing the "morbific accumulations" to the surface and providing an additional outlet for draining off the bad humors of the disordered system. Physician, patient, and family could observe the "signs" that such therapies were having an effect on the system. Bloodletting and various drugs produced copious perspiration, reduced fever and pulse rate, relieved pain, and brought relaxation and sleep. Physicians might also use medicines to stimulate the system, strengthen the pulse, improve appetite and digestion, and produce other outward manifestations of interior events. These physical effects demonstrated the power of the treatment and the doctor's ability to modify or "regulate" the secretions and other bodily processes.[9]

French versus Anglo-American Modes of Treatment

In the late eighteenth and early nineteenth centuries when yellow fever first began its summer appearances in New Orleans, physicians treated the malady as they treated other fevers, with whatever traditional measures seemed appropriate in each case. The recurring epidemics and the city's population growth allowed doctors to accumulate therapeutic experience. They also began to compare and analyze their observations collectively in newly formed professional societies, with French and Anglo-American practitioners initially organized in separate groups. During the early 1800s, French Louisianian and Anglo-American practitioners were beginning to exhibit different modes of treating fevers, emphasizing different aspects of the shared theoretical system.

This therapeutic divergence had already occurred between French and British physicians in the West Indies during the widespread epidemics of the 1790s. French physicians, especially in dealing with yellow fever, saw their healing role as supportive rather than combative, and they emphasized attentive nursing to keep the patient quiet, clean, and comfortable, with a minimum of medical intervention. This medical "laissez-faire" policy relied largely on the powers of nature to expel the disease and restore the patient to a state of health. The French physician's task was to assist nature without getting in the way of the healing process. Moderate assistance included giving the patient cool drinks in quantity such as lemonade or various teas, tepid sponging of the body, warm foot baths, cool applications, massage, and mild laxatives or emollient enemas. Following traditional theory, these mild therapeutic measures were designed to reduce fever and excitation, promote perspiration, and keep the bowels open and the kidneys functioning. While the French relied on nursing and nature, the British military physicians in the West Indies assaulted their patients' disease with such powerful weapons as bleeding, blistering, showering with buckets of cold water, and generous dosing with calomel, opium, camphor, cinchona bark, wine, and brandy.[10]

Inspired by Dr. Benjamin Rush's advocacy of aggressive bleeding and purging to overcome fevers, Anglo-American physicians in Louisiana and throughout the South until the mid-nineteenth century pursued a course even more "heroic" than the British doctors in the Caribbean. Their job, as American physicians saw it, was to wage a vigorous fight, not to stand idly by and let the disease take its natural course to a fatal conclusion. While they also had a holistic view of the diseased system, unbalanced by humoral corruption or vascular and nervous tension, the Americans believed that violent inflammatory disorders such as yellow fever required prompt, active intervention to calm the overexcited system, alter the course of the morbid process, and rescue the patient from death's door.

Competing Modes of Treatment 297

The doctor had to be courageous enough to employ harsh therapies against powerful disorders such as yellow fever which tended toward malignancy. Left to nature, the patient would die, they believed, but not if the doctor could take control of the disease process and disrupt it by vigorous bleeding and by very large doses of mercurials, especially calomel (mercurous chloride), which produced violent purging and salivation. Ptyalism, the excessive salivation that indicates mercurial poisoning, was considered a sign that the mercury was "working" to overcome the disease. With such potent "alterative" measures the physician presumably could break up the morbid, disorderly process (as one might break up a rebellion), and with auxiliary symptomatic treatments, followed by stimulants and tonics, the medical commander might gradually restore order to the patient's system and bring about full recovery.

During the epidemic of 1796 when New Orleans was still a Spanish property, Masdevall, physician to the king of Spain, recommended an "official remedy." Opposing blisters and bloodletting, he prescribed for all the fevers of Spain and America a mild emetic, followed by a compound of tarter emetic, wormwood, and Peruvian (cinchona) bark mixed in honey or syrup, and finally an emollient enema.[11]

Whatever the "official remedy," the French physicians of New Orleans used emetics, blisters, and venesection in treating yellow fever in the 1790s and early 1800s. Some condemned these traditional practices as useless and harmful, however, after experiencing the 1817 epidemic. The report on that epidemic prepared by the French physicians' *Société Médicale* discussed the successes and failures of various remedies. Experience had demonstrated the uselessness of both bleeding and emetics (*la saignée et vomatifs*), measures widely employed at the beginning of the epidemic. The best results had come from mild laxatives, soothing enemas, and acidulated drinks such as orange or lemonade. Cold baths, highly praised by some, were tried without success, but tepid bathing effectively "diminished irritation and excited a gentle perspiration," as did mustard poultices and frictions (rubbing). Although commonly used, cinchona tended to irritate the stomach and produce vomiting, and vesicatories on the epigastrium (blisters over the stomach) had not been effective in controlling the vomiting. Doses of opium sometimes stopped vomiting, as did "sulphuric ether in frictions on the epigastrium." Second stage vomiting, however, was generally unaffected by anything the physician tried. The society's report stressed the importance of gaining the patient's confidence and encouraging hope for recovery, especially in the last stage of the disease, "the desperate period" when the outcome was uncertain.[12]

After the 1819 epidemic, the report of the *Société* set forth a similar pattern of preferred treatment, which included mild laxatives, lemonade, fomentations (warm, moist poultices) on the stomach, foot baths, tepid bathing, vinegar frictions, decoction of cinchona bark, champagne, and diuretic drinks. While bleeding and blistering had not been effective, the French physicians were not willing to repudiate these measures altogether, retaining them in the therapeutic arsenal for occasions when they might be useful.[13] While it is impossible to determine from such reports what most physicians actually did, the evidence from a variety of sources suggests that Louisiana's French practitioners during this period, and with few exceptions thereafter, rejected the American extremes of bleeding, blistering, and purging with mercurials, believing that these methods irritated the system and further aggravated the disordered state.

An article on the "prevailing fever" in 1817 published in a New Orleans newspaper and signed "Philanthropy" provides a view of the aggressive American mode *à la Rush* based on "prompt decisive depletion by the most active means." The writer claimed that bleeding immediately "at the dawn of the fever" would save nine out of ten cases, all other therapies being "mere auxiliaries of the lancet." "Bleeding to syncope" (until the patient fainted), usually taking sixteen to thirty ounces, was to be "speedily followed by a *complete scouring of the stomach and bowels*, with 10 or 15 grains of Calomel and 20 of Jallap." Unless the patient had an easily irritated stomach, tartar emetic could also be given, followed by large quantities of water and other cool drinks. No food was allowed in the early stages of the disease, but after a few days the patient might be given chicken or beef broth and toast. The bowels were to be "kept open" by "small doses" of calomel, three to five grains every two or three hours as needed.[14] More aggressive therapy than the French doctors recommended, this advice was moderate compared to the "heroic" plan some American physicians claimed to follow and others found excessive.

Dr. Jabez Heustis, an army surgeon in Louisiana, described his plan of treatment in 1817, which included bleeding (16 to 20 ounces), ipecac to induce vomiting, calomel and jalap for purging, cold water for drinking and sponging, laudanum injections (enemas), and sometimes cinchona. While he accepted calomel as useful in reasonable doses, he opposed its widespread overuse by some physicians. He recalled that many soldiers had died in New Orleans during the pestilence of 1812, suffering from "the effects of mercury" as well as yellow fever, calomel being "given to the patient in a cup; and he was directed to eat it by the spoonful, like so much sugar."[15]

The Physico-Medical Society of New Orleans, the association of Anglo-American physicians, published a committee report on yellow fever in 1820, which included an evaluation of their members' therapeutic measures. The committee concluded that bloodletting had been effective in the first stage of the disease and early in the epidemic, but later in the season it failed to alter the disease, which had also happened in 1817 and 1819. Cathartics (strong purgatives) had been almost universally employed, the most common being calomel, jalap, castor oil, and magnesia. The medical committee praised cold water as a "powerful auxiliary," in the form of drinks, applications to the body, and clysters (enemas). Blisters proved beneficial only in the first few days, but in the "worst form" of yellow fever they were useless at any time. Cinchona lacked efficacy, and opinions varied on the value of opium, but champagne, wine, and brandy had served well as stimulants. It was now generally recognized that emetics should not be used, having a "pernicious tendency" in yellow fever. Reporting that confidence in mercury had been greatly underminded by therapeutic experience in 1820, the committee still considered calomel a valuable medicine but admitted that it had no effect on the most serious cases.[16]

While some American practitioners in New Orleans might have moderated their practice of bleeding, blistering, and mercurial purging in the 1820s, others throughout the city and region continued in traditional ways. Dr. Lyman Cronkrite, after the epidemic of 1829, spoke out for those who "dared to use the lancet freely." In his experience, bloodletting at the beginning of "febrile symptoms" made the disease "mild and manageable." It prompted sweating and relieved headache, backache, delirium, nausea, and "torpor of bowels." Cronkrite was contemptuous of a New Orleans physician who gave up bloodletting after having drawn eight or ten ounces in several yellow fever cases only to see them all die. "Surely this was a great stretch of human courage! The abstraction of eight or ten ounces of blood can have but little effect in a disease of such violence as yellow fever," he declared.

Cronkrite noted that Dr. Rush had often saved patients by taking as much as ninety ounces during the illness and that Dr. Samuel Cartwright of Natchez (later of New Orleans) had extracted sixty ounces at one time and cured his patient. Cronkrite said that during the 1829 epidemic, he had usually drawn thirty to sixty ounces from patients, and immediately thereafter dosed them with fifty to sixty grains of calomel, followed by castor oil or Epsom salts and frequent enemas, with cold applications to reduce their heat.[17] Heroic practice had its defenders as well as its critics and would advance on several fronts for decades to come before retiring altogether from the battle against yellow fever (although not from all others).

In 1833, Dr. Edward H. Barton criticized several modes of yellow fever treatment competing for ascendancy in New Orleans: (1) the mercurial plan; (2) purgatives, with moderate bleeding; and (3) the "West Indian or French mode," using "ptisans" (lemonade, teas, and other drinks) and diaphoretics (to cause sweating). The French mode, being harmless, was "infinitely preferable," but insufficient therapy, in Barton's judgment, because "its activity is not proportioned to the severity of the disease." He also rejected the excessive use of mercury and other harsh remedies, advocating a moderate course between extremes.[18]

Another New Orleans physician, in retrospect, categorized the treatments of the 1820s and 1830s as two "opposing plans": (1) the *antiphlogistic* or anti-inflammatory mode, consisting mainly of bloodletting, large doses of mercurial compounds, and other evacuants; and (2) the *expectant* plan, which employed "milder means" such as gentle laxatives, warm or hot baths, mustard poultices, and cool drinks, supporting the patient while waiting for nature itself to eliminate the "morbid material."[19]

Calomel, Bloodletting, and Quinine

The publication of the *New Orleans Medical and Surgical Journal*, beginning in 1844, offered a means for sharing knowledge and airing opinions. The journal's first issue included a lengthy essay in English on yellow fever treatment that had been presented in French to the bilingual Medico-Chirurgical Society in September, 1843, by the Paris-trained Dr. J. F. Beugnot. Troubled by the lack of agreement, Beugnot believed that medical societies should work to reduce "those scientific differences of opinion, which embarrass us, and which are so fatal to humanity."[20] He offered an extended discussion and evaluation of the principal therapies then employed against yellow fever: purgatives, bloodletting, and quinine. Purgatives, both strong and mild, he said, had long been accepted as a standard treatment for yellow fever, to relieve pain and reduce fever and stomach irritability. Dr. Benjamin Rush had sometimes prescribed as much as one hundred grains of calomel within three days. Many doctors believed yellow fever could be "arrested" if they could "obtain the desired salivation at a reasonable period." Others used milder mercurials; some prescribed magnesia, olive oil, and citron juice, avoiding mercury entirely.[21]

Because of their presumed successes in 1839, advocates of purgatives used the same harsh therapy in the 1841 epidemic but lost most of their patients. Yellow fever that year, being highly "inflammatory," did not respond well to "irritating remedies." Beugnot asserted that purgatives could not be considered an appropriate general treatment for yellow fever. "Shall I dwell . . . upon those terrible secondary symptoms which too frequently accompany the convalescence of those patients who had been gorged with calomel, as is too often done by American practitioners? Shall I mention those abominable salivations which are so painful, so distressing . . . [and] frequently followed by the destruction of all the teeth. . .?" He recommended enemata instead.[22]

Dr. P. H. Lewis of Mobile, Alabama, referring to the recent fashion of condemning mercury, reminded his colleagues that "an abuse of an article, constitutes no good reason why it should not be valuable if properly and judiciously directed."[23] Physicians treating yellow fever in Woodville, Mississippi, in 1844, still relied on calomel "in the maximum dose," some fifty or sixty grains given at first, then fifteen grains every three hours, then ten grains, and finally five.[24] Clearly, practitioners continued to use calomel, some in heroic measure, whatever reservations Beugnot and others expressed.

In rejecting purgatives and mercurials, Beugnot might at first appear to belong to that category of French Louisiana physicians who in contrast to "*les Américains*" favored mild, non-interventionist therapies—but not so. His preferred method was syncopal bleeding, a relatively new (or recycled) "abortive" therapy, quite as aggressive and heroic as anything that preceded it. Beugnot credited Dr. Charles A. Luzenberg, founder and president of the Louisiana Medico-Chirurgical Society, with developing this method in 1829 and using it successfully ever since.[25] Bloodletting was "the most energetic therapeutic agent," although highly controversial, as

Beugnot admitted. New Orleans physicians had always been divided over the question, he observed, and some twenty years before, the practice had been widely condemned as harmful and "employed with great timidity," if at all.[26]

Explaining and justifying his advocacy of bold phlebotomy, Beugnot argued that yellow fever, a disease characterized by "excitation," required measures "calculated to subdue these forces, and to calm that preternatural excitement." Since emetics, purgatives, and diaphoretics failed to achieve the desired effect, "what then have we left . . .?" he asked. "Nothing, save the loss of blood." Beugnot set forth as a fundamental principle: "In all cases of Yellow Fever, either severe or mild, it is invariably good practice to resort to the abstraction of blood in the first stage of the disease—varying it however, according to the nature and violence of each individual case." He disagreed with the view that bleeding conferred no benefit after the third or fourth day of the disease: "Bleeding cannot jeopardize the life of a patient who is already considered as lost; on the contrary, it offers, in these desperate cases, a chance of safety, slender, it is true, but one of which we may sometimes avail ourselves with advantage."[27]

Quoting various authorities who suggested taking 24 to 44 ounces or who recommended five or six bleedings of 12 to 16 ounces each time, Beugnot pointed out that bleeding to syncope, whatever the amount required to achieve it, was the appropriate measure. Only the "timid" proposed small amounts, "better calculated to waste the strength of the patient than to subdue the disease." He described the procedure as he thought it should go:

> Take a case of ordinary severity in the very commencement, sit the patient up in bed and make a large orifice in one of the veins of the arm; twelve ounces of blood shall have hardly been drawn, when a more favorable change in all the external phenomena, will take place. The face loses its colour, the eyes their redness, and their unnatural brilliancy, the patient declares that he can see better, and that the head is relieved. By allowing the blood to flow, the patient soon grows pale and feeble; he yawns at intervals, and states that he feels faint, and that the *cephalalgia*, pains in the loins, and limbs, are entirely dissipated. —Soon nausea manifests itself, and is succeeded by vomiting; then a profuse perspiration gushes from every pore, first appearing on the extremities, and finally spreading over the whole body. At this moment, the pulse, which before the bleeding, beat one hundred or one hundred and twenty per minute, gradually falls and sinks in force and frequency to its normal type. If we continue the flow of blood at this critical period, the patient will swoon, and when he recovers his speech, declare that he is infinitely better.

What influenced the disease was not the simple loss of blood, Beugnot explained, but the systemic "perturbation which supervenes when syncope is produced." It was often necessary, he said, to bleed several times at six to eight hour intervals, with the objective of "incipient syncope" each time, whatever the quantity required. "Nothing is here so dangerous as temporizing, which many physicians decorate with the false name of prudence. Sound prudence consists in speedily curing the patient, and not in waiting until the disease becomes stronger than the remedies." Beugnot described his own experience as a yellow fever patient in 1839, when he was bled to syncope, had one hundred active leeches applied to the epigastrium the same day, and another thirty leeches the next day. By the fourth day, he felt better, and within a week was able to resume his work.[28]

Leeching and cupping must have been widely employed in New Orleans during the epidemic of 1839. A newspaper editor commented in August on the need for more cuppers and leechers in the city, having observed that most seemed to have more calls than they could handle. As the process was simple and so beneficial in the early stage of yellow fever, the editor urged that "our young men . . . acquire a knowledge of the operation and render their assistance. It would be well if some of the ladies would also learn the practice."[29]

Syncopal bleeding as an "abortive" therapy probably had more opponents than supporters, among both French- and English-speaking physicians. According to Dr. Erasmus Darwin Fenner, the advocates of this plan included Luzenberg, Beugnot, and a few other "bold practitioners."[30] Speaking to the Medico-Chirurgical Society in 1843, Dr. P. A. Lambert questioned the excessive resort to phlebotomy in yellow fever treatment. While general bleeding might help to eliminate "the miasmatic poison," Lambert doubted its therapeutic value.[31] Dr. John Harrison thought leeches and cups safer than the lancet, more gradual in effect, and sometimes useful in relieving pain in the head and loins.[32]

A graphic description of cupping was provided by a member of the Howard Association in his account of an incident during the 1853 epidemic when he called in a professional cupper, "Eanes, a colored man," to bleed one of the patients under his care. First, the cupper shaved the back of the patient's neck, rinsed a glass cup with alcohol and set fire to it, applying the cup to the man's neck. In a few minutes, the cup was removed and the scarifying instrument placed on the reddened skin. The click of the spring released the blades, making superficial incisions, and bringing a loud cry and a curse from the patient, who had to be persuaded to allow the next step. More alcohol was poured into the cup and set afire (creating a vacuum), and the cup was quickly applied to the scarified area to draw out blood through the cuts in the skin. This patient jumped out of bed, pulled the cup from his neck and broke it, shouting and cursing as he did so, thus refusing to tolerate any further treatment.[33]

Another "abortive" plan of treatment, the quinine practice, was introduced in the late 1830s and employed with claims of great success in the epidemics of the 1840s. Like syncopal bleeding, it was a bold, heroic technique designed to cut short the disease process, and it attracted more widespread support than phlebotomy. From the beginning, the practice had its "warm advocates and violent opponents." Opponents insisted "that the blood requires a certain time to be rid of its poison, ... and that, by checking the effort of nature to work it off in violent agitation of the blood, we invite a more precarious disease."[34]

According to Dr. Harrison, the quinine treatment had been adopted at Charity Hospital and in private practice in 1839. He believed that Dr. J. M. Mackie of New Orleans had first employed the method, suggested to him by Dr. Thomas Hunt, who was influenced by an article in the *British and Foreign Medical Review*. Quinine had long been considered appropriate as a tonic in the latter stages of yellow fever, but this "new mode" used sulphate of quinine as soon as possible after the attack, from twenty to eighty grains in cold water, following the use of the lancet. Appearing to act directly on the "nervous substance," quinine was *not* appropriate for all cases of yellow fever, Harrison warned, but the drug could be highly effective under the right circumstances.[35] General interest in the quinine treatment in 1839 is suggested by an editorial in the New Orleans *Bee*, proclaiming this "novel curative method" to be a "most important and incalculably beneficial discovery."[36]

During the epidemics of 1847, 1848, and 1849, Dr. Erasmus Darwin Fenner had employed the "abortive method by quinine" in treating yellow fever, and he believed Drs. Harrison and Beugnot also supported the method. After ordering the hot mustard foot bath and purgative enema, Fenner prescribed twenty or thirty grains of quinine with twenty-five to thirty drops of laudanum or one or two grains of opium, followed by calomel. This plan, according to Fenner, generally calmed the "vascular and nervous excitement," brought on perspiration, relieved pain, and allowed the patient to sleep. In the later stages, the physician had little to do, he said, other than ordering rest, quiet, and bland nourishment for the patient, and using blisters, sponging, antacid mixtures, and gentle stimulants as needed.[37]

Until he learned from experience, Dr. Beugnot had accepted other's opinions of quinine as "the *definitive* and *supreme* remedy in Yellow Fever." By 1843, in his revised view, it was "an excellent remedy" in some conditions but "useless and sometimes hurtful" in others. When circumstances called for it, he prescribed two grains every hour until the system was "saturated, which may be recognized by a species of intoxication and partial deafness." Administered soon after syncopal bleeding in several of his cases, the large doses of quinine had brought on "a profound perturbation" and succeeded in breaking up "that morbid chain on which the disease depends." Beugnot concluded that this treatment seemed "rational," but had not yet been sufficiently tested for "unqualified recommendation." He hoped that physicians would continue to test this method, cautiously, avoiding its use in patients of "nervous temperament."[38]

In his work on southern diseases, published in 1849, Thompson McGown included a short section on yellow fever, praising the recent improvement in treatment, the "eminently successful" abortive method using large doses of quinine.[39] The editors of the *New Orleans Medical Journal* in 1844 had also referred to a major change in the treatment of southern fevers during the previous decade, involving moderation in the use of purgatives and emetics and more general use of tonics, especially sulphate of quinine. "Quinine, instead of calomel, is now considered in the South, the Sampson of the Materia Medica; and we congratulate our brethren and the community, on the change. The doses of this medicine have been increased from 2 grains, up to 10, 20, and upwards; and its beneficial effects are often truly wonderful."[40]

By the mid-1840s some Louisiana physicians began to express concern about the toxic effects of overdosing with quinine. Dr. J. B. Wilkinson, while accepting the drug as a specific for intermittent fever, criticized its excessive use and doubted its value in yellow fever. Wherever appropriate, a moderate dosage was sufficient, he said, but in twenty to forty grain doses, quinine was a dangerous medicine.[41] The same issue of the *New Orleans Medical Journal* in 1844 that praised quinine as the "Sampson of the Materia Medica" included a note from the *British and Foreign Medical Review* describing the harmful effects "distinctly observed to follow the immoderate use of quinine." The list included delirium and coma, hematuria, deafness, loss of vision, diarrhea, paralysis, and death.[42] Negative reviews of the quinine practice and reports of its damaging effects would increase greatly in the 1850s.

As physicians debated the relative merits of the "abortive" techniques and other measures, they reached agreement that emetics should be "generally stricken from the list of therapeutic means" as dangerous and useless in treating yellow fever. According to Dr. Beugnot, opium and other narcotics were appropriate only in "exceptional circumstances," for treating "feeble, irritable and nervous subjects, such as females in general." And opium (1/6 to 1/8 grain of morphine in water) "on rare occasions" might be used to control vomiting and calm the nervous system. Many physicians employed diuretics and sudorifics as "auxiliary means," but Beugnot considered them useless.[43]

Dr. Fenner summarized yellow fever therapeutics in the 1840s under two general modes of theory and practice: (1) the abortive methods, by syncopal bleeding, or by quinine (his practice at this time), and (2) the rational or eclectic method. As he described it, the rational or eclectic method was based on "experience and rational observation, but independent of scientific induction." Its objective was not to abort disease or take control from nature, but to help the patient through the stages of fever and employ appropriate symptomatic remedies. Diversity of practice resulted because each doctor used remedies he had "found by experiment" suitable to relieve the symptoms.[44] Empiricism and rationalism were at work in both methods, whatever their labels. What Fenner referred to as the rational-eclectic mode resembled the expectant approach (associated with creole physicians), whose advocates observed the natural progression of the disease and provided symptomatic treatment as needed. After 1853, many southern practitioners, at least among those who wrote for journals, became more interested in the healing power of nature and inclined toward the eclectic-expectant approach to treatment.

The Great Epidemics and Therapeutic Reformation

The Great Epidemic of 1853, followed by other major outbreaks in 1854, 1855, and 1858, challenged every tenet of yellow fever theory, every element of practice. Abortive therapy, whether phlebotomy or quinine, disappointed practitioners who had found these methods effective in the 1840s. Many came to doubt the efficacy of past practices, while others confidently continued their time-honored routines. One New Orleans physician reported that the abortive treatment was soon abandoned in 1853 by the "most judicious physicians," but others persisted in administering huge doses of quinine which left patients in a "wretched condition," suffering from deafness, blindness, and even insanity. Cupping, venesection, calomel, and other standard remedies, although widely employed, had little effect on the disease. "All violent, or 'heroic' medication, after the disease was fully developed, was found to be more injurious than beneficial; and more deaths were no doubt caused by over-anxiety to give medicine, than by the want of medicine." This doctor concluded that "Good nursing, reliance upon the defensive and recuperative powers of nature, and hygienic management, . . . saved more lives than medicine."[45] This theme would be repeated in journals, lecture halls, and clinics for the next forty years until most of the old guard were converted, found ways to incorporate the revised thinking into their practice, or simply died off, and new generations trained in new ways gradually took their place.

After the epidemic, Dr. T. A. Cooke of Washington, Louisiana, declared yellow fever therapeutics a disgrace to the profession, revealing "profound ignorance." Yellow fever actually required little medication, he wrote, yet one aggressive therapy after another had been hurled against it.

> Mercury has had its day, but is now remembered only in connexion with its victims. A few years since and quinine was enthroned. . . . After a short reign it has been deposed; but the throne is left vacant. Bloodletting boldly practiced, active emetics, purgatives, etc., have had their advocates and their opponents; the former lauding their beneficial effects, the latter condemning them as dangerous.

In the absence of knowledge, Cooke thought practitioners should rely mainly on "adjuvants" such as mustard pediluvia, warm drinks, and sponging, since strong medicine often aggravated the condition.[46]

Reviewing the therapeutic experience of 1853, Dr. Fenner stated that practitioners had employed every conceivable treatment from "doing nothing at all" to the "most potent remedies in heroic doses," and that some recovered and some died under every form of treatment. Without suggesting the necessity of a uniform treatment, Dr. Fenner wanted more agreement among physicians, which could only be achieved through observation and study. Learning more about the fever's natural course without medication would provide guidance, he thought, in selecting appropriate remedies and in deciding when to assist nature and when not to intervene. When yellow fever patients were admitted to his wards at Charity Hospital on the fourth day of their illness without having had medication, Fenner left them to the powers of nature. He simply put them to bed, prescribing mild enemas and sponging with warm vinegar or whiskey and water. "A number of these cases recovered," and Fenner concluded that after the first stage, the patient's recovery depended on nature, careful nursing, and cautious medication.[47]

From 1847 until 1853, Fenner and several other physicians had apparently enjoyed success with an abortive method, cutting short virtually all cases treated in the early stage with large doses of quinine and opium, or so it seemed. The "more malignant type" of fever in 1853, however, did not yield to such therapy. Fenner then began to use smaller doses of quinine without opium, and with better results. He blamed the popular prejudice that had arisen against quinine on those who lacked the knowledge "to prescribe it judiciously."[48]

Even before the 1853 experience, some Louisiana physicians spoke out against the use of quinine as a panacea. Dr. R. L. Scruggs, complaining in 1852 of the "ultraism in medicine," blamed physicians who routinely prescribed a cure-all for shaming the profession and encouraging quackery. Scruggs had other concerns as well: "Ask the Planter why he trusts the lives of his valuable slaves to the medical skill of his overseer, and his answer is, '. . . the Doctors say that Quinine can cure all disease, and my overseer can give *that* as well as a Doctor.'"[49]

The *New Orleans Medical and Surgical Journal* published a letter in 1853 from a local physician praising quinine as his "most effective agent" against yellow fever, in doses of thirty to sixty grains within the first twelve hours. The editors thought it necessary to note that the "quinine practice" had not worked as well in 1853 as it had in 1847. While ten or fifteen grains of quinine might be useful at the start, large doses of twenty or thirty grains given repeatedly could act as a "powerful sedative poison," depressing the heart, injuring the nervous system, and reducing the "vital forces" beyond repair. Although not opposing its "prudent use," the journal did object to 'monstrous doses."[50]

Revisionism in therapeutic doctrine occupied much attention in medical societies and in the pages of medical journals throughout the 1850s—before, during, and after yellow fever epidemics. By 1851, Dr.

Edward Hall Barton had noticed a major change in medical opinion regarding the use of calomel. In his analysis, the "clash of the ultraists" brought about investigations and improvements in "practical physic" as well as the "firm establishment of eclectic medicine, where there is no predominance of any dogma."[51]

The 1850s epidemic experiences shattered the faith of many practitioners (and patients) in the standard remedies.[52] Dr. Morton Dowler wrote of yellow fever late in 1854: "It is not a disease for blood-letting, cupping, leeching, mercurialization, vesication, antimonials, or rattling cathartics." From his years of experience, he rejected them all, his favored treatment being the frequent use of cool sponging for fever and opium as a sedative.[53] In an account of the epidemics of the 1850s in Lafourche Parish, published in French in 1863, Dr. D. Durac declared it impossible, given the present limited state of knowledge, to set forth a precise, "rational" treatment of yellow fever, although one could establish a symptomatic therapy. Emetics and opium were useless, he said, and mercurial frictions, calomel, cold baths, and quinine all failed to produce the desired result.[54]

In 1855, Dr. Nott of Mobile also rejected aggressive medication for treating yellow fever. "Bleeding and active purgation or emetics are worse than useless," he asserted, "and more good is effected by good nursing and constant attention to varying symptoms than by violent remedies."[55] The importance of nursing had long been acknowledged among New Orleans practitioners, especially in the creole tradition. In 1858, according to the *New Orleans Medical News and Hospital Gazette*, the best yellow fever treatment consisted of careful nursing, giving as little "perturbating medicine as possible, and only attacking when symptoms of localization of disease arise."[56]

Expressing concern that the reaction against heroic treatment of yellow fever would lead to the opposite extreme of "non-medication," Dr. Bennet Dowler challenged the position of medical skeptics and their theory of "self-limited" disease. "It may be well to throw a little cold water on the too ardent zeal of those who profess ability to cut up the disease root and branch," he admitted, referring to the extremes of the "abortive" treatments. On the other hand, ". . . the alleged doctrine of the self-limitation of fevers as a reason for not attempting to control or cure them, is in itself an affected hypothesis, being withal calculated to bring despair to the practitioner and to fill the public mind with an unwarrantable distrust in regard to the efficiency and utility of the medical profession."[57]

Experimentation

After a certain amount of failure with orthodox remedies during the epidemics of the 1840s and 1850s, the search for something better through trial and error was inevitable—especially with the availability of patients in the New Orleans Charity Hospital and similar dependent cases elsewhere.[58] Sometimes physicians tried a drug not previously employed in yellow fever, but drawn from the age-old pharmacopeia of minerals and botanicals and known to produce a particular physiological effect. Sometimes doctors developed new strategies by modifying or combining elements from traditional practice, raising or lowering dosages to produce different effects.

An editorial in the *Louisiana Courier* in the summer of 1820 noted that a "Mr. Eudes de Gentilly" had been claiming for some time that he possessed a "specific" for yellow fever. Now that the disease was present in the city with a number of cases at Charity Hospital, the editor thought the authorities should "let Mr. Eudes try his experiment."[59] The authorities probably did not grant this privilege to a layman, but it was widely accepted that physicians would test new remedies on charity patients, experiments considered unacceptable in private practice. Not unaware of this tendency toward experimentation, the sick poor at times expressed fear and distrust by their resistance to being hospitalized.[60]

In the *Charleston Medical Journal*, Dr. Josiah C. Nott described a successful experimental treatment he tried on two prostitutes in Mobile during the epidemic of 1843. When every one of the first fifteen cases of fever in the city died, Nott investigated and found that the standard remedies had been employed: some patients had been bled, all had been purged, all had received some form of mercury, and all had died. He then decided to try something different "as no method could be worse than those which failed in every case." Nott chose creosote for its antiseptic properties, dissolved it in alcohol and spirits of ammonia, and administered the medicine to "two girls, of easy virtue, in the same house," in doses of one tablespoonful every two hours during the first stage of the disease. Both prostitutes recovered, "and they were the first this season who survived the disease." Nott went on to use this remedy with great success for about a month, thinking he had found a specific for yellow fever. When he learned that other physicians, using a variety of treatments, were by that time also curing most of their patients, he concluded that the disease must have declined in potency from its early virulent form.[61]

An example of "last resort" experimentalism occurred in 1858, when Dr. N. B. Benedict of New Orleans, in consultation with five other physicians, decided to try a blood transfusion on a female patient, hemorrhaging for some time and near death. The doctors gathered at the bedside, and using a transfusion "apparatus" Benedict had obtained from England, injected into one of her veins about two and one-half ounces of blood from the arm of a healthy "young gentleman" who had recovered from yellow fever in 1853. According to Benedict, the treatment worked like a miracle, turning the dying patient toward recovery,[62] more than a bit of good luck for all concerned since nothing was known at the time about blood typing.

Dr. Erasmus D. Fenner, as editor of the *New Orleans Medical News and Hospital Gazette,* published his own articles in 1858 on two new remedies for yellow fever, chlorine and veratrum viride. While accepting the empirical nature of most yellow fever therapy, Fenner argued that "A correct theory is absolutely necessary to scientific and successful practice; and the physician, if there be one, who has *no theory*, is a mere empiric." In yellow fever, he theorized, the "conservative powers of the body" are engaged in battle with a "lethific agent"—whatever its nature, and treatment attempted to combat the poison and its effects.

Fenner encouraged further experimentation with two new remedies that he had tried with considerable success in yellow fever. First he had experimented with chlorine, which worked well in reducing fever and maintaining action of the kidneys. Later, another physician approached him in Charity Hospital and asked if Fenner had ever tried veratrum viride (a powerful cardiac sedative) in yellow fever. "He begged me to try it in the Hospital, as he did not like to experiment on patients in private practice, yet felt the necessity of our endeavoring to find out some more valuable remedies than any we now have." Although he had not tried this botanical remedy, Fenner had recently read of its successful use in treating fevers. He began his experiments at Charity Hospital with two Irishmen and a German. Observing that both chlorine and veratrum viride worked well together, he continued to use the combination for treating yellow fever, giving a mild purgative at the outset, and otherwise prescribing only mustard foot baths, enemata, and warm teas. As always, caution was in order because these potent therapeutic agents could produce prostration,

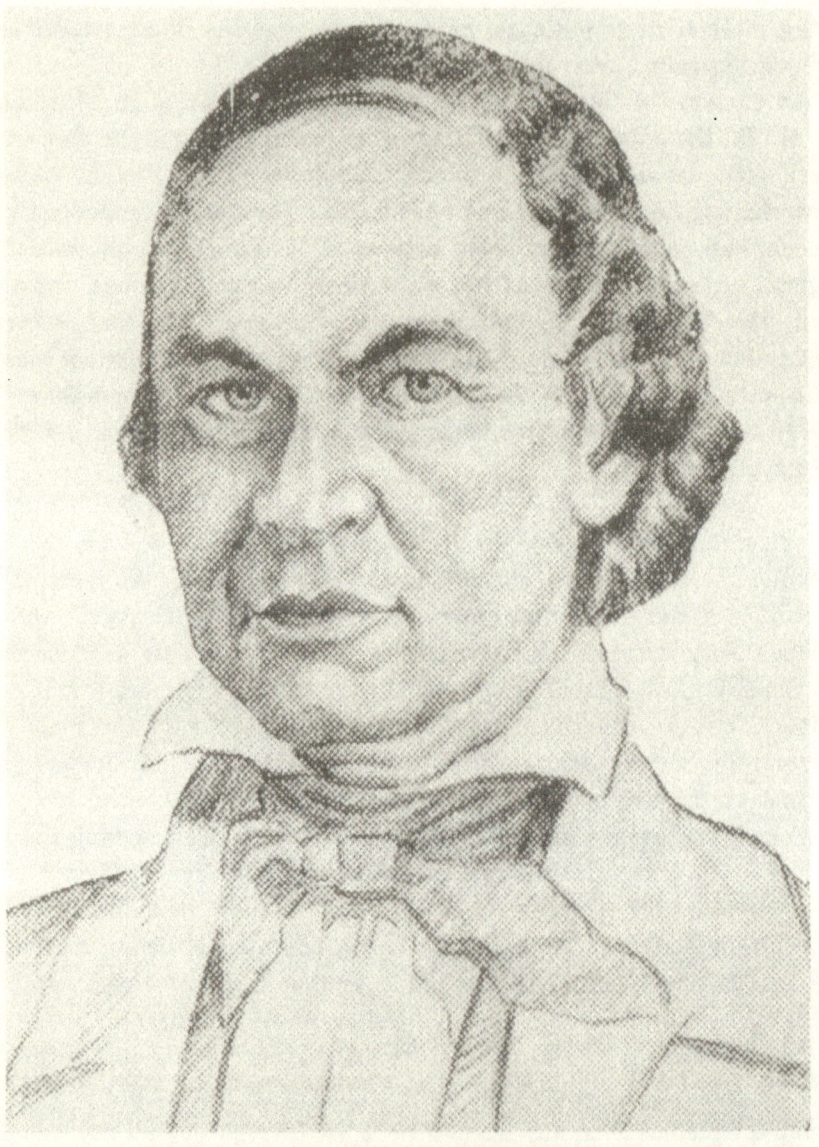

Bennet Dowler (1797-1878).
Courtesy Rudolph Matas Library, Tulane University Medical Center.

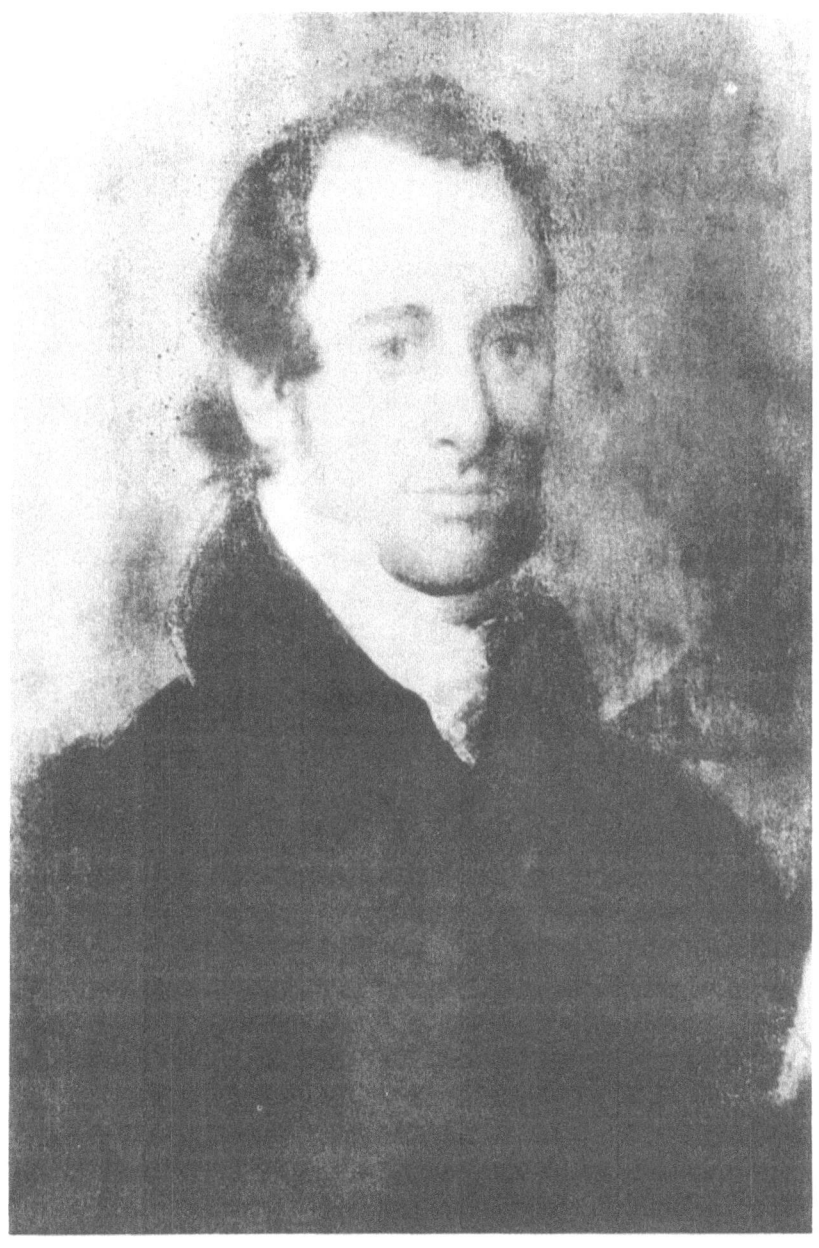

Edward Hall Barton (1796-1859).
Courtesy Rudolph Matas Library, Tulane University Medical Center.

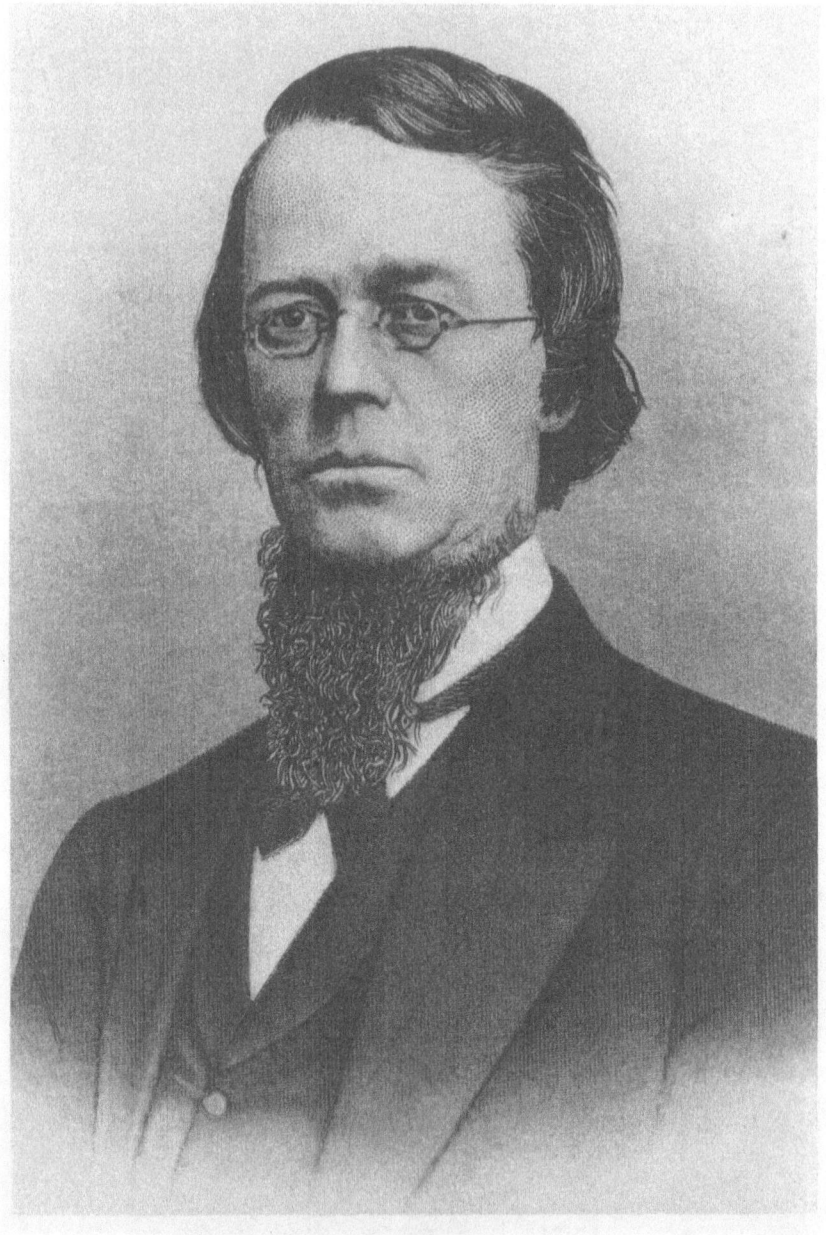

William H. Holcombe (1825-1893)—homeopathist.
Courtesy Rudolph Matas Library, Tulane University Medical Center.

restlessness, and a "peculiar wild delirium." Fenner called attention to the new remedies in 1858 so that physicians might test them during "this terrible Southern pestilence."[63]

Dr. Bennet Dowler, with his usual rhetorical excess, summed up the changing fashions of yellow fever therapeutics in 1858 after the fourth major epidemic within a six-year period. "Every epidemic develops some new remedial combination or phase of these, or revives others almost forgotten. Panaceas wax and wane more rapidly than the moon. Some favorite prescription for large, small, or medium doses which glimmers for a time in the reigning darkness, goes out like a meteor before the steady advance of the invisible foe whose victims fall by the thousands just as before," he expounded. The great diversity of treatments "from the slops called ptisans to the most concentrated preparations—from infinitesimal to heroic doses, show that a rational therapy of this disease . . . [is] yet unachieved, perhaps, unachievable." Rejecting further speculation as a waste of time under present conditions, Dowler believed that keeping detailed case histories provided the best foundation for deducing what treatments worked best and when they should be administered. Until the etiology and pathology of yellow fever were more clearly understood, he acknowledged that practitioners had to rely on empiricism and experimentalism.[64]

Hydropathy and Homeopathy

In antebellum America, the dissatisfaction with orthodox medicine that impelled some physicians toward experimentation also drove many patients to seek other options, giving rise to a popular health reform movement and several "irregular" systems of practice. The 1820s and 1830s saw the beginnings of a "patients' revolt" against heroic therapies. Every man could be his own physician, according to Samuel Thomson, a self-taught New England botanic practitioner, whose book and remedies became widely popular, especially in rural areas. In Louisiana, the most influential "irregular" systems, however, were hydropathy and homeopathy, both of European origin. Both arrived in Louisiana in the 1840s, an era of epidemics, suffering patients, and frustrated practitioners.[65]

Although the use of water for therapeutic purposes has an ancient history, hydropathy as a medical sect emerged from the ideas and practices of a nineteenth-century Austrian layman, Vincent Priessnitz, whose cures brought him fame and attracted a following in Europe and America. In his system, water was not merely one among many therapeutic weapons, but the only one. A true hydropath would reject the standard *materia medica* entirely, utilizing only water, externally and internally: for drinking in large and small amounts, cold, hot, or warm; for vaginal injections and enemas by the gallon; for bathing all over, soaking various parts of the body, showering, sponging, enveloping in a wet sheet from neck to ankles, and other variations. The emphasis on nature's healing power and the rejection of harsh therapies proved appealing to many in search of an alternative to bleeding and calomel.[66]

In treating yellow fever, some of Louisiana's regular physicians utilized "hydropathic" remedies, without rejecting other medications. Dr. S. W. Dalton tried the wet sheet with cold water on his patients in the 1847 epidemic with excellent results, but he also gave castor oil.[67] In 1843 Dr. J. F. Beugnot expressed interest in this new mode of treatment then spreading across Europe, which seemed to him "very rational." He encouraged New Orleans physicians to give it a trial, although he did not expect it to replace all other yellow fever remedies.[68]

Another French physician, Dr. A. J. F. Cartier, employed hydropathy in conjunction with his homeopathic remedies during the epidemic in 1853 and found it a powerful means of "aiding without disturbing the plan or action of fundamental treatment." In treating "*une dame américaine*" suffering from intense fever and delirium, Cartier decided to completely envelop the patient in a wet sheet "following the method of Priessnitz." Finding it effective, he combined the wet sheet with homeopathy in other cases with excellent results. Whether hydropathy would work in the absence of other medicines he could not say. The only doctor he knew who intended to apply the method pure and simple had died early in the 1853 epidemic. When Cartier's combination of methods failed to work well after 1853, he went back to the "exclusive usage of homeopathic remedies," convinced that this mode of treatment for yellow fever was far superior to regular practice.[69]

Theodore Clapp, a New Orleans clergyman, commented in the 1850s that since "our physicians" had recently substituted "gentle remedies" for heroic practice, the city's prevailing therapeutic system was quite similar to that of the homeopaths and more effective than it used to be.⁷⁰ Despite the hostility homeopathy inspired in most regulars, this competitive "irregular" practice made its influence felt in New Orleans, directly and indirectly.

Homeopathy was the conception of Samuel Hahnemann, a German physician who lost faith in traditional medicine. By the early nineteenth century he established a new practice based on two principles: (1) a drug that produces certain symptoms in a healthy person will cure them in a sick person—the doctrine of similars (like cures like); and (2) drugs must be diluted to an infinitesimal degree for their greatest effectiveness—the doctrine of infinitesimal dosage. Hahnemann and others tested drugs on themselves and recorded the symptoms they experienced in order to learn what drug to use in treating these symptoms. Some of his disciples brought homeopathy to the United States, and by the 1840s it began to attract an educated, urban following of both patients and practitioners.

In competition with the harsh practices of the regular physicians (or allopaths), homeopathic practitioners trusted the "vital powers" of the human body to fight off disease, aided by the stimulus of their properly diluted medicines. They enjoyed remarkable success. Their minute doses (containing little if any of the original drug) did no harm, and their supportive care gave the patient a chance to recover without the damaging effects often associated with mercury, quinine, and other drastic therapies. Some regulars broke ranks and joined the competition, or at least adopted and modified the method to suit their own uses. Homeopathy attracted considerable support among Louisiana French practitioners, and several French-language homeopathic journals enjoyed a brief existence in New Orleans during the 1850s. Other regulars, while ridiculing and ostracizing their rivals, proceeded to examine and moderate their own practice, if they had not already done so.⁷¹

Dr. Morton Dowler denounced homeopathy as "devoid of curative capacity," and "wholly unworthy of serious attention or examination." Infinitesimal dosage seemed to him expecially irrational: ". . . it is quite as philosophical to propose as diet the decillionth part of a roasted potato . . . to rescue an individual from death by starvation, as to propose the decillionth part of a grain of any medicine for the cure of any disease." Some regulars had credited homeopathy with revealing the natural course of disease and demonstrating that recovery could occur without medicine, homeopathic dilutions being a "mere therapeutic nullity." Dowler disagreed with this judgment, pointing out that not all homeopathists strictly followed their "creed," but that many also used "active medications."[72]

Louisiana's leading spokesman for the homeopathic cause in the 1850s, Dr. William Holcombe of Waterproof published several pamphlets explaining the theory and the method of preparing drugs for infinitesimal dosing. For example, ipecac, a well-known emetic, usually given to induce vomiting, could be used in its diluted form to relieve vomiting. One drop of tincture of ipecac in one-half glass of water and five or six drops of that dilution into the same amount of water produced the proper potency, of which one teaspoonful was given as needed. (Hahnemann's dilutions were far more "infinitesimal." By the third step the drug was diluted to 1/1,000,000 of its original strength, and Hahnemann proposed thirty dilutions.) Drugs commonly used by homeopaths for treating yellow fever included aconite, belladonna, arsenic, nitrate of silver, opium, quinine, hyoscyamus, and others from the standard *materia medica*, diluted two or three times in water, then administered by the spoonful.[73]

Holcombe's recommended homeopathic treatment for yellow fever in the 1850s also incorporated the elements long associated with the creole method: the mustard foot bath, bed rest, hot orange-leaf tea, cold water, soapsuds enema rather than purgatives, tea and toast if desired. Careful attention to the stages of the disease and the patient's condition determined which of the several homeopathic preparations was needed and when. Holcombe also advised that the patient be kept quiet, not overheated or oversweated. "Make him comfortable in every respect," he urged.[74]

Because of their "reputed success," homeopathists received many calls for assistance during the 1878 epidemic from families in New Orleans and the interior communities. Local practitioners and their supporters organized the New Orleans Homeopathic Relief Association to raise money and provide free treatment to those in need. Lacking enough physicians to send to all the towns requesting aid, the association established a "corps of homeopathic laymen," gave them some quick training and a printed guide book, and sent them forth. Medicines and circulars outlining treatment were also provided to hundreds of families requesting them.

The circular, prepared by Dr. James G. Belden, made it possible for laymen to treat yellow fever homeopathically in the absence of a physician. The initial medication was four drops of aconite in half a glass of water given by the teaspoonful at half-hour intervals, alternating with belladonna in a similar dilution, during a twenty-four hour period; thereafter, bryonia in the same dilution and dosage, until the fever abated. Mustard foot baths, lemonade, and other liquids were included in the treatment of virtually all practitioners, whatever their theory. Other homeopathic medicines (in similar dilution and dosage) might be necessary depending on specific symptoms: arsenicum for nausea, champagne or brandy (also highly diluted) for weakness, stramonium and cantharides in alternation for suppression of urine, and opium for retention of urine. Not unlike the regulars, homeopathic practitioners considered the "early attendance of a physician always desirable" because of the variability of yellow fever's effects and the need for expert advice.[75]

Medical historians have generally agreed with the judgment of nineteenth-century regulars who credited homeopathy and hydropathy with clearly demonstrating that no medicine was often the best medicine, especially in yellow fever. Both irregular practices offered a strong critique and an alternative to heroic therapeutics; both attracted patients and converted some physicians from the regular school; both were derived from and further contributed to the forces already at work against traditional therapeutics. By the end of the nineteenth century, the generally accepted yellow fever treatment would reflect the combined influence of creole nursing, expectant medicine, and some aspects of homeopathic and hydropathic practice, preserving an active role for the physician but a less active role for medicines.

Self-Treatment: Patent Remedies, Preventives, and Free Advice

Sharp operators, in every age, manage to profit from the fear and credulity of those who hope to avoid painful treatment or the doctor's fee. The inadequacies of medical practice in antebellum America that led to the rise of "irregulars" also encouraged resort to self-treatment. From the 1830s on, newspaper advertisements for yellow fever remedies proliferated, sometimes appearing in print before the journals had reported the presence of the disease.

Brandreth's Vegetable Universal Pills, Holt's Prescription and Remedies for Yellow Fever, Longley's Western Indian Panacea, and numerous other preparations could be purchased for self-treatment in the 1830s and 1840s.[76] Some advertisements ran on for two or three newspaper columns, detailing cases allegedly cured by the medicine, quoting from physicians' letters of praise, offering a monistic theory of disease, and warning against the dangerous and useless heroic practice of the times. The promoters wrote good copy that offered a simple appealing alternative to the extremes of regular therapeutics while preserving the traditional explanatory framework of systemic disorder (imbalance of body fluids or nervous forces), long embedded in popular culture as well as regular medicine.

Dr. Brandreth's Vegetable Universal Pills could only be purchased from his advertised agents or from his office on Old Levee near Canal Street. A lengthy advertisement in the New Orleans *Picayune* in 1838 included an account of "YELLOW FEVER CURED, WITH BRANDRETH'S PILLS ALONE!" As soon as the fever attacked, the person took five pills, followed by ten every hour for seven hours. Thereafter, fifteen pills each night and morning resulted in full recovery within ten days, according to the story. The pills cost twenty-five cents a box, but the ad did not specify how many pills each box contained.[77]

In 1840, another medical entrepreneur, Dr. Truman Stillman, set forth three columns of advertising for his original "Highly Concentrated Compound Syrup of Sarsaparilla and Purifying Alterative Blood Pills," a medicine to prevent as well as cure "yellow fever, or any other epidemic of equally dangerous or fatal character" by cleansing the blood of "all impurities" and eliminating from the stomach and bowels "all morbific matters that may have accumulated in the system by inhaling *impure air*, or from eating *unwholesome food*." Available wholesale and retail at the Southern Chemical Works on Customhouse Street in New Orleans, the medicine included directions for use and explanation of "its medical virtues on the human constitution" in English, French, Spanish, German, Portuguese, and Dutch.[78]

At the time, Stillman's explanations of disease and therapeutic objectives were not very different from the traditional views of regular physicians, but the claim for one specific remedy with universal effects was the mark of quackery. The truly professional practitioner was expected to use careful judgment in selecting from a large number of available drugs those measures appropriate to each individual case. Panaceas continued to appear in the marketplace, however, appealing to human hopes and fears in the absence of effective treatment. In the late 1850s, for example, Dr. Radway's Ready Relief, Regulating Pills and Resolvent allegedly would prevent and cure not only yellow fever but "all diseases or complaints incidental to the human race."[79]

Patent medicine advertising was remarkably adaptive to the changing times in the late nineteenth century, combining elements of the new germ theory and the emerging authority of "science" with the tradition of systemic "cleansing" and claims of universal efficacy.[80] The emphasis on disinfection by health authorities in the postebellum era also gave rise to numerous products such as Darby's Prophylactic Fluid in 1867, to be added to drinking water or bath water. Since "no offensive effluvia can exist in its presence," lodgings could also be disinfected by placing a saucer of Darby's Fluid in every room. In 1897, "Formozone, the ideal disinfectant," available from all druggists, was advertised as having the power to "destroy yellow fever germs" and halt contagion.[81]

After the discovery of the yellow fever mosquito, another advertising angle appeared. During the 1905 epidemic, this restrained, if slightly misleading, notice appeared in the New Orleans *Picayune*:

> TO THE PUBLIC:
> Mosquito Bites Rendered Harmless
> by the use of Dr. G. H.
> TICHENOR'S ANTISEPTIC
> rub in well[82]

Other products were displayed more flamboyantly that summer as specific yellow fever preventives. Disinfectine, "the modern toilet Soap," which "opens and searches the pores—destroys and removes the germs," was also guaranteed to heal mosquito bites and prevent yellow fever. Littell's Liquid Sulphur, taken internally and added to bath water, "absolutely" prevented mosquito bites and rendered the user immune to "all contagious or infectious diseases."[83]

New Orleans newspapers frequently published letters from well-meaning persons, local and distant, offering gratuitous advice on the prevention or cure of yellow fever, especially during epidemics. In 1853, for example, the New Orleans press reported that an American diplomat in Venezuela had informed the State Department of an effective yellow fever remedy: juice from the leaves of the verbena plant, taken three times a day and in "injections" (enemata) every two hours. Like so many proposed remedies, nothing more was heard of this South American "discovery." In

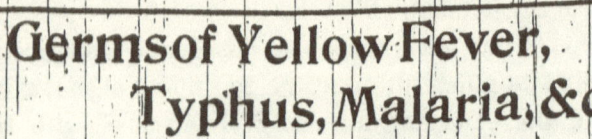

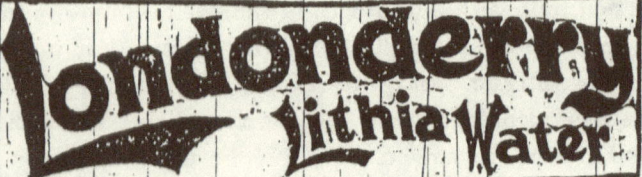

Londonderry Lithia Water.
Don't Wait Until You Have Yellow Fever.
(From New Orleans *Times-Democrat*, September 18, 1897.)

The Terrible Scourge Yellow Fever

will make no inroads in the system kept properly cleansed.

Hunyadi János

the natural laxative mineral water, will move the bowels regularly every day and keep the body free from poisonous germs. Now, if ever, it's the ounce of prevention that counts. Drink half a glass on arising.

The Terrible Scourge Yellow Fever.
(From New Orleans *Item*, August 26, 1905.)

JACK FROST "VERSUS" BRONZE JOHN

"TWO TUFF NUTS," but the match has been declared off by the combined efforts of Wyman, Blanchard and Behrman, who positively declare that the fight shall never be pulled off on Louisiana soil.

BRONZE JOHN is already packing his suit case and begging transportation, on the "SULPHUR AND SALTPETER LINE," for himself and MRS. STEGOMYIA, to PANAMA or PERNAMBUCO, where it is supposed they still have some friends.

Nothwithstanding this great disturbance in health circles, the "ORLEANS" enrolled last week five hundred and eighty new members at the usual rate, ten cents per week, which guarantees a "ONE HUNDRED DOLLAR FUNERAL" at time of DEATH.

ORLEANS UNDERTAKING CO., Ltd.
1164 to 1178 Camp Street.   ALBERT E. BRIEDE, Manager.
WRITE OR PHONE MAIN 580.

Jack Frost versus Bronze John.
(From New Orleans *Item*, September 17, 1905.)

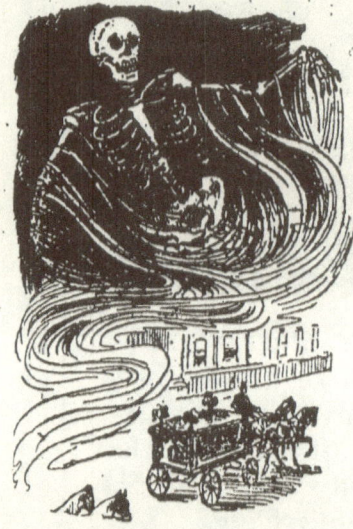
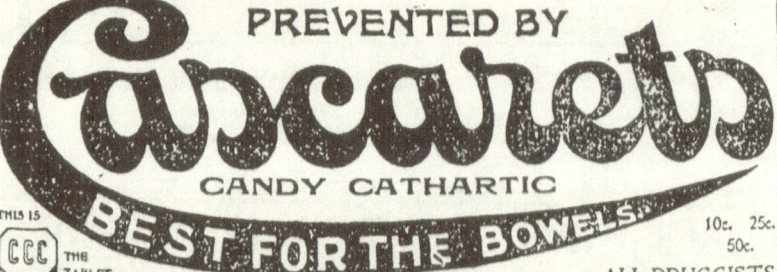

Yellow Jack.
(From New Orleans *Item*, September 17, 1905.)

1858, the *Picayune* reported that "some kind person" had given the Howard Association a bale of the "citronelle" plant for treating yellow fever, presumably as a tea. Citing the ancient theory "that in every country where specific diseases prevail, nature has provided a specific vegetable or mineral remedy," the editor speculated that some plant from "our forests and swamps" might eventually be found to cure yellow fever. The citronelle was available at the Howard Association office for anyone who wanted to try it. During the epidemic of 1867, a Texan visiting in London sent the *Picayune* a "communication" from an "eminent and philanthropic" Englishman, recommendng pulverized charcoal as preventive and cure.[84]

Not only the laity but some physicians also wrote letters to editors outlining a course of treatment for yellow fever, especially in the 1850s. The *Picayune* published a letter in 1858 from Dr. J. J. Hayes to the laborers of New Orleans, advising them to leave their crowded, ill-ventilated lodgings and camp out along the river. Theorizing that yellow fever was the result of "a deficiency of atmospheric air in the lungs," Hayes deduced that a plentiful supply of air would *prevent* the fever. Furthermore, abstaining from all food and labor for four days and four hours would *cure* the fever, he explained, by "reestablishing the balance of air in the system" and eliminating the bile produced by vegetable foods. Hayes was still promoting these ideas in the late 1870s.[85]

Dr. Fred B. Page of Donaldsonville, Louisiana, wrote the *Picayune* in August, 1853, detailing a "simple course" for treating yellow fever, probably the best advice available that year. At the first signs of illness (fatigue, chill, headache, back pain, dizziness), he recommended that the patient take a mustard foot bath, go to bed, keep warm, drink sage or orange-leaf tea, "send for a reliable physician," and in the meantime, employ "some good Creole nurse," likely to be safer and more effective than nine-tenths of the doctors out to test their latest theory. "Better to abandon disease to nature than submit to inefficient and injurious modes of practice usually adopted in this disease."[86]

A doctor employed by the Howard Association during the 1858 epidemic wrote a note to the *Picayune*, believing that the community would be interested in "almost everything" relating to yellow fever. After several weeks of disappointing results from the "ordinary plan of treatment," he had decided to begin each new case with a mild emetic and had lost no patient thus treated. "At present I only wish to make a statement of the facts which I have observed, and facts are much more valuable just now than the most learned theories," he declared.[87]

Not all physicians agreed that the community had any need to know the details of treatment or the uncertainties of practice, and some scolded their colleagues for therapeutic discussions in the popular press. The editors of the *New Orleans Medical News and Hospital Gazette* wondered who these misguided doctors intended to help by their letters in the papers. Certainly not other professionals, and "surely not . . . the people, for it is just as impossible that every man can be his own doctor as it is that he can be his own watchmaker, shoemaker, tailor, etc." The medical editors denounced as "utter madness" the efforts of physicians "to popularize medicine," and they chastised the press for cooperating in such a questionable practice.[88] Physicians at mid-century, with their limitations exposed to public view, feeling threatened by "irregular" practitioners, patent remedies, quacks offering "specific cures," and popular manuals of domestic medicine, were especially outraged by their regular colleagues who spelled out a simple course of treatment *gratis* in the daily newspapers, or openly discussed the trial-and-error aspects of medical practice.

Acknowledging the Limits of Medication

After the series of devastating epidemics in the 1850s, Yellow Jack was a less common visitor and although a recurring threat, only on three or four occasions during the last four decades of the nineteenth century did the disease spread in serious epidemic form. For a time, Civil War and Reconstruction occupied the attention of physicians and laity, and debates over quarantine and commerce in the late nineteenth century overshadowed the earlier concern with treatment. Medicine itself was in a state of transition. The centuries-old concept of disease as general systemic imbalance manifested variously in specific patients was being replaced by a view of diseases as specific entities with specific microscopic causes. In a remarkable cognitive reversal, diseases had become specific and patients had become generalized.

Yellow fever was increasingly described as a self-limited disease. During the 1860s and thereafter, the therapeutic tradition of *la médicine expectante*, whereby nature was accorded the major healing role, seems to have merged with an attenuated version of the activist mode. This synthesis gradually became an inclusive new orthodoxy for the treatment of yellow fever. Some physicians still referred to bloodletting (mainly cupping), quinine, and calomel as appropriate means for occasional use, in small amounts only, to manage various symptoms; but not in heroic quantities to jolt the system and break up the "morbid imbalance," as previously rationalized. Almost everyone who wrote on the subject advocated mild treatment for yellow fever and repeatedly warned against heroic medications. That such warnings continued for decades suggests that many practitioners outside the circles of urban academic medicine found it difficult to relinquish their aggressive tradition.

A pamphlet published in New Orleans in 1862 for the use of federal army surgeons in the Department of the Gulf offered "Some Practical Observations on Yellow Fever," including advice on treatment for the instruction of the northern doctors who lacked experience with the southern scourge. Moderation was the key, and rest and quiet essential. The pamphlet advised that "there is not much room for active interference of the physician, except to relieve any complication; or direct the nursing of the patient." Treatment was clearly symptomatic, even when traditional medicines were suggested.[89] Except for the references to cupping, calomel, and quinine (each of which was only one among several options proposed for treating a specific symptom), the pamphlet's course of treatment closely resembled the expectant practice attributed to creole practitioners and nurses since the early nineteenth century. Other commentators on yellow fever therapeutics during the rest of the century offered similar advice.[90]

After Shreveport's worst experience with yellow fever, in 1873, a committee of physicians prepared a report on the epidemic, in which they noted "the detrimental influence exerted by mercurials and quinine." All agreed that general phlebotomy was inappropriate, and they knew of no case of its use. The most effective treatment included a mild cathartic (castor oil or magnesia), a hot mustard foot bath, crushed ice and lemonade, cool sponging, and mild diuretics.[91] According to Dr. Henry Smith, in his account of the epidemic, "Every physician of the present day must acknowledge that good nursing is half the battle. . . ." He viewed the disease as a "a self-limited one . . . destined to run its course, [and one which] cannot be arrested or cured by drugs." Emphasizing rest, diet, and liquids, Smith treated "very few with calomel" and seldom used any strong purgatives; sometimes he employed cupping in the first stage, but always cautiously.[92]

Dr. Lassalinière Chérot, a native of Guadeloupe, had practiced medicine in Lafourche Parish since the 1850s with remarkable success in treating yellow fever. His "Celebrated Treatment," according to an 1878 report, included bed rest, the mustard foot bath, enemas, mild purgatives, lemonade, careful nursing, and keeping the patient in good spirits.[93] Moderation seemed to be winning out in the 1870s, but the dialectic continued.

Writing after the 1878 epidemic, Dr. Joseph Jones exhibited a somewhat more interventionist approach, believing that yellow fever could be "modified and controlled, if not arrested," by "judicious" treatment, good nursing, and certain drugs administered at the appropriate time. His treatment included ipecac at the start, then calomel and quinine (ten grains each), followed by castor oil, along with the common auxiliary measures.[94] Around the same time, Dr. Henry D. Schmidt, Charity Hospital Pathologist, asserted that yellow fever "will not bear much of what the profession calls 'meddlesome practice'; and it is for this reason that the most simple treatment will ever prove the most successful." He pointed out, however, that the patient required "constant" attention, "for certain conditions will arise . . . when the withdrawal of the attention for only half an hour may lead to a fatal issue."[95]

As late as the 1880s, some physicians cherished the old remedies despite the clear trend in the profession against them. Few were as bold, however, as Dr. R. H. Day of Baton Rouge. Writing in the *New Orleans Medical and Surgical Journal*, Day advocated bleeding to relieve delirium in spite of all the "authorities." He dismissed the warnings in recent years about the danger of bloodletting as "the sheerest nonsense . . . , [serving] only to make cowards of the timorous. . . ." He claimed successful use of quinine in every epidemic from 1853 through 1878. Day's prescription for yellow fever included calomel (20 grains) and quinine (30 to 40 grains), given in four equal doses at four-hour intervals; he also recommended the long-outmoded blisters on the epigastrium for nausea.[96] By 1890, however, Dr. George M. Sternberg, U. S. Army Surgeon, pioneer bacteriologist and yellow fever authority, could report that "the majority" of physicians had rejected active medication and adopted the expectant or symptomatic treatment, with good nursing, as the best management of yellow fever.[97]

Continuity and Change

From the 1890s on, virtually all discussions of yellow fever therapeutics emphasized the limits of medication and encouraged symptomatic treatment and attentive nursing care. From 1879 until 1897, the South had been relatively free of yellow fever. Although widespread and terrifying, the 1897 epidemic turned out to be a pale version of the old scourge in terms of mortality. The editors of the *New Orleans Medical and Surgical Journal* made this point in 1898, commenting that the decline in virulence together with the efficacy of modern "non-meddlesome" medication made this disease no more to be dreaded than any ordinary malady.[98]

After the 1897 epidemic, Surgeon-General Walter Wyman, U. S. Marine Hospital Service, arranged for the publication of a set of papers on yellow fever by several of his experienced officers. Writing on treatment, Surgeon R. D. Murray claimed that 75 percent of yellow fever cases "need only to be let alone by the extra-attentive nurse or friend and heroic physician." These would recover regardless of treatment. Among the remainder, "some will need formal attention and careful procedure; others will die in spite of all reasonable aid."[99]

Murray and another officer, H. D. Geddings, each wrote papers detailing what they considered the best treatment of the time. Both men supported the prevailing symptomatic approach and agreed on almost all points. They proposed much more intervention and drug use, however, than the "non-meddlesome" management then being advocated in New Orleans. Their recommendations included a number of newly developed antipyretics and analgesics such as acetanilid, antipyrine, phenacetin, or other coal-tar derivatives. Other drugs offered for various symptoms included citrate of caffeine taken with antipyretics; cinchonidia, a form of quinine, for cases where malaria might also be present; cocaine in tablet form for nausea; hypodermic morphia for chronic vomiting; sulfonal, bromide, and chloral for sleeplessness; and hypodermic strychnia for collapse.

Along with the newer medicines, the Marine Hospital surgeons also described the appropriate stages and symptoms requiring the use of the mustard foot bath, castor oil, magnesia, cathartic pills containing small amounts of calomel and jalap, high enemata made with soapsuds and molasses or a little whisky or turpentine, mustard plasters or small blisters, carbonated drinks, dry cupping, massage, tisanes of orange leaves or watermelon seeds (credited to New Orleans creoles), beverage alcohol as a stimulant, and a few other suggestions for remedial action.[100]

Since the 1870s, the work of Pasteur, Koch, and others had focused medical attention on pathogenic microorganisms as causes of infectious diseases. While no new treatments immediately resulted, germ theory began to influence the way some physicians thought and wrote about therapeutics and perhaps affected their practice as well. Dr. Just Touatre commented in 1898 that practitioners, recognizing that they had no means as yet of directly attacking the yellow fever "microbe" or its "toxin," were turning away from therapies that had dominated practice for the past century and almost to the present, such as purgatives, emetics, bleeding, cupping, blisters, and quinine.

"Drugs are dying out," he declared, and yellow fever treatment, like that of other infectious diseases, "tends to rid itself from day to day of remedies that are nearly always useless when they are not harmful." Touatre outlined what the doctors could do, however, to help the patient in fighting the toxin. His own method included (1) calomel, not as a purgative but as an "intestinal antiseptic," in a three-grain dose, plus enemata; (2) warm mustard foot bath "à la créole," to produce sweating and relaxation; (3) cold sponging all over, repeatedly, to reduce temperature; (4) cold bath, if temperature 105 degrees or more; (5) no food for about three days; only vichy water (or soda water) in generous quantity, to dilute the "icteroid toxin" and eliminate the poison through the urine. In cases with black vomit, Touatre judged the commonly employed astringents and coagulants as useless, but hot vinegar frictions, hot baths, and rectal injections of hot coffee with brandy might be tried; some patients would recover and some would die, no matter what.[101]

Some drugs might have been "dying out," as Touatre believed, but new ones were being born in the laboratory, the new center of pharmaceutical and physiological, as well as bacteriological, research. These new synthetic drugs and new forms of older drugs, administered hypodermically, found a prominent place in the prescriptions of Marine Hospital Surgeons Murray and Geddings. Murray mentioned at least a dozen new medications and more than a dozen old ones in his course of treatment, while describing his remedies as "limited" in number. Some practitioners were adding new weapons to the arsenal while retaining the tried-and-true auxiliary measures and reducing the dosage or finding new uses for other potent drugs in treating yellow fever.

A Louisiana State Board of Health pamphlet prepared in 1898 by its president, Dr. Edmond Souchon, gave detailed advice on the management of yellow fever. One set of instructions for "the lay nurse who may have to treat yellow fever patients in default of a physician" advised bed rest and quiet, no medicine whatsoever, enemas, sponging, mustard poultices on the stomach, and no food or drink except cold water for several days. The pamphlet encouraged the lay nurse to use a thermometer, an instrument only rarely used by physicians themselves as late as the 1880s. If the temperature exceeded 103 degrees, cold baths and cold enemas were needed to reduce the fever. After a few days, the nurse could offer milk and broth, a spoonful or two every few hours, slowly increasing the amount. After nine or ten days, the patient might gradually resume a normal diet.

Dr. Souchon's advice to inexperienced physicians outlined even less for them to do, beginning with a clear warning against the use of "strong medicines." A "mild" purgative was to be given at the start—a small dose of calomel, salts, or castor oil—only once. For headache or backache, a five-grain dose of phenacetin could be administered–only once. In case of extreme debility after the fever went down, a cardiac tonic such as digitalis or strychnine might be given hypodermically, but cautiously. "Use no other medicines," concluded these firm directions to the inexperienced.[102]

In a meeting of the Orleans Parish Medical Society during the epidemic of 1905, one physician remarked that the "specific" for yellow fever, if it had one, was "water, water, water."[103] This comment came in response to an earlier presentation by Dr. Lucien F. Salomon, a voice representing the past, challenging those who opposed active medication and those who doubted the existence of a yellow fever "specific." On the contrary, he believed yellow fever to be a "curable disease" and potassium nitrate a specific "antidote for the Yellow Fever poison." According to Salomon, the potassium nitrate not only acted as a diuretic but had a "specific effect as an anti-toxin." He supported the widely accepted simple measures for managing symptoms, but he continued to advocate creosote and ergot for the black vomit, taking issue with Dr. Rudolph Matas. Salomon also warned against the "so-called anti-pyretics" such as phenacetin, which he found "positively vicious" in effect. He asked his colleagues to "cut loose from the dicta and dogmas of those who have little faith in the efficacy of drugs, even when properly and intelligently applied," and give his method a fair trial.[104]

Representing what had become the new orthodoxy in New Orleans, a bulletin offering "First Aid Advice," signed by Dr. Quitman Kohnke of the city health board, appeared in the *Picayune* in the midst of the 1905 epidemic, New Orleans' final encounter with Yellow Jack. Kohnke provided instructions to the laity for managing yellow fever until a physician could be obtained: cold compresses for headache and fever; hot foot bath (mustard optional); water, vichy, seltzer, or watermelon juice in small amounts, given frequently to keep kidneys active; bits of ice to relieve nausea; no solid food whatsoever for several days; complete bed rest. According to Kohnke, the essence of treatment was "to avoid doing harm." He advised those administering this "First Aid" to call a physician quickly and expect from him "much advice and little medicine."[105]

Since 1905, North American physicians have not had to deal with yellow fever epidemics, and discussions of treatment ceased to consume the pages of medical periodicals, pamphlets, and reports. The disease remains endemic in the forests of South America, Central America, and Africa, and serious outbreaks have occurred in recent decades, mainly in Africa.[106] Treatment described in current texts and manuals resembles the symptomatic approach of the early twentieth century, with emphasis on bed rest and nursing care. Maintenance of fluid intake and electrolyte balance is important, while various drugs, as well as intravenous glucose saline and blood plasma transfusions, are used to relieve symptoms and treat complications as they arise. In most respects, current treatment is more "expectant" and supportive than "heroic" or "abortive." There is still, as always, an important arena in which the physician's expertise may be applied, monitoring the signs and administering medications to combat headache, fever, nausea and vomiting, dehydration, hemorrhage, shock, and renal failure.[107]

Yet despite the advances in knowledge about the virus, its vectors, and its epidemiological and immunological relations (including studies at the molecular level), yellow fever resists understanding and rational treatment: "At present, the complex pathophysiologic interrelationships of yellow fever cannot be specified, and directions for specific therapeutic interventions are consequently undetermined."[108] Texts reflect the emphasis on laboratory studies seeking basic knowledge and on prevention through immunization and mosquito control, devoting relatively little attention to therapeutics. Animal experiments in recent decades using antiviral agents and other measures have not been encouraging. Emphasis on prevention seems to offer a better chance of success relative to effort and cost than therapeutics, which remains as uncertain as it was a century ago. In the absence of urban epidemics in wealthy countries, there is also little pressure to attend to therapy. Reappearance of the disease in Central or South American cities (which some authorities predict) could pose a serious threat to the southern United States. Such epidemics would probably change research emphasis as well as afford more clinical material. For now, yellow fever treatment is still in a sense experimental. *Plus ça change, plus c'est la même chose.*

XIV

SOCIAL AND CULTURAL IMPACT OF YELLOW JACK

Yellow fever, wherever it appeared, affected almost every aspect of human affairs, disrupting the routines of individual and family life and community institutions as well as the larger patterns of social and economic activity. Epidemics created special medical and welfare needs that had to be met by organized effort: caring for the sick, feeding the families of the sick poor and others unemployed because of the epidemic, burying the dead, comforting the survivors, providing for orphans, and maintaining social order. In New Orleans and elsewhere in the nineteenth century, a combination of private and public endeavors provided minimal medical and welfare services; charitable societies functioned with the sanction of local government and received occasional public subsidy for epidemic relief.

Epidemics placed extraordinary demands upon doctors, nurses, clergy, police, volunteer relief workers, and graveyard sextons for essential services. Hospitals overflowed, temporary infirmaries and orphan shelters filled to capacity, schools postponed opening, small newspapers suspended operation because of staff illness, and coffins piled up at graveyard gates. The jobless, the hungry, and the sick sought relief. Mutual aid societies mushroomed in antebellum New Orleans, an attempt by occupational and ethnic groups to provide for themselves a form of "social insurance" in time of epidemics. Functioning as a quasi-governmental agency, the New Orleans Howard Association from 1837 through 1878 collected donations from the nation at large and dispensed aid to the sick and the poor in the Crescent City and many other afflicted towns throughout the state and region.

The scourge left its scars, visible and invisible, on behaviors, social relations, attitudes, feelings, mentality. Yellow fever heightened an awareness of class, race, and other social distinctions in nineteenth-century New Orleans. The influence of recurring epidemics was manifested in the contrasting extremes of indifference and altruism, fatalistic outlook and reformist vision, prayers for deliverance and bizarre epidemic humor. Yellow fever also contributed to the formation of an "insider" mentality shared by comfortable "acclimated" New Orleanians who felt no affinity for the "outsider" elements associated with disease and poverty. As "insiders," the political and business leaders constructed a distorted image of health and prosperity in antebellum New Orleans. That illusion was dispelled (in part) only in response to economic pressures in the new national marketplace after the Civil War.

An epidemic or the threat of an epidemic produced reactions of panic and lingering memories in small interior towns. Attitudes were somewhat different in the coastal cities where Yellow Jack was familiar and "acclimation" common. But whatever the variations in community responses to yellow fever's appearance, the deadly disease made its presence felt in countless ways, influencing the society and culture of all those within its path.

Insider-Outsider Mentality

One medical historian has claimed that "Yellow fever was a powerful (if not the most important) factor in the affective history of nineteenth century New Orleans."[1] Because of its differential impact along the lines of class, race, and ethnicity, yellow fever intensified class consciousness, race prejudice, and the potential for ethno-cultural conflict. Because of the apparent immunity of the native as opposed to the vulnerability of the newcomer, the disease contributed to an insider-outsider mentality. To become an insider, the newcomer had to survive an attack of the fever and become "acclimated," a process sometimes actually referred to as "naturalization" or "creolization."[2]

The native-born and the survivors perceived themselves as the true citizens of New Orleans. Yellow fever immunity provided one secure foundation for identity and social cohesion within the unstable, expanding, diverse, and fragmented urban society. Outsiders, who helped define the insiders, were "the strangers," blamed for bringing the disease upon themselves and upon the city: first the Americans (until they became creolized by survival or nativity), then mainly the German and Irish immigrants before the Civil War, and finally the Italian immigrants in the late nineteenth century.

Class divisions roughly followed ethnic lines, or so it seemed, as most nineteenth-century immigrants began in the ranks of the poor. Hence, the "better element" found little reason to sympathize with those they defined as a troublesome, foreign lower class, who came to New Orleans, indulged in their undisciplined, "imprudent" ways of living, fell sick, and died—a burden to the city and its reputation. New Orleans was always healthy, *except* for this group or that. On the other hand, survivors could displace their guilt, if necessary, by relief work among the sick poor during epidemic crises.[3] The voluntary benevolent associations also helped to define community (or a variety of communities) within the broken-up society of the nineteenth-century American city.

Black resistance to the disease aroused white fears of slave rebellion in the antebellum years, but with one or two exceptions it is difficult to determine whether the rumors had any real basis other than the anxiety of whites during epidemic crisis. Certainly blacks were aware of their presumed immunity. What some whites perceived as a "spirit of insubordination" during epidemics might have been inspired by a sense of black strength and superiority when faced with the saffron scourge. Ironically, one medical authority in the 1850s referred to the "inferior susceptibility" of blacks to yellow fever.[4] This distinction in racial vulnerability to the disease could have fueled lower class white resentment against blacks and reinforced the existing racial prejudice among all whites. The apparent immunity of blacks, however, made them especially useful and desirable during epidemics as nurses, hearse drivers, and grave diggers—the latter so greatly in demand that they received extraordinary wages.[5] The postwar epidemics, especially that of 1878, coming on the heels of Reconstruction and economic depression, exacerbated old class, racial, and religious hostilities.[6]

Yellow fever epidemics in the antebellum years sometimes served as an occasion for the venting of sectional antagonisms between North and South, even while northerners were sending contributions for the relief of afflicted communities. Some abolitionists pointed to yellow fever as a punishment for slavery, and southerners responded that black exemption from the disease was a powerful argument supporting slavery because of the high mortality among working class whites. The yellow fever zone in the United States had virtually the same boundaries as the southern slave states; the disease was defined as a southern malady to which the northern states were no longer subject. Not until 1878 when yellow fever traveled extensively along rivers and rails to points previously considered beyond the zone would the disease be accorded national status in the reunified and increasingly interdependent United States.[7]

Thus yellow fever made it possible for acclimated New Orleanians to define themselves as insiders, reinforced class and racial divisions and social power relations, and added another distinction between North and South. The same process would have obtained in other southern coastal cities where yellow fever was a common phenomenon. The disease also aggravated urban-rural antagonisms and heightened competition between southern cities, especially in the post-Civil War era. Primarily an urban disease, more precisely a disease identified with New Orleans, yellow fever was one of the many components of southern city life that the people of the hinterland feared and wanted to protect themselves against. In this case, the residents of interior communities were the "insiders" who declared quarantine "against the world," as it was sometimes phrased, to keep out the pestilence which might be introduced by merchandise or "outsiders" from the city.

Charges and counter-charges of deception, denial, exaggeration, and falsehood on the subject of yellow fever flew back and forth between city and country newspapers, reflecting different perspectives and views of the world: rural against urban, hinterland against New Orleans, and vice versa. Small towns and rural areas had plenty of complaints and reservations about the wicked but fascinating Crescent City in the nineteenth century, and yellow fever added one more prominent "evil" to the long list.

City and Country Attitudes Toward Epidemics

Antebellum New Orleanians developed an attitude toward the comings and goings of Yellow Jack that differed in some important respects from the reaction in small towns of the interior. Reflecting on these differences in 1854, Dr. T. A. Cooke of Washington, Louisiana, declared that "the effect of a fatal pestilence in towns of the country cannot well be conceived by those who have not witnessed it. It spreads alarm; the people are panic-stricken; and every death adds to the consternation, which sweeps over the land." Country folk long retained an intense memory of the epidemic with its terrors and suffering, while the large urban populace rapidly fell back into the "coldest apathy" and soon forgot the past. In small towns the majority of the dead were known by the survivors; in New Orleans, while many grieved over lost family and friends, the thousands of fatalities might represent little more to an individual than an impersonal item of mortality statistics.[8] Frequent epidemics since the 1790s had led to the acceptance of yellow fever as a regular summer visitor in New Orleans. But country towns suffered only occasional outbreaks, and some remained exempt for years. When yellow fever did arrive, almost everyone was susceptible to attack, whether old resident or newcomer, native or foreign, well-to-do or working class.

In contrast, most of the literature on yellow fever in nineteenth-century New Orleans emphasized the city's passive acceptance of epidemics. According to Charles Gayarré, nineteenth-century Louisiana historian, yellow fever had no more terrors for New Orleanians "than had for the ancients the skull which used to figure among the roses and other luxuries that adorned their banqueting tables."[9] Another nineteenth-century Louisiana writer, George Washington Cable, reported that the French creoles, usually enjoying immunity, worried little about the large numbers of strangers dying of yellow fever; after all, nobody asked them to come to New Orleans. As for busy Americans, whether creole or newcomer, their primary interest was the immediate monetary gain from the city's commerce, and although the summer brought the pestilence, the winter brought trade and prosperity![10]

During the severe epidemic of 1858, the editor of the New Orleans *Daily Delta* remarked that the outsider undoubtedly would be interested to know that "everywhere he would find but comparatively little attention paid to the scourge on the part of the great body of citizens." The first announcement of the fever created panic among the uninitiated, and the exodus began. But, the editor claimed, the acclimated (whether native or long-term resident) felt no fear whatsoever. In fact, "they seem to take the matter as cooly as if it was something expected annually, and about which it were idle to become alarmed." Even the unacclimated persons who found it necessary to stay in the city quickly fell into "this prevailing state of indifference."[11] On one occasion, a minister allegedly commented, "I like the people of New Orleans; they are not afraid of epidemics, and when they die, do not whine about it."[12]

The bulk of yellow fever victims—immigrants and others among the lower classes—were not included among the articulate self-defined citizenry, and the manuscript and printed sources reveal little about their feelings or opinions. Perhaps they considered the disease simply one more gamble among the countless other risks of their existence. Despite its growing reputation as the great southern graveyard, antebellum New Orleans continued to attract newcomers from Europe and other parts of America, and its population increased from less than 10,000 in 1803 to 170,000 in 1860, making it the sixth largest American city.[13]

During the first half of the nineteenth century, pestilential visitations were common, ordinary, expected, and accepted in New Orleans as apparently unavoidable disasters. When epidemics declined in frequency in the postbellum years, the disease became less familiar and more frightening, to many New Orleanians as well as to their small town neighbors in the interior. The expansion of southern railroads as part of a national transportation network in the late nineteenth century introduced the disease to many small communities previously protected by their relative isolation. After 1878, a report or rumor of a single case in New Orleans was sufficient to set off a panic throughout the gulf states and Mississippi Valley, prompting local and state authorities to erect quarantine barriers for the protection of their territory against the city's dreadful infection.[14]

The Medical Profession

In the grim battles against epidemics waged repeatedly in the towns of Louisiana and the South, the medical profession was necessarily on the front line. Physicians had to cope with the burden of duty and frustration as they tried to save lives from a deadly disease that spread unpredictably and ran its course in seeming defiance of all forms of therapy. No doctor who practiced any length of time in the deep South could ignore the yellow fever enigma. And probably no other disease in the nineteenth century provoked as much controversy, diversity of opinion, and professional antagonism.

Yet the saffron scourge seems to have been one of the principal forces influencing the French physicians of New Orleans to establish a professional organization, La Société Médicale de la Nouvelle-Orléans. The epidemic of 1817, the most destructive up to that time, apparently convinced the French-speaking doctors that it was necessary to pool their intellectual resources against the disease. One of the first official actions of the society was the appointment of a committee to inquire into the causes and treatment of the recent epidemic fever. In 1820 when the English-speaking physicians in New Orleans organized the Physico-Medical Society, they also began to study the recurring pestilence. These medical societies and their successors in nineteenth-century Louisiana continued to be preoccupied with yellow fever epidemics and the related issues of quarantine and sanitary reform, serving as a forum for debate and seldom showing consensus among their members.[15]

During the long war against yellow fever, the medical profession in southern coastal and river ports lost many practitioners to the disease, especially among the "unacclimated" doctors who had come from other parts of the country.[16] Like the physician in Camus' *La Peste*, most doctors labored on day after day, week after week, for several months, powerless against the disease, yet exerting all their energies toward alleviating the suffering and anxiety of as many patients as possible, sometimes with success, often with failure. A New Orleans physician wrote to an out-of-state acquaintance in 1808, describing the "fever of this year" and the large number of cases ending with the black vomit. He admitted that he would like to "forsake this scene of trouble and anxiety," but honor and good faith compelled him to stay "until this eventful period is past."[17]

One antebellum observer wrote: "I have always sympathized with the physicians in New Orleans. Their duties in a sickly season are most arduous and responsible. Often have I seen them in a few weeks reduced to their beds by anxiety, toil, watchings, and disappointment. . . ." Making matters even worse, "multitudes, instead of thanking them, have cursed them, because they did not at once expel the epidemic from the city, which they could no more control than they could raise the dead."[18] During epidemics some physicians ran notices in newspapers offering to "attend gratuitously" to the indigent sick. In 1853 Dr. Erasmus Fenner commented on this practice: "There is, perhaps, no place in the world where more *charity service* is done by the medical profession than in New Orleans . . . but I am sorry to add, that I know of no place where these benevolent services are more lightly appreciated than here."[19]

Throughout the decades of epidemics, New Orleans physicians generally received high praise for their courage, generosity, and tireless labors. As in all human activity, however, one can find examples of ignorance, greed, and callousness. A member of the Howard Association in the 1850s criticized those physicians who would "wring the last dollar from suffering humanity in advance of every service performed, and, when no more can be exacted, abandon them for nature to do the rest." Some doctors offered their services to the Howard Association, accepted the salary provided, then proceeded to extort additional payment from the association's patients. "If they did not succeed in obtaining money from our patients," one member complained, "they would divide with the apothecary the bill of expensive prescriptions."[20]

The Clergy

Like physicians, clergymen of every denomination were called on for an unusual performance of services during epidemics. They were in constant demand day and night to "soothe the last hours of the dying," to administer last rites, and to comfort the surviving family. In the chaos of a severe epidemic it was impossible for the clergy to perform all services at the grave, but they conducted brief services in the homes of the deceased or in the chapels. Many persons were buried without benefit of clergy. In some cases friends, family, or strangers said the final prayers over the grave.[21]

Although it was reported in New Orleans and elsewhere that Protestant ministers sometimes fled in panic along with other terrified émigrés, these clerical deserters seem to have been the exception rather than the rule. Most clergyman of all faiths stayed to face the danger, and some of them died of yellow fever while performing their pastoral duties.[22] At least thirteen Roman Catholic priests, four Sisters of Charity, and two Protestant ministers died of yellow fever in New Orleans in 1853.[23]

Joseph B. Stratton, a Presbyterian minister in Natchez, wrote in his diary after the 1853 epidemic that the rumored flight of all the Protestant clergy was entirely false. From the beginning of the outbreak, he had felt "no other purpose than to remain at my post prepared to perform whatever duties might arise under the new and distressing aspect of affairs." In the early weeks of the epidemic, he wrote, "there was little call for the services of Protestant clergymen. The greater part of those who died were foreigners, many were Jews and many Catholics." Beginning in September, however, his work increased and his journal entries stopped until late November when he began an account of the "extraordinary chapter" in his experience: "After more than three months I resume my diary, three months that seem like an awful dream, three months that have been spent mostly amidst the pain of the sick chamber and homes of deathbeds and the shadows of eternity. The pestilence came and swept over us like a hurricane."[24]

The customary duties of the clergy—performing last rites and funeral services, visiting the sick, sometimes acting as doctor and nurse—were multiplied and magnified during epidemics with the hundreds, or thousands, of yellow fever casualties requiring attention. Their work did not end when the epidemic subsided. In small communities the minister's residence sometimes served as relief headquarters for the collection and distribution of food and clothing for the needy, and the epidemic-scarred populace often turned to the clergy for leadership in reconstructing their lives and their social order.[25]

In New Orleans' final battle against yellow fever in 1905, Catholic priests and nuns of Italian background accepted an additional assignment as propagandists for the new "mosquito doctrine" and as assistants to the health authorities in dealing with the frightened Italian immigrant population. They tried to persuade Italian families to report cases and to allow their sick members to be taken to an isolation hospital. At least one priest told his parishioners they could not be "good Catholics" if they failed to obey the authorities.[26]

For much of the nineteenth century when yellow fever was popularly viewed as a scourge beyond explanation or control, religious rhetoric linked the pestilence with sin, and the frightened people of an afflicted community often prayed for forgiveness and the cessation of what they considered to be God's wrathful punishment. In 1853 the Presbyterian ministers of New Orleans called for a "Union Meeting for humiliation and prayer" to be held at 5 p.m. daily throughout the epidemic.[27] Bishop Leonidas Polk prepared a special prayer in 1853 for use in all churches in the Protestant Episcopal Diocese of Louisiana, acknowledging "that by our sins we have most justly provoked thy wrath and indignation against us."[28] In August, 1853, at the height of the awful epidemic, the mayor of New Orleans proclaimed a special day "for the general voice to rise in supplication to Almighty God, that he may be pleased to lighten the heavy burthen of grief, sickness and death."[29]

At least one dissenting voice was raised in protest against viewing God as the source of the epidemic in 1853. In a statement published in the *Picayune*, Theodore Clapp, Unitarian minister, rejected the proposition that "the epidemic ravaging our city is a display of God's anger." Were New Orleanians any more "deserving at present of Heaven's wrath" than the people of London, Paris, Boston, New York, or any other city? Dr. Clapp did not think so. The afflictions of human life might be "a test of moral character," he affirmed, but to attribute to God such indiscriminate wrath and vengeance visited upon the faithful and the wicked alike was to place the deity beyond all love and respect.[30]

Clapp and others like him remained a minority as long as the disease remained a mystery. Following the precedent set in earlier epidemics, Governor Francis T. Nicholls proclaimed October 9, 1878, as a day of "fasting, humiliation, and prayer" and requested that all Louisianians "join in a concern of devout petition to the Almighty to stay his severe chastisement and to spare an afflicted people."[31] As late as 1897 some persons still considered the wrath of God a factor in pestilential outbreaks, despite the scientific developments that had begun to demystify certain diseases and that offered so much promise for eventual success in cracking the codes of disease processes.

Although consistently serving up supportive editorials and headlines for "science" and "modernity" in 1897, the *Picayune* also published the full text of a sermon delivered by the minister of the evangelical Lutheran Church, describing the current epidemic as God's "chastisement" of New Orleans, "a warning for our citizens to repent." While many New Orleanians under the influence of germ theory (including newspaper editors) were advocating comprehensive sanitary reform, the Lutheran minister called for "moral sanitation," insisting that the city's impure moral atmosphere required as thorough a cleansing as its filthy streets and gutters.[32] Covering all bases that year, the *Picayune* reprinted Bishop Polk's prayer of 1853.[33]

During the 1905 epidemic which occurred after yellow fever's agent of transmission had been positively identified, the New Orleans clergy participated actively in the anti-mosquito campaign, preaching from their pulpits the crusade against the *Aedes aegypyi*. Apparently, nothing further was said about God's anger in that last epidemic. One of the black churches of New Orleans, Central Congregational, did call a "special prayer service for the city and the yellow fever epidemic," the first church to do so. The congregation not only prayed for the sufferers, but organized the Colored Sanitary Association to cooperate with white New Orleanians in a campaign against yellow fever.[34] Other churches, white and black, also seem to have mixed prayer with collective purposive action once they had a specific target and a well-defined strategy for fighting the disease with some hope of success.

Benevolent Associations and Relief Work

Severe epidemic conditions required the labor of countless volunteer relief workers and sizeable contributions of funds and supplies. The problem of caring for the sick poor and their families grew with the expanding population of New Orleans. In the early nineteenth century, the municipal government appropriated funds for medicine and food, established temporary hospitals, and appointed and paid physicians and apothecaries during epidemics to attend to the indigent sick.[35] As the city expanded, its municipal administration as well as its population and culture became fragmented. American privatism and commercial values gradually displaced old traditions of French and Spanish paternalism. At various times in the nineteenth century the city council contributed to the Howard Association and provided funds for the care of orphans, medicines needed by the poor, and other services. Nevertheless, for most of the century the task of epidemic relief was assumed largely by private organizations and charitable individuals.

Dozens of societies were organized in New Orleans and other communities to provide emergency relief during epidemics. Without such organized effort, starvation would have increased the mortality lists, and thousands of yellow fever patients would have suffered without attention of any kind. The Masons, Odd Fellows, Young Men's Christian Association, labor organizations, and other professional, social, and religious groups established special relief committees to assist their members or to extend charitable services to the sick poor and their families.[36]

Ethnic and occupational groups began to establish associations in the 1840s and 1850s to provide a form of sickness and burial insurance for their members. New Orleans city directories and other sources listed Spanish, Portuguese, French, Irish, German, Swiss, Italian, and Jewish associations, the United Laborer's Benevolent Association, and the Firemen's Charitable Association. Especially important during epidemics, these societies offered financial aid to any member who became ill, and if he died, made some provision for his widow and children. For example, the Iberia Benevolent Association, organized by Spanish-born residents of New Orleans, was designed "to provide for and assist those of its members who through sickness or other . . . circumstances, may become destitute, and also to inter with proper cermonies, the bodies of such as demise." Only a native Spaniard might become president, but any person "of irreproachable character" could join the society by paying an initiation fee of three dollars and monthly dues of fifty cents. Although not stipulated, it seems clear that all of these insurance associations were composed of men only, except for groups organized by women and specifically designated "female" or "ladies" societies.[37]

A mutual aid society called the Young Men's Crescent and Star Benevolent Association was organized during the epidemic of 1867 by "the elite of the Second and Third Districts" of New Orleans. Membership requirements included "an unstained character," a five dollar initiation fee, and dues of one dollar per month. The group promised to provide medical attention and drugs to any sick member, seven dollars per week during the period of his illness, and proper burial and assistance to the widow and orphans of any deceased member.[38]

After the Civil War, black benevolent associations offering similar benefits began to appear in New Orleans. The Young Female Benevolent Association, for black women, offered a form of mutual medical and burial insurance for an admission fee of two to five dollars and monthly payments of twenty-five to fifty cents. *Les Jeunes Amis*, organized in 1867, and *La Concorde*, in 1878, provided similar services for their French-speaking black members.[39] In 1878 black leaders also organized relief associations in New Orleans and Baton Rouge to collect donations and dispense relief to the sick and the poor among their people.[40]

The Sisters of the Holy Family, a black religious community, performed valuable services in several New Orleans yellow fever epidemics. Henriette Delille, the first mother superior, having acquired experience and skill in nursing yellow fever patients in 1841, was believed to possess special knowledge of remedies. In 1853 she and the other "colored sisters" responded to many calls for their help in nursing the sick. They also provided temporary shelter and care for orphans, both black and white, brought to them during the epidemic. In 1905 the motherhouse was located on the corner of St. Ann and Bourbon streets, near the original focus of the yellow fever outbreak. The health authorities, after having been refused by all the commercial laundries, asked the Sisters of the Holy Family if they would wash the bed linens, gowns, and doctors' coats from the yellow fever isolation hospital. Mother Austin agreed to accept the task if the hospital would disinfect the bedding and clothing before sending it out. From August until the end of the epidemic in November, wagons transported the dirty linens to the sisters and returned clean ones to the hospital several times each day.[41]

Middle and upper class white women in nineteenth-century New Orleans participated in epidemic relief work through such groups as the Ladies' Benevolent Society, the Ladies' Physiological Society, and Les Dames de la Providence. They collected funds and provisions, called on the sick, and offered kindness and encouragement along with food, clothing, and medicine.[42] Les Dames de la Providence, an association of "married ladies belonging to the most respectable class of our Creole population," went about in groups of three or four, attending to the needs of female yellow fever patients, and dispensing relief with funds collected from generous donors of their class.[43]

Unless becoming ill themselves, women of all classes generally nursed the sick in their own families as they had traditionally done. In institutions or in households, paid nurses might be male or female, black or white, their degree of skill depending mainly on experience and intelligence. The Sisters of Charity managed several New Orleans hospitals (including Charity Hospital) and supervised the nursing of the sick, coping with stress, risk, and frustration no less than that of the doctors.[44]

The Howard Association

Unquestionably the most important of the New Orleans societies established to relieve the sick and destitute was the Howard Association, named after the eighteenth-century English philanthropist, John Howard. Organized during the yellow fever epidemic of 1837, the Howard Association was incorporated in 1842 and granted a twenty-five year charter by the Louisiana legislature. The association was reincorporated in 1867, and again in 1893, but its work was largely concluded with the epidemic of 1878.[45]

Initially made up of young men who believed themselves "acclimated," the first Howards were mostly clerks from mercantile firms and members of the Protection Hose Fire Company. They actively sought out those in need of medical care, and they solicited contributions to finance their work, providing food for the poor as well as paying for physicians and medicines. In the first few epidemics the Howards did most of the nursing themselves. Each member was responsible for a certain section of the city, which he was able to cover on foot. As the city expanded in area by mid-century, the Howards had to use horse-drawn cabs to make their rounds. When their "case loads" also expanded in the 1840s and 1850s, they served more as organizers, fund-raisers, and supervisors, hiring and assigning physicians and nurses, managing infirmaries and orphanages, arranging for burial of the dead, and dispensing relief to the needy. New members had to be recruited for each outbreak since a large majority dropped out after working in only one epidemic. Over the years the group included men from a variety of ages, national and religious backgrounds, and occupations, although they remained "predominantly bourgeois."[46]

The Howard Association went into action whenever "an unusual amount of sickness prevailed" in New Orleans, specifically during yellow fever or cholera epidemics. Sometimes they organized and began their relief work before the epidemic had been officially acknowledged. The Howards left slates at various pharmacies on which those needing help could write their names and addresses. Members checked these lists regularly and called on the applicants later the same day. Advertisements in newspapers and placards at street corners gave the names and addresses of all the Howard Association members. Before breakfast and before dinner each member was supposed to be available at his residence to interview applicants for relief who gathered there. After recording the names and addresses of newly reported yellow fever cases and persons requesting emergency relief, the "samaritan" set out on his daily and nightly rounds; visiting patients, checking on families requesting relief, visiting new cases, purchasing and sometimes administering medicines, assigning the new cases to physicians employed by the association, hiring and assigning nurses, sometimes acting as a nurse himself, and so on, day after day, night after night throughout the epidemic.

In addition to making home visits and providing medical care and outright relief to the poor, the Howards also established and supervised temporary hospitals, convalescent infirmaries, and orphan asylums. They issued printed cards known as *bons* worth a dollar or less for the purchase of ice, medicines, or groceries. Knowing the cards would be promptly redeemed by the association, merchants readily accepted them as cash.

Active participants in eleven epidemics during more than four decades, the New Orleans Howard Association served at least 130,000 persons, providing medical care and subsistence and spending more than three-quarters of a million dollars in the process. Twenty-nine other Howard Associations were formed in nine states between 1853 and 1878, modeled after the New Orleans group and often receiving direct assistance from the parent organization. The New Orleans Howards on many occasions sent a few members in person to assist other communities in organizing relief work, and throughout its history the association shared supplies, medicines, nurses, and money with other plague-stricken towns. In 1847 the Howards attended to some 1,200 yellow fever cases in New Orleans; in 1853, 11,000; and in 1878 more than 21,000 in the city and nearly 11,000 in other towns. In 1878 they spent almost $400,000. In New Orleans that year, $107,000 went for relief, $73,000 for nurses, $25,000 for doctors, and $60,000 for medicines. Their funds always came from both local and nationwide contributions.[47]

So extensive was the epidemic in 1878 that the Howards, having fewer members than usual and only four with previous epidemic experience, soon found it necessary to concentrate on the provision of medical care. They turned over the relief work and some of their funds to the Peabody Subsistence Association, an auxiliary body organized to receive donations and to dispense provisions to the destitute.[48] Poverty was so widespread and demands on the resources so great that rations were eventually limited to the families of yellow fever sufferers, certified by the Howards and one or two other approved charitable societies working specifically with epidemic casualties. The restrictive policies and procedures led to criticism, and both the Peabody Association and the Howards were charged with racial and religious discrimination by various sectarian and black societies that felt excluded from the charity.

The Howards were also accused of financial mismanagement during the 1878 epidemic. Their financial difficulties came mostly from the unprecedented demands placed upon the organization and the unpredictability of the needs from one week to the next as calls for Howard assistance kept coming in from towns throughout the region. In September the association made the mistake of assuming that it had received sufficient funds for the duration of the epidemic and announced that no additional contributions were needed. Within a short time, more than eighty towns requested help. Attempting to meet these needs, the Howards renewed their appeal to northern cities for additional funds, a reversal that suggested bad management or poor judgment. When the New Orleans Howards had to cut off aid to some of their small-town auxiliaries, those groups charged the parent society with misuse of funds and discriminatory treatment. New Orleans physicians hired by the Howards also expressed dissatisfaction with the payment they received. Some persons questioned why the association would call a halt to outside donations and at the same time turn down the many requests for assistance from poverty-stricken New Orleanians, both black and white.

The small band of amateur social workers and their volunteer assistants were simply not equal to the enormity of the task in 1878 when faced with the magnitude of disease and poverty in a city population of 200,000, not yet having recovered from the economic depression of the 1870s. The sick and the needy in an entire region of the country also looked to the Howards for help. Overwhelmed by organizational and financial burdens, the Howard Association made mistakes and enemies and went into debt. Although it paid the debt and accounted for all its receipts and expenditures in the official report for 1878, the association had lost the confidence of a more diverse and demanding public. This "early Red Cross" continued to exist on paper until the early twentieth century, but the 1878 epidemic was its final mission.[49] Within the national communication network then taking shape, newspaper reports and telegraphic exchange of "news" could stir sympathy and support for epidemic sufferers among a nationwide reading public; these channels could also carry a flow of information and commentary causing widespread criticism and concern about the problems of relief-management, problems which might have passed without notice by a less-informed populace in an earlier day.

Local, state, and federal health officials began to assume a more active role in epidemics toward the end of the century, taking responsibility for locating and isolating yellow fever cases. The Howard Association's traditional medical aid services were no longer required, but the need for charitable relief work among the destitute persisted. New Orleans' Charity Organization Society was established in the 1890s as an attempt at centralized, efficient management of philanthropy. During the epidemics of 1897 and 1905, it functioned as the principal agency for the receipt and distribution of contributions to relieve those determined by its "investigators" to be the "truly needy" and the "worthy poor."[50]

Schools and Colleges

Yellow fever epidemics, usually lasting from July until early November, made it necessary to postpone for six to eight weeks the opening of public and private schools.[51] Sometimes during major epidemics New Orleans officials authorized the use of public school buildings as temporary hospitals or orphan asylums under the supervision of the Howard Association, the state board of health, or the Charity Hospital administrators.[52]

Colleges and medical schools also postponed the beginning of regular sessions until epidemics subsided.[53] Yellow fever caused illness and death among faculty and local students and discouraged the attendance of some out-of-state students while quarantine barriers hindered the arrival of others. The epidemic of 1905 ruined Tulane's football season. Since the players were scattered throughout the state, quarantine restrictions made it impossible to bring them together for practice until the season was almost over.[54] At least two black institutions of higher education, Tougaloo University in Mississippi and Straight University in New Orleans, announced in October, 1905, that the fall term would not begin until "the departure of the yellow fever."[55]

Yellow fever had a "retarding effect" on the growth of the Charity Hospital Training School for Female Nurses established in 1894. In her report of 1905, Sister Agnes, "Directress" of the school, stated that the epidemic had deterred many applicants and had raised the question of the "advisability" of accepting non-immunes. Of some 300 application forms sent out on request that season, only fifty-two were returned. According to the faculty chairman, the school had not yet reached its full capacity, "owing to circumstances over which we had no control, and which forbade entrance of non-immunes into this city. . . ."[56]

During the final epidemic of 1905, the public schools opened by early October and participated in the city-wide crusade against the yellow fever mosquito. Children heard lectures on the new "mosquito doctrine" and carried home pamphlets containing simple instructions for fumigating houses and oiling and screening cisterns as part of the war against the disease-bearing mosquito.[57]

Disorder, Negligence, and Police

Having witnessed many New Orleans epidemics, Dr. Theodore Clapp was always impressed by the organized benevolence and the relative lack of disorder during the crises. In contrast, he noted that pestilence, especially the plagues of ancient and medieval times, traditionally resulted in "wild, frantic excesses, neglect of the sick and dying, the plunder of houses, murder, and other atrocities too awful to mention."[58] Epidemic conditions in New Orleans (or perhaps any other nineteenth-century American community), no matter how terrible, failed to match this description of social disintegration.

One of the most critical accounts of epidemic behavior was provided by Perrin du Lac, a French traveler in Louisiana in the early 1800s, who found little to praise in the province. He wrote that "the fear and horror which this disease inspires break the most sacred ties of society, and cause all ideas of humanity to vanish." In flight from the city, parents abandoned their sick children, and children their sick parents, leaving the afflicted with black caretakers, who, according to the French visitor, "often dispatch the patient in order to get possession of his property; certain to escape punishment when the courts are shut and the officers fled." No major epidemic occurred during his sojourn in the colony, 1800 through 1803; this description must have been derived from local informants recounting for the traveler their "stories" about the first yellow fever outbreak in 1796 or the one in 1799.[59]

While some officials at times did leave their posts during antebellum epidemics, other persons stepped forward to offer leadership and assistance. After a series of epidemics in the 1820s and 1830s, many New Orleanians who were safe and secure by "acclimation" had no need to flee the city, and some even felt inclined to engage in relief work. Nevertheless, instances of neglect, plunder, drunkenness, extortion, and profiteering undoubtedly occurred in every epidemic, even as they occurred every day in New Orleans, a city as notorious for its drinking, fighting, gambling, and violent crime as for its epidemics.

William L. Robinson, a member of the New Orleans Howard Association, described a scene of disorder and negligence in an infirmary under his supervision during the great epidemic of 1853. Arriving late one night, he found patients calling for assistance, their neglected waste matter fouling the air of the rooms, and not an attendant to be seen except one "old colored nurse." Robinson found the other nurses, both male and female, passed out "beside the dead and dying," intoxicated from consuming three gallons of brandy. Even when awakened, the nurses were unable to perform the tasks of the infirmary. The next day all but two of them were fired. Some tried to justify their actions, arguing that the strain of caring for the sick and handling the dead was so awful that they needed the stimulant to keep going. The Howard Association managers refused to accept these excuses. It also came to light that one of the male nurses had stolen money and jewelry from the pockets of patients, not an uncommon problem. The association obtained nurses by advertising for experienced male and female attendants, paying them thirty to forty dollars a month.[60] Since formal training for nurses was nonexistent in Louisiana until the late nineteenth century, most nurses employed by the Howards were recruited from the lower class and sometimes did not share the middle-class view of discipline exhibited and expected by the Howards.

According to an article in *DeBow's Review* detailing the epidemic of 1853, "Crime was very prevalent, if we judge from the lengthened police reports in the journals . . . ." Manifestations of the "moral epidemic" included the "utter thoughtlessness and indifference to even the most horrid things in life," such as the morbid curiosity of crowds gathered around the cemeteries to watch the work of burial, apparently undisturbed by the ghastly sights and putrid fumes. As additional evidence of prevailing immorality, the author cited the "songs and obscene jests of the grave-diggers," the presence of the "huxter-women vending their confections" outside the cemetery gates, and the cursing and disrespectful whistling of the men who drove the hearses.[61]

Epidemics in the 1870s and after provoked a form of widespread panic and disorder throughout the hinterland where shotgun quarantines and the threat of violence (including an occasional bridge-burning) disrupted regional and national transportation systems. One newspaper in 1897 suggested the possibility of requesting federal troops to prevent interference with the flow of interstate commerce and the U. S. mail. Increased fear of yellow fever in New Orleans also gave rise to a neighborhood riot in 1897 protesting the opening of an isolation hospital in a local school building.[62]

In describing epidemic behaviors, some observers emphasized the stability, courage, generosity, and altruism exhibited during New Orleans epidemics, while others focused on episodes of panic, negligence, insensitivity, and greed. One writer who witnessed the New Orleans epidemic in 1853 noticed the diversity and the extremes of human responses. He wrote: "There are few events in history which afford more striking illustrations of the good and bad qualities of humanity . . . and present more impressive and startling pictures of virtue and vice, or sorrow and suffering, of generosity and selfishness, of true courage and cowardice, of charity and meanness, than the visitation of a destructive pestilence."[63]

New Orleans police patrolled the streets and performed a variety of social services during epidemics that placed them in danger of infection, not unlike the risks of others who worked closely with the sick. Policemen delivered the sick poor in city carts to Charity Hospital or one of the infirmaries, took orphans to the shelters, and in various ways assisted the health authorities. At one time during the combined epidemic of yellow fever and cholera in 1832, sickness incapacitated almost one-third of the force, and many died, including the captain. In the 1820s and 1830s, German and Irish immigrants, highly susceptible to yellow fever, constituted an increasing proportion of the New Orleans police; like their compatriots elsewhere in the city, they contributed heavily to the epidemic casualty list. Beginning in the 1870s, a special sanitary police force was assigned to carry out the instructions of the state board of health: taking the sick to hospitals, inspecting houses, fumigating and disinfecting the premises—sometimes over the protests of householders. In providing both formal and informal social services as well as the maintenance of order during epidemics, the police force played a dual role in community survival.[64]

Cemeteries and Funeral Processions

One of the most horrible and demanding features of any yellow fever epidemic involved the burial of the dead. Fatalities increased daily in July, August, and September, during the extreme heat and frequent rains of summer, and gradually declined in October and early November until cold weather ended the epidemic. In 1817 the New Orleans city council found it necessary to authorize the use of four "chain gang negroes" to help dig graves at the Protestant cemetery as it was difficult to keep up with demand. In later epidemics the city officials again supplemented the supply of gravediggers by using prisoners and by paying high wages.[65]

At the height of the epidemic of 1853 with more than a thousand deaths a week, the task of prompt interment became impossible. One observer wrote of the unbroken line of vehicles crowding the roads to the cemeteries, morning and evening. "The city commissary's wagon, and the carts of the different hospitals, with their loads of eight or ten coffins each, fell in with the cortege of citizens."[66] The public and private cemeteries were simply overwhelmed by the volume of traffic and the cargo of corpses delivered to their gates. In August, 1853, a reporter for the *Daily Crescent* sketched a scene at one of the overloaded public cemeteries, which is a classic of extravagant nineteenth-century epidemic description:

> At the gates, the winds brought intimation of the corruption working within. Not a puff but was laden with the rank atmosphere from rotting corpses. Inside they were piled by fifties, exposed to the heat of the sun, swollen with corruption, bursting their coffin lids, and sundering, as if by physical effort, the ligaments that bound their hands and feet. . . . What a feast of horrors! Inside, corpses piled in pyramids, and without the gates, old and withered crones and fat huxter women . . . dispensing ice creams and confections, and brushing away . . . the green bottle-flies that hovered on their merchandise, and that anon buzzed away to drink dainty inhalations from the green and festering corpses.[67]

There is no reason to doubt the conditions the journalist described. Other sources painted a similar picture, although in less vivid hues.

Most families who could afford it arranged for burial in brick or stone vaults above ground. For the poor, the city provided free burial underground (or, more accurately, under water). In 1878 one of the New Orleans health inspectors reported to the state board that the old Potter's Field in his district had coffins so near the surface they warped in the sun and split open, exposing the corpses and giving off a powerful stench. Boards from coffins were often broken up and taken away for use as firewood or for fences "by certain degraded whites and negroes in the district." The new "pauper graveyard" adjoining the old Potter's Field was no better. It was described as "a low marsh, wherein the sexton performs his heavy task faithfully and as best he can; sometimes floating to their graves the dead and weighting them into their homes, the whole graveyard being often a foot under water." The health officer considered these conditions "an outrage upon the living, a disgrace to our humanity, to our morals and to our city; an indecency perpetrated upon the dead, because they died poor!"[68]

Throughout the years doctors complained that the sounds of funeral processions disturbed the sick and sometimes brought on convulsions and death. In 1817 the city council requested that the clergy stop the singing and funeral rituals along the streets until the end of the epidemic. In 1853, and again in 1867, when physicians complained that bell-ringing and loud music of marching bands in funeral ceremonies had a dangerous effect on patients, the mayor requested that such practices be suspended "until the health of the city improves."[69] When city authorities tried to counteract the epidemic atmosphere in 1853 by firing cannons and burning tar, doctors reported that the noise of the explosions was injurious to the sick, and the mayor stopped the practice. Added to all the other horrors of black vomit, delirium, and death, the booming cannon and the rising columns of smoke must have made the city seem even more the headquarters of the "King of Terrors."[70]

Humor, Satire, and Poetry

Even in the worst of epidemics, some persons always managed to find something to laugh about, making jokes based on exaggeration of current conditions. According to one epidemic "tall tale" that circulated around New Orleans in 1853, "the fever was so bad at the St. Charles Hotel, that as soon as a man arrived and registered his name they immediately took his measure for a coffin, and asked him to note down in which cemetery he desired to be interred." Another story declared that "as soon as a man arrived on one of the steamboats, the office of the Board of Health immediately took his name and entered it in their books as *deceased*, to save all trouble in calling upon him again."⁷¹ One visitor to New Orleans in the 1840s was disturbed that the familiarity with epidemic disease caused some men to "laugh & jest about these yearly visitations of death as if he were a welcome guest.... It makes me sick at times to hear men joke about 'Yellow Jack' & about old companions who as they say were in a hurry & went to breakfast in the graveyard."⁷²

Mayor Martin Behrman considered it "astonishing" during the epidemic of 1905 how many New Orleans citizens "found something in it to laugh about." One man told the mayor he had bet ten dollars that next week's mortality would be higher than last week's. Others made jokes about the epidemic and "seemed to think yellow fever was close to a sporting event." The mayor saw nothing amusing about the epidemic, but he did march in the Elks Club parade where all were dressed in costumes made of cheesecloth with hats designed to look like screened cisterns. The parade was part of the Diamond Festival held during the epidemic to raise money for the anti-mosquito campaign and to show the rest of the world that yellow fever was no longer a disease to be feared.⁷³

Yellow fever epidemics stimulated the production of a number of poems and at least one satirical novel. In an amusing narrative with a serious purpose, *Doctor Dispachemquic: A Story of the Great Southern Plague of 1878*, author James Dugan of New Orleans satirized the attitudes and activities of "so-called physicians" and some of the benevolent associations in New Orleans during the 1878 epidemic. The three principal characters were Drs. Dispachemquic, Kwarantenus, and Kancurum. Dr. Dispachemquic was a recent graduate of a "cold-water medical institution in a distant state," employed by the "_____ Association," which set him loose "to experiment with his acqueous theories to his heart's content." Pompous, pedantic, arrogant, and superficial, this doctor hastened most of his patients to their final destiny. The fatalities were neither his fault nor the fault of his medical regimen, he explained, but simply nature's will. Dr. Kwarantenus was Dispachemquic's colleague, friend, and echo.

Dr. Kancurum, in contrast to the others, had spent a lifetime studying yellow fever and was skillful in treating his patients. Observing that many "nurses" hired by a certain benevolent association were persons of low character, interested only in easy money, neglecting their duties, and consuming the brandy and champagne provided for the yellow fever patients, Dr. Kancurum commented at length on the serious need for a nurses training school in New Orleans. Highlighting the inadequacy of most medical education of that time, the conflicts among competing medical systems, and the deficiencies of the Howard Association, Dugan also ridiculed some of the female benevolent societies. In the novel, "the Ladies Good Samaritan, Christian Flower Mission and Theological Association of New Orleans" visited the poor and sick, offered gratuitous advice, and distributed flowers among the lower classes to arouse them to an appreciation of beauty. Dugan portrayed these "charitable" ladies as doing their duty with determination and distaste, their noses in the air.[74]

According to Dr. Bennet Dowler, the "contrast between the beauty and repose of nature and the march of death" in 1853 provided inspiration for "several poetical contributions." Some of the poems, he said, had been cut short by the very "pest-king" whose destructive effects the writers were attempting to describe.[75] The epidemic experience of 1878 gave rise to several long "poetical" works, such as "Dorothy—Gift of God, A Ballad of the New Orleans Plague of 1878" by Paul H. Hayne; "Andromeda Unchained" by Henry Guy Carleton; and "The Welded Link" by Judge J. F. Simmons.[76]

In "The Welded Link" Judge Simmons, of Sardis, Mississippi, claimed that northern generosity and kindness toward the South during its disastrous regional epidemic in 1878 had accomplished "what arms never could have done. It conquered the Southern people and the Southern heart." That sentiment was apparently shared by others, including the editor of the New Orleans *Picayune*. Believing that the outpouring of northern contributions and concern had relieved "the Southern heart" of much of the lingering bitterness of war and reconstruction, the editor wrote: "In the name of that philanthropy which has overswept all geographical and party lines, we declare that the war is over, now at last and forever." Simmons also composed numerous short poems based on epidemic themes, including "The Little Faded Dress," "Minnie's Farewell," and "I am Ready."[77]

Although none of these sentimental endeavors inspired by epidemics approached the level of great (or even good) poetry, they serve as additional examples of Yellow Jack's ubiquitous influence on intellect and imagination, along with its impact on emotions, attitudes, and behaviors throughout a broad range of social and cultural phenomena.

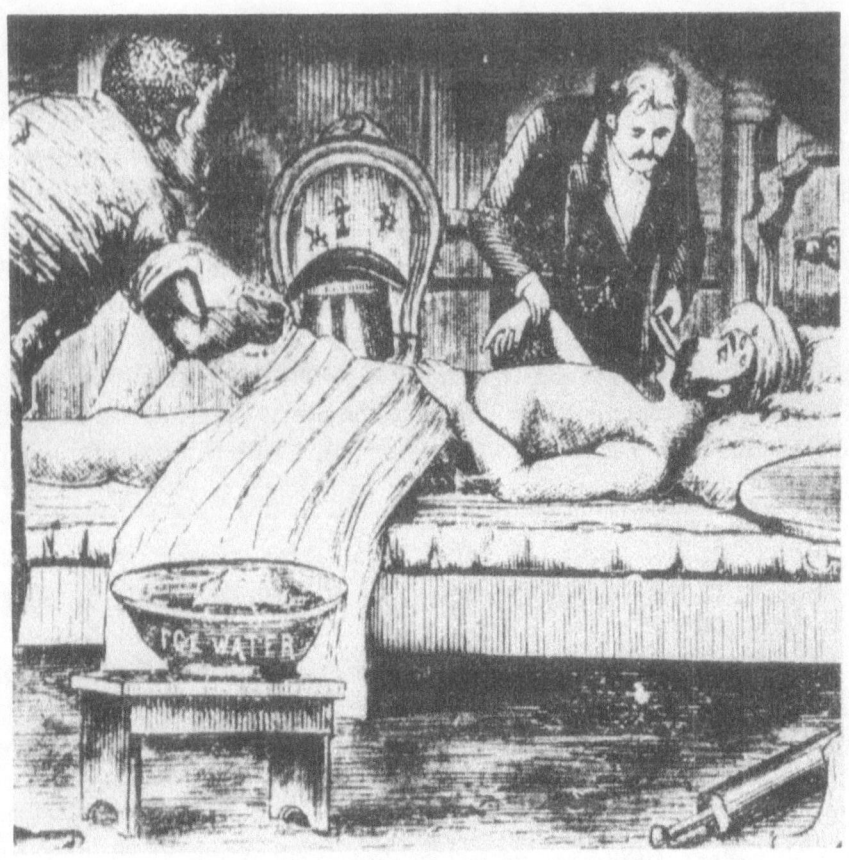

Yellow Fever, 1878.
(From *Doctor Dispachemquic*.) Courtesy The Historic New Orleans Collection, Museum/Research Center, Acc. No. 1974.25.11.128.

XV

ECONOMIC AND POLITICAL CONSEQUENCES OF EPIDEMIC YELLOW FEVER

Antebellum New Orleans was a boomtown, a thriving port attracting people by the thousands as well as enormous quantities of sugar, cotton, tobacco, and grain crops shipped downriver from the increasing number of farms and plantations of the interior. The city's boosters were convinced that its location near the mouth of the great Mississippi made it the natural trade outlet for much of the country and that nothing could halt its progress or alter its destiny.

Epidemics were troublesome, and epidemics did indeed interfere with commerce, but yellow fever was a summer complaint, and nobody expected much business in the summer. As the population grew in pre-Civil War decades, so did the virulence, extent, and notoriety of the city's yellow fever epidemics; the more immigrants, the more potential victims for the scourge, and still they came. And the river continued to bring a huge and ever-expanding volume of agricultural products to the Crescent City's docks for export on the ocean vessels waiting there to be loaded. It seemed that New Orleans was simply "too busy with gainful pursuits to concern itself much about the fever, which was looked on rather as an established institution."[1] This attitude prevailed among the established residents, the so-called "acclimated." As yellow fever epidemics recurred two or three times in each decade before the Civil War, New Orleanians insisted repeatedly that their community was a healthy place and that the local epidemic fevers affected only the indigent immigrants and the intemperate.

Yellow fever epidemics always disrupted commercial connections with the interior and delayed the start of the fall trade. Yet despite the adverse influences of the disease upon the New Orleans economy, each epidemic setback appeared to be only temporary—at least in the short-range view. When cool weather arrived and the epidemic subsided, the business season opened, river steamers and ocean vessels arrived and departed, and crops of the interior poured into the city along with orders for supplies and goods of all kinds. New Orleans filled up with thousands of newcomers and visitors as well as the returning summer absentees. The gaiety of social life and the profitable business activity soon replaced the distress associated with the recent epidemic.[2]

Viewed from the insider's perspective as an occasional setback with temporary effects, yellow fever epidemics could be fatalistically dismissed as a nuisance but not a serious obstruction to the continued growth and prosperity of New Orleans. The disease could be discounted as a cost of doing business in a semitropical climate but a cost easily borne in a booming economy, a risk that newcomers were apparently willing to take for the benefits of the city. Only a few negative voices appeared in the antebellum years, and newspapers did their best to contradict all criticism and to present the Crescent City as a healthy place with no more disease than any other large population center.

Yellow fever continued to afflict New Orleans after the Civil War, and more medical observers began to point to the disease as the "chief drawback" to the city's economic advancement. In the long-term perspective, and especially from the viewpoint of outsiders, the damage caused by nineteenth-century yellow fever epidemics was neither temporary nor negligible, but cumulative, lasting, and of major importance in the relative decline of New Orleans among the nation's cities.

In the political arena, major epidemics stimulated public demand for governmental action of some kind, even when medical opinion was divided on the appropriate course to follow. State and local legislation providing for quarantine and sanitation might be enacted, but if implementation required raising taxes or if strict enforcement of quarantine was deemed injurious to commerce, the laws brought little change. Widespread and destructive epidemics that aroused intense public fears and also damaged powerful interstate as well as local economic interests eventually generated support for quarantine legislation, sanitary improvements, and state and national institutions designed to safeguard the free flow of commerce while calming public fears and limiting the spread of disease.

Short-Term Effects on Business and Labor

During severe epidemics, New Orleans business activity declined to a fraction of its normally slow summer pace. Many commercial establishments closed down entirely or remained open only during part of the day. Dread of the fever kept rural inhabitants from going anywhere near the plague-stricken city until the first frost, and most country merchants and planters refused to accept goods from New Orleans while yellow fever prevailed. The spread of disease to towns and large plantation communities along the rivers and bayous interfered with the harvesting of crops and the shipment of cotton and other produce, disturbing the process of exchange. Not only did epidemics suspend intercourse with the interior, they also kept northern and European vessels away from the infected port city. Ships already loaded with cargo at New Orleans docks found it necessary to postpone their departure because of strict quarantine rules in northern ports.[3]

The extensive epidemics of the 1850s brought a greater awareness of the economic liabilities imposed on New Orleans by its old familiar fever, even on a short-term basis. Exhibiting a concern felt by many New Orleanians, the editor of the Bee commented in 1858: "Everyone is aware that the prevalence of yellow fever in our city is the chief drawback to our prosperity; that but for this haunting apprehension our summer population would not be materially reduced, nor would the tide of business recede from our shores." The progress of New Orleans would be at least ten times greater if the threat of epidemics could be eliminated, the editor declared, and it was time to seek ways of preventing the pestilence—for the good of humanity as well as the city's commercial benefit.[4]

Epidemics in the post-Civil-War era continued to disturb the processes of commerce and finance. In September, 1867, the Bee reported that business was "in a state of stagnation" because of the obstacles to trade and travel. In October the *Picayune* complained of the commercial deadlock and the scarcity of money. Although payment was due on notes held by northern firms for goods purchased months before by New Orleans merchants, the editor hoped that the northern creditors would recognize "the difficulties . . . caused by the dreadful scourge paralyzing the arm of trade" and would wait until cool weather and the revival of commerce before demanding payment.[5]

When the city was almost sealed off from its hinterland by quarantine in 1878, one merchant complained that "the present state of affairs is fairly killing business in New Orleans."[6] Even without an epidemic, a few cases of fever would trigger the interior quarantines, especially after 1878. These barriers halted or limited the exchange of goods, diverted the flow of commerce to rival centers, and postponed for many weeks the customary brisk trade based on the late summer harvest. The resulting damage to the New Orleans economy, when deprived of the inland trade, caused some local business leaders to come out in favor of sanitary improvements and a more rigorous quarantine—to improve the image of the city as well as its health.[7]

Yellow fever epidemics always resulted in severe distress among the laboring classes. The economic slowdown brought unemployment and hard times, even among families otherwise unaffected by yellow fever. Disease and death further augmented the list of the destitute, leaving broken families and orphaned children behind. The hardship occasioned by the spread of yellow fever in 1878, for example, necessitated an appeal for relief to the "Chambers of Commerce and the Charitable of the Chief Cities of the Union." Signed by the president of the New Orleans Chamber of Commerce and by others representing Mississippi and Alabama, the appeal requested that a central headquarters to receive donations be established in cities around the country. Transportation lines had volunteered to ship all donations without charge to New Orleans; from there the relief could be distributed to other desperate towns.

Because of the disruption of commerce on the Mississippi River south of Memphis, more than fifty steamboats were tied up and their crews laid off. Laborers engaged in handling freight were out of work, and four railroad lines ceased to function, leaving their employees idle. According to the published appeal, at least 15,000 heads of households were unemployed in New Orleans, 8,000 in Memphis, and thousands more in scattered small towns, representing a total of more than 100,000 persons in dire need by September, 1878. "For them there is no labor, no wages, no bread—nothing but death, or starvation; and this condition must last at least for fifty days

. . . until frost." Funds were needed for food, clothing, medicines, care of the sick, and burial of the dead.[8]

The field of insurance offers another example of yellow fever's influence on financial decisions. In 1848 *DeBow's Review* protested against northern ignorance regarding the health of southern states: "Their insurance companies exact a higher premium if the party, being a southerner, remained at *home during summer* . . . yet permit him to *spend his winter in New-England*, where, perhaps, his chances of life would be diminished one half!" The southern journalist further complained, "For New-Orleans many of the companies refused to insure altogether! Sapient statisticians these." Residents of New Orleans, unless they could supply evidence of having survived an attack of yellow fever, were definitely at grave risk. In fact, they were probably poor risks under any circumstances, given the high mortality rate of New Orleans, with or without yellow fever.[9]

The increased demand for certain goods during an epidemic encouraged shrewd and unscrupulous entrepreneurs to take advantage of the situation. During the epidemic of 1839, the *Picayune* editor angrily reported an incident relating to traffic in coffins. "Speculation in wooden nut-megs, bass-wood hams and horn flints we look upon as 'fair business transactions,'" he declared, "but the man who can look complacently forward to a season of epidemic and mortality, and prepare to turn a time of death and mourning to profitable account, we view as a soulless, unsympathising scoundrel. . . ." Early that summer a New York speculator had made a large shipment of coffins under a false bill of lading to a New Orleans mercantile house. Coffins of assorted sizes had been packed one inside another in nine cases labeled "Pianos—With Care." The New Yorker's letter to the New Orleans firm stated: "As the taste for music appears to be making rapid strides in the South, and as instruments *such as I send you*, must inevitably increase in value, I would advise, that at present you merely take them into your warerooms, permitting them to remain in the cases, subject to my future directions." According to the *Picayune*, the New Orleans merchants, on discovering the nature of the merchandise, had been outraged by the "endeavor to make them a tool in so disreputable a 'commission business'" and had sold the coffins to Charity Hospital for one dollar each.[10]

Others had better luck in profiteering. Monopolizing the importation and sale of ice in New Orleans, the Crescent City Ice Company raised the price during the epidemic of 1878. The mayor and the board of health became concerned and began making inquires about buying and shipping ice from several northern cities. Hearing of this action, representatives of the ice company then called on the mayor and agreed to reduce the price immediately to forty dollars per ton. They also promised another reduction with the arrival of shipments then on the way, and the mayor decided to take no further action. Considering that ice could be purchased from a firm in Maine for two dollars per ton and shipped to New Orleans for three dollars per ton, the *Picayune* editor felt that the company's high charges were inexcusable, especially during an epidemic.[11]

During the city's worst epidemic, in 1853, newspapers reported numerous complaints against druggists who charged exorbitant prices for medicines. In ordinary times the drugs would have been considered expensive at one-half or one-third the price charged during the crisis. Also in 1853 the Howard Association discovered several cases of collusion between druggists and physicians to share profits from expensive and unnecessary prescriptions paid for by the benevolent society.[12] Certainly in every epidemic some greedy individuals turned a calamity into an opportunity for unreasonable gain. For most businessmen, however, Yellow Jack brought losses rather than profits, but the booming trade of the winter season more than made up for the summer deficits, and most saw no cause for worry.

The menace of yellow fever did not seem to discourage the great hordes of persons who moved to antebellum New Orleans each year, swelling the city's population by more than 900 percent between 1810 and 1860. In the last days of the epidemic of 1817, one resident compared New Orleans to a plate of honey where thousands of insects came to eat their fill and die. But, he added, "where one dies, a thousand visit the delicious repast. So it is with men—where their interests lie, they'll come to the place, tho' death may stare them in the face."[13] Apparently, not even the prospect of disease and early death could interrupt "the forward march of the city" during the antebellum years, wrote Grace King in *New Orleans: The Place and the People*. On the contrary, the Crescent City enjoyed "more emigrants, more imports, more exports, more trade, more cotton, sugar, plantations, slaves; and to off-set, the more death, the more life, the city's gayety, like the city's gold, mounting in the flood tide over it."[14]

Even in the midst of the paralyzing epidemic of 1853, the editor of the *Daily Crescent* discounted the notion that the epidemic would ruin the city.

He expected the population to increase rather than decrease as newcomers would rush in to seek the positions left vacant by yellow fever's victims. The death of one man would attract two to fill his job, and business would become more active than ever. The pestilence did not drive people away, the editor insisted; it attracted those adventurers who would brave any danger. Concluding with an optimistic but callous reflection, he predicted, "There is a good time coming for the fortunate who live to see it."[15] Assuming that the threat of the fever did discourage some prospective residents, and considering the thousands who died there each year (not only from yellow fever but from the other common maladies), one can only speculate about what the growth of New Orleans might have been without its unhealthy influences.

Long-Range Economic and Demographic Impact

That epidemic yellow fever had serious economic and demographic consequences is undeniable, whether as a single outbreak in one community, or as a handicap to New Orleans' development for more than a century, or as a negative influence in other southern coastal cities and in the region as a whole. It is impossible to calculate precisely the long-term cost of yellow fever to New Orleans, or the South, or the nation at large, although every commentator noted its damaging effects on commerce and labor, and some attempted to assess the damages. Estimates of the cost to New Orleans of the 1878 epidemic ranged from twelve to one hundred million dollars, depending on the values assigned to human lives, days of labor, medical care, supplies, burials, charity, crop spoilage, investment losses, and the general disturbance to business. During the yellow fever "panic" of 1897, one railroad alone, the Southern Pacific, claimed that its losses in Texas and Louisiana amounted to more than a million dollars.[16] New Orleans suffered at least thirty yellow fever epidemics from 1796 to 1905, and many more if one included all those outbreaks that were mild only in comparison with the terrible ones.

In 1850 Dr. J. C. Simonds calculated that the city's monetary losses attributable to all diseases during four and one-third years, from January, 1846, through April, 1850, totaled $45,437,700, or an average annual cost of $10,485,623. For the same period (during which only one severe yellow fever epidemic had occurred, in 1847), he found the average yearly mortality rate of New Orleans to be 8.1 percent (or 1 in 12), while most other cities had rates between 2 and 3 percent.[17]

An article in *DeBow's Review* in 1846 acknowledged yellow fever as the "one retarding cause" to the city's development. The disease had been absent for several years, however, and in view of its comings and goings in other cities, the writer expected that "this eccentric visitor" would soon disappear from New Orleans altogether. In any case, he believed New Orleans would be the "greatest city in the Union" within fifty years. After a severe epidemic the following year, another local booster insisted that nothing could interrupt the city's progress "toward its highest destiny." And even after 1853, *DeBow's Review* continued to project New Orleans' "glorious future . . . which cannot be checked by pestilential chastenings."[18]

Despite the bravado of these journalists who scoffed at the notion that yellow fever could hinder New Orleans, other voices, mainly from the medical community, began to express grave concern in the 1840s and 1850s over the immediate and long-range demographic and economic costs of the disease. In 1845 Dr. John Harrison, professor of physiology and pathology in the Medical College of Louisiana, referred to yellow fever as "the pestilence of the South—the great obstacle to increase of population in her cities, and, of course, to all other advantages which increase of population brings with it."[19] An editorial in the *New Orleans Medical and Surgical Journal* in 1846 expressed the opinion that New Orleans' future development largely depended on getting rid of yellow fever, hence the importance of keeping up the search for its cause and a means of prevention.[20]

After the epidemic of 1847, Dr. William P. Hort of New Orleans considered the costs of epidemic disease and advocated the expenditure of public funds to improve New Orleans' sanitary condition. Benevolent societies spent thousands of dollars in 1847, and the "great alarm" in neighboring states had kept an estimated fifty to one hundred students from attending the university in New Orleans. Hort also reminded his readers that the list of yellow fever victims included many of "our most valuable citizens, ornaments of society," as well as the newly arrived immigrants and the poor. According to his sources, a false alarm of yellow fever in 1845 had caused at least two million dollars worth of produce destined for New Orleans to be diverted to eastern cities.[21]

In the report of the New Orleans Board of Health for 1849, Dr. Edward H. Barton and the other board members confronted the ruling powers with the truth about the city's high death rate and the price of disregarding the unhealthy conditions. The board argued that no matter what the cost of water supply, drainage, sewerage, street cleaning, and garbage removal systems, such an investment in public improvements would pay off in future benefits: the reduction of disease and mortality rates, expansion of population and commerce, and increased real estate values.[22] In its 1850 report the board of health granted that New Orleans could boast of its progress and prosperity but wondered what the city's development might have been if the fear of yellow fever had not caused the annual departure of "probably one-third of the most enterprising, active, intelligent and wealthy part of the community."[23]

In an article on vital statistics and hygiene published in 1850, Dr. Barton calculated the mortality of New Orleans for the previous decade as 5.5 percent annually. He believed that the causes of sickness could be eliminated "by determination, enterprise, science and capital," and he contended that health was a necessary basis for prosperity: ". . . a sickly country is the main cause of that absenteeism which not only deprives the State of the services of a large portion of her citizens, but abstracts from profitable use and investment at home, millions of her natural resources; retards the advancement of the permanent population of the city; [and] keeps down the value of city property. . . ." Barton called attention to the fact that other cities were outpacing New Orleans and urged that the city invest in sanitary improvements as a matter of self-interest. New Orleans' high death rate was a serious handicap, he said, because "capitalists, proverbially timid, will not invest permanently where the mortality is double what it is elsewhere," and the middle class will not settle permanently "where there is not as fair an average of health as can elsewhere be procured in our country."[24]

Published in 1850, in the *Daily Delta* as well as in several medical journals, Dr. Simonds' articles on the city's vital statistics and sanitary conditions struck at the myth of New Orleans salubrity. He stressed the high cost of denial, and he called for sanitary reform, "the question which is agitating other civilized communities, [and] must take place here, whether the movement commences now, or at some future time." His painstaking statistical computations and comparisons had found the mortality of New Orleans to be double or triple that of other cities. Having appealed to the medical profession, "which elsewhere has taken the lead on this subject," Simonds also directed his message "to the other classes of the community,—to the city authorities, and to all who, being identified in interest with the city, desire its welfare."[25]

Mayor A. D. Crossman in his annual address in 1852 called yellow fever "one of the greatest drawbacks to the prosperity of New Orleans." Because of the continuing progress of swamp drainage in back of the city, however, the mayor believed the disease would soon be eliminated along with the miasmatic poisons—not knowing that the worst epidemic was yet to come. The editors of the *New Orleans Medical and Surgical Journal* commended the mayor's work and expressed hope that yellow fever might soon be brought under control. They noted that the "terrible epidemics" of previous years had "destroyed a large portion of our population—crippled our commerce—checked the growth of our city and paralyzed every species of trade and manufacture."[26]

In the first report of the Louisiana State Board of Health in 1855, its president, Dr. Samuel Choppin, discussed the benefits to be achieved from the recently established state quarantine system. Pointing to the "incalculable" losses suffered by the city and the state because of disease, he attributed "the transient character of much of our population" to the frequency of epidemics. Valuable resources were drained out of New Orleans each year "by a system of absenteeism which is a curse to any country." Fifty thousand dollars had been appropriated by the state for the new quarantine system, a small sum, Choppin believed, considering the value of the work. Without the diversion of commerce caused by the yellow fever epidemics of the past four years, the total trade of Louisiana, by his estimate, would have been at least 30 percent greater. According to Choppin, only 21 of the 1149 vessels examined at the three Louisiana quarantine stations in 1855 had to be detained because of their unsanitary condition or because of disease on board, and these were mostly small vessels from the West Indies. To show how little of Louisiana's trade would be subject to interruption by quarantine, Choppin noted that the total value of goods brought into New Orleans annually from the interior and from the sea amounted to $166 million, whereas the value of imports from yellow fever centers in the West Indies, Mexico, and Central America was only about $2.6 million. Of the total commerce, $46 million was seaborne, including $30 million from domestic sources and only $16 million from foreign ports. The board president thought it would be worthwhile to completely exclude the trade from yellow fever areas if necessary to preserve the far more valuable domestic commerce, as well as the "happiness and prosperity" of New Orleans. But he believed that careful inspection and detention of unsanitary and infected vessels would suffice to prevent the entry of yellow fever.[27]

As early as 1850, in reviewing the city's mortality and the costs of disease, Dr. Simonds had asked, "Is it, then, surprising that New Orleans has not progressed more rapidly? What other city has had to encounter such losses, and what other city could stand them?"[28] Perhaps yellow fever played a larger role in retarding New Orleans' growth and development than has generally been recognized. In 1840 New Orleans was the third largest city in the Union and the first city in exports, handling a greater volume than New York and twice as much "western produce" as all other American ports combined.[29] *Hunt's Merchant's Magazine* designated New Orleans as the "only city in America that can run a close race with New York, and the ratio of its past increase is such that it bids fair to be the empire city of America."[30] Although the volume of the city's trade continued to increase, New Orleans suffered a relative decline between 1840 and 1860 when an increasing proportion of the products of the upper valley flowed eastward on the railroads rather than southward on the river. By 1860 the city had also dropped from third to sixth place in population.[31] New Orleans' failure to develop railroad connections early enough to compete with the east for the upper valley trade has usually been cited as one of the main reasons for the city's falling behind in the nineteenth-century race for metropolitan empire. Scarcity of manufacturing enterprises also ranks high on the list of explanatory factors for New Orleans' economic backsliding. And of course the Civil War had an impact, both economic and demographic, requiring many years for the city to recover from altered trade patterns and debt.[32]

Yellow fever itself influenced the antebellum diversion of trade from New Orleans to the east—contributing to, but independent from, the attractive power of the east-west railroad connections.[33] Even if New Orleans had been able to develop a vast railroad network to complement the river trade before 1860, yellow fever would have continued to create problems for the city. The disease undoubtedly would have spread along the rail lines, provoking shotgun quarantines (as it did in the 1870s), and still causing the shift of commerce toward the eastern centers. If New Orleans had been able to develop more industries, the immigrant or "unacclimated" labor force would have increased, providing more fuel for the fever. As long as the saffron scourge was a regular visitor to New Orleans, railroads and factories would probably *not* have prevented the city's relative decline. A massive investment in sanitary improvements and a stringent quarantine against the tropical trade might have done more for New Orleans' growth and development than any other projected changes in its antebellum history, but such expenditures did not appear to be "cost-effective" in the short-range business view.

New Orleans experienced further relative population decline in the postbellum years—falling from sixth to twelfth ranking city in size by 1900. Immigration, disrupted by the Civil War, never resumed its earlier volume; if it had done so, the vulnerable foreign population might have sparked more frequent and virulent epidemics as in the 1850s. The Crescent City suffered the effects of economic depression as well as disease in the 1870s, and its postwar recovery proceeded somewhat more slowly than other towns with better health conditions.[34] The threat of yellow fever continued to cast its shadow over New Orleans, and internal quarantines plagued the city's commerce and often enhanced that of its rivals.

The epidemic of 1878 focused the eyes of the nation on New Orleans and the South because the disease spread so extensively and proved so disruptive to trade and transportation in a large area of the nation's expanding capitalist economy. Thereafter, yellow fever was viewed as a problem of national dimensions, the epidemic having cost the country an estimated one hundred to two hundred million dollars. President Rutherford B. Hayes discussed the strong public sentiment favoring "national sanitary administration" in his annual message to Congress, and legislation on health and quarantine was approved by June, 1879.[35]

Newspaper Policy

Until the late nineteenth century, New Orleans newspapers failed to provide prompt or accurate reporting on yellow fever, always attempted to discount the severity of an epidemic, and routinely praised the city as an extraordinarily healthy place. The direct influence of commerical interests often dictated that policy. In 1819 architect Benjamin Latrobe asked an editor why the journals avoided the subject of yellow fever even when knowledge of the epidemic was general throughout the city. The editor answered "that the principal profit of a newspaper arising from advertisements, the merchants, their principal customers, had absolutely forbid the least notice of fever, under a threat that their custom should otherwise be withdrawn. . . ." In Latrobe's judgment, merchants and editors were guilty of "sacrificing to commercial policy the lives of all those who, believing from the silence of the public papers that no danger existed, might come to the city."[36]

Before the news of yellow fever's presence was published in 1853, the Howard Association had already begun its relief work among the indigent sick in New Orleans. The notice of the Howards' initial meeting published in the papers did not even mention the words "yellow fever." In fact, the members had been "requested by *editors* and *merchants* to withhold publication of our acts, as the report of an epidemic—which might yet be checked—would entail severe loss on merchants and shopkeepers."[37] An article in *DeBow's Review* outlining the epidemic of 1853 noted the reluctance of New Orleans journals to provide information on yellow fever. Not until the daily mortality was too great to ignore and alarm was general throughout the city did the newspapers include any reference to the disease. The first news of fever in the city came to some of its residents through the country papers. "New-Orleans being an entirely commercial city, the love of money and self-interest prevail there as much as in other commercial communities," the article stated, "and it is a standing maxim in the commercial world that nothing must be said that might injure trade."[38]

In its annual report for 1873 the state board of health revealed that as soon as yellow fever appeared in New Orleans that year, a deputation of merchants called upon the policy-makers of the city newspapers and requested that the weekly mortality reports supplied by the health board not be published. All agreed except the editor of the *German Gazette*. As the board had predicted, exaggerations then spread throughout the country, and no official information was readily available to "control the public imagination."[39] While refusing to publish information furnished by the board of health, New Orleans papers went to great pains to correct the so-called exaggerations and erroneous opinions appearing in the journals of the interior and the North.

In April, 1852, for example, the *Picayune* editor complained of reports in northern papers that the Crescent City was anxiously "expecting the near approach of the plague." To the editor, it seemed that the outsider's conception of life in New Orleans consisted of "cotton bales and yellow fever, balls, duels, operas and cholera." In 1867, the *Bee* castigated several northern journals for reporting that New Orleans authorities and newspapers were in collusion to withhold information on the severity of the pestilence. Such a statement, the *Bee* editor declared, was nothing less than an "abominable lie."[40]

People in other Louisiana communities and in other states had learned not to trust New Orleans journalists on matters relating to the city's health. They listened instead to reports supplied by persons in flight from the pestilence, or they relied on information provided by correspondents in the city. The New Orleans press protested bitterly against what they considered rumors of imagined epidemics or exaggerations of existing ones in country newspapers.[41] Sometimes the newspapers of England received a share of criticism for "distorting" the picture of New Orleans' health. In 1853 the *Picayune* editor lashed out at several English journals for their allegedly unfair treatment of the disease-ridden city: "They find the ordinary sanitary, physical, and moral condition of New Orleans to be horrid." He thought it strange indeed that outsiders always professed to know so much more about the affairs of the city than those present on the scene.[42]

In the late nineteenth century when improved transportation and communication knit the country ever more closely together, it became impossible to conceal the presence of disease—especially with *New York Times* correspondents everywhere and with increasing federal involvement in public health and quarantine matters. After the outbreak of 1878 assumed national importance, the New Orleans papers abandoned the attempt at deception and provided extensive coverage of epidemic events. When yellow fever appeared in 1897, the editor of the *Times-Democrat* remarked that the traditional policy of not reporting on the disease until it became undeniably epidemic had "brought New Orleans to the verge of ruin." The *Picayune* made a similar declaration that the concealment of disease was not only unwise but impossible and could result only in ultimate exposure and harsh criticism.[43] Nevertheless, the city's journals continued to follow the cautious lead of the state board of health through the last epidemic, reporting yellow fever's presence only when the board made its first official statement in 1905, ten days after the first suspicious cases had been reported, and weeks after the disease had first arrived in the city.

Economic & Political Consequences 373

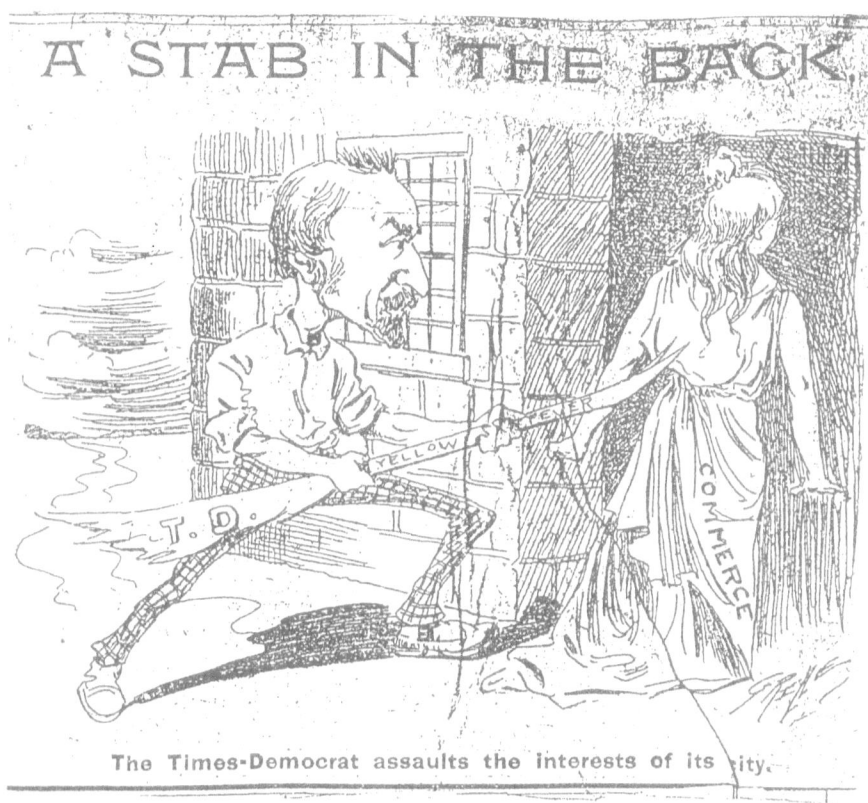

Cartoon: "A Stab in the Back."
A cartoon in the New Orleans *Item* attacking the New Orleans *Times-Democrat* for reporting cases of yellow fever in the city. The *Times-Democrat*'s editorial response the next day defended its policy against criticism for telling the "whole truth" and denounced concealment of disease as bad for New Orleans. (From New Orleans *Item*, September 14, 1897).

New Orleans' Greatest "Drawback"

New Orleans physicians continued to single out the disease as one of the principal causes of the city's failure to fulfill its economic promise. Dr. Choppin, first president of the Louisiana State Board of Health, and president again in 1877-1879, offered his judgment of yellow fever's enduring impact on New Orleans: Despite its great "natural advantages as a mart of trade . . . the [city's] growth in population, business and wealth, has hitherto been inconceivably retarded by these visitations of yellow fever. . . . But for this one great drawback to its progress . . . New Orleans at this hour might aspire to be considered the first commercial city of the Union." According to Choppin, at least 100,000 "of the flower and strength of the land" had died of yellow fever in New Orleans since the first major epidemic in 1796. Mortality from the same disease "in neighboring towns and the country" added 75,000 to the total. "The people who have died here of yellow fever would have built up a State," he wrote.[44]

The next two presidents of the state board of health also pinpointed yellow fever as New Orleans' chief handicap. Dr. Joseph Jones stated in the board's report for 1881 that except for yellow fever, New Orleans would be the leading American city in imports and exports.[45] His successor, Dr. Joseph Holt, in an address to the American Public Health Association in 1885, raised these questions: "Why is New Orleans as it is? why not more progressive? why not a manufacturing . . . as well as a commercial city? Why does not her commerce sweep the circle of the world at all times? and, considering her age in relation with the age and growth of other American cities, why has she not a million of inhabitants? I would promptly answer you in a compound word—*Yellow Fever!*"[46]

Dr. Stanford E. Chaillé, professor in the medical department of the University of Louisiana, who later achieved prominence in national public health circles and as Dean of the Tulane Medical School, published a study in 1870 of the vital statistics of New Orleans. Twenty years had passed since the pioneering studies of Barton and Simonds, yet Chaillé still had to cover much of the same ground. Like other frustrated nineteenth-century health reform agitators, Chaillé also asked, "Are we like children to go on wondering . . . why our city has comparatively languished in the race of progress, when we rate human life so cheaply, and cause by our negligence an extravagant waste of not only the foreign importation, but also of the home production of it?" At that time, 25 per thousand, or 2.5 percent annual mortality, was considered "a fair standard of health." His examination of New Orleans data for 1856-1860, the five healthiest years on record, yielded an annual mortality rate of 46.3 per thousand, or 4.6 percent.[47] Only one severe yellow fever epidemic had occurred during those years. Yellow Jack was simply the most notorious contributor to the city's high death rate, not its only cause—as would become clear after 1905.

But the disease was notorious, and to think of New Orleans was to think of yellow fever throughout the nineteenth century. The New Orleans *Times-Democrat* in July, 1882, reprinted an article from the Nashville *American* entitled "What New Orleans Might Be." The article pointed out that the Southern Pacific Railway from California to the Crescent City would soon be completed and that steamers were about to begin running between New Orleans and European ports. According to the Nashville editor, New Orleans had an opportunity to become one of the richest cities in modern history because of its postwar railroad system and its geographical position relative to Texas, Mexico, the West Indies, and South America. The article concluded that New Orleans might become a "great city" if it would only rid itself of yellow fever.[48]

When New Orleans had no epidemics and only a few cases of yellow fever during the 1880s and much of the 1890s, Dr. Joseph Holt's innovative quarantine system based on disinfection received the credit, and it seemed that the city might indeed be safe at last. A promotional volume issued in 1894 by the New Orleans Chamber of Commerce and Industry praised Louisiana's quarantine system which had "barred out the plague of yellow fever for many years now, and has shown, by that very fact, that the disease does not originate here." The boosters also noted the decline of the old custom of summer absenteeism and the expansion of "all-the-year-round business."[49] Advertisements in New Orleans newspapers for hotels, summer resorts, and reduced railway fares to "all popular Northern points" during the epidemic of 1905, however, suggest that some outsiders believed the old custom of absenteeism could be quickly revived in time of crisis.[50]

In 1905, as the epidemic was waning and health officials had demonstrated the practical effects of the "mosquito doctrine," Dr. E. B. Craighead, president of Tulane University, declared that ". . . New Orleans and the South are at the end of a hundred years war." Referring to yellow fever by its time-worn label, "the greatest drawback the South ever had," Craighead praised the successful campaign against the New Orleans epidemic as "the greatest scientific triumph the South has ever witnessed."[51]

In trying to judge the long-term effects of yellow fever on the economy of New Orleans and the South in general, one must allow for some measure of rhetorical exaggeration in the testimony, as well as the bias of physicians involved in the work of public health and quarantine. Consciously or unconsciously, physicians might have exaggerated the importance of yellow fever in their articles and reports—their jeremiads—as a way of bolstering their importance, diagnosing New Orleans' economic problems in medical terms with remedies prescribed by the doctors. Divided on most issues and faced with serious competition from "irregular" practitioners, M.D.s had little power and influence during much of the nineteenth century. By asserting authority as analysts, prophets, and advisors about matters concerning the future wealth and prosperity of the city, physicians might have hoped to gain status and social power.

But whatever the rhetoric of physicians (and others) may reveal about their own self-interest, yellow fever was an undeniable fact of life and death in the nineteenth-century, a recurrent presence, a constant threat, an image of terror. The disease left its mark not only in the impressionistic accounts of memoirs, letters, diaries, newspapers, and in the special genre of medical literature, but also in the quantitative, cumulative evidence of census data, hospital records, death lists, cemeteries, and monetary losses however calculated. Although yellow fever was certainly not the only "drawback" to New Orleans' economic development, many nineteenth-century commentators judged it to be the city's worst handicap. One could make an even stronger case for the crucial disadvantage inherent in nineteenth-century New Orleans' overall pattern of disease and high mortality, including but not limited to yellow fever. Common endemic diseases such as tuberculosis, typhoid fever, dysentery, and infant disorders claimed far more lives over the years than yellow fever did.[52] Nevertheless, the saffron scourge was the dramatic deviation that captured public attention and symbolized for the outside world the dreadful insalubrity of New Orleans.

Politics of Health and Quarantine

As a life and death matter and the object of great public fear, yellow fever inevitably became a political issue. Whether as a peripheral or central concern, as a current epidemic, or as a memory of the past and a threat for the future, the disease was always there—in the foreground or the background, making its presence felt and influencing thought and behavior in small ways as well as large. For example, the convention to draft Louisiana's first constitution in preparation for statehood met in New Orleans in early November, 1811, but the representatives in attendance agreed to adjourn until November 18 because of the city's unhealthy condition. Many of the "country members" of the convention, apprehensive about entering New Orleans with a yellow fever epidemic still in progress, had failed to arrive on the opening date.[53]

In 1845 at the convention assembled to revise Louisiana's constitution, the question of a suitable time for holding general elections became a matter for debate. Some delegates proposed that elections be held during the summer when yellow fever generally prevailed, thereby denying the vote to strangers who left New Orleans annually to escape the pestilence. They contended that these "birds of passage . . . having only temporary interest and residence" in the city did not deserve the vote. Other delegates pointed out that such a provision would prevent at least half the *"resident"* population from voting because many natives and long-term residents also left the city each year during the sickly season.[54]

During the epidemic of 1853, some New Orleanians engaged in a discussion about which political party, Whig or Democrat, would lose more of their voters to the fever. The *Daily Crescent* reported that the "vile Whigs" were rejoicing at the "thinning of the ranks of the democracy by the great leveller, death." The large majority of those leaving the city for the Gulf coast or northern resorts belonged to the Whig Party, while most of the people remaining in New Orleans, including many "unacclimated" residents, were Democrats, according to the *Crescent* editor. He considered it "horrible . . . that men should cooly reason, in the midst of a pestilence, on the probable good or bad fortune to befall a political party in consequence of a terrible mortality. . . ."[55]

Far beyond its influence in delaying conventions, setting election dates, and calculating partisan advantages, yellow fever had wide-ranging political clout in stimulating public demand for government protection against disease. Under pressure from a public aroused by epidemics, local and state (and eventually national) representatives repeatedly found it necessary to pass laws dealing with quarantine, sanitation, and public health, even in the absence of medical knowledge sufficient to frame effective legislation.

In 1855 Louisiana established the first state board of health in the United States as a direct response to the widespread epidemics of 1853 and 1854. Residents of many small Louisiana communities had suffered severely for the first time. Believing yellow fever to be contagious, transportable, and foreign, the voters demanded legislation to protect the state from its importation. Although the majority of physicians still considered yellow fever a product of locally generated miasmatic poisons, a few doctors had decided the disease was imported and believed that quarantine should again be tried. Despite the dominant medical opinion to the contrary and the opposition of shipping interests, Louisiana legislators provided for maritime quarantine and created a board to protect the health of the state. Largely based on trial and error, additional laws in later years gradually expanded the board's functions and powers and revised and improved the quarantine system—always reflecting the chronic concern with yellow fever.[56]

While statewide popular pressure could obtain quarantine legislation, it could not insure enforcement. The strength of commercial interests in New Orleans and elsewhere made it impossible for the board of health to apply a consistent set of regulations. Board members were bombarded with requests by companies for special treatment such as suspension of the rules or reduction of the detention period for particular vessels. Loopholes here and there made the quarantine a less effective screen than it might have been. After 1878, New Orleans' domestic business interests recognized that *not* having a strong maritime quarantine was more destructive to their trade than having one. An effective quarantine was needed to retain the confidence and the trade of the Mississippi Valley. Even so, corporations most directly affected by quarantine restrictions continued to use their influence to obtain special consideration, and New Orleanians continued to have doubts about the benefits of quarantine relative to the cost and delays affecting commerce.

The first president of the Louisiana State Board of Health, Dr. Samuel Choppin, was again board president during the 1878 epidemic. His experience convinced him that the only certain barrier was "absolute nonintercouse" with yellow fever ports from April to November. In a post-epidemic address to the American Public Health Association, Choppin argued that no "conditional" quarantine could ever be enforced because of "the cupidity of commercial men having large interests at stake, who will always move heaven and earth to evade all quarantine laws and regulations." When Dr. Joseph Jones became president of the state board of health in 1880, he found that "the Quarantine laws of the State were openly violated by rich and powerful steamship and railroad corporations."[57]

The value of New Orleans' tropical trade was slight compared to that of its domestic commerce in 1879 when Dr. Choppin suggested an absolute ban on trade with yellow fever ports. Even then he found little support for his proposal. During the 1880s and 1890s, however, the city's Latin American trade expanded greatly, especially the fruit trade with Central America. Because of the growing value of this commerce, the state board of health considered it necessary to alter the quarantine rules to accommodate the needs of the fruit companies. To avoid injury to the cargo, the board allowed the fruit boats to unload bananas in New Orleans prior to fumigation and disinfection. Sometimes the board dispensed with the disinfection procedure altogether if other conditions were met.[58]

In the 1890s the state board began to appoint port inspectors to reside in Honduras, Guatemala, Nicaragua, Costa Rica, and other places from which yellow fever might be transported to New Orleans. Inspectors were instructed to arrange for the fumigation of the "fruiters" prior to loading, and they were to inform the board if cases of yellow fever appeared in the port. By special arrangement with United Fruit, Morgan Steamship Lines, and others, the state board appointed marine medical inspectors to travel on company vessels engaged in the New Orleans traffic. Although the companies paid their salaries, these medical appointees were expected to carry out state board regulations, perform regular inspections, and certify the health status of the steamer and its crew upon arrival at the Mississippi River Quarantine Station. Under these special provisions, fruit boats and other steamers were allowed to proceed upriver to New Orleans after inspection, but without detention or fumigation.[59]

Even after the Reed Commission announced its findings, the state board took no special measures in the early 1900s to destroy mosquitoes on fruit boats. When Dr. Kohnke of the city health agency suggested that the state quarantine authorities should take into account the "mosquito theory" and "adopt measures to meet the danger," the state board responded that it would "continue its tried and reliable methods of quarantine."[60]

Regulatory measures in the interest of health were impossible to enforce if perceived to be in conflict with powerful economic interests. On the other hand, when complaints registered by large corporations happened to coincide with public demand for health protection as in 1878, legislation at the national level quickly followed. Congress created the National Board of Health (NBH) in response to pressure from a frightened public and from commercial and transportation interests adversely affected by the 1878 epidemic.

Authorized to assist state and local officials with maritime quarantine and to aid in combating the interstate spread of epidemic disease, the NBH was an experiment that failed, lasting only from 1879 to 1883. Its inspection and certification services did prove useful in keeping open trade along rivers and rails, and it had the support of many state officials, commerical exchanges, and health organizations, especially in the Mississippi Valley states. The NBH had many other assignments, however, and it soon encountered formidable opponents in rival bureaus—the Louisiana State Board of Health and the U. S. Marine Hospital Service. The NBH also had an unwieldy administrative structure and a lack of certainty about the extent of its legal authority, given the awkwardly drafted legislation defining its duties. Because of its complicated rules and regulations and the elaborate procedures required of states that requested aid, the NBH generated hostility among state and local officials not yet accustomed to the ways of modern bureaucracy.[61]

After the demise of the NBH, Congress reassigned limited functions in quarantine and public health to the Marine Hospital Service (MHS). As its duties and powers were gradually expanded, the MHS evolved into the U. S. Public Health Service by the early twentieth century. These uniformed federal medical officers had cooperated with state officials and provided important services to commercial interests during the yellow fever panic in 1897, inspecting railroad freight and passengers, operating detention camps, issuing health certificates, and fumigating the U. S. mail. They opened a path for trade and travel through interstate and intrastate quarantine barriers, and they made it possible for New Orleans laborers to reach the sugar plantations where they were needed for the harvest. In 1905, at the request of Louisiana's governor, the U. S. Public Health and Marine Hospital Service took charge of the campaign against yellow fever in New Orleans, working with state and local authorities to curb the spread of the disease. Since the 1905 outbreak, no yellow fever epidemic has occurred in the United States.

After that epidemic, the federal government assumed full control of all maritime quarantine operations in 1906. Martin Behrman, mayor of New Orleans at the time, later wrote of the injuries to the city from quarantines imposed by other states. "Our commercial rivals had in former years established quarantine at the slightest excuse." But, "we stopped them by getting the federal government to take charge"; and, he boasted, "as I remember it, we started the movement for federal control of quarantine."[62] When centralized federal control of maritime quarantine seemed to offer protection from the costly disruptions of state quarantines, it was clearly the lesser of the evils.

Like wars and depressions, epidemics disrupt normal routines, produce a sense of crisis, and create the need as well as the opportunity for an extension of government power through new agencies and regulations. By stirring popular fears and interrupting the profits of powerful railroad and steamship corporations and other interstate commercial interests, yellow fever became a problem of national proportions which the federal government had to address. Most of the concerned interest groups cared little whether it was the NBH or the MHS that provided the desired services during epidemics as long as some agency kept the trains and steamboats running and halted the spread of disease—without great expense or delay. In fact, when several years went by without epidemics in the 1880s and 1890s, the concern of the public and the commercial interests almost evaporated altogether, only to surface again in another wave of panic whenever the disease reappeared. On the positive side—if there is a positive side—yellow fever was a primary influence in shaping public health consciousness and institutions in Louisiana, in other southern states, and at the national level.

One among the many burdens of southern history, the disease weighed most heavily on the coastal and river cities, damaging Mobile, Memphis, and other communities, as well as New Orleans. Perceived as a southern disease, yellow fever added another component to the region's bad reputation, and nineteenth-century observers considered the disease a hindrance to population growth, capital investment, and commercial expansion. A major villain in Louisiana history, Yellow Jack killed thousands of the state's residents, consumed energies and wasted millions of dollars that might have been used more productively, disrupted and diverted commerce, and destroyed the hopes and prospects of New Orleans for becoming the nation's leading city, the metropolis of the Western Hemisphere.

NOTES

Introduction to 2015 Edition

[1] Jim Murphy, *An American Plague: The True and Terrifying Story of the Yellow Fever Epidemic of 1793* (New York: Clarion Books, 2003). Another non-fiction work for elementary and junior high school, part of a series on epidemic diseases, consists of 64 pp. of yellow fever's history and information about causes and modern methods for prevention and control: Holly Cefrey, *Yellow Fever* (New York: Rosen Pub. Group, 2002).

[2] Laurie H. Anderson, *Fever, 1793* (New York: Simon & Schuster Books for Young Readers, 2000).

[3] Sarah Masters Buckey *et al.*, *Marie-Grace Makes a Difference*, and *Marie-Grace and the Orphans* (Middleton, WI: American Girl Pub., 2011); Denise Louis Patrick *et al.*, *Troubles for Cecile*, and *Cecile's Gift* (Middleton, WI: American Girl Pub., 2011).

[4] Anna Myers, *Graveyard Girl* (New York: Walker, 1995).

[5] Josh Russell, *Yellow Jack* (New York: W. W. Norton, 1999).

[6] James D. Brewer, *No Escape* (New York: Walker and Co., 1998).

[7] Taylor Polites, *The Rebel Wife* (New York: Simon & Schuster, 2012); (Waterville, Maine: Thorndike Press, 2012).

[8] Barbara Hambly, *Fever Season- Benjamin January, Book 2* (New York: Bantam, reprint ed., 1999). Another book entitled *Fever Season* about the 1878 Memphis epidemic, by historian Jeanette Keith, was published in Oct. 2012—about which more later.

[9] Benjamin H. Trask, *Fearful Ravages: Yellow Fever in New Orleans, 1796-1905* (Lafayette: Center for Louisiana Studies, University of Louisiana at Lafayette, 2005).

[10] Henry M. McKiven, Jr., "The Political Construction of a Natural Disaster: The Yellow Fever Epidemic of 1853," *Journal of American History* 94 (Dec. 2007): 734-42. See also Patrick Brennan, "Getting out of the Crescent City: Irish Immigration and the Yellow Fever Epidemic of 1853," *Louisiana History* 52 (Spring 2011): 189-205, which relates another aspect of the 1853 epidemic to Katrina experience.

[11] Jonathan B. Pritchett and Isan Tunali, "Strangers' Disease: Determinants of Mortality in 1853 New Orleans," *Explorations in Economic History* 32, no.4 (1995): 517-39; Tunali & Pritchett, "Cox Regression with Alternative Concepts of Waiting Time: The New Orleans Yellow Fever Epidemic of 1853," *Journal of Applied Econometrics* 12, no. 1 (1997): 1-25.

[12] Jerah Johnson, "Yellow Fever and the Louisiana-Mississippi War of 1905," *Louisiana Cultural Vistas* 11 (Fall 2000): 70-79; Horace Knowles, "Long-Forgotten Letters of Hero [Eugene Augustus Woodruff] of Shreveport's Yellow Fever Epidemic of 1873 Found," *North Louisiana Historical Association Journal* 27 (Spring-Summer 1996): 63-82; Margaret Johnson, "The Great Yellow Fever Epidemic of 1873 in Shreveport," *North Louisiana History* 30 (Fall 1999): 106-8.

[13] http://www.caddohistory.com/yellow_fever.html.

[14] http://www.oaklandcemeteryla.org/History/Historical-Overview.aspx.

[15] http://www.c-spanvideo.org/program/304647-1;http://www.youtube.com/watch?v=CN8KJDcJVOM.

[16] http://freepages.family.rootsweb.ancestry.com/~ltrichel/History/YellowFever1873/htm

[17] Wesley Bradshaw [Charles Wesley Alexander], *Angel Agnes* (Shreveport: Ritz Publications, 2005); for online text see http://www.gutenberg.org/dirs/1/7/2/0/17200/17200.txt.

[18] Eric J. Brock, Review, http://www.ritzpublications.com/angel-agnes-book-review.html (all 1873 Shreveport online items accessed 10/14/2012).

[19] I am indebted to Martha Fitzgerald, Shreveport journalist and independent scholar, for bringing to my attention Father Seelos and the websites about his life and work. http://www.redemptorists.net/saints-seelos.cfm;http://www.seelos.org/lifeBiography.html; http://www.seelos.org/beatification1.html; http://www.seelos.org/shrineAssumption1.html; http://www.seelos.org/Heibel_Case_Closure_Statement_Nov_2011.pdf (all accessed 12/28/2012).

[20] Carrigan, *Saffron Scourge*, 120-125, 346-350.

[21] Deanne Stephens Nuwer, *Plague Among the Magnolias: The 1878 Yellow Fever Epidemic in Mississippi* (Tuscaloosa: University of Alabama Press, 2009); quotation, 54. Public health crises such as severe epidemics and concern with human resources for economic self-sufficiency were key influences in the building and strengthening of the modern nation-state. European historians trace the beginnings of this development back to the seventeenth and eighteenth centuries. The United States, however, followed a significantly different path, with localization and fragmentation of health policy instead of centralization, limited by the federal-state structure and prevailing resistance to central authority. See Dorothy Porter, *Health, Civilization, and the State* ... (London: Routledge, 1999). While U.S. institutional structures developed in different ways, major epidemics and other public health concerns, here as elsewhere, prompted the creation of state and federal agencies and health regulations that expanded the scope and power of both state and national governments.

[22] Edward J. Blum, "The Crucible of Disease: Trauma, Memory, and National Reconciliation during the Yellow Fever Epidemic of 1878," *Journal of Southern History* 69 (November 2003): 791-820; and "The White Flag Waves ...," Chap. 5 in Blum, *Reforging the White Republic: Race, Religion, and American Nationalism, 1865-1898* (Baton Rouge: Louisiana State University Press, 2005), 146-73; quotation, 147. See also 248-49.

[23] Blum, *Reforging the White Republic*, 167-170, quotation, 15-16.

[24] See Conevery Bolton Valencius, "Mudslides Make Good History," *Journal of the Early Republic* 24 (Summer 2004): 252-59. This remarkably insightful article suggests "ways to write good history that engages public interest." Although not specifically about yellow fever, her ideas about the use of narrative, drama, and visual images in environmental history are broadly applicable. Epidemics and other disasters, she says, "make good copy," and "histories that tell good stories ... get read and remembered." (quotations, 252-53, 257).

[25] Deanne Stephens Nuwer, "The 1878 Yellow Fever Epidemic in Mississippi: 'For God's Sake, Send Us Some Nurses and Doctors,'" in Barbra Mann Wall & Arlene W. Keeling (eds.), *Nurses on the Front Line: When Disaster Strikes, 1878-2010* (New York: Springer Publishing Company, 2011), 1-15.

[26] Linda E. Sabin, "Unheralded Nurses: Male Caregivers in the Nineteenth Century South," in Patricia D'Antonio et al. (eds.), *Nurses' Work: Issues Across Time and Place* (New York: Springer Publishing Company, 2007), 49-64. See also Charles McGraw, "Mammy at MacClenny, Jezebel in Jacksonville: Southern Fever Nursing in History and Memory," *Labor: Studies in Working-Class History of the Americas* 9 (Summer 2012): 95-112, which challenges the stereotypes in early professional nursing histories and provides an important account of the "range of experienced practitioners—black and white, female and male—that public officials actually employed during the Jacksonville fever epidemic." (p.112).

[27] Linda E. Sabin, "Sweating, Purging, and a Passion for Care: The Yellow Fever Nurse in the Deep South in the Early Nineteenth Century," in Patricia D'Antonio and Sandra B. Lewenson (eds.), *Nursing as Evidence: Nursing Interventions through Time* (New York: Springer Publishing Company, 2011), 3-16.

[28] A. S. Melissinos, "From Houston to Memphis: The Kezia Payne DePelchin Letters and the Yellow Fever Epidemic of 1878" (Ph.D. dissertation, Texas Woman's University, 2010).

[29] Kathryn Keller, "Racing Immunities: How Yellow Fever Gendered a Nation" (Ph.D. dissertation, University of Washington, 2000).

[30] Michael D. Thompson, "Working on the Dock of the Bay: Labor and Life along Charleston's Waterfront, 1783-1861" (Ph.D. dissertation, Emory University, 2009).

[31] John R. Pierce and Jim Writer, *Yellow Jack: How Yellow Fever Ravaged America and Walter Reed Discovered its Deadly Secrets* (Hoboken, N.J.: John Wiley & Sons, Inc., 2005).

[32] World Health Organization, "Yellow Fever," Fact Sheet No. 100, January 2011, http://www.who.int/mediacentre/factsheets/fs100/en/ (accessed 10/08/2012).

[33] James L. Dickerson, *Yellow Fever: A Deadly Disease Poised to Kill Again* (Amherst, New York: Prometheus Books, 2006); Molly Caldwell Crosby, *The American Plague: The Untold Story of Yellow Fever, the Epidemic That Shaped Our History* (New York: Berkley Books, 2006).

[34] See for example, Lyle R. Peterson, Review of Dickerson, *Yellow Fever*, in *Nature Medicine* 13 (January 2007): 23, http://www.nature.com/naturemedicine (accessed 10/12/2012); Alan D. T. Barrett, Review of Dickerson, in *Journal of Clinical Investigation* 116, no.10 (October 2006): 2566, http://www.ncbi.nlm.nih.gov/pmc/articles/PMC1578627/ (accessed 11/19/2012); Mariola Espinosa, Review of Crosby, *The American Plague*, in *Bulletin of the History of Medicine* 82 (Fall 2008): 734-35.

[35] For another opinion similar to Dickerson's warning, see Jeffrey A. Lockwood, *Six-Legged Soldiers: Using Insects as Weapons of War* (New York: Oxford University Press, 2009), 310-13.

[36] See Paul Reiter, "Climate Change and Mosquito-Borne Disease," *Environmental Health Perspectives* 109, Supplement 1 (March 2001): 141-161; quotation, 158.

[37] Dickerson, *Yellow Fever*, 232-36; quotation, 250.

[38] Kenneth F. Kiple (ed.), *Plague, Pox & Pestilence* (London: Weidenfeld & Nicolson, 1997); quotations, 6, 92.

[39] Richard Platt; John Kelly (illus.), *Plagues, Pox, and Pestilence* (New York: Kingfisher, 2011).

[40] A recent article deserving special notice here relates southern railroad development in the 1870s and 1880s, major yellow fever epidemics, panic-stricken southern towns, shot-gun quarantines, and the disruption of trade and travel: R. Scott Huffard Jr., "Infected Rails: Yellow Fever and Southern Railroads," *Journal of Southern History* 79 (Feb. 2013): 79-112.

[41] In my digging around in the University of Nebraska-Omaha library among actual "hard copy" journals, I accidentally came across a highly significant article which is relevant here for medical-military history and deserves widespread attention: J. David Hacker, "A Census-Based Count of the Civil War Dead," *Civil War History* 57 (December 2011): 307-48. Using census data and statistical techniques, Hacker makes a strong case that the figure long accepted for estimated total Civil War mortality from diseases and battle wounds (both North and South) should be adjusted upward from 620,000 to 750,000. See also Sarah Richardson's interview with Hacker in *Civil War Times* 51 (August

2012): 26-27. For the most comprehensive and recent treatment of Civil War health issues, public and private, military and home-front, see Margaret Humphreys, *Marrow of Tragedy: The Health Crisis of the American Civil War* (Baltimore: Johns Hopkins University Press, 2013).

[42] Andrew McIlwaine Bell, *Mosquito Soldiers: Malaria, Yellow Fever, and the Course of the American Civil War* (Baton Rouge: Louisiana State University Press, 2010); quotation, 118.

[43] Jim Downs, *Sick from Freedom: African-American Illness and Suffering during the Civil War and Reconstruction* (New York: Oxford University Press, 2012); quotations, 12, 32, 56.

[44] Benjamin F. Butler, *Autobiography and Personal Reminiscences of Major-General Benj. F. Butler: Butler's Book* . . . (Boston, 1892), 394-413.

[45] Christopher Wills, *Yellow Fever, Black Goddess: The Coevolution of People and Plagues* (Reading, Mass.: Helix Books, Addison-Wesley, 1996); quotations, 49, 254, 163n. Seminal works by historians in this developing field with special value for medical history are William McNeill, *Plagues and Peoples* (Garden City, NY: Anchor/Doubleday, 1976); Alfred W. Crosby, *The Columbian Exchange: Biological and Cultural Consequences of 1492*, 30th Anniversary Edition (Westport, Conn.: Praeger, 2003; first ed., 1972); and Crosby, *Ecological Imperialism: The Biological Expansion of Europe, 900-1900* (Cambridge: Cambridge University Press, 1986). See also Donald Worster, *The Ends of the Earth: Perspectives on Modern Environmental History* (Cambridge: Cambridge University Press, 1989).

[46] J. R. McNeill, *Mosquito Empires: Ecology and War in the Greater Caribbean, 1620-1914* (New York: Cambridge University Press, 2010); quotations, 264, 313. See also reviews that provide extensive discussion and assessment of McNeill's work: Matthew Mulcahy, Review of *Mosquito Empires*, in *William and Mary Quarterly* 67 (October 2012): 788-91, http://www.jstor.org/stable/10.5309/willmaryquar.67.4.0788 (accessed 11/08/2012); Bonham C. Richardson, Review of *Mosq. Empires*, in *American Historical Review* 116 (February 2011): 133-35, http://www.jstor.org/stable.10.1086.ahr.116.1.133 (accessed 8/11/2012); and Shawn W. Miller, "Flying the Yellow Jack: Microbes in Defense of America," in *Reviews in American History* 40 (March 2012): 1-5.

[47] Mariola Espinosa, *Epidemic Invasions: Yellow Fever and the Limits of Cuban Independence, 1878-1930* (Chicago: University of Chicago Press, 2009); quotation, 119. On the issue of credit for the mosquito "discovery," see also Pierce & Writer, *Yellow Jack*, 212-14.

[48] Jeanette Keith, *Fever Season: The Story of a Terrifying Epidemic and the People Who Saved a City* (New York: Bloomsbury Press, 2012); quotations, 197.

[49] Keith, 8; see Carrigan, *Saffron Scourge*, 10-11, 238-39, 242-45, *passim*.

[50] J. Worth Estes and Billy G. Smith (eds.), *A Melancholy Scene of Devastation: The Public Response to the 1793 Philadelphia Yellow Fever Epidemic* (Philadelphia: Science History Publications/USA, 1997).

[51] Margaret Humphreys, "Appendix II: Yellow Fever Since 1793: History and Historiography," in Estes and Smith (eds.), *A Melancholy Scene of Devastation*, 183-98; quotation, 195.

[52] Simon Finger, *The Contagious City: The Politics of Public Health in Early Philadelphia* (Ithaca and London: Cornell University Press, 2012); quotations, 162, xi, 5.

[53] John McKiernan-Gonzalez, *Fevered Measures: Public Health and Race at the Texas-Mexico Border, 1848-1942* (Durham and London: Duke University Press, 2012); quotations, xi-xii, 158.

[54] Kenneth Kiple (ed.), *Cambridge World History of Human Disease* (New York: Cambridge University Press, 1993), 1100-1107; Kiple (ed.), *Cambridge Historical Dictionary of Disease* (New York: Cambridge University Press, 2003), 365-69.

[55] See Kenneth F. Kiple and Virginia H. King, *Another Dimension to the Black Diaspora: Diet, Disease, and Racism* (New York: Cambridge University Press, 1978); Kiple, *The Caribbean Slave: A Biological History* (New York: Cambridge University Press, 1984); Sheldon Watts, *Epidemics and History: Disease, Power and Imperialism* (New Haven: Yale University Press, 1997).

[56] John Ellis, *Yellow Fever and Public Health in the New South* (Lexington: University Press of Kentucky, 1992), 57; Keith, *Fever Season*, 6, 220n5; Carrigan, *Saffron Scourge*, 192, 255-56.

[57] Sheldon Watts, "Yellow Fever Immunities in West Africa and the Americas in the Age of Slavery and Beyond: A Reappraisal," *Journal of Social History* 34 (Summer 2001): 955-67; Kenneth F Kiple, "Response to Sheldon Watts," 969-74; Watts, "Response to Kenneth Kiple," 975-76.

[58] McNeill, *Mosquito Empires*, 46.

[59] Recently I met and have since enjoyed an amiable exchange of ideas with a historian who argues that there is no basis for the "belief in black immunity" and historians should give it up. See: Mariola Espinosa, "The Question of Racial Immunity to Yellow Fever in History and Historiography," *Social Science History* 38 (Winter 2014). While bold and provocative, her arguments conflate "complete immunity" and "resistance to lethal effects of yellow fever," and do not, in my judgment, explain away the voluminous historical record (about "resistance") that I and others have encountered. Her article is an attempt to put an end to the issue, raised by Sheldon Watts and others. It is indeed a complicated matter, but I am not yet persuaded that Espinosa's work has settled it once and for all. Even so, the article is important, for it forces one to think carefully about the complexity of explaining and interpreting historical materials and clarifying concepts that require both contemporary and current medical/scientific theory and knowledge for analysis and context.

[60] Margaret Humphreys, *Intensely Human: The Health of the Black Soldier in the American Civil War* (Baltimore: Johns Hopkins University Press, 2008), 38-45, 48-50.

[61] Andrew Spielman and Michael D'Antonio, *Mosquito: A Natural History of Our Most Persistent and Deadly Foe* (New York: Hyperion, 2001), 30-35.

[62] Art Chimes, "New Yellow Fever Vaccine Shows Promise," *Voice of America* (April 6, 2011), http://www.voanews.com/articleprintview/171436.html (accessed 12/28/2012); Thomas Monath *et al.*, "An Inactivated Cell-Culture Vaccine against Yellow Fever," *New England Journal of Medicine* 364 (April 7, 2011): 1326-33, http://www.ncbi.nlm.nih.gov/pubmed/21470010 (accessed 12/28/2012). See also J. Gordon Frierson, "The Yellow Fever Vaccine: A History," *Yale Journal of Biology and Medicine* 83 (2010): 77-85.

[63] Centers for Disease Control and Prevention, "Yellow Fever Vaccine: Recommendations of the Advisory Committee on Immunization Practices, 2002," *MMWR* 51: RR-17 (November 8, 2002): 1-10, http://www.cdc.gov/mmwr/PDF/rr/rr5117.PDF (accessed 12/28/2012).

[64] WHO, "Yellow Fever—Fact Sheet," http://www.who.int/mediacentre/factsheets/fs100/en/ (accessed 10/08/12).

[65] World Health Organization, "Dengue and Severe Dengue--Fact Sheet," November 2012, http://www.who.int/mediacentre/factsheets/fs117/en/ (accessed 1/12/2013); Thomas P. Monath, "Dengue and Yellow Fever—Challenges for the Development and Use of Vaccines," *New England Journal of Medicine* 357 (November 29, 2007): 2222-2225.

[66] Monath, 2223.

[67] Monath, 2222-2225. See also Stephen Higgs *et al.*, "Growth Characteristics of Chimerivax-Den Vaccine Viruses in *Aedes Aegypti* and *Aedes Albopictus* from Thailand," *American Journal of Tropi-*

cal Medicine and Hygiene 75 (November 2006): 986-993; and Cameron P. Simmons *et al.*, "Current Concepts: Dengue," *New England Journal of Medicine* 366 (April 12, 2012):1430.

[68] "Fight fever with 'Franken-skeeters'?" Omaha *World-Herald*, December 7, 2012, article about dengue and the controversy regarding possible release of transgenic mosquitoes in Key West, Florida, under consideration by FDA.

[69] Michael Specter, "The Mosquito Solution," *New Yorker* (July 9, 16, 2012): 38-46.

[70] Specter, 40.

[71] Specter, 42-46. See also Amy Maxmen, "Florida Abuzz Over Mosquito Plan," *Nature /News* (July 17, 2012), http://www.nature.com/news/florida-abuzz-over-mosquito-plan-1.11023 (accessed 12/28/2012); and *GM-Free Brazil Campaign* (July 2012), http://aspta.org.br/campanha/fly-away-with-transgenic-mosquitos/ (accessed 12/28/2012).

[72] Specter, 43-44; Kiera Butler, "Can GMO Mosquitoes Save You From Dengue?" *Mother Jones* (May/June 2012), http://www.motherjones.com/environment/2012/04/genetically-engineered-mosquitoes-oxitec (accessed 1/14/2013); Andrew Pollack, "Concerns Are Raised About Genetically Engineered Mosquitoes," *New York Times*, October 30, 2011, http://www.nytimes.com/2011/10/31/science/concerns-raised-about-genetically-engineered-mosquitoes.html?pagewanted=all&_r=0 (accessed 1/12/2013); Mae-Wan Ho, "Transgenic Mosquitoes **Not** a Solution," *Institute of Science in Society* (July 3, 2012), http://www.i-sis.org.uk/Transgenic_Mosquitoes_Not_a_Solution.php (accessed 12/28/2012).

[73] Oxitec FAQs, http://www.oxitec.com/faqs/ (accessed 1/12/2013); Chris Sweeney, "Study Shows Oxitec GM Mosquitoes Work," Broward/Palm Beach *New Times*, September 10, 2012, http://blogs.browardpalmbeach.com/pulp/2012/09/study_shows_oxitec_gm_mosquito.php (accessed 1/12/2013).

[74] Susan Milius, "Mosquitoes REMADE," *Science News* 182 (July 14, 2012): 22-26, http://www.sciencenews.org/view/feature/id/341843/description/Mosquitoes_Remade (accessed 10/13/2012). Milius discusses research underway on malaria's mosquito vectors, and she describes the two major strategies dealing with *A. aegypti*: Oxitec's genetically modified RIDL (Release of Insects carrying a Dominant Lethal genetic system), and the Australian team's *Wolbachia*-infected mosquito.

[75] Milius, 22-26. See also Ed Yong, "Defeating dengue by releasing mosquitoes with virus-blocking bacteria," *Discover: The Magazine of Science, Technology, and the Future* (August 24, 2011), http://blogs.discovermagazine.com/notrocketscience/?p=6281 (accessed 12/30/2012); Mae-Wan Ho, "Non-transgenic Mosquitoes to Combat Dengue," *Institute of Science in Society* (December 3, 2012), http://www.i-sis.org.uk/Non-transgenic_Mosquitoes_to_Combat_Degue.php (accessed 12/28/2012).

[76] Charles C. Choi, "Prickly Problem: Engineering Mosquitoes to Spread Less Disease without Boosting Virulence," *Scientific American* (August 21, 2009), http://www.scientificamerican.com/article.cfm?id=transgenic-mosquitoes (accessed 12/29/2012).

[77] Some scientists have not given up on "classical SIT" (Sterile Insect Technique) by radiation. In Italy and Austria they are having some success with *A.albopictus* and one of the malaria vectors (*Anopheles arabiensis*). *A. aegypti* will probably be next in line. It remains to be seen whether transgenic or classical SIT proves better in the long run in actually limiting disease. http://www.malariaworld.org/blog/are-transgenic-mosquitoes-beating-old-school-sterile-insect-technique (accessed 12/28/2012).

[78] Chris Swanson, Linda Pratt, Robert Harms, David Sutherland, and Yvonne Rucker read various drafts of this new chapter, or parts thereof, and all offered helpful suggestions, for which I am most grateful. Thanks also to Ada Bello for suggesting Michael Specter's article in the *New Yorker*,

and to Amy Hay for calling my attention to McKiernan-Gonzalez's work on the "Texas-Mexican Borderlands."

Chapter 1

[1]Charles E. Lyght, et al., eds., *The Merck Manual of Diagnosis and Therapy*, 9th ed. (Rahway, N.J., 1956), 966-67, hereafter cited as *Merck Manual*, 9th ed.; Richard P. Strong, *Stitt's Diagnosis, Prevention and Treatment of Tropical Diseases*, 7th ed., 2 vols. (Philadelphia, 1944), II, 872-73, 879-82; Loring Whitman, "The Arthropod Vectors of Yellow Fever," in George K. Strode, ed., *Yellow Fever* (New York, 1951), 233-61; Richard M. Taylor, "Epidemiology," in ibid., 445-47. For a clear, detailed, and beautifully illustrated account of the *Aedes aegypti* ("The most dangerous of all the species of mosquitoes"), its life cycle, and the anatomy and physiology of its feeding system, see Jack Colvard Jones, "The Feeding Behavior of Mosquitoes," *Scientific American*, 238 (June, 1978): 138-48. For a brief but comprehensive discussion of arbovirus (*arthropod-borne* virus) infections, including yellow fever, with attention to etiology, epidemiology, pathology, immunology, clinical features, diagnosis, treatment, and control, see Charles Wilcocks and P. E. C. Manson-Bahr, eds., *Manson's Tropical Diseases*, 17th ed. (Baltimore, 1972), 355-83.

[2]Taylor, "Epidemiology," in Strode, ed., *Yellow Fever*, 427-538. Although the virus is the same in both forms, a distinction is now usually made between urban and jungle yellow fever because of differences in transmission patterns. Researchers and public health workers in the early twentieth century had believed the *Aedes aegypti* to be the only vector for the virus, and humans the only host. The Rockefeller Foundation in 1915 set out to rid the world of the virus by eradicating, or at least controlling, the *Aedes aegypti*. By the 1930s and 1940s it was recognized that vast reservoirs of the yellow fever virus were maintained in certain jungles or forests of Central and South America and Africa, propagated through a transmission cycle involving several types of forest mosquitoes and monkeys. When forest mosquitoes infect humans with the virus acquired from monkeys, the disease is referred to as jungle yellow fever. Such human cases may then become the source of infection for the *Aedes aegypti* and a classic urban epidemic can result. Although the disease remains endemic (or at least enzootic) in those forest areas, the International Health Division of the Rockefeller Foundation, in cooperation with the governments of fourteen countries on three continents, was remarkably successful in eliminating urban yellow fever through mosquito control programs. The Foundation also funded long-term research which led to many advances, including the development of an effective yellow fever vaccine in 1937. The Foundation's work continued over a period of thirty-two years at a cost of almost fourteen million dollars. Andrew J. Warren, "Landmarks in the Conquest of Yellow Fever," in ibid., 12-20, 24-37; and George K. Strode, "Costs and Man Power," in ibid., 631-39. See also John P. Fox, Carrie E. Hall, and Lila R. Elveback, *Epidemiology: Man and Disease* (New York, 1970), 270-71, 286-88.

[3]Robert Berkow, ed., *The Merck Manual of Diagnosis and Therapy*, 15th ed. (Rahway, N.J., 1987), 192, hereafter cited as *Merck Manual*, 15th ed. In its 9th edition, published in 1956, the *Merck Manual* stated that the case fatality rate might run as high as 85 percent. (p. 968.)

[4]Quoted in J. Austin Kerr, "The Clinical Aspects and Diagnosis of Yellow Fever," in Strode, ed., *Yellow Fever*, 398. See also 389-90, 397.

[5]Phillip H. Manson-Bahr, ed., *Manson's Tropical Diseases: A Manual of the Diseases of Warm Climates*, 8th ed. (London, 1925), 174; *Merck Manual*, 9th ed., 968. The case fatality rate varied greatly from one epidemic to another, from place to place, and among different groups.

[6]Kerr, "The Clinical Aspects and Diagnosis of Yellow Fever," in Strode, ed., *Yellow Fever*, 391-97; *Merck Manual*, 9th ed., 967-68; *Merck Manual*, 15th ed., 189-93.

[7]John Duffy, ed., *Parson Clapp of the Strangers' Church of New Orleans* (Baton Rouge, 1957), 95-97.

[8]Kerr, "The Clinical Aspects and Diagnosis of Yellow Fever," in Strode, ed., *Yellow Fever*, 397.

[9]George Augustin, *History of Yellow Fever* (New Orleans, 1909), 70-84. According to Augustin (p. 84), the term yellow fever was first applied to the disease in 1750 by Griffith Hughes in a publication entitled *Natural History of Barbadoes*. From the mid-eighteenth century onward, English and American writers generally used the label yellow fever, and French and Spanish authors (and others) eventually adopted the term in translation. At least some Anglo-American colonials had been using the term yellow fever for decades before Hughes published his volume. See John Duffy, *Epidemics in Colonial America* (Baton Rouge, 1953), 148-60, *passim.*, for several direct quotations from the writings of physicians and laymen of Charleston, Philadelphia, and Boston in the late 1720s, 1730s, and 1740s, referring to a "distemper" generally called "the yellow" or "the Yellow Fever." *Mal de Siam*, one of the oldest names for the disease, was first used in the late seventeenth century when it was believed that a ship from Siam had introduced the fever to the West Indies. Some writers later argued that yellow fever was already epidemic in Brazil and that the vessel from Siam, having stopped there, simply transported the malady from Brazil to Martinique; hence, Siam was not the point of origin after all. In one form or another the tradition persisted, and *mal de Siam* was a synonym for yellow fever among French medical writers well into the nineteenth century. *New Orleans Medical and Surgical Journal*, 6 (January, 1850): 530-31, hereafter cited as *NOM&SJ*; Elisha Bartlett, *The History, Diagnosis, and Treatment of the Fevers of the United States*, 4th ed. (Philadelphia, 1856), 447; A. J. F. Cartier, *La Fièvre Jaune de la Nouvelle-Orléans* (Paris, 1859), 1; D. Durac, *De La Fièvre Jaune et des Epidémies de 1853, 1854 et 1858 dans la paroisse Lafourche* (Nouvelle-Orléans, 1863), 4.

[10]Fielding H. Garrison, *John Shaw Billings: A Memoir* (New York, 1915), 177-78.

[11]As Charles E. Rosenberg has stated so succinctly in his history of cholera epidemics, "A disease is no absolute physical entity but a complex intellectual construct, an amalgam of biological state and social definition." *The Cholera Years: The United States in 1832, 1849, and 1866* (Chicago, 1962), 5n. See John H. Ellis, "The New Orleans Yellow Fever Epidemic in 1878: A Note on the Affective History of Societies and Communities," *Clio Medica*, 12 (1977): 189-216, for an insightful discussion of the psychological impact of yellow fever on nineteenth-century New Orleans, especially the intensification of class consciousness and the tendency of the dominant elements to blame the "strangers" for New Orleans' unhealthy reputation and indeed to define them as outside the community altogether.

[12]Susan Sontag, *Illness as Metaphor* (New York, 1978).

[13]*NOM&SJ*, 15 (November, 1858): 731; William L. Robinson, *The Diary of a Samaritan* (New York, 1860), 77-78; Erasmus Darwin Fenner, *History of the Epidemic Yellow Fever, at New Orleans, Louisiana, in 1853* (New York, 1854), 57-58; Strode, ed., *Yellow Fever*, 417-22; *Manson's Tropical Diseases*, 8th ed., 174-75; *Merck Manual*, 13th ed., 58. Quotation is from Kerr, "The Clinical Aspects and Diagnosis of Yellow Fever," in Strode, ed., *Yellow Fever*, 417.

[14]William H. McNeill, *Plagues and Peoples* (Garden City, N.Y., 1976), 211-15; Macfarlane Burnet and David O. White, *Natural History of Infectious Disease*, 4th ed. (Cambridge, 1972), 242, 245; Josiah C. Trent, ed., "The Men Who Conquered Yellow Fever," in Ashbel Smith, *Yellow Fever in Galveston, Republic of Texas, 1839* . . . (Austin, 1951), 85-86; Charles-Edward A. Winslow, *The Conquest of Epidemic Disease: A Chapter in the History of Ideas* (Princeton, N.J., 1943), 193; Augustin, *History of Yellow Fever*, 85-130, 649. See especially Strode, ed., *Yellow Fever*, 529-33, and Henry Rose Carter, *Yellow Fever: An Epidemiological and Historical Study of its Place of Origin*, edited by L. A. Carter and W. H. Frost (Baltimore, 1931), for the careful reasoning from medical and historical data which led to the conclusion in favor of Africa. See also Kenneth F. Kiple and Virginia H. Kiple, "Black Yellow Fever Immunities, Innate and Acquired, as Revealed in the American South," *Social Science History*, 1 (Summer, 1977): 419-36.

[15]Duffy, *Epidemics in Colonial America*, 138-63; Wilson G. Smillie, *Public Health, Its Promise for the Future: A Chronicle of the Development of Public Health in the United States, 1607-1914* (New York, 1955), 33-38; McNeill, *Plagues and Peoples*, 213-14.

[16] In many cases it is impossible to identify the specific disease in question from the ambiguous and obscure terms used in the records. For example, a disease referred to as "Calenture" erupted in 1779 in the interior of Spanish Louisiana and made great ravages in the settlement of Galveztown on the Amite River. Like yellow fever (and dengue), this disease did not decline until cool weather. According to an army surgeon writing in 1899, *calentura* was a name applied by Cubans to a specific fever, symptomatically similar to yellow fever and often confused with it, but essentially different. George Augustin, on the other hand, listed *calentura* as one of yellow fever's many synonyms. Meaning heat or fever, the term could have referred to any one of a number of infectious diseases characterized by high fever. The exact nature of the illness in 1779 remains a mystery. See V. M. Scramuzza, "Galveztown, A Spanish Settlement of Colonial Louisiana," *Louisiana Historical Quarterly*, 13 (October, 1930): 576-77; *NOM&SJ*, 52 (September, 1899): 144-45; Augustin, *History of Yellow Fever*, 73; John Duffy, ed., *The Rudolph Matas History of Medicine in Louisiana*, 2 vols. (Baton Rouge, 1958-1962), I, 200, hereafter cited as Duffy, *Medicine in Louisiana*.

[17] The concept of specificity of diseases, each as a separate and distinct clinical entity with a specific cause, was not elaborated and convincingly demonstrated until the second half of the nineteenth century. For further discussion of the emergence and impact of the "specificity" concept, see Richard Harrison Shryock, *Medicine in America: Historical Essays* (Baltimore, 1966), 15-17, 315-25; and Morris J. Vogel and Charles E. Rosenberg, eds., *The Therapeutic Revolution: Essays in the Social History of American Medicine* (Philadelphia, 1979), especially the essays by Rosenberg, 3-25, and by Edmund D. Pellegrino, 245-66.

[18] *NOM&SJ*, new series, 7 (July, 1879): 132-33, 146.

[19] Alcée Fortier, *Louisiana*, 3 vols. (Madison, Wis., 1914), II, 661.

[20] Duffy, *Medicine in Louisiana*, I, 11-12.

[21] Bennet Dowler, "Tableau of the Yellow Fever of 1853, with Topographical, Chronological and Historical Sketches of the Epidemics of New Orleans," in *Cohen's New Orleans Directory . . . of 1854* (New Orleans, 1854), 7; *NOM&SJ*, new series, 7 (July, 1879): 132; Alcée Fortier, *A History of Louisiana*, 4 vols. (New York, 1904), I, 51. According to Fortier (I, 48-49), and most other historians of Louisiana, yellow fever was the disease that took the life of Pierre le Moyne, Sieur d'Iberville, founder of French Louisiana. Iberville had ample opportunity to contract the infection during his West Indies expeditions in the summer of 1706; he died aboard ship at Havana. See also Edwin Adams Davis, *The Story of Louisiana* (New Orleans, 1960), 43.

[22] François-Xavier Martin, *The History of Louisiana, From the Earliest Period . . .* (reprint edition, New Orleans, 1963), 177-78; Fortier, *History of Louisiana*, I, 126; Charles Gayarré, *History of Louisiana*, 4 vols. (reprint edition, New Orleans, 1965), I, 507.

[23] J. F. H. Claiborne, *Mississippi, As a Province, Territory and State . . .* (reprint edition, Baton Rouge, 1964), 64-85.

[24] Louboey to the Minister, October 12, 1739, Archives Nationales, Paris, Colonies C13A, volume 24, folio 204. Maurepas was Minister of the Marine and Colonies at the time. In most Louisiana histories Louboey is referred to as Loubois, *lieutenant du roi* in New Orleans. See Gayarré, *History of Louisiana*, I, 516, and Fortier, *History of Louisiana*, I, 117. Winston DeVille, Louisiana genealogist, historian, and publisher, deserves credit for calling my attention to this document as described in an inventory of colonial correspondence. Barbara Allemand in Paris obtained a copy for me, and DeVille provided assistance in translating the relevant portions. A study of French Louisiana commerce, published in 1916, stated that yellow fever "was raging" in the colony in 1739 and that some persons claimed the "great swarms of mosquitoes" were related to the malady. N. M. Miller Surrey, *The Commerce of Louisiana during the French Regime, 1699-1763* (New York, 1916), 194. This passage caught my attention only after I had read the Louboey letter. I have since obtained some of the documents Surrey cited as sources for the epidemic, but have not yet located the reference to the mosquitoes.

25See note 9 above.

26David Geggus, "Yellow Fever in the 1790s: The British Army in Occupied Saint Domingue," *Medical History*, 23 (1979): 38-44; John Blake, "Yellow Fever in Eighteenth Century America," *Bulletin of the New York Academy of Medicine*, 44 (June, 1968): 673-77. Blake concluded that the disease had actually disappeared from most of the islands for some thirty years after 1762. Geggus, on the other hand, doubted that the long period without epidemics meant the total absence of the virus. In those areas lacking sufficient population to maintain the disease on a year-round endemic basis, Geggus postulated that yellow fever had been "effectively endemic" through regular reintroduction by infected mosquitoes from the West African slave trade and by commercial contact with other Caribbean centers of infection. Blake also noted the occasional reintroduction of the disease to some of the islands from Africa and from the Spanish mainland colonies, and he stressed the role of wartime conditions in the various outbreaks that affected the entire region and extended to the Atlantic ports of British North America.

27See Duffy, *Epidemics in Colonial America*, 162-63, and Smillie, *Public Health, Its Promise for the Future*, 33-38, for the chronology and location of seventeenth- and eighteenth-century yellow fever epidemics. Blake, "Yellow Fever in Eighteenth Century America," 674-76, and John Duffy, "Yellow Fever in the Continental United States during the Nineteenth Century," *Bulletin of the New York Academy of Medicine*, 44 (June, 1968): 697-98, both discussed the correlation between colonial wars and the extent and magnitude of yellow fever outbreaks.

28An unidentified "sickness" in 1740 wiped out almost 10 percent of New Orleans' population, according to John G. Clark, *New Orleans, 1718-1812: An Economic History* (Baton Rouge, 1970), 49.

29One historian has suggested that "the sugar connection" may be an important explanatory factor in the chronological and epidemiological patterns of yellow fever activity in Caribbean and North American port cities, patterns which have seemed at times more like puzzles than solutions. See James D. Goodyear, "The Sugar Connection: A New Perspective on the History of Yellow Fever," *Bulletin of the History of Medicine*, 52 (Spring, 1978): 5-21. In the areas he studied, Goodyear found that yellow fever became a major problem only after the introduction and rapid expansion of cane culture and sugar refining. A number of yellow fever outbreaks in ports where the *Aedes aegypti* was not ordinarily present can be linked to shipments of raw sugar and molasses. Cane culture and sugar processing apparently enhanced the breeding conditions and augmented the food supply (cane juice) for a vastly expanded vector population of *Aedes Aegypti*, one of the necessary elements in a large-scale epidemic. Louisiana's yellow fever history lends support to the hypothesis; the worst epidemics coincided with a rapidly expanding sugar industry beginning in the 1790s.

30There is no census for 1739. These figures are simply my estimate based on a census of 1744 which counted 300 adult slaves and 800 white adult males in New Orleans. According to one nineteenth-century source, the total in 1744 was probably at least 3,000. George E. Waring, Jr., "The Southern and Western States," *Report of the Social Statistics of Cities, Tenth Census, 1880*, XIX, pt. 2 (Washington, 1887), 220, hereafter cited as Waring, *Social Statistics of Cities*.

31Clark, *New Orleans, 1718-1812*, 50, 127-28; see also Martin, *History of Louisiana*, 176. Imported slaves would probably have already acquired immunity to yellow fever before arriving in Louisiana, either from a childhood case in Africa or in the West Indies. During the colonial period, the larger the proportion of imported blacks in the population, the smaller the proportion of persons likely to be vulnerable to yellow fever.

32Geggus, "Yellow Fever in the 1790s," 39-41.

33*NOM&SJ*, new series, 7 (July, 1879): 146; Gayarré, *History of Louisiana*, II, 133; George W. Cable, *The Creoles of Louisiana* (New York, 1884), 291; John Smith Kendall, *History of New Orleans*, 3 vols. (Chicago, 1922), I, 174.

[34] *DeBow's Commercial Review*, 2 (July, 1846): 73; *NOM&SJ*, new series, 7 (July, 1879): 132, 146; Dowler, "Tableau of the Yellow Fever of 1853," 8; Joseph Jones, *Medical and Surgical Memoirs*, 3 vols. in 4 (New Orleans, 1876-1890), III, pt. 1, cxxxi-cxxxvi. According to Edwin Davis, *The Story of Louisiana*, 147, there could be "little doubt that a calenture first appearing in 1769 and reaching epidemic proportions in 1779, 1791, and from 1793 to 1795" was in fact the same yellow fever that attacked New Orleans in 1796.

[35] Duffy, *Medicine in Louisiana*, I, 206.

[36] Erasmus Darwin Fenner, "The Yellow Fever Quarantine at New Orleans," *Transactions of the American Medical Association*, 2 (1849): 624; Berquin-Duvallon, *Vue de la Colonie Espagnole du Mississippi ou des Provinces de la Louisiane ... en l'année 1802* (Paris, 1803), trans. by John Davis as *Travels in Louisiana and the Floridas, in the year, 1802* (New York, 1806), 114, 118. It is possible that a different strain of the yellow fever virus, more virulent than usual, prevailed in the 1790s and made the disease seem unlike any in previous experience. More likely, the local population was simply not accustomed to seeing the disease in epidemic form. See Geggus, "Yellow Fever in the 1790s," 43.

Chapter 2

[1] Davis, *The Story of Louisiana*, 130-31; Waring, *Social Statistics of Cities*, 220, 232, 238; Jones, *Medical and Surgical Memoirs*, III, pt. 1, cxxxiii-cxxxv.

[2] Alcée Fortier, *History of Louisiana*, edited with commentary by Jo Ann Carrigan, 2nd ed. (Baton Rouge, 1972), II, 149-69, 395-99, 433-36, hereafter cited as Carrigan, ed., *Fortier's History of Louisiana*; Harold Sinclair, *The Port of New Orleans* (Garden City, N.Y., 1942), 56-105, *passim*.

[3] Geggus, "Yellow Fever in the 1790s," 38-44, 56, 58. Imported from the West Indies, the disease spread through New York in 1798, causing almost 2,600 fatalities in a population reduced to 20,000 when another 20,000 fled to escape the city's worst yellow fever epidemic. Harry Bloch, "Yellow Fever in City of New York: Notes on Epidemic in 1798," *New York State Journal of Medicine*, 73 (October 15, 1973): 2504. The death toll from the Philadelphia epidemic of 1793 had been even greater: more than 4,000 deaths among 24,000 persons remaining in the city; at least 13,000 had left during the epidemic. Smillie, *Public Health, Its Promise for the Future*, 36-37.

[4] See Goodyear, "The Sugar Connection: A New Perspective on the History of Yellow Fever," 5-21. At the very least, it is an interesting coincidence that New Orleans' first notable yellow fever epidemic finally happened the year immediately following the first successful processing of sugar in the province, the achievement of Etienne de Boré aided by West Indian experts in 1795. By 1800 more than 60 estates had a combined yield of 4 million pounds of sugar; by 1802 New Orleans marketed 5 million pounds of sugar and 250,000 gallons of molasses. Production continued to expand throughout the antebellum years. Gayarré, *History of Louisiana*, III, 436; Waring, *Social Statistics of Cities*, 231-32. It is puzzling that New Orleans did not have a major epidemic earlier in the 1790s inasmuch as the city already had a sizeable susceptible population and the same opportunities for the introduction of disease through the usual Caribbean shipping and the extraordinary influx of refugees that had begun well before 1796. Perhaps it was indeed the availability of sugar that caused a population explosion among the *Aedes aegypti*, bringing it finally to the "critical number" required for an epidemic. Perhaps the vector population in New Orleans had not previously reached the necessary density relative to the susceptible human population for propagating a widespread epidemic. As Goodyear has pointed out, the sugar business can provide a favorable environment for the feeding and breeding of an enlarged mosquito population; by 1796, New Orleans had it all—including the sugar. In the course of this study, the "sugar connection" with yellow fever will be noted wherever it is found in the context of Louisiana's epidemic experiences.

[5] Gayarré, *History of Louisiana*, III, 375; "Letters of Joseph X. Pontalba to his Wife, 1796" (W. P. A. trans. typescript, Louisiana State University Archives, Baton Rouge), September 6, 11, 24, 30, November 3, 1796,

pp. 274, 284, 312, 323, 393, hereafter cited as Pontalba Letters.

[6] Pontalba Letters, September 6, 11, 1796, pp. 274, 284; Records of the City Council of New Orleans, Book 4079, Document 259, October 21, 1796 (W. P. A. trans. typescript, Louisiana State Museum Library, New Orleans).

[7] Pontalba Letters, September 19, 24, October 30, 1796, pp. 300, 312, 385; Gayarré, *History of Louisiana*, III, 375.

[8] See John H. Powell, *Bring Out Your Dead: The Great Plague in Philadelphia in 1793* (Philadelphia, 1949).

[9] Pontalba Letters, September 15, October 15, 1796, pp. 291, 358. One American acquaintance, according to Pontalba, was so frightened that he was unable to urinate. When he did come down with a mild case of fever, he was so "awe-stricken" that his physicians feared the effects of "his own imagination" more than the disease itself. Ibid., October 13, 1796, p. 353.

[10] Ibid., September 28, October 30, 1796, pp. 321, 386. A tea made of cinchona bark was a common prescription for all kinds of fever, but it was actually effective only in the treatment of malaria. The alkaloid quinine was isolated from the bark in 1820. Erwin H. Ackerknecht, *A Short History of Medicine* (rev. ed., New York, 1968), 125-26, 169.

[11] Pontalba Letters, October 10, 1796, p. 344; Gayarré, *History of Louisiana*, III, 375. The description of Masdevall's remedy came from Dowler, "Tableau of the Yellow Fever of 1853," 9.

[12] Pontalba Letters, September 14, 15, 1796, pp. 290-91; Records of the City Council of New Orleans, October 21, 1796.

[13] Pontalba Letters, September 19, 21, 22, 28, 30, October 7, 13, November 6, 7, 1796, pp. 300, 305-7, 321, 323, 338, 353, 399, 402.

[14] Records of the City Council of New Orleans, October 21, 1796; Gayarré, *History of Louisiana*, III, 375.

[15] Dowler, "Tableau of the Yellow Fever of 1853," 9; *NOM&SJ*, 15 (November, 1858): 818. A New Orleans census in 1769 counted 468 households with a total population of 3,190. Dr. Joseph Jones in his *Medical and Surgical Memoirs*, III, pt. 1, cxxxv, gave New Orleans a population of 8,756 with a total annual mortality of 638 in 1796 (or 72.86 deaths per thousand). He did not reveal the source of the population or mortality figures, and one may assume it was his own estimate based on various fragments as no census was taken in 1796. It could also have been an error in transcription as the figure he cited for the New Orleans population in 1803 was 8,056—exactly 700 less than his figure for 1796. It does not seem likely that New Orleans population suffered such a decline in those years. See also Gayarré, *History of Louisiana*, III, 374, for Governor Carondelet's reference to New Orleans in 1796 as "a city of six thousand souls."

[16] These figures have been extrapolated from census records of years before and after 1796 and from estimates made by various historians. Between 1769 and 1788 the New Orleans population grew from 3,190 to 5,338, mainly it seems from natural increase, although the Spanish did promote immigration. New Orleans was beginning to attract American and European merchants, but the Creoles, or native-born, constituted the overwhelming majority of the white population and continued to do so in the early nineteenth century. By 1806 the English-speaking residents of the city numbered less than 20 percent of the white population, or about 12 percent of the total. In the 1760s the proportion of blacks in the New Orleans population was about two-fifths, or 40 percent, as it was also in 1806. See the historical sketch of New Orleans by George W. Cable, in Waring, *Social Statistics of Cities*, 220, 232, 237-38, 243-44. Some estimates for 1803, when the United States acquired New Orleans, set the total population at 8,000 to 13,000 with one-third to two-fifths black. Of the white population, approximately one-half was French Creole, one-fourth Spanish or Spanish Creole, and the remaining one-fourth American, British, German, and other foreign nationals. See Davis, *The*

Story of Louisiana, 143. If the proportions were roughly the same in 1796 as in 1803, New Orleans' white population would have been about 3,600 of the 6,000 total, and yellow fever mortality almost 10 percent of their number. Virtually all of the fever victims were white. The attorney general had observed in 1796 that blacks, as well as Spaniards, seemed immune to the disease. In all later epidemics yellow fever cases among blacks were generally mild in effect and the case fatality rates exceedingly low relative to whites.

[17] Pontalba Letters, September 12, 15, 22, 24, October 13, November 3, 1796, pp. 285, 291, 307, 312, 353, 393.

[18] Ibid., October 13, 1796, p. 353.

[19] Ibid., October 9, 1796, p. 342.

[20] Ibid., October 15, 1796, p. 358.

[21] Ferdinand de Feriet described the activities that took place in his home on the outskirts of New Orleans during the epidemic of 1822: "To pass away the time, the neighborhood assembles sometimes at our house and play[s] a comedy in a little theater which I have had arranged." There were two "troupes" of actors, "the children and company for the French pieces, and some American neighbors for the English pieces." He considered "this little distraction . . . an antidote against the cursed yellow fever." Ferdinand de Feriet to Janica de Feriet, October 7, 1822, Ferdinand de Feriet Letters, Volume I, 1816-1825 (Manuscripts Section, Howard-Tilton Memorial Library, Tulane University, New Orleans).

[22] Pontalba Letters, September 21, 22, October 7, 30, 1796, pp. 306-7, 338, 385-88.

[23] Ibid., September 22, October 7, 1796, pp. 307, 338. In early October the governor "finally consented to yield to the importunities of his ladies, and he will stay on the other side."

[24] Carrigan, ed., *Fortier's History of Louisiana*, 412-14.

[25] Sometime during the Spanish era New Orleans finally "gained an identity of self" which had failed to develop under French rule, according to John Clark, *New Orleans, 1718-1812*, 250-51.

[26] Recognizing particular clusters of symptoms and labeling the "prevailing" malady, however, was not incompatible with the generalized pathology of the times, which defined disease in terms of body responses to environmental influences of various kinds, a singular process with many individual variations. At least fifty years would pass before medical theorists began to develop a different conception in which the unity of disease was transformed into the plurality of diseases, specific clinical entities with specific causes, each entirely separate from the other and not simply variations or gradations of bodily dysfunction. In 1796 Pontalba described the epidemic in terms of "the maladies" or "the fevers"—that is, the process manifested in many individuals, with worse effects in some than in others. And in 1799, reporting the death of Louisiana's Governor Gayoso—probably from yellow fever, Intendant Morales said that he "died of a malignant fever [una calentura maligna], of the nature of those which prevail in this country during the summer. . . ." Gayarré, *History of Louisiana*, III, 404-5. For many years, yellow fever would be viewed as the most malignant grade of a general class of "bilious" fevers. The doctrine of specificity was yet to come.

Chapter 3

[1] Records of the City Council of New Orleans and Documents Pertaining to the Government of Louisiana, 1800 to 1803, Book 4088, Document 337, pp. 9-16 (W. P. A. trans. typescript, Louisiana State Museum Library, New Orleans).

[2] Augustin, *History of Yellow Fever*, 771-75, 868; *NOM&SJ*, 15 (November, 1858): 818-19; 23 (January, 1870): 25. The years of relatively mild outbreaks were 1800, 1801, 1802, 1803, 1808, 1812, and 1818.

³Clark, *New Orleans, 1718-1812*, 212-20; Davis, *The Story of Louisiana*, 165; Waring, *Social Statistics of Cities*, 213.

⁴Quoted in Henry E. Chambers, *A History of Louisiana*, 3 vols. (Chicago & New York, 1925), I, 394. See also Minter Wood, "Life in New Orleans in the Spanish Period," *Louisiana Historical Quarterly*, 22 (July, 1939): 645-46; and Edward H. Barton, "Sanitary Report of New Orleans, La.," *Transactions of the American Medical Association*, 2 (1849): 591-97.

⁵William C. C. Claiborne to James Wilkinson, August 10, 1804, Dunbar Rowland, ed., *Official Letter Books of William C. C. Claiborne, 1801-1816*, 6 vols. (Jackson, Mississippi, 1917), II, 306; Joseph Briggs to James Madison, August 25, 1804, ibid., 306-7; Claiborne to Albert Gallatin, August 31, 1804, ibid., 314; Claiborne to Madison, September 8, 17, 1804, ibid., 328, 337; Claiborne to Thomas Jefferson, August 29, 30, September 13, 27, 1804, Clarence E. Carter, ed., *The Territory of Orleans, 1803-1812*, 9th vol. of *The Territorial Papers of the United States* (Washington, 1940): 279-80, 286, 294.

⁶Claiborne to Jefferson, October 5, 1804, Carter, ed., *Territory of Orleans*, 309; Dr. O. H. Spencer to Nathaniel Evans, October 5, 1804, and James Sterrett to Nathaniel Evans, October 23, 1804, Nathaniel Evans Family Papers (Louisiana State University Archives, Baton Rouge).

⁷Claiborne to Madison, October 16, 1804, William C. C. Claiborne Letterbook, 1804-1805 (Louisiana State University Archives, Baton Rouge).

⁸Sterrett to Nathaniel Evans, October 29, 1804, Nathaniel Evans Family Papers; Claiborne to Jefferson, September 13, November 4, 1804, Carter, ed., *Territory of Orleans*, 294, 319.

⁹Claiborne to Jefferson, September 18, 1804, Carter, ed., *Territory of Orleans*, 298. During the epidemic of 1837 in Alexandria, a slave uprising was planned; when the plot was discovered, a vigilante group lynched the alleged leaders. R. F. McGuire, Diary (Louisiana State University Archives, Baton Rouge), September-October, 1837.

¹⁰This journalistic practice can also be found in the colonial period. See John Duffy, "A Sidelight on Colonial Newspapers," *The Historian*, 18 (Spring, 1956): 230-48. For New Orleans examples, see *NOM&SJ*, 1 (October, 1844): 216; *Picayune*, June 6, August 4, 19, 31, September 2, 25, October 16, November 10, 1837; June 24, August 19, September 20, 26, 1838; September 13, 15, October 6, 22, November 5, 1839; June 27, August 4, 31, October 3, 8, 9, 20, 26, 1841; August 28, September 12, 19, October 3, 10, 19, 1847; New Orleans *Bee*, July 20, August 3, 9, November 3, 1841; August 5, 1847; New Orleans *Price-Current and Commercial Intelligencer*, September 9, 23, October 2, November 4, 1837; July 29, August 19, September 9, November 4, 1843. Almost any New Orleans newspaper during the months of June or July through October or November from the 1830s to the end of the century revealed a preoccupation with matters of health, whether an epidemic actually developed or not.

¹¹Fox, Hall, and Elveback, *Epidemiology: Man and Disease*, 16.

¹²*Louisiana Gazette* (New Orleans), August-November, 1804; September 28, 1804. At least part of the explanation for the lack of attention given the epidemic could be the general neglect of local news in the weekly or semi-weekly papers of the early 1800s. Not until the 1830s with the expansion of daily newspapers in size and number did it become a common practice to provide extensive coverage of local affairs in the growing towns and cities of the nation.

¹³Gayarré, *History of Louisiana*, IV, 36-37; Duffy, *Medicine in Louisiana*, I, 348. Having been responsible for the Louisiana Purchase in 1803, President Jefferson concerned himself with matters relating to its principal city. Jefferson had serious reservations about cities because of his observations in Europe. He considered them sores on the body politic—centers of disease, disorder, and corruption. His plan for checkerboard development was an attempt to reduce population density and provide trees and country-like

fresh air in the midst of the urban setting. Yellow fever in Philadelphia had led him to propose such a plan in 1800 as "the best means of preserving the cities of America from the scourge of yellow fever." See Morton and Lucia White, *The Intellectual Versus The City* (Cambridge, Mass., 1964), 28-29.

[14]David Bradford to David Redick, July 1, 1805, David Bradford Letters (Louisiana State University Archives, Baton Rouge).

[15]*NOM&SJ*, new series, 7 (July, 1879): 152; Waring, *Social Statistics of Cities*, 213, 243-44; Gayarré, *History of Louisiana*, IV, 214-20.

[16]Gayarré, *History of Louisiana*, IV, 220-22.

[17]Sterrett to Nathaniel Evans, December 2, 1809, Nathaniel Evans Family Papers.

[18]Claiborne to Madison, December 17, 1809, Carter, ed., *Territory of Orleans*, 859-60. There are some indications that the disease was actually more virulent the previous year, but it arrived so late in the season that the city escaped a major epidemic. See letters from Dr. Oliver Spencer to Nathaniel Evans, November 5, 13, 1808, Nathaniel Evans Family Papers; and Samuel Philips to John M. Pintard, November 13, 20, 1808, John M. Pintard Papers (Louisiana State University Archives, Baton Rouge).

[19]*Louisiana Courier* (New Orleans), October 2, November 6, 1811; Lt. E. Prebble to Nathaniel Evans, August 28, 1811, Nathaniel Evans Family Papers; Claude Dejan to James Monroe, October 12, 1811, Rowland, ed., *Claiborne Letter Books*, V, 363.

[20]Claiborne to Albert Gallatin, August 19, 1811, Carter, ed., *Territory of Orleans*, 944; Claiborne to James Madison, October 8, 1811, ibid., 948; Claiborne to James Monroe, August 27, 1811, Rowland, ed., *Claiborne Letter Books*, V, 343; Claiborne to Paul Hamilton, September 9, 1811, ibid., 356.

[21]Claiborne to Paul Hamilton, October 28, 1811, Rowland, ed., *Claiborne Letter Books*, V, 369; Mather to Claiborne, September 9, October 12, 1811, Carter, ed., *Territory of Orleans*, 946, 949; Duffy, *Medicine in Louisiana*, I, 350.

[22]*Louisiana Courier*, October 2, November 6, 1811; *Louisiana Gazette*, November 5, 1811.

[23]James Mather to Claiborne, September 9, 1811, Carter, ed., *Territory of Orleans*, 947.

[24]*Louisiana Courier*, August 29, 1817; see also Jones, *Medical and Surgical Memoirs*, III, pt. 1, cxli-cxlii. The *Louisiana Gazette*, October 4, 1817, labeled the prevailing disease "this high charged bilious fever."

[25]A. A. Gros et N. V. A. Gérardin, *Rapport fait a la Société Médicale sur la Fièvre Jaune qui a regné d'une Manière Epidémique pendant l'eté de 1817* (Nouvelle-Orléans, 1818), 5-6, 59-62.

[26]See Jones, *Medical and Surgical Memoirs*, III, pt. 1, cxliv-cxlix.

[27]*Rapport publié au nom de la Société Médicale de la Nouvelle-Orléans sur la Fièvre Jaune, qui y a regné Epidémiquement, durant l'Eté et l'Automne de 1819* (Nouvelle-Orléans, 1820), 7, 35-36. Not to be outdone, the Anglo-American physicians organized their own English-speaking group, the Physico-Medical Society, and published a report on the yellow fever outbreak of 1820. *Report of the Committee of the Physico-Medical Society of New Orleans, on the Epidemic of 1820* (New Orleans, 1821).

[28]Jones, *Medical and Surgical Memoirs*, III, pt. 1, cxliv.

[29]Benjamin Latrobe, *Impressions Respecting New Orleans*, edited by Samuel Wilson, Jr. (New York, 1951), xxii, 146. Latrobe himself died of yellow fever in 1820.

30*Louisiana Courier*, November 15, 1819.

31*Yellow Fever Statistics* (undated pamphlet, Tulane University Medical Library, New Orleans), 57; Jones, *Medical and Surgical Memoirs*, III, pt. 1, cxliv; Duffy, *Medicine in Louisiana*, I, 360. New Orleans' suburbs, with a population almost as great as the city proper, would have contributed additional fever victims, which may account for some of the estimates of 2,000 or more.

32*NOM&SJ*, 15 (November, 1858): 818-19; 22 (January, 1870): 25; Pierre Frederick Thomas, *Essai sur la Fièvre Jaune d'Amérique . . . avec l'Histoire de l'Epidémie de la Nouvelle-Orléans en 1822 . . .* (Paris, 1823), 110; *Niles' Weekly Register*, October 26, 1822. Dr. Thomas arrived at a total of 1,400 for 1822, a figure supported also by the *Louisiana Gazette*. See Duffy, *Medicine in Louisiana*, I, 367. For 1829 yellow fever mortality, see *NOM&SJ*, new series, 6 (March, 1879): 699.

33Ferdinand de Feriet to Janica de Feriet, September 15, 1822, Ferdinand de Feriet Letters, I, 1816-1825.

34Thomas, *Essai sur la Fièvre Jaune d'Amérique*, 111, 113.

35*Louisiana Gazette*, September 14, 1822.

36*Louisiana Courier*, July 10, 11, 13, August 12, September 7, 23, October 5, 12, 1829.

37Duffy, ed., *Parson Clapp*, 95.

38Jones, *Medical and Surgical Memoirs*, III, pt. 1, cccvi; *NOM&SJ*, new series, 6 (March, 1879): 699; 5 (September, 1848): 203-6. Yellow fever mortality was 1.7 percent of New Orleans' population in 1833, 1.9 percent in 1837, 1.1 percent in 1839, 2.3 percent in 1841, and 2.8 percent in 1847. See population and mortality data in Dana G. Ketchum, "Yellow Fever in New Orleans: A Study of the Decline in Incidence of Yellow Fever in the Crescent City from 1861 to 1905" (M.A. Thesis, Johns Hopkins University, Baltimore,1983), 62 (a).

39*Louisiana Courier*, September 29, October 20, 27, 1832; Jones, *Medical and Surgical Memoirs*, III, pt. 1, cccvi; see also Leland A. Langridge, "Asiatic Cholera in Louisiana, 1832-1873" (M.A. Thesis, Louisiana State University, Baton Rouge, 1955).

40Edward Hall Barton, *Account of the Epidemic Yellow Fever, which prevailed in New Orleans during the Autumn of 1833* (Philadelphia, 1834), iii, 7, 9. See also *Louisiana Courier*, August 31, 1833.

41New Orleans *Daily Picayune*, July 25, 1837.

42*Bee*, August 24, September 5, 1837; *Picayune*, August 4, 31, September 13, 1837.

43*Picayune*, September 23, 1837.

44*Price-Current*, September 6, 1837.

45*Picayune*, October 26, 1841. On another occasion, the *Picayune* cutely warned strangers not to come to the city "till *White* Jack Kills off *Yellow* Jack." (October 1, 1843).

46*Bee*, November 3, 1841.

47Population percentages were computed from U. S. census data. See Ketchum, "Yellow Fever in New Orleans," 51-52. The demographic trends have also been noted in other contexts in Louisiana historical sources. See Robert C. Reinders, *End of an Era: New Orleans, 1850-1860* (New Orleans, 1964), 17-28; Jones, *Medical and Surgical Memoirs*, III, pt. 1, cclxxiii-cclxxv, ccxcvi; Dennis Rousey, "The New Orleans

Police, 1805-1889: A Social History" (Ph. D. Dissertation, Cornell University, 1978), 10-13, 82, 117, 120.

[48]See Chapter 1, note 29, and Chapter 2, note 4. From the early 1800s cane cultivation expanded northward along the Mississippi. In the 1820s the development of cold-resistant varieties of cane and the use of steam power in processing made possible even greater production, increasing from 10 million pounds in 1810 to 75 million pounds in 1830, 120 million pounds in 1840, and reaching the all-time high of 495 million pounds in 1853, also the year of Louisiana's worst yellow fever epidemic. Davis, *The Story of Louisiana*, 204; Jones, *Medical and Surgical Memoirs*, III, pt. 1, cxxxvi; J. Carlyle Sitterson, *Sugar Country: The Cane Sugar Industry in the South, 1753-1950* (Louisville, Ky., 1953), 23-30.

[49]*Report of the Committee of the Physico-Medical Society of New Orleans, on the Epidemic of 1820*, 7; Thomas, *Essai sur la Fièvre Jaune d'Amérique*, 111, 113; Robert C. Randolph, "Remarks on the Endemic Yellow Fever of New-Orleans during the summer and autumn of 1822," *Medical Repository* (New York), new series, 8 (1824): 169-70.

[50]*Picayune*, August 19, 1837.

[51]Fortier, *Louisiana*, I, 515. See also Peggy Bassett Hildreth, "Early Red Cross: The Howard Association of New Orleans, 1837-1878," *Louisiana History*, 20 (Winter, 1979): 49-75. The work of the Howard Association and other benevolent societies will receive more extensive treatment later; see especially Chapter 14.

[52]*Picayune*, July 13, 24, 26, August 6, 9, 11, 1839; *Bee*, August 3, September 3, 10, 1839.

[53]*NOM&SJ*, new series, 6 (March, 1879): 699; *Price-Current*, October 9, 1841; *Picayune*, October 3, 8, 12, 1841.

[54]*Picayune*, August 1, 3, 1847.

[55]*NOM&SJ*, 4 (September, 1847): 274; *Bee*, August 31, 1847; *Picayune*, August 29, 1847; Jones, *Medical and Surgical Memoirs*, III, pt. 1, cccxxv; *NOM&SJ*, 5 (September, 1848): 204-6.

[56]Charles Harrod to Mrs. S. B. Evans, October 23, 1847, Nathaniel Evans Family Papers; *Picayune*, September 5, 1847; Robinson, *Diary of a Samaritan*, 86.

[57]*NOM&SJ*, 4 (January, 1848): 535; 5 (September, 1848): 202-6.

[58]Ibid., 4 (September, 1847): 274.

[59]Ibid., 4 (January, 1848): 540-41.

[60]Ibid., 5 (September, 1848): 205; *DeBow's Commercial Review*, 3 (March, 1847): 250; *Picayune*, August 1, 1847.

[61]*NOM&SJ*, 4 (September, 1847): 274.

[62]*NOM&SJ*, new series, 6 (March, 1879): 699.

[63]Gordon E. Gillson, *Louisiana State Board of Health: The Formative Years* (Baton Rouge, 1967), 30-32, hereafter cited as *Formative Years*.

[64]See *Monthly Journal of Medicine* (Hartford, Conn.), 3 (January, 1824): 60.

[65]See Gillson, *Formative Years*, 15-34, for a concise account of the numerous boards and their vain attempts

to function without adequate official or popular support.

⁶⁶Reinders, *End of an Era*, 51-54.

⁶⁷Augustin, *History of Yellow Fever*, 899.

⁶⁸Lists of Louisiana communities and the years when each experienced yellow fever epidemics can be found in J. M. Toner, "Reports upon Yellow Fever: The Distribution and Natural History of Yellow Fever as it has Occurred at Different Times in the United States," *Reports and Papers of the American Public Health Association, 1873*, 1 (New York, 1875): 369-73, hereafter cited as *Reports and Papers, APHA*; and Augustin, *History of Yellow Fever*, 844-902. For the 1820s and earlier, see also *NOM&SJ*, 5 (September, 1848): 227; G. P. Whittington, "Rapides Parish, Louisiana—A History," *Louisiana Historical Quarterly*, 16 (July, 1933): 431; Erasmus Darwin Fenner, "Report on the Epidemics of Louisiana, Mississippi, Arkansas, and Texas in the year 1853," *Transactions of the American Medical Association*, 7 (1854): 512; McGuire Diary, 41; *St. Francisville Asylum and Feliciana Advertiser*, September 12, October 17, 24, 1822; *Louisiana Courier*, October 5, 1827.

⁶⁹See for example, *Louisiana Herald* (Alexandria), September 17, 1823; *Planter's Banner* (Franklin), quoted in *Picayune*, October 15, 1839; *Red River Republican* (Alexandria), October 9, December 4, 1847; and *Democratic Advocate* (Baton Rouge), October 6, 1847. Sampling various journals in towns along the rivers or bayous between July and October readily reveals the standard controversies in almost any year, but especially during New Orleans' epidemic years.

⁷⁰*Louisiana Herald*, September 7, 1822.

⁷¹Toner, "Reports upon Yellow Fever," 369-73; Augustin, *History of Yellow Fever*, 844-902; Edwin A. Davis, ed., *Plantation Life in the Florida Parishes of Louisiana, 1836-1846, as Reflected in the Diary of Bennet H. Barrow* (New York, 1943), 163-69; François Charles Deléry, *Précis Historique de la Fièvre Jaune* (Nouvelle-Orléans, 1859), 20-21; *Picayune*, October 3, 1839. The cultivation and milling of sugar cane, which can provide favorable conditions for an enlarged mosquito population, expanded into the same general areas of the state that yellow fever would soon claim as its territory. The 1820s and 1830s witnessed tremendous growth in the number of sugar plantations and volume of production, with land under cultivation along Bayous Lafourche and Teche and on Red River as far north as Natchitoches. Yellow fever appeared in Natchitoches and in the Teche region for the first time in 1839. Of course "the sugar connection" may be that the growth in sugar culture simply brought more commercial contact between the metropolis and various parts of the hinterland than ever before, and that the geographical areas suitable for growing sugarcane are also favorable to the *Aedes Aegypti* with heat, humidity, and many frost-free months. See also note 48 above.

⁷²A. D. Gove to Lewis Gove, November 8, 1839, A. D. Gove Letters (Louisiana State University Archives, Baton Rouge).

⁷³Deléry, *Précis Historique de la Fièvre Jaune*, 21.

⁷⁴*NOM&SJ*, 3 (July, 1846): 30-31, 37-40.

⁷⁵Davis, ed., *Plantation Life in the Florida Parishes*, 306; Fenner, "Report on the Epidemics . . . in the year 1853," 512; Corrine L. Saucier, *History of Avoyelles Parish, Louisiana* (New Orleans, 1943), 112; *NOM&SJ*, 5 (September, 1848): 216; see also note 68 above.

⁷⁶*NOM&SJ*, 4 (November, 1847): 409; 5 (September, 1848): 216.

⁷⁷Ibid., 5 (September, 1848): 213; *Red River Republican*, October 9, 16, December 4, 1847. Alexandria's population had been about 500 in 1819 when the first yellow fever epidemic occurred; by 1847 it was probably about 1,000.

Chapter 4

[1] John Duffy, *Sword of Pestilence: The New Orleans Yellow Fever Epidemic of 1853* (Baton Rouge, 1966), vii. This work provides a detailed picture of the 1853 episode in New Orleans and in other southern towns. See also Jo Ann Carrigan, "Yellow Fever in New Orleans, 1853: Abstractions and Realities," *Journal of Southern History*, 25 (August, 1959): 339-55.

[2] Dowler, "Tableau of the Yellow Fever of 1853," 31, 60.

[3] *Picayune*, August 21, 1841; New Orleans *Daily Delta*, August 10, 1858; see also Duffy, *Sword of Pestilence*, 22-23. According to Edward Hall Barton, *The Cause and Prevention of Yellow Fever, Contained in the Report of the Sanitary Commission of New Orleans* (Philadelphia, 1855), 41-42, the permanent population in 1853 was approximately 154,000, an increase of about 45,000 since 1847. Barton then added a conservative estimate of 5,000 to cover the "floating population" of the city. The 50,000 unacclimated newcomers, largely Irish and German immigrants, served to fuel the fever in 1853 once it started.

[4] *NOM&SJ*, 8 (May, 1852): 819; 9 (November, 1852): 415-16.

[5] Fenner, *Epidemic Yellow Fever*, 72; New Orleans *Daily Crescent*, July 6, 1853.

[6] Fenner, *Epidemic Yellow Fever*, 25. For a detailed description of the earliest cases and the various localities where the fever first appeared, see ibid., 15-31.

[7] Ibid., 35; *Picayune*, June 28, 1853; *NOM&SJ*, 10 (September, 1853): 275.

[8] Barton, *Cause and Prevention of Yellow Fever*, 42; Duffy, *Sword of Pestilence*, 27, 85, 105, 167.

[9] New Orleans *Weekly Delta*, June 12, 1853.

[10] New Orleans *Daily Crescent*, June 22, 1853.

[11] *Weekly Delta*, July 3, 1853; see also *Daily Crescent*, June 24, 1853; and *Picayune*, June 28, 1853.

[12] *Daily Crescent*, June 25, July 1, 6, 1853; *Picayune*, June 28, July 1, 6, 15, 1853.

[13] Fenner, *Epidemic Yellow Fever*, 35, 48; *DeBow's Review*, 15 (December, 1853): 603.

[14] *Picayune*, July 21, 26, 1853.

[15] *DeBow's Review*, 15: 609-11, 620.

[16] Robinson, *Diary of a Samaritan*, 150-52; *DeBow's Review*, 15: 614.

[17] Coroner's Office, Record of Inquests and Views, 1844-1904 (New Orleans Public Library), 7 (July-October, 1853).

[18] *NOM&SJ*, 10 (November, 1853): 310.

[19] Fenner, *Epidemic Yellow Fever*, 38-46.

[20] *DeBow's Review*, 15: 621.

[21] Leonard V. Huber and Guy F. Bernard, *To Glorious Immortality: The Rise and Fall of the Girod Street*

Cemetery, New Orleans' First Protestant Cemetery (New Orleans, 1961), 13; *History of the Yellow Fever in New Orleans, During the Summer of 1853 . . . By a Physician of New Orléans* (Philadelphia and St. Louis, 1854), 50, 53, 67-69.

[22]*NOM&SJ*, 5 (March, 1849): 648.

[23]Robinson, *Diary of a Samaritan*, 151.

[24]*History of the Yellow Fever in New Orleans, During the Summer of 1853*, 68; *DeBow's Review*, 15 (December, 1853): 620-21.

[25]*Daily Crescent*, August 9, 11, 1853; see also *Picayune*, August 8, 1853; and *DeBow's Review*, 15 (December, 1853): 615, 629. Unskilled workers ordinarily earned about a dollar for a day's work of ten or twelve hours; a skilled laborer, around two dollars per day. See Roger W. Shugg, *Origins of Class Struggle in Louisiana: A Social History of White Farmers and Laborers during Slavery and After, 1840-1875* (Baton Rouge, 1939), 113. The Howard Association paid its infirmary nurses $30 to $40 per month in 1853. See Chapter 14.

[26]*DeBow's Review*, 15: 626-28; see also Fenner, *Epidemic Yellow Fever*, 38.

[27]*Daily Crescent*, August 2, 8, 1853; *DeBow's Review*, 15 (December, 1853): 599-601; 16 (May, 1854): 463-66. See also Chapter 10.

[28]*Weekly Delta*, October 2, 1853.

[29]Ibid., August 14, 1853; *NOM&SJ*, 10 (November, 1853): 313.

[30]Fenner, *Epidemic Yellow Fever*, 57-58, 61; Durac, *De La Fièvre Jaune*, 17-20; *NOM&SJ*, 10 (September, 1853): 249; (March, 1854): 650-51; *Picayune*, August 30, 1853; *DeBow's Review*, 19 (October, 1855): 445. See also Duffy, *Sword of Pestilence*, 151-52, 163.

[31]*DeBow's Review*, 15: 607.

[32]Fenner, *Epidemic Yellow Fever*, 64, 69; *Picayune*, August 6, 1853.

[33]*DeBow's Review*, 15: 626, 633; Robinson, *Diary of a Samaritan*, 125-26, 132; see also Hildreth, "Early Red Cross: The Howard Association of New Orleans, 1837-1878," 58-64.

[34]Robinson, *Diary of a Samaritan*, 184-85, 208-85.

[35]Fenner, *Epidemic Yellow Fever*, 42-43; *DeBow's Review*, 15: 633-34.

[36]*Report of the Howard Association of New Orleans, Epidemic of 1853* (New Orleans, 1853), 3, 23-26; *DeBow's Review*, 16 (February, 1854): 213.

[37]*Daily Crescent*, August 31, 1853; *DeBow's Review*, 15: 629; *Gardner & Wharton's New Orleans Directory, for the Year 1858 . . .* (New Orleans, 1857), 389-90.

[38]*Weekly Delta*, August 28, 1853.

[39]Fenner, *Epidemic Yellow Fever*, 45-47.

[40]Barton, *Cause and Prevention of Yellow Fever*, 41-44; table in *Report of the Sanitary Commission of New Orleans on the Epidemic Yellow Fever* of 1853 . . . (New Orleans, 1854).

⁴¹Fenner, *Epidemic Yellow Fever*, 71-72; Duffy, *Sword of Pestilence*, vii, 167.

⁴²Fenner, "Report on the Epidemic of Louisiana, Mississippi, Arkansas, and Texas in the year 1853," 424. Sugar plantations especially had a sufficiently dense population of humans and mosquitoes to support an outbreak of yellow fever. In 1854 an outbreak occurred on Judge Baker's plantation on Bayou Teche a few miles below Centreville. Of the 190 slaves, 130 came down with the fever but only 6 died. *New Orleans Medical News and Hospital Gazette*, 2 (November 1, 1855): 406-9.

⁴³*DeBow's Review*, 15: 631-32; *History of the Yellow Fever in New Orleans, during the Summer of 1853*, 30.

⁴⁴*Report of the Louisiana State Board of Health for 1888 and 1889*, 39; Duffy, *Sword of Pestilence*, 117-18. The reports of the state board of health vary slightly in title from year to year, but will be cited uniformly herein with the year or years covered. Publication occurred the year after the report was made, in New Orleans or Baton Rouge.

⁴⁵*NOM&SJ*, 10 (March, 1854): 670-72; *New Orleans Medical News and Hospital Gazette*, 2 (January 1, 1856): 483-85. Pattersonville, some twelve miles below Centreville, also had an epidemic about the same time, as did other points in the southern part of the parish.

⁴⁶Toner, "Reports Upon Yellow Fever," 369-73; Augustin, *History of Yellow Fever*, 844-902; *DeBow's Review*, 15: 631-32; Dowler, "Tableau of the Yellow Fever of 1853," 26-27.

⁴⁷Dowler, "Tableau of the Yellow Fever of 1853," 26; John McGrath, Scrapbook (Louisiana State University Archives, Baton Rouge), 32 left, 39 right.

⁴⁸*DeBow's Review*, 15: 631-32; Dowler, "Tableau of the Yellow Fever of 1853," 26-27; Frederick Law Olmsted, *The Cotton Kingdom*, edited by Arthur M. Schlesinger (New York, 1953), 278.

⁴⁹Barton, *Cause and Prevention of Yellow Fever*, comparative table, preceding p. 1.

⁵⁰Thomas K. Wharton, Diary (Louisiana State University Archives, Baton Rouge), September 21, November 6, 1854.

⁵¹*Picayune*, August 4-December 4, 1854; *NOM&SJ*, 11 (November, 1854): 416.

⁵²Wharton Diary, October 4, 1854.

⁵³Toner, "Reports Upon Yellow Fever," 369-73; Augustin, *History of Yellow Fever*, 778-79, 844-902; *Picayune*, September 29, 1854. Among the places revisited were Bayou Sara, Franklin, Pattersonville, Washington, Thibodaux, Alexandria, and Cloutierville. Locations experiencing yellow fever for the first time included Jeanerette and Judge Baker's plantation in St. Mary Parish, and several small villages in Plaquemines Parish below New Orleans.

⁵⁴*Picayune*, August 11, 1853.

⁵⁵Ibid., September 25, 1853.

⁵⁶Ibid., March 9, 14, 18, 19, 1854; *Acts Passed by the Second Legislature of the State of Louisiana, at Its Second Session . . . 1855* (New Orleans, 1855), 471-77; see also Gillson, *Formative Years*, 58-63.

⁵⁷*Report of the Louisiana State Board of Health for 1855*, 10. The Act of 1855 provided for three quarantine stations: on the Mississippi River at least seventy miles below New Orleans; at the mouth of the Atchafalaya River; and at the Rigolets, the entrance from the gulf to Lake Pontchartrain.

[58] *NOM&SJ*, 12 (September, 1855): 285; 12 (November, 1855): 432; *Report of the Louisiana State Board of Health for 1856*, 25.

[59] Wharton Diary, September 30, 1855. In 1855 the disease spread up the Mississippi to Baton Rouge, Plaquemine, and Pointe Coupée Parish; up the Red to Alexandria; all along the Ouachita and Black Rivers; to Pattersonville, Centreville, St. Martinville, and New Iberia on the Teche. See Toner, "Reports Upon Yellow Fever," 369-73; Augustin, *History of Yellow Fever*, 844-902; *Picayune*, September 20, 25, 1855.

[60] *Report of the Louisiana State Board of Health for 1856*, 34; *New Orleans Medical News and Hospital Gazette*, 5 (March, 1858): 42.

[61] *New Orleans Medical News and Hospital Gazette*, 5 (August, 1858): 390-91; (September, 1858): 481; Wharton Diary, August 6, 30, 1858.

[62] *Picayune*, October 10, November 16, 23, 1858.

[63] Toner, "Reports Upon Yellow Fever," 369-73; Augustin, *History of Yellow Fever*, 844-902; *NOM&SJ*, 15 (November, 1858): 811.

[64] *Bee*, September 4, 1858.

[65] For a detailed account of the early quarantine system, the governor's proclamations, and the variations in requirements as the board employed its "discretionary powers," see Gillson, *Formative Years*, 60-99.

[66] *Report of the Louisiana State Board of Health for 1858*, 20, 28-32; *Acts passed by the Fourth Legislature of Louisiana, at its First Session . . . 1858* (Baton Rouge, 1858), 187-89.

[67] *DeBow's Review*, 15: 632.

Chapter 5

[1] *Report of the Louisiana State Board of Health for 1861*, 4.

[2] Wharton Diary, July 28, 1861.

[3] Benjamin F. Butler, *Butler's Book* (Boston, 1892), 396.

[4] Benjamin F. Butler, "Some Experiences with Yellow Fever and its Prevention," *North American Review*, 147 (November, 1888): 530.

[5] *NOM&SJ*, 23 (1870): 568.

[6] Howard Palmer Johnson, "New Orleans under General Butler," *Louisiana Historical Quarterly*, 24 (April, 1941): 478.

[7] Elisabeth Joan Doyle, "Civilian Life in Occupied New Orleans, 1862-65" (Ph. D. dissertation, Louisiana State University, Baton Rouge, 1955), 56-57.

[8] *Butler's Book*, 398-400.

[9] Ibid., 400-401, 407-8.

[10] Ibid., 401.

11 Ibid., 403, 408-10. Writing on another occasion, Butler mentioned only one case of yellow fever imported from Nassau. See Butler, "Some Experiences with Yellow Fever," 531, 536-37, and *Medical and Surgical History of the War of the Rebellion*, Part III, Vol. I (Washington, 1888): 675-76.

12 James Parton, *General Butler in New Orleans* (New York, 1864), 295.

13 *Butler's Book*, 403-4.

14 Ibid., 400, 406-7; Butler, "Some Experiences with Yellow Fever," 536.

15 *Butler's Book*, 404-6.

16 New Orleans *Daily True Delta*, August 20, 1862.

17 Johnson, "New Orleans under General Butler," 478.

18 *Some Practical Observations on Yellow Fever, Published for the Use of Surgeons of the Volunteer Forces in The Department of the Gulf* (New Orleans, 1862); *Butler's Book*, 398.

19 *NOM&SJ*, 23 (July, 1870): 569.

20 Parton, *General Butler in New Orleans*, 605.

21 *Picayune*, November 14, 1867.

22 Elisha Harris, "Hygienic Experience in New Orleans during the War: Illustrating the Importance of Efficient Sanitary Regulations," *Southern Journal of the Medical Sciences*, 1 (May, 1866): 25-30; Doyle, "Civilian Life in Occupied New Orleans, 1862-65," 66-67.

23 *NOM&SJ*, 23 (July, 1870): 569-74.

24 *Report of the Louisiana State Board of Health for June 1866-January 1867*, 3-4.

25 *Picayune*, July 24, 1866.

26 Harris, "Hygienic Experience in New Orleans during the War," 30.

27 *Report of the Louisiana State Board of Health for June 1866-January 1867*, 6, 12-13; *Report of the Louisiana State Board of Health for 1867*, 18, 20.

28 E. D. Fenner, "Remarks on the Sanitary Condition of the City of New Orleans, during the period of Federal Military Occupation, from May 1862 to March 1866," *Southern Journal of the Medical Sciences*, 1 (May, 1866): 22-25.

29 *NOM&SJ*, 23 (July, 1870): 589-92. See also Gillson, *Formative Years*, 108.

30 *NOM&SJ*, 23 (July, 1870): 563-64.

Chapter 6

1 See tables, "Yellow Fever Mortality in New Orleans, 1867-1905" and "Yellow Fever in Louisiana Outside of New Orleans, 1867-1898," following Chapter 8. Memphis, Tennessee, suffered severely from yellow fever in 1873 and 1878, and had the worst epidemic in the country in 1879, while New Orleans that year had a

limited outbreak.

²See Gillson, *Formative Years*, 111-241; John Ellis, "Businessmen and Public Health in the Urban South During the Nineteenth Century: New Orleans, Memphis, and Atlanta," *Bulletin of the History of Medicine*, 44 (May-June, 1970): 197-212; (July-August, 1970): 346-70; Dennis East II, "Health and Wealth: Goals of the New Orleans Public Health Movement, 1879-84," *Louisiana History*, 9 (Summer, 1968): 245-75; Margaret Warner, "Local Control versus National Interest: The Debate over Southern Public Health, 1878-1884," *Journal of Southern History*, 50 (August, 1984): 407-28; Peter Bruton, "The National Board of Health, 1879-1893" (Ph. D. dissertation, University of Maryland, 1974); Joy J. Jackson, *New Orleans in the Gilded Age: Politics and Urban Progress, 1880-1896* (Baton Rouge,1969), 170-87.

³Kelly, *Walter Reed and Yellow Fever*, 115-24; Margaret Warner, "Hunting the Yellow Fever Germ: The Principle and Practice of Etiological Proof in Late Nineteenth-Century America," *Bulletin of the History of Medicine*, 59 (Fall, 1985): 361-82.

⁴Exploding gunpowder, burning tar or sulphur, exposing materials to sunlight, and using lime or charcoal to combat noxious odors were all common methods of disinfection in the antebellum era, some having been used for hundreds of years to fight the invisible "miasmatic influences" believed to produce epidemics. Some of the materials actually had germicidal effects, but others were mere deodorants. Steam heat, carbolic acid, chlorine gas, sulphur dioxide, and various mineral salts were increasingly used in the mid-nineteenth century, especially from the 1870s onward, as health officials tried to limit the spread of infectious diseases with fumigants, powders, and liquids known to destroy germs. Although limited in effectiveness, a grand strategy of disinfection and fumigation was adopted by many late nineteenth-century sanitation and quarantine authorities in their war against disease. More precise understanding of infectious diseases, their specific causative microorganisms, and various modes of transmission eventually rendered much of the fumigators' work obsolete in the early twentieth century. Smillie, *Public Health: Its Promise for the Future*, 69, 363-68.

⁵See table, "Yellow Fever Mortality in New Orleans, 1859-66," following Chapter 5. Asiatic cholera struck New Orleans as an epidemic in 1866, claiming some 2,000 victims before its disappearance in 1867. Duffy, *Medicine in Louisiana*, II, 444; *Report of the Louisiana State Board of Health for June 1866-January 1867*, 6, 12-13; *Report of the Louisiana State Board of Health for 1867*, 18, 20.

⁶*Picayune*, May 26, 1867.

⁷Ibid., July 30, 31, August 3, 7, 14, 1867.

⁸Ibid., August 23, 27, 1867. According to the *Picayune* editor, "At no time have the deaths from yellow fever exceeded the total number of deaths from other diseases during any given period, and until such is the case, physicians do not speak of the fever as epidemic." And when reporting the weekly mortality on August 27, the editor again stated: "Notwithstanding this increase, we do not think the disease can yet be pronounced an epidemic. When the number of deaths from yellow fever are in excess of the number of deaths from all other causes, then, and only then, is it regarded as epidemical."

⁹*NOM&SJ*, 20 (September, 1867): 284-86; Gillson, *Formative Years*, 116. Although not officially declaring an epidemic in progress until early September, the board of health later stated in its annual report that yellow fever was epidemic by the middle of August. *Report of the Louisiana State Board of Health for 1867*, 5.

¹⁰*Picayune*, September 16, 21, 22, 24, October 8, 21, 28, November 1, 3, 6, 1867.

¹¹*Report of the Louisiana State Board of Health for 1867*, 18; *NOM&SJ*, 21 (April, 1868): 413-14.

¹²Augustin, *History of Yellow Fever*, 872; *NOM&SJ*, 20 (September, 1867): 196-98; see also Ketchum, "Yellow Fever in New Orleans," 81-83.

[13] *Report of the Louisiana State Board of Health for June 1866-January 1867*, 4-5; *Report of the Louisiana State Board of Health for 1867*, 4-5; *Picayune*, May 8, June 1, 1867; Gillson, *Formative Years*, 111-15, 117, 119.

[14] See Duffy, *Medicine in Louisiana*, II, 461. According to Gordon Gillson, "Possibly the most extensive functions performed by the [Louisiana] State Board of Health during the post-Civil War years were those connected with disinfection." *Formative Years*, 135. Indeed, some felt that the board went too far with its disinfection policy in 1867. Some physicians complained that the use of disinfectants in patients' rooms had a damaging effect. Patients became frightened when sanitary police charged in and sprinkled carbolic acid all over their rooms, and in some cases the patients took a turn for the worse. A committee recommended that the board wait until the sick either recovered or died before disinfecting rooms. *Picayune*, August 21, 1867.

[15] *NOM&SJ*, 20 (November, 1867): 419; *Report of the Louisiana State Board of Health for 1867*, 6.

[16] *Gardner's New Orleans Directory for 1868* (New Orleans, 1868), 9, 11.

[17] The Howard Association's low case fatality rate (about 8 percent) was attributed to the "mild character" of the fever that year as well as to a "more rational treatment," described as "the most careful nursing with very little medication." *NOM&SJ*, 21 (April, 1868): 414; 20 (November, 1867): 420; New Orleans *Bee*, September 22, 1867.

[18] Toner, "Reports Upon Yellow Fever," 371-73; Augustin, *History of Yellow Fever*, 861, 893, 902; *Picayune*, September 15, 18, October 16, 31, 1867; *Iberville South* (Plaquemine), October 19, 26, December 21, 1867; *Report of the Louisiana State Board of Health for 1867*, 7-8.

[19] *Picayune*, August 6, 10, 12, 13, 29, September 3, 1867. See also *Report of the Louisiana State Board of Health for 1867*, 7.

[20] *Picayune*, September 3, 1867.

[21] *Iberville South*, September 7, 1867.

[22] Robert Hilliard to Charles McVea, August 25, September 1, 1867; Hilliard to Lucy Hilliard McVea, September 3, 1867, in Hilliard-McVea Letters, private collection of Mrs. Jac Chambliss, Lookout Mountain, Tennessee. I am indebted to Glenn R. Conrad, Center for Louisiana Studies, University of Southwestern Louisiana, Lafayette, for providing excerpts from these letters and for his estimate of the New Iberia mortality based on church records and other local data.

[23] *Picayune*, October 28, 1867.

[24] *NOM&SJ*, 23 (April, 1870): 398; *Picayune*, August 10, 24, 1868; July 20, 1869.

[25] *Report of the Louisiana State Board of Health for 1870*, 74, 80.

[26] *NOM&SJ*, 23 (October, 1870): 874-76. See Toner, "Reports Upon Yellow Fever," 369-73, and Augustin, *History of Yellow Fever*, 844-902, for lists of towns affected by the disease.

[27] *Report of the Louisiana State Board of Health for 1871*, 98; *Report of the Louisiana State Board of Health for 1872*, 135.

[28] *NOM&SJ*, 50 (May, 1898): 636; *Report of the Louisiana State Board of Health for 1873*, 9, 19, 23-24, 66, 73, 158. In New Orleans in 1873 smallpox killed 505 and cholera 241, compared to the 226 yellow fever deaths. (p. 9).

[29] *NOM&SJ*, new series, 1 (November, 1873): 338-41. See also Gillson, *Formative Years*, 136-37.

30"Two-hundred and Fifteen Years of Sanitation in New Orleans," *Vox Sanitatis*, 2 (November, 1933): 28. This bulletin, published for a time in the 1930s by the New Orleans Board of Health, is located in the vertical file, Louisiana Collections, Tulane University Library, New Orleans.

31*Report of the Louisiana State Board of Health for 1873*, 55.

32*Report of the Committee appointed by the Shreveport Medical Society on the Yellow Fever Epidemic of 1873 at Shreveport, Louisiana* (Shreveport, 1874), 12-13; Henry Smith, *Report of the Yellow Fever Epidemic of 1873, Shreveport, Louisiana* . . . (New Orleans, 1874), 1, 3.

33Smith, *Report of the Yellow Fever Epidemic of 1873*, 3; *Picayune*, September 17, 18, 1873.

34*Picayune*, September 19, 20, 1873.

35Ibid., September 23, 26, 27, 1873.

36Ibid., September 28, 30, October 1, 4, 1873.

37Ibid., October 7, 11, 1873. Other sources suggest that criminal incidents were relatively few during the ten-week epidemic. See Steven Alan Honley, "A History of the 1873 Yellow Fever Epidemic in Shreveport, Louisiana," *Journal of the North Louisiana Historical Association*, 13 (1982): 90-96.

38Smith, *Report of the Yellow Fever Epidemic of 1873*, 11; *Picayune*, October 30, November 4, 1873.

39*Picayune*, September 10, 15, 1873.

40Ibid., September 23, 1873.

41*Report of the Committee . . . on the Yellow Fever Epidemic of 1873 at Shreveport*, 10, 12, 14, 20. Among the Shreveport victims in 1873 were five Catholic priests, three nuns, four physicians, one of the publishers of the *Shreveport Times*, and a city judge. See R. J. Miciotto, "Shreveport's First Major Health Crisis: The Yellow Fever Epidemic of 1873," *Journal of the North Louisiana Historical Association*, 4 (1973): 116.

42*NOM&SJ*, new series, 1 (January, 1874): 626-28; *Picayune*, October 10, 16, 1873.

43*Picayune*, October 2, 1873.

44*NOM&SJ*, new series, 1 (May, 1874): 791-93; 50 (May, 1898): 636.

Chapter 7

1*Picayune*, July 24, 1878.

2*Report of the Louisiana State Board of Health for 1878*, 1, 9-10, 20-23; *Report of the Louisiana State Board of Health for 1881*, 116; *Picayune*, July 24, 25, 26, 27, 1878; John Ellis "The Southern Yellow Fever Epidemic of 1878" (unpublished manuscript; copy provided by author), 4-5; Ellis, "The New Orleans Yellow Fever Epidemic in 1878," 191-92; Ellis, "Businessmen and Public Health in the Urban South during the Nineteenth Century," part II, 346.

3*Picayune*, July 26, 1878. (Italics added.) Contrary to Choppin's view, Dr. William Austin, one member of the board, told a *Picayune* reporter he believed the case on the *Souder* to be the source of the outbreak.

[4]Joseph Jones, "Yellow Fever Epidemic of 1878 in New Orleans," *NOM&SJ*, new series, 6 (March, 1879): 689-90, 694; *Report of the Louisiana State Board of Health for 1881*, 116-18.

[5]Ellis, "The Southern Yellow Fever Epidemic of 1878," 3-7; Ellis, "The New Orleans Yellow Fever Epidemic in 1878," 191-92, 208-10. Contemporary records contain inconsistent data and conflicting testimony. Whether by deliberate deception, faulty perception, or flawed memory, reports left by observers and interpreters of epidemics, like most other "primary sources," present less than a clear view for the historian.

[6]Ellis, "The New Orleans Yellow Fever Epidemic in 1878," 192-93.

[7]*Picayune*, July 25, 26, 27, August 2, 9, September 6, 1878.

[8]Thomas C. Porteous to J. Levois, August 3, 1878, Thomas C. Porteous Letter Book (Louisiana State University Archives, Baton Rouge).

[9]Ibid., August 6, 9, 1878.

[10]Ibid., August 23, 30, September 3, 10, 1878.

[11]Ibid., October 15, November 2, 5, 15, 22, 1878.

[12]*Report of the Louisiana State Board of Health for 1878*, 13, 158-59; *Picayune*, November 10, 1878; Ketchum, "Yellow Fever in New Orleans," 5, 62(d).

[13]Jones, "Yellow Fever Epidemic of 1878 in New Orleans," 698.

[14]Ellis, "The Southern Yellow Fever Epidemic of 1878," 27-28, 37; Ellis, "The New Orleans Yellow Fever Epidemic in 1878," 198, 211-12.

[15]U. S. Board of Experts, *Proceedings of the Board of Experts Authorized by Congress to Investigate the Yellow Fever Epidemic of 1878* . . . (New Orleans, 1878), 31-35.

[16]*Report of the Louisiana State Board of Health for 1878*, 13.

[17]See *Report of the Louisiana State Board of Health for 1867*, 6, 18; *NOM&SJ*, 20 (November, 1867): 419-20; 21 (April, 1868): 413-14.

[18]Ketchum, "Yellow Fever in New Orleans," 116.

[19]From 1860 to 1880, the New Orleans population increased only 28 percent, compared to 65 percent for the period from 1840 to 1860. See *Report on Population of the United States at the Eleventh Census: 1890*, Part 1 (Washington, D.C., 1895): 370-71, 374-75; Ketchum, "Yellow Fever in New Orleans," 114-16; Jackson, *New Orleans in the Gilded Age*, 11-22. Death rates generally exceeded birth rates in large American cities during most of the nineteenth century. In 1880 the New Orleans population included 5,041 children under one year of age; that year the city's mortality from all causes was 5,623. See Table 19, p. 244, in John W. Blassingame, *Black New Orleans, 1860-1880* (Chicago, 1973).

[20]C. B. White, "The Yellow Fever Epidemic at New Orleans in 1878," *Reports and Papers of the American Public Health Association*, 7 (1881): 201-4. See also Ellis, "The New Orleans Yellow Fever Epidemic in 1878," 193, 212.

[21]Ellis, "The New Orleans Yellow Fever Epidemic in 1878," 193. The epidemic seems to have intensified existing class, racial, and religious antagonisms in southern cities. Ellis, "The Southern Yellow Fever Epidemic of 1878," 21.

²²*Report of the Howard Association of New Orleans, of Receipts, Expenditures, and Their Work in the Epidemic of 1878* . . . (New Orleans, 1878), 18; Howard Association Memorandum Books, 1 & 2, 1878, John B. Vinet Papers, Addendum (Louisiana State University Archives, Baton Rouge); *Report of the Louisiana State Board of Health for 1878*, 178.

²³*American Missionary*, 32 (October, 1878): 291. The *Louisianian*, a black newspaper published in New Orleans, suspended publication for more than three months because of the 1878 epidemic. The paper's business manager, Henry Adams Corbin, died of yellow fever in September, and other staff members suffered severe cases of the disease. Corbin's brother John, who was principal of one of the McDonough schools in New Orleans, also died of yellow fever. See New Orleans *Weekly Louisianian*, November 30, 1878.

²⁴Kenneth F. Kiple and Virginia H. Kiple, "Black Yellow Fever Immunities, Innate and Acquired, as Revealed in the American South," *Social Science History*, 1 (Summer, 1977): 428; *Report of the Louisiana State Board of Health for 1878*, 158-59; Jones, *Medical and Surgical Memoirs*, III, pt. 1, cccxviii. See also Dennis C. Rousey, "Yellow Fever and Black Policemen in Memphis: A Post-Reconstruction Anomaly," *Journal of Southern History*, 51 (August, 1985): 357-74, for a brief account of the black experience with the disease in Memphis in the 1870s. Their relative resistance to yellow fever appears to have prompted the employment of blacks on the Memphis police force during the epidemic of 1878. Radical Reconstruction was over, and other southern cities with an integrated force since the early days of Reconstruction were dismissing blacks and returning to an all-white force when Memphis hired black police for the first time.

²⁵From 1860 to 1880, the annual black mortality rate in New Orleans was higher than the white rate every year except 1867 and 1878 when yellow fever was epidemic. See Blassingame, *Black New Orleans, 1860-1880*, Table 17, pp. 242-43, and Jones, *Medical and Surgical Memoirs*, III, pt. 1, cccxvi-cccxviii.

²⁶*American Missionary*, 32 (October, 1878): 332.

²⁷*Picayune*, September 7, 14, 22, 1878; *Report of the Orleans Central Relief Committee to all Those who have so Generously Contributed to the Yellow Fever Sufferers of New Orleans, from the Great Epidemic of 1878* (New Orleans, 1879), 3-4. See also Baton Rouge *Weekly Advocate*, November 29, 1878, for a report on various organizations, black and white, male and female, which provided relief in that community during the epidemic.

²⁸*Picayune*, August 16, 17, 1878; *Report of the Howard Association of New Orleans . . . 1878*, 12-20.

²⁹*Picayune*, August 31, September 5, 14, October 29, 1878; *Report of the Howard Association of New Orleans . . . 1878*, 25.

³⁰The Howards did provide funds to the Peabody group, at least $20,000. *Report of the Howard Association of New Orleans . . . 1878*, 25-27. Blacks in Memphis also considered the Howard Association hard to deal with. A black minister, recently recovered from yellow fever, wrote a letter of thanks to the American Missionary Association for a fifty-dollar contribution, which he intended to use "among the people." The Memphis Howard Association and Relief Committee had adequate supplies on hand, he said, "but there is such a routine imposed upon the poor colored people that many of them get out of heart before they reach the end." *American Missionary*, 32 (October, 1878): 332. According to one study of the New Orleans Howards, the 1878 epidemic marked the end of any effective role for the association, given the size of the city, the demands for relief, and the extent of the epidemic. "Besides organizational and servicing problems, the group got into debt and lost the public's faith in their stewardship." Peggy Bassett Hildreth, "Early Red Cross: The Howard Association of New Orleans, 1837-1878," *Louisiana History*, 20 (Winter, 1979): 67-68.

³¹*Picayune*, September 14, 1878.

³²Ibid., September 22, 1878.

³³The Army also provided medicines, rations, and tents to other Mississippi Valley communities in distress during the epidemic. *Report of the Orleans Central Relief Committee*, 3-4, 60, 68, 74; *Picayune*, August 28, September 24, 27, October 3, 4, 5, 1878.

³⁴Ellis, "The New Orleans Yellow Fever Epidemic in 1878," 211; Hildreth, "Early Red Cross," 72.

³⁵*Picayune*, September 7, 1878.

³⁶*Picayune*, August 25, 27, 1878; *Sugar Bowl* (New Iberia), September 12, 19, 26, October 3, November 14, 1878 (transcriptions of articles made available through the kindness of Glenn R. Conrad, University of Southwestern Louisiana, Lafayette). See also *Report of the Howard Association of New Orleans . . . 1878*, 28-59, for list of contributors.

³⁷*Picayune*, September 4, 1878.

³⁸J. P. Dromgoole, *Yellow Fever Heroes, Honors, and Horrors of 1878* (Louisville, Ky., 1879), 21.

³⁹*Picayune*, September 6, 1878.

⁴⁰*Commercial and Statistical Almanac, Containing a History of the Epidemic of 1878 . . .* (New Orleans, 1879), 56; Augustin, *History of Yellow Fever*, 844-902; *NOM&SJ*, new series, 6 (November, 1878): 410; n.s., 11 (September, 1883): 162; 57 (October, 1906): 291-92; Baton Rouge *Advocate*, November 15, 1878; *Thibodaux Sentinel*, September 14, October 5, November 30, 1878; *Picayune*, August 24, September 10, 20, 21, October 11, 1878.

⁴¹Police Jury Minutes, Caddo Parish, August 23, 1878; Avoyelles Parish, September 3, November 11, 12, 1878; Rapides Parish, August 26, 27, October 9, 1878 (W. P. A. transcriptions of Parish Records of Louisiana, Louisiana State University Archives, Baton Rouge); *Sugar Bowl* (New Iberia), September 5, 12, 19, 26, October 3, 10, 17, 24, November 14, 21, 1878. See also *Lafayette Advertiser* (Vermillionville), August 3, September 7, 1878, for a report of that town's quarantine against New Orleans and other infected places as early as July 30, designed to prevent a repetition of the local experience of 1853 and 1867.

⁴²Dr. Andrew Neel Carrigan to William A. Carrigan, September 10, October 9, 1878, William A. Carrigan Papers (Darlington County Historical Society, Darlington, South Carolina.)

⁴³*Report of the Louisiana State Board of Health for 1878*, 13-14.

⁴⁴Ibid., 14; *Report of the Louisiana State Board of Health for 1881*, iv, 109-15.

⁴⁵*Commercial and Statistical Almanac, Containing a History of the Epidemic of 1878*, 56; *Report of the Louisiana State Board of Health for 1878*, 158-59; *Proceedings of the Board of Experts Authorized by Congress . . . 1878*, 31-35.

⁴⁶Ellis, "The Southern Yellow Fever Epidemic of 1878," 25.

⁴⁷Gillson, *Formative Years*, 175-98; Jo Ann Carrigan, "The National Board of Health, 1879-1893: A Significant Failure" (unpublished manuscript).

⁴⁸See Chapter 12, on "Specificity, Germs, and Mosquitoes."

⁴⁹Waring, *Social Statistics of Cities*, 286; Smillie, *Public Health: Its Promise for the Future*, 321-30.

⁵⁰J. C. LeHardy, "The Yellow Fever Panic," *Atlanta Medical and Surgical Journal*, 5 (1888-89): 609-14. LeHardy claimed that the chief cause of the fear was "ignorance among the masses" who had come to

believe the disease contagious and transportable, persuaded by all the national political agitation and publicity given to the quarantine issue.

[51]East, "Health and Wealth: Goals of the New Orleans Public Health Movement, 1879-84," 256-60, 267-72; Ellis, "Businessmen and Public Health in the Urban South During the Ninteenth Century," 352-56.

[52]Joseph Jones referred to the "hostile attitude of mercantile men" and concluded that Louisiana's quarantine had failed to hold back disease or to win the confidence of other state authorities "because it has been uniformly opposed by the commercial interests, and has been alternately advocated and condemned by members of the medical profession. . . ." *Report of the Louisiana State Board of Health for 1881*, iv, 109-10. See also Official Records, Louisiana State Board of Health, 1883 (Historical Collections, Rudolph Matas Library, Tulane University Medical Center), 99, 111, 117, 129, 175, containing letters of complaint, petitions, requests for special favors, clippings, and board decisions; and *Report of the Louisiana State Board of Health for 1878*, 12; *NOM&SJ*, new series, 2 (May, 1875): 960-63; 3 (November, 1875): 444-46.

[53]East, "Health and Wealth," 249. See also Gillson, *Formative Years*, 187, 196-97.

[54]*NOM&SJ*, new series, 11 (September, 1883): 198; *Report of the Louisiana State Board of Health for 1879*, 8; Gillson, *Formative Years*, 193.

[55]*NOM&SJ*, new series, 7 (October, 1879): 495.

[56]See *Reports of the Louisiana State Board of Health*, 1880 through 1896.

[57]Among the places reporting a few cases or an outbreak of yellow fever in the 1880s were Key West (1880, 1887), Galveston (1882), Brownsville, Texas (1882), Pensacola (1882, 1884), Biloxi (1886), Tampa (1887, 1888), Jacksonville, Florida (1888), and Jackson, Mississippi (1888). Augustin, *History of Yellow Fever*, 780; *Report of the Louisiana State Board of Health for 1882-83*, 211, 281; *Picayune*, September 22, 1882, September 3, 1886, October 9, 1887, September 21, 22, 1888; *NOM&SJ*, new series, 14 (November, 1886): 371-88; 15 (August, 1887): 141-42; (May, 1888): 900-902; (September, 1888): 223-24; LeHardy, "The Yellow Fever Panic," 603-16.

[58]Louisiana State Board of Health, *Outbreak of Yellow Fever at Biloxi, Harrison County, Miss. & Its Relation to Inter-State Notification* (New Orleans, 1886), 3-51; *NOM&SJ*, new series, 8 (October, 1880): 382, 391-92; (November, 1880): 476-82; 10 (September, 1882): 194-205, 227-33; 14 (October, 1886): 273-95, 298; (November, 1886): 371-88; "Proceedings and Discussions at the Eighth Annual Meeting, New Orleans, La., December 7-10, 1880," *Reports and Papers, APHA, 1880*, VI, 471; Gillson, *Formative Years*, 211-14.

[59]*Picayune*, September 24, 1880; *NOM&SJ*, new series, 11 (May, 1884): 876-77; 12 (July, 1884): 26-29; 16 (September, 1888): 223; *Report of the Louisiana State Board of Health for 1886-87*, 7, 10; LeHardy, "The Yellow Fever Panic," 611-12.

[60]George E. Waring, Jr., "The National Board of Health," *Nation*, 29 (August 21, 1879): 123-24; James L. Cabell, "A Review of the Operations of the National Board of Health," *Reports and Papers, APHA, 1882*, VIII, 71-73; J. S. Billings, "National Public Health Legislation," *American Journal of the Medical Sciences*, 78 (October, 1879): 475-78. See *Annual Report of the National Board of Health, 1883* (Washington, 1884), Appendix D, 148-49, for the exact language of the two congressional acts creating and assigning duties and limited powers to the NBH.

[61]Cabell, "A Review of the Operations of the National Board of Health," 89-99; Robert D. Leigh, *Federal Health Administration in the United States* (New York, 1927), 368-69. The *Annual Reports of the NBH* (1879-1885) included hundreds of pages of appendices reporting on the results of scientific investigations, sanitary surveys, and other research projects conducted under board sponsorship. The weekly *Bulletin of the National Board of Health* (1879-1882) also published reports on some of the projects.

⁶²*Annual Report of the National Board of Health, 1883* (Washington, 1884), 20-55, provided a summary of its work under the quarantine act of 1879. See also Cabell, "A Review of the Operations of the National Board of Health," 74-88.

⁶³Published and unpublished materials relating to Joseph Jones' campaign against the NBH are voluminous. For a sample, see Stanford E. Chaillé, *The Louisiana State Board of Health in its Annual Report for 1881 versus the National Board of Health, Reply in Behalf of the Latter* (New Orleans, 1882); Louisiana State Board of Health, *Investigation and Refutation of Certain Statements and Charges made . . . by the National Board of Health in its Annual Report for the Year 1882* (New Orleans, 1883). For a detailed narrative account of the conflict, see Gillson, *Formative Years*, 175-241. East, "Health and Wealth," 245-75, and Warner, "Local Control versus National Interest," 407-28, both offer brief insightful interpretations of the encounter between state and national authorities. Warner's work outlined the different responses of interior and coastal health officers to the NBH.

⁶⁴*NOM&SJ*, new series, 9 (May, 1882): 841; East, "Health and Wealth," 262, 264; Warner, "Local Control versus National Interest," 425.

⁶⁵Cabell, "A Review of the Operations of the National Board of Health," 100-101; Smillie, *Public Health, Its Promise for the Future*, 336-39; Leigh, *Federal Health Administration in the United States*, 481-83; Carrigan, "The National Board of Health, 1879-1893."

⁶⁶Morton Keller, *Affairs of State: Public Life in Late Nineteenth Century America* (Cambridge, Mass., 1977), 85, 122-24, 234, 285-86, 499-500; Stephen Skowronek, *Building a New American State: The Expansion of National Administrative Capacities, 1877-1920* (New York, 1982), 10, 13, 46.

⁶⁷Leigh, *Federal Health Administration in the United States*, 294-97; Robert Straus, *Medical Care for Seamen: The Origins of Public Medical Service in the United States* (New Haven, 1950); Ralph Chester Williams, *The United States Public Health Service, 1798-1950* (Washington, 1951); Laurence F. Schmeckebier, *The Public Health Service: Its History, Activities and Organization* (Baltimore, 1923); *Annual Report of the Supervising Surgeon-General of the Marine Hospital Service of the United States for the Fiscal Year 1897* (Washington, 1899), 580-676, hereafter cited as *USMHS Annual Report, 1897*.

⁶⁸See note 61 above, and Chapter 12, notes 48, 50, 67.

⁶⁹See Chapter 12 for discussion of government-sponsored investigations of yellow fever.

⁷⁰Joseph Jones, *The Relation of Quarantine to Commerce in the Valley of the Mississippi River . . . 1880-1887 . . .* (New Orleans, 1889), 13-18; *Picayune*, July 20, 1883; *Report of the Louisiana State Board of Health for 1888-1889*, 8-9.

⁷¹*Report of the Louisiana State Board of Health for 1879*, 16-21; *Report of the Louisiana State Board of Health for 1881*, iv, 109-10; Official Records, Louisiana State Board of Health, 1883, 87, 117, 123, 217; *Picayune*, August 3, 10, 17, September 7, 1883. For an excellent brief review of Louisiana's highly variable quarantine requirements (altered from year to year, sometimes week to week, with exemptions and evasions more the pattern than consistent enforcement), see Quitman Kohnke, "History of Maritime Quarantine in Louisiana against Yellow Fever," *NOM&SJ*, 56 (September, 1903): 167-80.

⁷²Joseph Holt, *Quarantine and Commerce, Their Antagonism Destructive to the Prosperity of City and State . . .* (New Orleans, [1884]), 1-15; *NOM&SJ*, new series, 12 (August, 1884): 147-50.

⁷³Dr. Alfred W. Perry must be credited with introducing the idea of replacing detention with disinfection and devising an apparatus to pump sulphurous acid vapor into a vessel to purify its cargo. While serving as quarantine physician at the Mississippi River Station in 1874, he initiated this system, including the liberal use of chlorine gas and carbolic acid solution to disinfect clothing, baggage, and the surfaces and contents of all

vessels from infected ports. Even before Perry, some effort had been made at disinfecting certain vessels with carbolic acid—at least since the late 1860s. The apparent success of Perry's method led to the legislation in 1876 leaving the matter of detention to the board's discretion. The board continued the use of fumigation and disinfection but lacked the resources to develop a well-equipped system until 1884 when Holt succeeded in obtaining state funds for his program of "Maritime Sanitation." See *NOM&SJ*, new series, 1 (January, 1874): 567-72; 2 (January, 1875): 597-99; *Report of the Louisiana State Board of Health for 1875*, 21; *Picayune*, October 3, 1876.

[74]Joseph Holt, *The Quarantine System of Louisiana, Methods of Disinfection Practiced* . . . (New Orleans, [1887]), 3-20; *NOM&SJ*, new series, 13 (August, 1885): 137-40; 14 (June, 1887), 977-81; 17 (July, 1889): 39-42; 18 (September, 1890): 241.

[75]Gordon E. Gillson, *Louisiana State Board of Health: The Progressive Years* (Baton Rouge, 1976), 22-24, hereafter cited as *Progressive Years*.

[76]Ketchum, "Yellow Fever in New Orleans," 92-93.

[77]*Report of the Louisiana State Board of Health for 1888-1889*, 32; *NOM&SJ*, new series, 17 (November, 1889): 342-46; (December, 1889): 393-98; 18 (September, 1890): 241; *Report of the Louisiana State Board of Health for 1890-1891*, 21.

[78]Gillson, *Progressive Years*, 16, 56; Kohnke, "History of Maritime Quarantine in Louisiana against Yellow Fever," 175-79.

[79]Ketchum, "Yellow Fever in New Orleans," 93-94.

Chapter 8

[1]*NOM&SJ*, new series, 18 (December, 1890): 483-84.

[2]Ibid., 50 (October, 1897): 263-64. Both dengue and yellow fever could have been present simultaneously. Clinically similar to mild yellow fever, dengue is also transmitted by the *Aedes aegypti*.

[3]*USMHS Annual Report*, 1897, 622-24; *Picayune*, September 7, 10, 1897.

[4]*Picayune*, September 18, October 9, 1897; Gillson, *Progressive Years*, 84-85.

[5]*Picayune*, October 3, 1897.

[6]Ibid., October 1, 2, 1897.

[7]Ibid., October 6, 1897.

[8]*New York Times*, October 26, 1897.

[9]See Gillson, *Progressive Years*, 84-87, for a description of board regulations of burial, management of infected premises, and other "repressive measures."

[10]*Picayune*, October 10, 1897.

[11]Ibid., October 22, 23, 28, 29, 31, November 1, 2, 12, 1897.

[12]Ibid., September 19, 1897. It is significant that "the professions" had been elevated in the rhetoric of the day

to the level of "labor" and "capital" as a special category deserving representation on committees advocating causes of "civic importance." Despite the rhetoric of consensus, the white representatives of capital and the professions dominated such "citizens committees," made decisions, determined policy, and often raised (or contributed) funds to hire laborers, black and white, to do the work the committee thought should be done.

[13]Ibid., September 19, 20, 28, 29, 1897.

[14]New Orleans *Times-Democrat*, September 22, 1897.

[15]*Picayune*, September 18, 19, 20, 21, 24, 1897.

[16]The following reconstruction of this incident is based almost entirely on articles in the *Picayune*, September 24, 25, 26, 1897. A few additional details on the temporary hospital itself were found in *NOM&SJ*, 50 (October, 1897): 262, and *Report of the Board of Administrators of the Charity Hospital to the General Assembly of the State of Louisiana for 1897* (New Orleans, [1898]), 11-12, 53.

[17]*Picayune*, September 17, 1897.

[18]*New York Times*, September 15, 1897.

[19]Correspondence from Shreveport revealed that the Vicksburg, Shreveport, and Pacific Railroad had closed down operations, as also had the southern section of the Kansas City line. New Orleans newspapers each day reported the establishment of additional quarantines as "country people" overreacted; the Illinois Central, the Northeastern, and the Louisville and Nashville railroads were now more than ever "fastened in a closer grasp of king quarantine." See *Times-Democrat*, September 13, 20, 1897, and *Picayune*, September 12, 1897.

[20]*Times-Democrat*, September 22, 1897.

[21]*USMHS Annual Report, 1897*, 627-30; *Picayune*, September 17, 1897. The federal agency that became the U. S. Public Health Service of the twentieth century, the Marine Hospital Service was originally established in 1798 and placed under the Treasury Department to provide medical care for American seamen. In 1870-71 the service was completely reorganized, and within the next few decades its powers and functions were expanded to include the assistance of states in maritime and interstate quarantine in order to prevent the spread of epidemic diseases. There was considerable overlapping of quarantine powers among local, state, and federal authorities in the late nineteenth century. Wilson G. Smillie, *Preventive Medicine and Public Health* (New York, 1946), 516-18; Leigh, *Federal Health Administration in the United States*, 296-301.

[22]*Times-Democrat*, September 26, 1897.

[23]*Picayune*, September 30, October 1, 1897.

[24]Baton Rouge *Weekly Advocate*, October 2, 1897; *USMHS Annual Report, 1897*, 628, 630.

[25]Baton Rouge *Weekly Advocate*, September 18, October 2, 23, 30, November 6, 1897.

[26]*Shreveport Evening Journal*, September 13, 1897.

[27]Ibid., September 6-November 17, 1897, *passim*.

[28]*Picayune*, September 29, 1897.

[29]Ibid., October 13, 1897.

[30]*Picayune*, October 22, 1897.

³¹Ibid., October 2, 1897.

³²*USMHS Annual Report, 1897*, 627, 638; *Picayune*, October 20, 21, 22, 24, 1897. Thousands of migrant laborers from southern Italy also came annually for the cane harvest, after which they returned to Italy. The *Picayune*, on October 24, reported that 1,100 Italians, expected to arrive that day on the steamer *Montebello*, would be held at the Port Eads quarantine station near the mouth of the Mississippi until arrangements could be made for transporting them to the sugar parishes.

³³*Picayune*, October 20, 25, 1897.

³⁴Ibid., October 24, 29, 1897. In an attempt to protect Jackson, Mississippi, against the introduction of yellow fever by railway passengers or freight, some local citizens burned a bridge on the Alabama-Vicksburg Railroad line in 1897. See Marshall Scott Legan, "The Evolution of Public Health Services in Mississippi, 1865-1910" (Ph. D. dissertation, University of Mississippi, 1968), 94-95; and *New York Times*, November 2, 1897.

³⁵Ibid., November 12, 15, 24, 1897.

³⁶See *USMHS Annual Report, 1897*, 580-676, for detailed reports on Marine Hospital Service activities in the southern states during the yellow fever epidemic of 1897.

³⁷Gillson, *Progressive Years*, 90-92.

³⁸*Report of the Louisiana State Board of Health for 1896-1897*, 85; *Picayune*, September 14, October 19, November 23, 1897; *NOM&SJ*, 50 (May, 1898): 635; Augustin, *History of Yellow Fever*, 845, 853, 894. One set of figures compiled by the Marine Hospital Service listed 4,289 cases in nine states, with a total of 446 deaths, making a case fatality rate of almost 10 percent. By this tally, Louisiana had 1,847; Mississippi, 1,625; and Alabama, 740 cases. A few cases were also reported in Tennessee, Kentucky, Illinois, Georgia, Florida, and Texas. The totals are probably too low as the number of cases listed for Louisiana was smaller than the number reported for New Orleans alone by the Louisiana State Board of Health. See *Picayune*, November 23, 1897.

³⁹*USMHS Annual Report, 1897*, 626.

⁴⁰*Picayune*, October 24, 1897.

⁴¹*NOM&SJ*, 50 (October, 1897): 258-59, 265; *Picayune*, September 13, 1897; Ketchum, "Yellow Fever in New Orleans," 95.

⁴²Gillson, *Progressive Years*, 121-23.

⁴³*Report of the Louisiana State Board of Health for 1898-1899*, 45-46; *NOM&SJ*, 51 (October, 1898): 209.

⁴⁴Gillson, *Progressive Years*, 123.

⁴⁵Ibid., 119-21, 125-26, 132-33.

⁴⁶*Report of the Louisiana State Board of Health for 1898-1899*, 47, 272.

⁴⁷See for example, *Picayune*, September 9, 13, October 10, 1897.

⁴⁸See Ketchum, "Yellow Fever in New Orleans," 69-122, for a careful analysis of the possible factors involved in yellow fever's decline in the late nineteenth century. Ketchum concluded that the virus was probably less virulent and that the decline in immigration diminished the likelihood of epidemics in Havana as

well as New Orleans. Other factors included the earlier establishment of Louisiana's quarantine (in April rather than June), the systematic use of sulphur fumigation to "disinfect" incoming vessels (which would also have destroyed the mosquitoes on board), and the replacement of sailing vessels by modern iron steamships with sealed water tanks, thereby reducing the opportunities for transporting mosquitoes.

[49]Fortier, *A History of Louisiana*, IV, 232-33; Gillson, *Progressive Years*, 129-30.

[50]*NOM&SJ*, 51 (October, 1898): 188. Official figures for New Orleans, which are by no means infallible, show about one yellow fever death in every three or four cases in 1853 (28%), and one in six cases (16%) in 1897. Barton, *Cause and Prevention of Yellow Fever*, 41-45; *Report of the Louisiana State Board of Health for 1896-1897*, 85.

[51]*USMHS Annual Report, 1897*, 639. Those physicians who insisted on the remarkable mildness of the 1897 fever argued that the house quarantine policy in New Orleans was known to have resulted in concealment of many cases, meaning a much lower case fatality rate than the one on record. Carter pointed out that the same policy that led to non-reporting of cases also would have encouraged false reporting of yellow fever deaths under some other disease label, bringing the rate back up.

[52]*Report of the Louisiana State Board of Health for 1867*, 18, 20; *NOM&SJ*, 21 (April, 1868): 413-14; *Report of the Louisiana State Board of Helalth for 1896-1897*, 85.

[53]Epidemic is defined as "unusually frequent occurrence of disease in the light of past experience" in Fox, Hall, and Elveback, *Epidemiology: Man and Disease*, 16. The phrase "excessive prevalence" is from Brian MacMahon & Thomas F. Pugh, *Epidemiology: Principles and Methods* (Boston, 1970), 2.

[54]New Orleans, with at least a quarter of a million population during the 1890s, was considered *the city* by an extensive region including Arkansas and Mississippi. After New Orleans, the next largest towns in Louisiana in 1890 were Shreveport with approximately 12,000 and Baton Rouge, the capital, with only 10,500. About a dozen other places in the state could claim a population numbering as many as 1,500 to 5,000. These figures suggest the dimensions of the urban-rural dichotomy and help explain why New Orleanians considered the rest of the state "the country." *Report on Population of the United States at the Eleventh Census: 1890, Part I* (Washington, D.C., 1895): 378-90, 532.

[55]See Richard Jensen, "Modernization and Community History," *Newberry Papers in Family and Community History* (January, 1978), and Richard D. Brown, *Modernization: The Transformation of American Life, 1600-1865* (New York, 1976), for general discussion of modernization theory and its use in historical explanation. See also Robert H. Wiebe, *The Search for Order, 1877-1920* (New York, 1967), for an account of professionalization, expertise, and the emergence of a "bureaucratic orientation" in shaping the new social order; and Herbert G. Gutman, "Work, Culture and Society in Industrializing America, 1815-1919," *American Historical Review*, 78 (June, 1973): 531-88, for analysis of the recurring conflict between traditional and modern ways as immigrant workers resisted industrial discipline and other aspects of "modernization."

[56]Jean Anne Scarpaci, "Immigrants in the New South: Italians in Louisiana's Sugar Parishes, 1880-1910," in Milton Cantor, ed., *American Workingclass Culture: Explorations in American Labor and Social History* (Westport, Conn., 1979), 377-95; originally published in *Labor History*, 16 (Spring, 1975): 165-83. A trickle of antebellum immigration from Sicily to New Orleans, following the citrus fruit trade, expanded greatly in volume in the 1880s and 1890s, encouraged by the state immigration bureau and the sugar planters association. South Italian peasants were viewed as cheap, productive workers who could supplement the black labor supply. Foreign-born Italian residents in Louisiana plus those of Italian parentage numbered almost 27,000 by 1900, concentrated mainly in the sugar parishes and in New Orleans. In addition, the sugar harvest and grinding season (October to January) attracted a migratory Italian labor force estimated at 30,000 to 80,000 who came and went each year—some all the way from Italy and back, others from Chicago and New York. Whether temporary or permanent residents, Italians in South Louisiana, wanting to preserve their "Old World traditions," maintained a strong sense of "group cohesiveness," family orientation, and

418   Notes to Pages 164-171

identification with their village of origin. In the United States as in Italy, this "*campanilismo*" or localism was sustained by various mutual benefit associations organized in such a way as to reflect and strengthen village or regional identification. Ibid., 377-79, 382-85, 388-89, 392-93. See also Belle Hunt, "New Orleans, Yesterday and Today," *Frank Leslie's Popular Monthly*, 31 (June, 1891): 642, for a description of the area near the French Market in New Orleans where slum housing sheltered Italians and others employed on the waterfront. A ten-room tenement with a filthy courtyard, for example, was inhabited by fifty families.

[57]Many of the folk, white and black alike, in my village of origin in Southwest Arkansas could have been similarly described as late as the 1930s and 1940s.

Chapter 9

[1]Andrew J. Warren, "Landmarks in the Conquest of Yellow Fever," in Strode, ed., *Yellow Fever*, 8-12; Aristides Agramonte, "The Inside Story of a Great Medical Discovery," *Scientific Monthly* (December, 1915), 209-37, reprinted in *Yellow Fever Studies*, Arno Press series, *Public Health in America*, edited by Barbara Gutmann Rosenkrantz *et al.* (New York, 1977); Winslow, *Conquest of Epidemic Disease*, 352-54; Howard A. Kelly, *Walter Reed and Yellow Fever* (New York, 1906).

[2]*NOM&SJ*, 53 (April, 1901): 595.

[3]*Report of the Louisiana State Board of Health for 1900-1901*, 77-79.

[4]Sir Rubert William Boyce, *Yellow Fever Prophylaxis in New Orleans, 1905* (London, [1906]), 8, 16; *Report of the Louisiana State Board of Health for 1900-1901*, 46-51; *Picayune*, August 30, 1901. Prior to 1898, the state board handled all matters relating to public health in New Orleans as well as having general responsibility for the state at large. The new constitution of 1898 together with measures passed by the legislature that year completely reorganized the state's health institutions. Although the state board retained control of maritime quarantine, New Orleans was provided with a city board to deal with local health-related matters. Parish or town health officials were made auxiliary and subordinate to the state board. Local quarantine restrictions that went beyond those set at the state level were explicitly prohibited to avoid the conflicts that characterized the 1897 outbreak. Commercial and transportation interests favored centralized authority that could establish uniform regulations. For a detailed account of the reorganization of Louisiana's public health system in 1898, see Gillson, *Progressive Years*, 99-117.

[5]*Report of the Louisiana State Board of Health for 1900-1901*, 7; Boyce, *Yellow Fever Prophylaxis*, 1.

[6]Rudolph Matas, "A Yellow Fever Retrospect and Prospect," *Louisiana Historical Quarterly*, 8 (July, 1925): 462-63; *Picayune*, July 23, 31, October 15, 1905; *NOM&SJ*, 58 (March, 1906): 744. The U. S. Marine Hospital Service had been renamed by act of Congress in 1902. The addition of "Public Health" to the agency's designation recognized its vastly expanded activities in health service far beyond the original purpose of marine hospital management.

[7]Augustin, *History of Yellow Fever*, 889-90; Gillson, *Progressive Years*, 179.

[8]*Picayune*, July 31, 1905.

[9]Gillson, *Progressive Years*, 179; *Report of the Public Health and Marine-Hospital Service*, 1906, 59th Cong., 2nd sess., 1906-1907, *House Documents*, Vol. 49, No. 199, pp. 128-30, hereafter cited as *USPH & MHS Report, 1906*; Boyce, *Yellow Fever Prophylaxis*, 17-18; *Picayune*, October 15, 1905; *New York Times*, July 29, 1905.

[10]Boyce, *Yellow Fever Prophylaxis*, 18-20.

[11] *Picayune*, July 23, 1905. In *L'Abeille de la Nouvelle-Orléans*, July 23, 1905, an article on page 4 was headlined: "Quelques cas de fièvre jaune constates en ville."

[12] *Picayune*, July 25, 27, 28, 29, 1905. For a detailed description of "volunteer work" in the well-to-do section of the Tenth Ward, see Henry Dickson Bruns, "Experiences during the Yellow Fever Epidemic of 1905," in Augustin, *History of Yellow Fever*, 1027-48. Residents of this area included Dr. Beverley Warner of Trinity Church; Dr. Louis G. LeBeuf, president of the Orleans Parish Medical Society; Dr. Joseph Holt, a former president of the state board of health; and other prominent physicians and businessmen. Dr. Bruns supervised the project, and a committee collected contributions and disbursed funds for workmen and supplies. During the height of activity, seventy-five laborers were employed at one time. Approximately $1,200 was spent for oiling and screening cisterns within an area of thirty-eight blocks.

[13] *Picayune*, July 27, 1905; *New York Times*, July 28, 1905.

[14] Augustin, *History of Yellow Fever*, 885; Boyce, *Yellow Fever Prophylaxis*, 19; *Picayune*, July 27, 28, 1905. Names usually mentioned as leaders in the Italian community were Anthony Patorno, Arturo Dell Orto, Father P. Scotti, E. Cavalli, and Charles Papini, the vice-consul for Italy. Patorno, president of the League of Italian Societies, had also been involved in organizing relief for the sick and the indigent during the epidemics of 1878 and 1897. At the beginning of the 1905 crusade against the fever, some of the leaders visited the mayor and Dr. Kohnke and offered to assist in every way possible. Mayor Behrman later recalled a story he heard during the epidemic: ". . . one of the Italian leaders had told some of his friends that inspectors were authorized to destroy their household goods and put them in jail if their cisterns were not oiled and screened by a certain day." John R. Kemp, ed., *Martin Behrman of New Orleans: Memoirs of a City Boss* (Baton Rouge, 1977), 138.

[15] Boyce, *Yellow Fever Prophylaxis*, 52-53; *Times-Democrat*, August 28, 1905; *Picayune*, July 23, 1905; *USPH & MHS Report, 1906*, 135-37.

[16] Boyce, *Yellow Fever Prophylaxis*, 21-27; Louis G. LeBeuf, "The Work of the Medical Profession of New Orleans during the Epidemic of 1905," in Augustin, *History of Yellow Fever*, 1062-63. The *Aedes aegypti* at that time was referred to as the *stegomyia*.

[17] *Picayune*, July 25, 27, 29, 31, August 4, 1905; Boyce, *Yellow Fever Prophylaxis*, 28, 59.

[18] *Picayune*, July 29, 1905.

[19] Ibid., August 17, 1905.

[20] Ibid., August 23, 1905. New Orleans' black population was approximately 85,000, more than one-fourth of the total. As previously noted, Africans and people of African ancestry, although susceptible to yellow fever, usually exhibited mild cases and relatively low fatality rates compared to other groups.

[21] Boyce, *Yellow Fever Prophylaxis*, 59; *Picayune*, August 3, September 3, 1905.

[22] *Picayune*, September 16, October 6, 1905.

[23] Ibid., August 15, 1905.

[24] Ibid., July 28, 1905.

[25] Ibid., July 25, 1905.

[26] Ibid., September 3, October 5, 15, 1905.

27Ibid., August 17, 21, 25, September 30, October 5, 15, 1905.

28Boyce, *Yellow Fever Prophylaxis*, 27; *Picayune*, July 26, 1905.

29*Picayune*, August 2, 3, 18, September 22, 27, 1905.

30Ibid., August 5, 1905.

31Boyce, *Yellow Fever Prophylaxis*, 25-26.

32Quitman Kohnke, "The Sanitary Prevention of Yellow Fever," in Augustin, *History of Yellow Fever*, 1135.

33*Report of the Louisiana State Board of Health for 1904-1905*, 26-27; *Picayune*, August 5, 1905.

34*Picayune*, August 5, 23, 1905.

35Augustin, *History of Yellow Fever*, 882-84; Boyce, *Yellow Fever Prophylaxis*, 37-44; *Picayune*, August 8, October 15, 1905. See *USPH & MHS Report, 1906*, 128-94, for a comprehensive account of the work carried out by the federal health service during the 1905 epidemic, not only in New Orleans but throughout the southern region wherever yellow fever appeared.

36Boyce, *Yellow Fever Prophylaxis*, 37, 42.

37Augustin, *History of Yellow Fever*, 886.

38*Report of the Louisiana State Board of Health for 1904-1905*, 30; Boyce, *Yellow Fever Prophylaxis*, 51; *Picayune*, October 11, 16, 1905.

39*Picayune* July 23, 24, 1905; *New York Times*, July 28, 1905. Passenger detention camps were located at Kenner, Avondale, Waveland, and Slidell. A six-day period of observation was required, according to the *USPH & MHS Report, 1906*, 135. For the first time, a quarantine barrier was erected against New Orleans by Havana, Cuba, a yellow fever center frequently quarantined in the past by New Orleans and other southern ports. The *Picayune* (July 24) called the Havana quarantine "one of the revenges of fate," but saw the Cuban city's success in eradicating yellow fever as encouragement to New Orleans.

40*Picayune* July 29, August 6, 9, 1905; Louisiana State Board of Health, *The Sanitary Code, 1899* (New Orleans, 1899), 8; Gillson, *Progressive Years*, 166-70.

41*Picayune*, August 10, 1905.

42Ibid., July 29, August 2, 3, 4, 5, 6, 1905.

43Ibid., October 22, 1905; Thibodaux *Lafourche Comet*, November 16, 1905.

44Augustin, *History of Yellow Fever*, 884-85; *Picayune*, August 6, 7, 11, October 15, 18, 22, 29, 1905; Boyce, *Yellow Fever Prophylaxis*, 60-62; Gillson, *Progressive Years*, 164, 172; Kemp, ed., *Martin Behrman of New Orleans*, 143-44.

45*Picayune*, July 28, 1905; Boyce, *Yellow Fever Prophylaxis*, 32.

46Eleanor McMain, "Behind the Yellow Fever in Little Palermo: Housing Conditions Which New Orleans Should Shake Itself Free From Along with The Summer's Scourge," *Charities*, 15 (1905): 152-59. McMain was president of the Women's League in New Orleans and "head-worker" at Kingsley House. Her article furnishes a detailed view (including photographs) of dilapidated housing and overcrowded conditions in the "infected district," a slum area near the riverfront and French Market populated mainly by Italian immigrants. In one lodging-house filled with workers on their way to the sugar plantations, who were delayed in New Orleans by the epidemic, McMain found that twenty to thirty persons often spent the night in a single room. Her article includes sketches of individuals and their epidemic experiences as told to her by a member of the Relief Committee. She also described other poverty-stricken areas of the city where family income was five to ten dollars per week, showing that "Little Palermo" was not unique in its need for attention and sanitary improvement.

[47]*Picayune*, October 11, 15, 1905.

[48]*USPH & MHS Report, 1906*, 141-42; *Picayune*, August 3, 1905.

[49]*Picayune*, August 5, 1905. Diet was viewed as an important factor in recovery because of yellow fever's effects on the stomach and liver. Physicians prescribed a liquid or soft diet during illness and convalescence, believing that heavy foods burdened the stomach and hastened the fatal effects of the disease. Modern supportive therapy includes a balanced, moderate diet of easily digestible foods, but cautions against overeating or use of alcohol. Ethnic foods appear so often in the nineteenth and early twentieth-century medical literature as targets of criticism, as a ready explanation for high mortality among certain population groups, that one may reasonably doubt that these foods caused all the fatalities attributed to them.

[50]McMain, "Behind the Yellow Fever in Little Palermo," 154; *Picayune*, August 14, 1905; Augustin, *History of Yellow Fever*, 1083.

[51]*Report of the Louisiana State Board of Health for 1904-1905*, 38-39, 50-57; *NOM&SJ*, 59 (October, 1906): 282-91; *Picayune*, July 25, 1905. Some parishes adopted regulations denying entry to all Italians from infected places, with or without federal health certificates. For example, see Transcriptions of Parish Records of Louisiana, No. 44, St. Bernard Parish Police Jury Minutes, 3 (1895-1914): 282-83.

[52]*Picayune*, September 3, 1905; see also *New York Times*, September 3, 1905.

[53]*Picayune*, September 3, 4, 1905.

[54]Ibid., September 12, 1905.

[55]Ibid., October 14, 15, 1905; Charles Chassaignac, "Some Lessons Taught by the Epidemic of 1905," in Augustin, *History of Yellow Fever*, 1055.

[56]*Picayune*, September 27, 1905; *Report of the Louisiana State Board of Health for 1904-1905*, 53; Thibodaux *Lafourche Comet*, September 21, 1905; Transcriptions of Parish Records of Louisiana, Lafourche Parish Police Jury Minutes, IV, pt. 2 (1892-1906): 748-49. The U. S. Public Health and Marine Hospital Service listed 430 cases and fifty-seven deaths for Leeville. *USPH & MHS Report, 1906*, 55.

[57]Chassaignac, "Some Lessons Taught by the Epidemic of 1905," 1051-55.

[58]*Lake Providence Sentry*, July 28, August 4, 25, 1905; *NOM&SJ*, 57 (October, 1906): 285-91; *USPH & MHS Report, 1906*, 147; *Report of the Louisiana State Board of Health for 1904-1905*, 46-47, 59-63.

[59]*Picayune*, September 22, October 15, 1905; *Report of the Louisiana State Board of Health for 1904-1905*, 65-66; Gillson, *Progressive Years*, 173-74.

[60]*Shreveport Journal*, July 22, 27, August 1, 2, 15, 26, 29, September 1, October 30, 1905; *Picayune*, October 15, 1905.

[61]*Report of the Louisiana State Board of Health for 1904-1905*, 45-48. Yellow fever also became epidemic in

Vicksburg, Natchez, Gulfport, and Pensacola. *Report of the Public Health and Marine Hospital Service, 1905*, 59th Cong., 1st sess., 1905, *House Documents*, Vol. 84, p. 11.

[62] Jules Lazard, "Statistical Review of the Yellow Fever Epidemic of 1905, New Orleans," in Augustin, *History of Yellow Fever*, 1083.

[63] *NOM&SJ*, 58 (March, 1906): 751.

[64] *Picayune*, October 3, 27, 1905.

[65] Kemp, ed., *Martin Behrman of New Orleans*, 148-50.

[66] Boyce, *Yellow Fever Prophylaxis*, 6.

[67] Augustin, *History of Yellow Fever*, 881.

[68] *USPHS & MHS Report, 1906*, 141.

[69] A front-page headline in the New Orleans *Picayune*, September 13, 1897, notified the public, "SEVEN CASES HERE, THE EXPERTS SAY . . . Science and Sanitation Keeping the Disease Down. . . ." For other references to the power of science and modernism see editorials in *Picayune*, September 9, October 3, 10, 1897; July 24, August 15, 1905; and almost any report on the 1905 epidemic.

[70] Augustin, *History of Yellow Fever*, 887-88. (italics added).

[71] Article by Rubert Boyce in *Southern Magazine* (October, 1905), quoted in Kelly, *Walter Reed and Yellow Fever*, 203.

[72] For examples of White's letters, orders, instructions, and forms, see Boyce, *Yellow Fever Prophylaxis*, 42-50.

[73] Ibid., 46, 48.

[74] *Picayune*, September 28, 1897. White's account of work in New Orleans in 1905 was summarized in the *USPH & MHS Report, 1906*, 145-46, as follows:

Population of city	325,000
Total area	196 sq. miles
Occupied area	44 sq. miles
Cases of yellow fever	3,404
Deaths from yellow fever	452
House inspections	269,128
Rooms disinfected	55,151
Miles of gutters salted	753
Cisterns screened & oiled	68,000
Freight cars fumigated	33,565
Lbs. of salt used in gutters	2,998,000
Gallons of oil	67,375
Lbs. of sulphur	448,000
Lbs. of pyrethrum	5,000
Total officers employed at one time	73
Total men employed at one time	1,323

[75] *Report of the Board of Administrators of the Charity Hospital to the General Assembly of the State of*

Louisiana for 1905 (Baton Rouge, 1906), 39.

[76]*NOM&SJ*, 59 (October, 1906): 253-73. In the summer of 1903 the *Picayune* polled New Orleans physicians and found that fifty-three of the sixty-one participants (87%) accepted the Reed Commission's view of the mosquito as sole transmitter of yellow fever. In another survey, the *New Orleans States* learned that 80 percent of the M.D.s interviewed found the mosquito doctrine convincing. Gillson, *Progressive Years*, 160. Most of the skeptical had their doubts removed in 1905, but a few others, like Faget, remained unconverted.

[77]*Report of the Louisiana State Board of Health for 1904-1905*, 7-9.

[78]*Report of the Louisiana State Board of Health for 1906-1907*, 15-18.

[79]Gillson, *Progressive Years*, 183-86; Augustin, *History of Yellow Fever*, 1188.

[80]*Report of the Louisiana State Board of Health for 1906-1907*, 21-28; see also *Weekly Iberian* (New Iberia), August 25, September 1, 15, 1906, and *Annual Report of the Surgeon-General of the Public Health and Marine-Hospital Service of the United States for the Fiscal Year 1907*, 60th Cong., 1st sess., 1907-1908, *House Documents*, Vol. 83, No. 456, pp. 65, 90.

[81]On August 18, 1906, the *Weekly Iberian* reported, "We have missed the yellow fever entirely this year so far, but typhoid is with us in pretty ugly shape." The Mouton boy came down with a fever on August 14, but it was not until the 19th that the doctors agreed on a diagnosis. The local newspaper in its next issue on August 25 provided a complete account of the previous week's developments. (I am indebted to Glenn R. Conrad, University of Southwestern Louisiana, for the material detailing the Mouton case.) On the matter of diagnostic confusion, see also Lazard, "Statistical Review of the Yellow Fever Epidemic of 1905, New Orleans," 1079-80, for a list of "suspicious" deaths and their assigned causes reported in New Orleans in 1905 during the month before yellow fever was officially recognized. Eighteen of the thirty-five fatalities had been attributed to typhoid and most of the rest to malarial or "hemorrhagic" fever.

[82]U. S. Public Health Service, *Yellow Fever: Its Epidemiology, Prevention, and Control*, Lectures delivered at the U. S. Public Health Service School of Instruction by H. R. Carter, Senior Surgeon, USPHS (Washington, D.C., 1914), 22, 27-28, reprinted in *Yellow Fever Studies* (New York, 1977).

[83]Matas, "A Yellow Fever Retrospect and Prospect," 468.

[84]Kendell, *History of New Orleans*, II, 525-26, 559, 575-79; see also Gillson, *Progressive Years*, 188-90.

[85]*Report of the Louisiana State Board of Health for 1906-1907*, 45-68.

[86]Gillson, *Progressive Years*, 198-99.

Chapter 10

[1]*NOM&SJ*, 3 (September, 1846), 165.

[2]Winslow, *Conquest of Epidemic Disease*, 182.

[3]The above discussion of epidemiological theory from Galen to Rush and Webster is based largely on Winslow, *Conquest of Epidemic Diseases*, 68-87, 193-235. See also Wesley W. Spink, *Infectious Disease: Prevention and Treatment in the Nineteenth and Twentieth Centuries* (Minneapolis, 1978), 3-27; Gillson, *Formative Years*, 3-7; Shryock, *Medicine in America: Historical Essays*, 233-58; Richard Harrison Shryock, *Medicine and Society in America: 1660-1860* (Ithica, N.Y., 1962), 71-76.

⁴Pontalba Letters, September 6, 11, 19, 24, 1796, pp. 274, 284, 300, 312; Gayarré, *History of Louisiana*, III, 375; Records of the City Council of New Orleans, Book 4079, Document 259, October 21, 1796.

⁵See for example, François Marie Perrin du Lac, *Voyage dans les Deux Louisianes . . . en 1801, 1802, et 1803 . . .* (Paris, 1805), trans. as *Travels Through the Two Louisianas . . . in 1801, 1802, & 1803* (London, 1807), 7; Amos Stoddard, *Sketches, Historical and Descriptive, of Louisiana* (Philadelphia, 1812), 171; Berquin-Duvallon, *Travels*, 115.

⁶See *Medical Repository* (New York), 1797-1809, *passim*. One of the more obscure abstractions advanced in the nineteenth century to explain the origin of yellow fever epidemics appeared in a pamphlet by an unnamed author, reviewed in the *Medical Repository* in 1803, VI, 417. Accepting the ancient doctrine of the four basic elements (earth, air, fire, and water) from which all things were made, the pamphleteer added two more from his own creative imagination: electrical fire and an entity that he called "Mother" and described as "the great agent of vegetable and animal life." Ordinarily "Mother" inhabited the earth's surface, but under certain circumstances, which remained unspecified, it was forced far down into the earth, eventually to rise again to the surface of its own power. Usually, this element emerged in a pure state, but sometimes on the way up to the surface it combined with putrefying matter, particularly in hot weather. Under such conditions "Mother" became "vitiated and venomous" and in its transformed state contaminated the earth and water through which it ascended, causing epidemic disease. The medical reviewer dismissed this theory as sheer nonsense, as nothing more than "an old woman's story." The concept of epidemic constitution, however, widely accepted by the early nineteenth-century medical profession, was no more open to investigation or analysis than this imaginative construction called "Mother."

⁷Colin Chisholm, *A Letter to John Haygarth . . . from Colin Chisholm . . . author of an Essay on the Pestilential Fever . . .* (London, 1809).

⁸*Louisiana Courier*, September 10, 1817.

⁹Jabez W. Heustis, *Physical Observations and Medical Tracts and Researches, on the Topography and Diseases of Louisiana* (New York, 1817), 113-14.

¹⁰Jones, *Medical and Surgical Memoirs*, III, pt. 1, cxlii.

¹¹*Report of the Committee of the Physico-Medical Society of New Orleans, on the Epidemic of 1820*, 5.

¹²Jean Louis Chabert, *Réflexions Médicales sur le Maladie Spasmodico-Lipyrienne des Pay Chauds Vulgairement Appelée Fièvre Jaune* (Nouvelle-Orléans, 1821), iii; Thomas, *Essai sur la Fièvre Jaune d'Amérique*, v, 65.

¹³For a comprehensive account of Louisiana's early quarantine legislation, see Jones, *Medical and Surgical Memoirs*, III, pt. 1, cxliv-cxlix.

¹⁴Ibid., cxlvii-cxlix.

¹⁵*New Orleans Medical Journal*, 1 (July, 1844): 94.

¹⁶Ibid., 31-41.

¹⁷Ibid., 42-44.

¹⁸Ibid., 1 (October, 1844): 178-80.

¹⁹Ibid., 1 (July, 1844): 4-5, 13.

[20]*NOM&SJ*, 3 (March, 1847): 580, 591-92.

[21]Ibid., 4 (January, 1848): 537, 540.

[22]Ibid., 9 (July, 1852): 35-40.

[23]Fenner, *Epidemic Yellow Fever*, 72-75.

[24]Considering the enormous cane crop in 1853, the leakage from hogsheads of sugar and molasses (considered by Barton as a source of miasma) could have served as a large-scale food supply for an expanding mosquito population, a phenomenon also noted by observers that fateful summer—and another bit of circumstantial evidence in favor of Goodyear's "sugar connection." See Chapter 2, note 4, and Chapter 3, note 49.

[25]Barton, *Cause and Prevention of Yellow Fever*, x, xv, 70, 134.

[26]Ibid., 49-51.

[27]Ibid., 52, 61-62.

[28]Ibid., 5-8. Speaking to the New York Academy of Medicine on yellow fever in 1856, Dr. Barton insisted that three ingredients were required to produce a yellow fever epidemic: high temperature, dampness, and miasms from filth. Local authorities had it entirely in their power, he said, to prevent the disease by draining and cleansing their city to remove the filth that served as "the electric spark which fires the other elements." *New York Times*, December 13, 1856.

[29]*DeBow's Review*, 15 (December, 1853): 599-600.

[30]New Orleans *Daily Crescent*, August 2, 8, 1853.

[31]*DeBow's Review*, 16 (May, 1854): 463-66.

[32]J. S. McFarlane, *A Review of the Yellow Fever, Its Causes, etc., and an Interesting and Useful Abstract of Mortuary Statistics* (New Orleans, 1853), vii, xii.

[33]*NOM&SJ*, 7 (September, 1850): 172-76. See also Duffy, *Medicine in Louisiana*, II, 85-86.

[34]*NOM&SJ*, 10 (May, 1854): 813-14.

[35]Ibid., 11 (July, 1854): 43-44, 47-50.

[36]Ibid., 11 (November, 1854): 429-30.

[37]Ibid., 11 (January, 1855): 503-5.

[38]Ibid., 16 (March, 1859): 173-74.

[39]*Report of the Louisiana State Board of Health for 1857*, 23.

[40]Barton, *Cause and Prevention of Yellow Fever*, 67.

[41]*NOM&SJ*, 10 (May, 1854): 814.

[42]Ibid., 10 (March, 1854): 571, 577-79.

⁴³Ibid., 4 (March, 1848): 563-601; 10 (March, 1854): 581.

⁴⁴Ibid., 10 (March, 1854): 606-8.

⁴⁵Ibid., 608-12.

⁴⁶*History of the Yellow Fever in New Orleans, during the Summer of 1853, with Sketches of the Scenes of Horror which Occurred during the Epidemic . . . by a Physician of New Orleans*, 38-39.

⁴⁷*NOM&SJ*, 7 (November, 1850): 362.

⁴⁸Duffy, ed., *Parson Clapp*, 84.

⁴⁹René La Roche, *Yellow Fever, Considered in its Historical, Pathological, Etiological and Therapeutical Relations*, 2 vols. (Philadelphia, 1855).

⁵⁰*NOM&SJ*, 12 (January, 1856): 555-74.

⁵¹William H. Holcombe, *Yellow Fever and its Homeopathic Treatment* (New York, 1856), 61-65.

⁵²See Gillson, *Formative Years*, xiii, 60-65.

⁵³*Report of the Louisiana State Board of Health for 1856*, 7-9. Originally, the term "virus" meant simply a poison of some sort, venom or slime. By the late nineteenth century it was used generally to refer to all disease-producing agents, including known microorganisms as well as those germs or toxins yet unidentified. Around the turn of the century the "virus" label became largely restricted to submicroscopic infective agents, known only by their effects and capable of passing through filters that stopped bacteria; these agents were conceived to be parasitic microorganisms that could multiply only within living cells. With technological developments and new paradigms in genetics and microbiology, the virus is now described as a complex structure of protein and nucleic acid; it is not a microorganism, having no metabolic mechanisms and requiring a host cell to reproduce itself. See Burnet and White, *Natural History of Infectious Disease*, 52-53; Spink, *Infectious Diseases*, 25-26; Rom Harre, *Great Scientific Experiments* (New York, 1983), 97-99.

⁵⁴*Report of the Louisiana State Board of Health for 1857*, 4-5. A New Orleans newspaper editor complained of the conflict between those arguing for importation and those who believed the fever indigenous. Why not cover all the opinions, the editor suggested, and establish both quarantine and sanitary measures? *Picayune*, September 25, 1853. "Either-or" thinking, however, usually seems more attractive to the human mind than "both-and."

⁵⁵Cartier, *La Fièvre Jaune de la Nouvelle-Orléans*, 46-47; Durac, *De la Fièvre Jaune*, 20-24, 65-72; Deléry, *Précis Historique de la Fièvre Jaune*, 52, 147.

⁵⁶Durac, *De la Fièvre Jaune*, 24, 65, 67, 69.

⁵⁷Duffy, ed., *Parson Clapp*, 105.

⁵⁸*NOM&SJ*, 3 (September, 1846): 174.

⁵⁹Ibid., 12 (November, 1855): 322.

⁶⁰*Report of the Louisiana State Board of Health for 1858*, 19-20.

⁶¹See Chapter 5 for a discussion of measures employed to prevent yellow fever in occupied New Orleans.

Chapter 11

[1] Berquin-Duvallon, *Travels*, 116.

[2] Heustis, *Physical Observations*, 113.

[3] See F. L. Hoffman, *Vital Statistics of New Orleans, 1787-1909* (New York, 1913); and Ketchum, "Yellow Fever in New Orleans," 48-61, 114-16, and tables. Ketchum's excellent work has provided a thorough analysis of the demographic and other factors contributing to the rise and decline of yellow fever in New Orleans.

[4] *NOM&SJ*, 2 (September, 1845): 130.

[5] Ibid., 5 (September, 1848): 206-7. See also La Roche, *Yellow Fever*, II, 27, 61, 765.

[6] *NOM&SJ*, 7 (July, 1850): 67. La Roche, *Yellow Fever*, II, 25, 38, also used the term "creolization" for the process of gradual adaptation to the climate whereby immunity was supposedly achieved, whether or not one actually suffered a yellow fever attack.

[7] New Orleans *Weekly Delta*, August 7, 1853.

[8] Clarissa E. Leavitt Town, Diary (Louisiana State University Archives, Baton Rouge), July 21, 1853, p. 202.

[9] Robinson, *Diary of a Samaritan*, 61, 88; see also *Weekly Delta*, July 24, 1853.

[10] Edward Hall Barton, *Introductory Lectures on Acclimation, Delivered at the Opening of the Third Session of the Medical College of Louisiana* (New Orleans, 1837), 13.

[11] Isaac H. Charles to John Edward Siddall, September 18, 1847, Isaac H. Charles Letters (Louisiana State University Archives, Baton Rouge).

[12] Ibid., November 18, 1847. Dr. J. C. Simonds, one of the first to make a careful study of New Orleans' available mortality records for comparison with other cities, calculated the average annual death rate of New Orleans, 1846-1850, as 8.1 percent; the long-term rate for Philadelphia, 1807-1840, was only 2.55 percent. During 1849, a year considered generally healthy in New Orleans, except for cholera, the city's mortality, excluding cholera deaths, was 5.7 percent. Philadelphia had three times the population and a mortality rate only half that of the Crescent City, even when cholera deaths were subtracted from New Orleans' death count. In 1850, a year without epidemics, 6.2 percent of New Orleans' population died, victims of the ordinary ailments that attracted so little attention or concern. J. C. Simonds, "On the Sanitary Condition of New Orleans, as Illustrated by its Mortuary Statistics," *Southern Medical Reports*, 2 (1850): 215-17.

[13] Charles to Siddall, November 18, 1847, Isaac H. Charles Letters.

[14] Gayarré, *History of Louisiana*, IV, 636.

[15] *NOM&SJ*, 2 (November, 1845): 397-98.

[16] Ibid., 12 (November, 1855): 432.

[17] *Picayune*, November 6, 1867.

[18] *NOM&SJ*, 10 (November, 1853): 312-15.

[19] McFarlane, *A Review of the Yellow Fever*, viii.

[20] Gerald Capers, *Occupied City: New Orleans Under the Federals, 1862-1865* (Lexington, Ky., 1965), 11.

[21] Harriet Martineau, *Retrospect of Western Travel*, 2 vols. (Cincinnati, 1838), I, 264-65.

[22] Ellis, "The New Orleans Yellow Fever Epidemic in 1878," 203, n.9; see also Latrobe, *Impressions Respecting New Orleans*, 146-47; *New Orleans Directory for 1842* (New Orleans, 1842), 15-16; *Report of the Louisiana State Board of Health for 1855*, 6; Ketchum, "Yellow Fever in New Orleans," tables and graphs.

[23] *New Orleans Bee*, September 10, 1839; Bartlett for Smith & Bro. to T. Smith & Co., August 12, 1847, T. Smith & Company Papers (Louisiana State University Archives, Baton Rouge).

[24] *NOM&SJ*, 5 (July, 1848): 52-53.

[25] Ibid., 6 (November, 1849): 407-9.

[26] James Mather to Claiborne, September 9, 1811, Carter, ed., *Territory of Orleans*, 947; *Louisiana Courier*, August 29, 1817; *NOM&SJ*, 58 (January, 1906): 551, 554.

[27] See notes 1 and 2 above; and *History of the Yellow Fever in New Orleans, during the summer of 1853 . . . by a Physician of New Orleans*, 37.

[28] *NOM&SJ*, 1 (May, 1844): 76-77; 4 (January, 1848): 535; 9 (November, 1852): 417; *Louisiana Herald* (Alexandria), September 7, 1822; *Picayune*, July 18, 1865; August 3, 5, 1905.

[29] See Geggus, "Yellow Fever in the 1790s," 52-53, for comments on the detrimental influence of alcohol in reducing prospects for recovery from yellow fever; and Strode, ed., *Yellow Fever*, 418-22, on the role of diet in treatment. Ketchum, "Yellow Fever in New Orleans," 109, suggests a possible influence of nutrition in resistance to the disease.

[30] Physicians, newspaper editors, merchants, travelers, and almost everyone who put pen to paper offered similar judgments about the lower class way of life as a cause of disease in the city, especially during the several decades of urban growth before the Civil War. See for example, *New Orleans Medical News and Hospital Gazette*, 6 (November, 1859): 698; *Picayune*, July 30, 1853; August 6, 11, 1839. Filthy, crowded lodging places were considered a source of disease-producing "miasmatic poisons" in the antebellum years; and as a source of disease-producing microorganisms after the development of germ theory in the 1870s.

[31] *New Orleans Monthly Medical Register*, 2 (August 1, 1853): 130; (September 1, 1853): 139-40. Todd Savitt found similar victim-blaming attitudes and explanations among whites in antebellum Virginia with regard to blacks and their susceptibility to cholera. Intemperance, imprudence, poor housing, eating habits that they refused to change "even when their lives depended on it," and delay in requesting medical aid—all these behaviors added up to a satisfactory explanation for whites of the high cholera mortality among blacks. As the New Orleans Italians were denounced for their macaroni and bananas, the Virginia slaves and free blacks had been charged with rejecting medical advice and refusing to give up watermelons, turnips, and other vegetables and fruits believed by physicians to have bad effects in cases of cholera. The whites in Virginia concluded that close supervision of black habits and manner of living was necessary in the interest of the larger community since blacks would not follow instructions. There is also a parallel between the myth of creole immunity to yellow fever and the perception of cholera as a disease to which the better element was simply not susceptible, a disease exclusive to blacks and poor whites, attributable to their unsanitary and intemperate habits. As yellow fever among creole children in New Orleans was called bilious, remittent, or hemorrhagic fever, or some other vague label, cholera among well-to-do Virginia whites was diagnosed as dysentery or bilious fever since it was inconceivable that they might suffer from diseases associated with the lower classes. Todd L. Savitt, *Medicine and Slavery: The Diseases and Health Care of Blacks in Antebellum*

Virginia (Urbana, Ill., 1979), 227-33.

³²*NOM&SJ*, 23 (April, 1870): 202-3.

³³See Carrigan, ed., *Fortier's History of Louisiana*, I, xxix-xxxi; and Joseph G. Tregle, "On That Word 'Creole' Again: A Note," *Louisiana History*, 23 (1982): 193-98, for a discussion of the definition and historical usage of "creole" (meaning native to Louisiana) and how a controversy in the 1870s and 1880s over the application of the term to "persons of color" led to an attempt in New Orleans by white descendants of Louisiana's French or Spanish colonials to redefine the label exclusively for themselves.

³⁴Ellis, "The New Orleans Yellow Fever Epidemic in 1878," 193-94.

³⁵*New Orleans Medical News and Hospital Gazette*, 5 (October, 1858): 553. See also *NOM&SJ*, 5 (September, 1848): 206-7.

³⁶Edward Larocque Tinker, *Pen, Pills, and Pistols: A Louisiana Chronicle* (New York, 1934), 7.

³⁷François Charles Deléry, *Memoire sur l'Epidémie de Fièvre Jaune, qui a Regné à la Nouvelle-Orléans et dans les Campagnes pendant l'Année 1867* (Nouvelle-Orléans, 1867), iii-iv, 7-10, 94.

³⁸*NOM&SJ*, new series, 8 (August, 1880): 11, 114, 122; see also 6 (November, 1878): 416; 51 (July, 1898): 56-57.

³⁹Latrobe, *Impressions Respecting New Orleans*, 146; *DeBow's Review*, 1 (April, 1846): 382; Gillson, *Formative Years*, 12-14. In almost any New Orleans newspaper during the summer months of any antebellum year, one can find assertions about the healthy condition of the city and the denial of all rumors and claims to the contrary.

⁴⁰E. H. Barton, "Annual Report of the New Orleans Board of Health [1849]," *Southern Medical Reports*, 1 (1849): 78, 85-86, 99; Gillson, *Formative Years*, 27-28; J. C. Simonds, "Report on the Hygienic Characteristics of New Orleans," *Transactions of the American Medical Association*, 3 (1850): 272.

⁴¹Simonds, "On the Sanitary Condition of New Orleans," 205, 229.

⁴²Stanford E. Chaillé, "Vital Statistics of New Orleans," *NOM&SJ*, 23 (January, 1870): 8.

⁴³Barton, "Annual Report of the New Orleans Board of Health [1849]," 86, 92, 94-95; *DeBow's Review*, 9 (August, 1850): 245.

⁴⁴Simonds, "On the Sanitary Condition of New Orleans," 219-20.

⁴⁵Ibid., 220-22. See also J. C. Simonds, "The Sanitary Condition of New-Orleans, as Illustrated by its Mortuary Statistics," *Charleston Medical Journal and Review*, 6 (1851): 677-745, a revised and considerably expanded version of the paper that originally appeared in *Southern Medical Reports*. See also his series of nine articles in the New Orleans *Daily Delta*, June 28, July 2, 3, 4, 9, 11, 12, 13, 18, 1850, commenting on the sanitary condition of the city, using mortality figures from the 1849 Board of Health Report to demonstrate that New Orleans was the unhealthiest city in the union, and trying to stimulate public opinion to demand hygienic reform. He was also attempting to cultivate popular appreciation for the importance of vital statistics in determining the salubrity (or insalubrity) of a city and making comparisons with other locations. His effort was obviously not very successful. See James H. Cassedy, *American Medicine and Statistical Thinking, 1800-1860* (Cambridge, Mass., 1984), for a good general account of the introduction of statistical methods into the various areas of medical activity during the antebellum years. Cassedy commented briefly on the work of Edward H. Barton and Bennet Dowler of New Orleans, but made no mention of J. C. Simonds, who was actually a better statistician than either Barton or Dowler.

⁴⁶Barton, "Annual Report of the New Orleans Board of Health [1849]," 85, 96-97.

⁴⁷James Stark, "Vital Statistics of New Orleans," *Edinburgh Medical and Surgical Journal* (January, 1851): 134-36, 138-41.

⁴⁸Fenner, *Epidemic Yellow Fever*, 56. La Roche, *Yellow Fever*, II, 64, wrote of the "inferior susceptibility" of blacks to the disease.

⁴⁹*NOM&SJ*, 10 (November, 1853): 312-13. See also New Orleans *Weekly Delta*, August 14, October 2, 1853, for other examples of the medical proslavery argument in relation to yellow fever.

⁵⁰*NOM&SJ*, 15 (March, 1858): 150.

⁵¹Ibid., 11 (November, 1854): 375.

⁵²Ibid., 20 (September, 1867): 286.

⁵³Kenneth F. Kiple and Virginia Himmelsteib King, *Another Dimension to the Black Diaspora: Diet, Disease, and Racism* (Cambridge, 1981), 45-46.

⁵⁴*Picayune*, July 29, August 17, 23, 1905.

⁵⁵Chassaignac, "Some Lessons Taught by the Epidemic of 1905," in Augustin, *History of Yellow Fever*, 1054-55.

⁵⁶Kiple & King, *Another Dimension to the Black Diaspora*, 27-28, 47-49; Kiple & Kiple, "Black Yellow Fever Immunities, Innate and Acquired," 419-36; Carter, *Yellow Fever*, 270; Trent, ed., "The Men who Conquered Yellow Fever," in Smith, *Yellow Fever in Galveston*, 85. See also Chapter 1, note 14, above.

⁵⁷*Picayune*, September 9, 1867; Edward H. Barton, "Sanitary Report of New Orleans, La.," *Transactions of the American Medical Association*, 2 (1849): 605.

⁵⁸Elisha Bartlett, *History, Diagnosis, and Treatment of the Fevers of the United States*, 4th ed. (Philadelphia, 1856), 509.

⁵⁹*Report of the Louisiana State Board of Health for 1878*, 83; *NOM&SJ*, new series, 8 (August, 1880): 115-22.

⁶⁰David T. Purtilo and John L. Sullivan, "Immunological Bases for Superior Survival of Females," *American Journal of Diseases of Children*, 133 (December, 1979): 1251.

Chapter 12

¹*NOM&SJ*, 23 (July, 1870): 568, 597.

²*Report of the Louisiana State Board of Health for 1878*, 10-14; Gillson, *Formative Years*, 179-85.

³Joseph Holt, *The Quarantine System of Louisiana, Methods of Disinfection Practiced . . .* (New Orleans, [1887]; *NOM&SJ*, new series, 18 (December, 1890): 483-84; Gillson, *Progressive Years*, 10-24.

⁴See Thomas Kuhn, *The Structure of Scientific Revolutions*, 2nd ed. (Chicago, 1970). Although Kuhn drew his specific examples from physics, his insights are useful in dealing with the "bacteriological revolution" of the late nineteenth century.

[5] Erwin H. Ackerknecht, *A Short History of Medicine* (New York, 1968), 175-85; Spink, *Infectious Diseases*, 18-27.

[6] *NOM&SJ*, new series, 8 (October, 1880): 315.

[7] Ibid., new series, 8 (December, 1880): 513.

[8] Winslow, *Conquest of Epidemic Disease*, 200, 214. See Shryock, *Medicine in America: Historical Essays*, 236-45, for more on Rush's monistic concept of disease.

[9] Heustis, *Physical Observations*, 114.

[10] *New Orleans Medical Journal*, 1 (October, 1844): 219.

[11] *Picayune*, August 21, 1841.

[12] *New Orleans Medical Journal*, 1 (July, 1844): 7-11, 23-24.

[13] *NOM&SJ*, 6 (July, 1849): 48.

[14] Erasmus Darwin Fenner, ed., *Southern Medical Reports*, 2 vols. (New Orleans, 1849-1850), I, 111-13.

[15] Ibid., II, 85.

[16] Barton, *Cause and Prevention of Yellow Fever*, 113-14.

[17] Cartier, *La Fièvre Jaune de la Nouvelle-Orléans*, 2-5.

[18] *NOM&SJ*, 10 (March, 1854): 625; 11 (September, 1854): 175-84; 15 (July, 1858): 500-17.

[19] Ibid., 10 (March, 1854): 625.

[20] See Shryock, *Medicine and Society in America: 1660-1860*, 123-30, for a discussion of the "Paris school" of clinical medicine and its contributions.

[21] "Yellow Fever Research Notebook, 1870-1872," Joseph Jones Papers (Louisiana State University Archives, Baton Rouge); see also *NOM&SJ*, new series, 4 (September, 1876): 159-65.

[22] "Composition and Character of the Urine in Yellow Fever," Joseph Jones Papers.

[23] "Yellow Fever Research Notebook, 1870-1872," 5-6, Joseph Jones Papers.

[24] *Merck Manual*, 13th ed., 57; Wilcocks & Manson-Bahr, eds., *Manson's Tropical Diseases*, 17th ed., 377.

[25] Jean Charles Faget, *Monographie sur le Type et la Spécificité de la Fièvre Jaune, Établis avec l'Aide de la Montre et du Thermomètre* (Nouvelle-Orléans, 1875); *NOM&SJ*, new series, 1 (September, 1873): 145-68.

[26] Durac, *De la Fièvre Jaune*, 65; Cartier, *La Fièvre Jaune de la Nouvelle-Orléans*, 7. See Duffy, *Medicine in Louisiana*, II, 18-19, for a reference to Faget's first announcement of his "sign" in an 1859 pamphlet. This publication was concerned primarily with establishing a distinction between malaria and yellow fever. Faget, a defender of the doctrine of creole immunity, argued that creole children had suffered from a malarial epidemic in 1858, not from yellow fever as many doctors had claimed.

[27] "Review of *Yellow Fever: Clinical Notes* by Dr. Just Touatre," *NOM&SJ*, 51 (July, 1898): 56. Although the

thermometer had been developed in Europe in the seventeenth century, physicians did not find it generally useful until the mid-nineteenth century. Spink, *Infectious Diseases*, 133-37. In Louisiana, as late as the 1880s the thermometer was still not routinely used by medical practitioners. Duffy, *Medicine in Louisiana*, II, 340.

[28]*NOM&SJ*, new series, 6 (September, 1878): 240-55.

[29]U. R. Milner, *Yellow Fever, not Imported, nor Contagious, but Indigenous, and Intrinsically Identical with our Paludal Fevers. Preventable by Well Determined and Wisely Executed Local Sanitary Measures. Quarantine a Wide-spread Calamity, and Should no longer be Tolerated. A Lecture before the Academy of Sciences of New Orleans . . . 1879*, in Miscellaneous Publications on Yellow Fever in Louisiana and Adjoining States, Howard-Tilton Memorial Library, Tulane University, New Orleans, 3-18, 22, 26.

[30]Gillson, *Formative Years*, 171.

[31]*Report of the Louisiana State Board of Health for 1871*, 20, 25, 51, 75.

[32]*Report of the Louisiana State Board of Health for 1878*, 10-13; *NOM&SJ*, new series, 6 (August, 1878), 179.

[33]Frederic P. Gorham, "The History of Bacteriology and Its Contribution to Public Health Work," in Mazyck P. Ravenel, ed., *A Half-Century of Public Health* (New York, 1921), 66-93; Spink, *Infectious Diseases*, 18-21; Ackerknecht, *A Short History of Medicine*, 175-85; Winslow, *Conquest of Epidemic Disease*, 291-310; René Dubos, *Pasteur and Modern Science* (Garden City, N. Y., 1960). See also John Farley, "The Social, Political, and Religious Background to the Work of Louis Pasteur," *Annual Review of Microbiology*, 32 (1978): 143-54.

[34]Smillie, *Public Health, Its Promise for the Future*, 385-88.

[35]*NOM&SJ*, new series, 2 (March, 1875): 645.

[36]Ibid., new series, 7 (October, 1879): 495.

[37]Garrison, *John Shaw Billings*, 178-80.

[38]Henry D. Schmidt, *The Pathology and Treatment of Yellow Fever with Some Remarks upon the Nature of its Cause and its Prevention* (Chicago, 1881), 151, 190, 197-212; H. D. Schmidt, "On the Pathology of Yellow Fever . . . ," *New York Medical Journal*, 29 (February, 1879): 151-54. See also Duffy, *Medicine in Louisiana*, II, 336, 346-48, 389.

[39]*NOM&SJ*, new series, 7 (May, 1880): 1019.

[40]Ibid., new series, 8 (January, 1881): 609-29.

[41]Ibid., new series, 16 (July, 1888): 2. See also ibid., new series, 13 (August, 1885): 129, for a letter in which a New Orleans physician said he had accepted the theory, "now generally received," that yellow fever's cause was a microorganism, animal or vegetable, which could reproduce itself and be carried in vessels, cargoes, and clothing.

[42]This analysis of the "hunt" and its obstacles is derived from Warner, "Hunting the Yellow Fever Germ," 365-67, 371-72, 375, 381.

[43]*NOM&SJ*, new series, 13 (January, 1886): 547-51; (February, 1886): 624-32, 641-63; (March, 1886): 712-28; (June, 1886): 964-72, 990-94; (August, 1886): 140-43; 15 (May, 1888): 894-95.

[44]Ibid., new series, 13 (January, 1886): 547-51; 14 (August, 1886): 141.

⁴⁵Ibid., new series, 13 (February, 1886): 642.

⁴⁶Ibid., 626-29. See also editorials in issue of March, 1886, 712-28.

⁴⁷Ibid., new series, 13 (February, 1886): 630-31.

⁴⁸Ibid., new series, 15 (May, 1888): 894-95; George M. Sternberg, *Report on Etiology and Prevention of Yellow Fever* (Washington, 1890), 13, 17-35, 97, 222; Jorge Boshell, *et al.*, *Yellow Fever: A Symposium in Commemoration of Carlos Juan Finlay* (Philadelphia, 1955), 6-7.

⁴⁹Warner, "Hunting the Yellow Fever Germ," 372-81.

⁵⁰*NOM&SJ*, 52 (October, 1899): 210-12; *Report of the Commission of Medical Officers* [U. S. Marine Hospital Service], *Detailed by Authority of the President to Investigate the Cause of Yellow Fever* (Washington, 1899), 3-10. Dr. Paul E. Archinard achieved positive results with Sanarelli's "serum diagnosis" (based on agglutination) and believed it would be useful in determining early or questionable cases. In other experiments at Charity Hospital with Sanarelli's "anti-amarylic serum," Archinard found no therapeutic benefits whatsoever, although the attenuated bacillus was supposed to be effective as both treatment and preventive. *NOM&SJ*, 50 (February, 1898): 456, 468; 52 (August, 1899): 85.

⁵¹Just Touatre, *Yellow Fever: Clinical Notes* . . . , trans. by Charles L. Chassaignac (New Orleans, 1898), 145, 153-55.

⁵²*NOM&SJ*, 52 (May, 1900): 617-36.

⁵³Augustin, *History of Yellow Fever*, 50-51.

⁵⁴*Rapport . . . de la Société Médicale de la Nouvelle-Orléans sur la Fièvre Jaune . . . 1819*, 7; Latrobe, *Impressions*, 141-43. The *Aedes aegypti*, having white bands on its legs and abdomen and white spots on the side of its thorax, has sometimes been called the "tiger mosquito." See Boyce, *Yellow Fever Prophylaxis*, 11-12.

⁵⁵Lyell, *A Second Visit to the United States*, II, 135-36.

⁵⁶*NOM&SJ*, 12 (September, 1855): 186-87.

⁵⁷See for example, New Orleans *Daily Crescent*, June 24, 1853; *Picayune*, June 28, 1853; *Weekly Delta*, July 3, 1853.

⁵⁸Wharton Diary, November 1, 1854. Homeopathic medical practice was based in part on the "doctrine of infinitesimal dosage," the belief that medicines were most efficacious in minute quantities. Homeopaths would not have resorted to cupping and bleeding (an orthodox, allopathic practice) in any amount, but the tiny amount of blood drawn by a mosquito might be facetiously labeled "homeopathic."

⁵⁹*NOM&SJ*, 4 (March, 1848): 563-64, 580-81, 601.

⁶⁰Augustin, *History of Yellow Fever*, 45.

⁶¹Trent, "The Men Who Conquered Yellow Fever," and Chauncey D. Leake's concluding note in Smith, *Yellow Fever in Galveston*, 100, 103, 126-27.

⁶²Nancy Stepan has argued persuasively that "political or economic factors were more important . . . than any supposed shortcomings in Finlay's science" in explaining why his work was ignored for almost twenty years. "The Interplay between Socio-Economic Factors and Medical Science: Yellow Fever Research, Cuba and

the United States," *Social Studies of Science*, 8 (1978), 397-423. See also J. A. Del Regato, "Carlos Finlay and the Carrier of Death" (reprint from *Americas*, May, 1968).

[63] Carlos Finlay, *El Mosquito Hipoteticamente Considerado como Agente de Transmission de la Fiebre Amarilla* (Habana, 1881), 3-4, 23.

[64] *NOM&SJ*, new series, 9 (February, 1882): 601-16.

[65] Ibid., new series, 12 (August, 1884): 116-17; 14 (November, 1886): 394-95.

[66] Boshell et al., *Yellow Fever*, iv, 8.

[67] Walter Reed et al., "The Etiology of Yellow Fever: A Preliminary Note," *Philadelphia Medical Journal*, 6 (October 27, 1900): 790-96; Walter Reed, "The Propagation of Yellow Fever: Observations Based on Recent Researches," *Medical Record*, 60 (August 10, 1901): 201-9; *Yellow Fever: A Compilation of Various Publications*, 61st Cong., 3rd sess. (1910-1911), *Senate Documents*, Vol. 61, No. 822 (serial set #5919); *NOM&SJ*, 54 (May, 1902): 711-14; 56 (May, 1904): 805-6; 61 (July, 1908): 4-5; Kelly, *Walter Reed and Yellow Fever*, 120-209; William B. Bean, *Walter Reed* (Charlottesville, Va., 1982), 103-80. See also François Delaporte, *The History of Yellow Fever: An Essay on the Birth of Tropical Medicine*, trans. by Arthur Goldhammer (Cambridge, Mass., 1991). Delaporte credits the English researchers with providing the crucial key to the yellow fever puzzle, although neglected by both Cuban and American historians. Without denying Finlay and Reed their due as contributors, he argues that the work of Patrick Manson probably influenced Finlay to begin investigating the mosquito, and that the Liverpool Commission in Havana suggested to Reed the probable connection of Carter's "extrensic incubation" period, Ronald Ross's concept of the mosquito as "intermediate host," and Finlay's old hypothesis. Delaporte denies conceptual continuity between the work of Finlay and the Reed Commission, insisting that Finlay viewed the mosquito only as "mechanical agent of transmission," not as "intermediate host," a concept supplied by Ross. See, however, Finlay's 1886 article in *American Journal of the Medical Sciences*, suggesting that the mosquito's sting or its sheath "may constitute an appropriate soil for the preservation or even for the culture of those germs; might it not indeed be the 'intermediate host' necessary for some phase of their development?" "Yellow Fever: Its Transmission by Means of the Culex Mosquito," 402.

[68] *NOM&SJ*, 54 (October, 1901): 231.

[69] See Winslow, *Conquest of Epidemic Disease*, 355; Spink, *Infectious Diseases*, 157; "Report of Maj. W. C. Gorgas, Medical Corps, United States Army, July 12, 1902," in *Yellow Fever: A Compilation of Various Publications*, 234-50.

[70] *NOM&SJ*, 55 (August, 1902): 102-4; 56 (May, 1904): 858-59.

[71] Ibid., 58 (July, 1905): 46-47. Thomas Kuhn also observed that the acceptance of new paradigms (or subparadigms) comes not solely through the power of rational argument but more as a matter of "conversion" to a new doctrine, a shifting of vision. *The Structure of Scientific Revolutions*, 111-35, 198-204.

[72] Burnet & White, *Natural History of Infectious Disease*, 242-49; Strode, ed., *Yellow Fever*, 39-136; *Manson's Tropical Diseases*, 17th ed., 355-65, 374-83. Vast reservoirs of the virus are maintained in monkeys and mosquitoes in African and South American forests, occasionally spreading to human communities where *Aedes aegypti* reside. The yellow fever mosquito, which also transmits dengue, is reinfesting areas of the Western Hemisphere where it had been wiped out. The Gulf Coast area of the American South is still *Aedes aegypti* territory, and imported cases of yellow fever or dengue could spark an outbreak. See Jonathan Leonard, "The Ghost of Yellow Jack," *Harvard Magazine* (March-April, 1981): 20-27; David Zimmerman, "The Mosquitoes Are Coming . . . ," *Smithsonian*, 14 (June, 1983): 28-37; Jean Slosek, "*Aedes Aegypti* Mosquitoes in the Americas: A Review of Their Interactions with the Human Population," *Social Science and Medicine*, 23 (1986): 249-57.

Chapter 13

[1] See John Harley Warner, *The Therapeutic Perspective: Medical Practice, Knowledge, and Identity in America, 1820-1885* (Cambridge, Mass., 1986), for a thorough untangling and "decoding" of therapeutic theory, principle, and practice, in relation to the major transformations that occurred during the nineteenth century. Warner and others have called attention to methodological problems in studying the history of therapeutics, not least of which has been the tendency for historians to accept physicians' rhetorical jousting and generalizations about therapeutics in journals and textbooks as evidence of actual practice—to confuse what they said with what they did. Hospital case records, prescription books, and physicians's case books must be utilized to discover what specific treatments doctors actually selected from the armamentarium available to them, in what measure, how often, and for what purpose. My chapter on therapeutics is not based on specific case records. I have used reports of medical societies, physicians' accounts of specific epidemics, textbooks, pamphlets, and journal articles, which reveal the general "plans" or "modes" of treatment advocated at various times, the diversity of remedies available for similar purposes, the rhetoric used in justifying certain practices and condemning others, and the recurring themes of continuity and change. This material is more indicative of what Warner describes as therapeutic *theory* and *principle* (and professional tensions) than actual therapeutic *practice*, although some "behavioral" reflections are surely there. The important task of locating and analyzing a large quantity of comparable case records kept by hospitals, pharmacies, and physicians regarding treatment of yellow fever patients from the early nineteenth through the early twentieth century remains for some future researcher.

[2] Kerr, "The Clinical Aspects and Diagnosis of Yellow Fever," in Strode, ed., *Yellow Fever*, 417.

[3] *NOM&SJ*, 2 (November, 1845): 323, 325; see also J. C. Nott, "Sketch of the Epidemic of Yellow Fever of 1847, in Mobile," *Charleston Medical Journal and Review*, 3 (January, 1848): 14-21, reprinted in Barbara Gutmann Rosenkrantz et al. eds., *Yellow Fever Studies* (New York, 1977).

[4] Robinson, *Diary of a Samaritan*, 77, 132.

[5] Ibid., 200.

[6] Pontalba Letters, October 15, 1796, p. 358.

[7] Robinson, *Diary of a Samaritan*, 269.

[8] John Harrison, "Remarks on Yellow Fever," *NOM&SJ*, 2 (November, 1845): 323.

[9] See Charles E. Rosenberg's pathbreaking essay, "The Therapeutic Revolution: Medicine, Meaning, and Social Change in Nineteenth-Century America," in Vogel and Rosenberg, eds., *The Therapeutic Revolution*, 3-25; Warner, *The Therapeutic Perspective*, 83-102; William G. Rothstein, *American Physicians in the Nineteenth Century: From Sects to Science* (Baltimore, 1982), 46-53, 61-62.

[10] Geggus, "Yellow Fever in the 1790s," 53-56. For an account of the "cold water" treatment used by "Dr. Flood" in New Orleans in 1801, see *DeBow's Review*, 6 (August, 1848): 156-58.

[11] Bennet Dowler, "The Tableau of Yellow Fever of 1853," in *Cohen's New Orleans Directory . . . of 1854*, 9. Quinine is a derivative of cinchona bark.

[12] Gros et Gerardin, *Rapport fait a la Société Médicale sur la fièvre jaune . . . 1817*, 20-22; see also Pontalba Letters, September 14, 1796, p. 290.

[13] Some society members had tried "la methode Anglaise par le mercure," but found it almost always useless. *Rapport . . . de la Société Médicale . . . 1819*, 10-12; See also Chabert, *Réflexions Médicales*, 209-23.

[14]*Louisiana Courier*, September 10, 1817.

[15]Heustis, *Physical Observations*, 115-18.

[16]*Report of the Committee of the Physico-Medical Society . . . 1820*, 11-14.

[17]Lyman Cronkrite, "An Inquiry into the Pathology and Treatment of Yellow Fever, as it Prevails at New Orleans at this Time, August, 1829," *Western Journal of the Medical and Physical Sciences*, 3 (1830): 385-89. This was the same year that Dr. Charles Luzenberg introduced syncopal bleeding to New Orleans, according to Dr. J. F. Beugnot. See note 25 below.

[18]Barton, *Account of the Epidemic Yellow Fever . . . 1833*, 14, 37, 49.

[19]*NOM&SJ*, new series, 14 (June, 1887): 923.

[20]*NOM&SJ*, 1 (May, 1844): 1-3.

[21]Ibid., 4-7.

[22]Ibid., 7-8.

[23]Ibid., 1 (March, 1845): 419-25.

[24]Ibid., 1 (October, 1844): 240.

[25]Ibid., 1 (May, 1844): 22. Luzenberg came from Italy to the United States as a youth, took his degree at the Jefferson Medical College in Philadelphia, and moved to New Orleans in 1828. The following year he suffered an attack of yellow fever and treated himself by syncopal bleeding, "to disembarrass the nervous centers of the excess of blood concentrated upon them by the morbific cause," according to his own explanation. Cupping seem to have been little used in New Orleans at that time as Luzenberg was unable to locate either a cucurbitula (bleeding cup) or a scarificator (spring-operated device to make superficial cuts in the skin). Luzenberg used a wine glass and a lancet instead and had a successful recovery. An abrasive personality, he criticized the therapies of experienced New Orleans practitioners and made more enemies than friends in his adopted city. See A. E. Fossier, "Charles Aloysius Luzenberg, 1805-1848: A History of Medicine in New Orleans During the Years 1830 to 1848," *Louisiana Historical Quarterly*, 26 (January, 1943): 49-50, 64.

[26]*NOM&SJ*, 1 (May, 1844): 11-12.

[27]Ibid., 14-16.

[28]Ibid., 17-19, 21-22.

[29]*Picayune*, August 30, 1839.

[30]*NOM&SJ*, 5 (September, 1848): 208.

[31]Ibid., 1 (July, 1844): 14-15.

[32]Ibid., 2 (November, 1845): 325-26.

[33]Robinson, *Diary of a Samaritan*, 95.

[34]Ibid., 22-23.

35*NOM&SJ*, 2 (November, 1845): 326, 331-33.

36New Orleans *Bee*, October 1, 1839.

37Fenner, ed., *Southern Medical Reports*, I, 117-18.

38*NOM&SJ*, 1 (May, 1844): 25-28.

39Thompson McGown, *Diseases of the South* (Philadelphia, 1849), 294.

40*NOM&SJ*, 1 (October, 1844): 247-48.

41Ibid., 3 (July, 1846): 50-51.

42Ibid., (October, 1844): 194-95.

43Ibid., 1 (May, 1844): 8-9.

44Ibid., 5 (September, 1848): 208-12. See Warner, *The Therapeutic Perspective*, 41-46, for a delineation of the multiple and contradictory meanings of the terms *empirical* and *rational* in therapeutic discourse, 1820 to 1860. Each could be used in a positive or negative sense in either a methodological or a professional context—four different meanings for each term. "Both could mean discriminating or mechanical, professional or quackish, scientific or ignorant; they were synonyms and antonyms of each other and of themselves." (p. 45).

45*History of the Yellow Fever in New Orleans, During the Summer of 1853 . . . by a Physician of New Orleans*, 40-41.

46*NOM&SJ*, 10 (March, 1854): 646-51.

47Fenner, *Epidemic Yellow Fever*, 57-58.

48Ibid., 59-61.

49*NOM&SJ*, 9 (July, 1852): 32-33.

50Ibid., 10 (November, 1853): 403-4; see also ibid., 10 (September, 1853): 279; and Cartier, *La Fièvre Jaune*, 25-27.

51Edward Hall Barton, *An Address Before the Louisiana State Medical Society* (New Orleans, 1851), 7.

52Yellow fever epidemics were not the only influence undermining traditional practice by mid-century. For several decades medical researchers in the Paris hospitals had been questioning speculative theory and routine practice, some rejecting virtually all standard therapies ("therapeutic nihilism") and gradually formulating a new kind of pathology, localized and specific rather than systemic and holistic. Symptoms, carefully observed and recorded, measured with new instruments such as thermometer and stethoscope, and correlated with postmortem dissections and microscopic studies of diseased tissue, gave rise to a new perception of specific disease entities, each with unique symptom patterns, each causing damage to specific organs or tissues. Such studies, while contributing to knowledge, did not immediately offer much therapeutic benefit to practitioner or patient. See John Duffy, *The Healers* (Urbana, Ill., 1979), 98-103; Shryock, *Medicine and Society in America, 1660-1860*, 123-30; Erwin H. Ackerknecht, *Medicine at the Paris Hospital, 1794-1848* (Baltimore, 1967).

53*NOM&SJ*, 11 (November, 1854): 368-69, 371.

⁵⁴Durac, *De La Fièvre Jaune* . . . *1853, 1854, 1858,* 17-20, 72-73.

⁵⁵*DeBow"s Review,* 19 (October, 1855): 445.

⁵⁶*N. O. Med. News & Hosp. Gazette,* 5 (September, 1858): 481-82; *Picayune,* September 4, 1839.

⁵⁷*NOM&SJ,* 15 (September, 1858): 718; see also ibid., 12 (September, 1855): 287.

⁵⁸Not all physicians felt so inclined to experiment. One of New Orleans "most eminent physicians," according to one account, left the city during the epidemic of 1853, "not having saved one patient, and determined not to experiment when his knowledge and experience had failed to produce expected results." Robinson, *Diary of a Samaritan,* 215.

⁵⁹*Louisiana Courier,* August 14, 1820.

⁶⁰See Savitt, *Medicine and Slavery,* 239-45. The fearful attitude of the poor, both black and white, toward charitable institutions treating infectious disease in antebellum Virginia, as described by Savitt, probably applies equally to New Orleans, although I found no precise record of how charity patients at this time felt about serving as experimental subjects. In the 1890s the records clearly show the intense fear, however unfounded, of Italian immigrants who resisted hospitalization, believing they would be poisoned.

⁶¹Nott, "Sketch of the Epidemic of Yellow Fever of 1847, in Mobile," 19-21.

⁶²*N. O. Med. News & Hosp. Gazette,* 5 (January, 1859): 721-27.

⁶³Ibid., 5 (October, 1858): 562-68, and (November, 1858): 625-28. See Warner, *The Therapeutic Perspective,* 227-31, for discussion of the passing fashion of veratrum viride (hellebore) as a general remedy for fevers in the 1850s and 1860s. Some doctors rationalized its use as a substitute for venesection, suited for diseases that had changed in nature, having become less "inflammatory" than the types prevailing in previous decades. The drug acted as a nervous, respiratory, and cardiac sedative, as well as a diuretic and diaphoretic, but too large a dose of this potent medicine could also kill. In previous years, it was sometimes used as an emetic.

⁶⁴*NOM&SJ,* 15 (November, 1858): 731, 739-71. See also *Picayune,* August 30, 1878, for front-page coverage of Dr. Samuel Choppin's successful "cold water experiment" on a dying patient in Charity Hospital. Choppin, state health board president, encouraged practitioners to engage in "experimentation guided by common sense and based on the principles of pathology and physiology," for only through such means could advances be made in knowledge of yellow fever and ways of treating it.

⁶⁵See Rothstein, *American Physicians in the Nineteenth Century,* 125-74, and Duffy, *Medicine in Louisiana,* II, 32-42, for more detail on "irregular" medical practice.

⁶⁶Joel Shew, *The Water-Cure Manual: A Popular Work* . . . (New York, 1850); Duffy, *Medicine in Louisiana,* II, 37-39.

⁶⁷*NOM&SJ,* 5 (September, 1848): 212-13.

⁶⁸Ibid., 1 (May, 1844): 9-11.

⁶⁹Cartier, *La Fièvre Jaune,* 28, 36-37, 41-45.

⁷⁰Duffy, ed., *Parson Clapp,* 106.

⁷¹See Martin Kaufman, *Homeopathy in America: The Rise and Fall of a Medical Heresy* (Baltimore, 1971),

23-47; Duffy, *Medicine in Louisiana*, II, 36-37, 283.

[72]*NOM&SJ*, 12 (July, 1855): 52-53.

[73]Holcombe, *Yellow Fever and Its Homeopathic Treatment*, 31, 35-40; see also Rothstein, *American Physicians in the Nineteenth Century*, 154-56, for a description of the dilution process to the decillionth level. One Louisiana layman, compiling a home guide to homeopathic treatment and not so concerned with super dilutions, recorded that yellow fever at the beginning called for aconite, two or three drops diluted in a glass of rain water. Joseph Beraud Manuscript, "Guide Homeopathique," 1876 (Louisiana State University Archives, Baton Rouge).

[74]William H. Holcombe, *On the Treatment, Diet, and Nursing of Yellow Fever* . . . (New York, n.d.), 2-4, 9-19.

[75]The New Orleans Homeopathic Relief Association provided treatment for 5,640 cases of yellow fever in the 1878 epidemic, 3,184 in New Orleans and the rest in seventeen Louisiana and Mississippi towns. *Report of the Homeopathic Relief Association, 1878*, 4-23; Ernest Hardenstein, *The Epidemic of 1878 and Its Homeopathic Treatment: A General History of the Origin, Progress, and End of the Plague in the Mississippi Valley* (New Orleans, 1879).

[76]See for example, *Picayune*, May 25, 1838, October 1, 1843; *Bee*, October 11, 1847.

[77]*Picayune*, May 25, 1838.

[78]Ibid., August 6, 1840.

[79]Ibid., December 7, 1859.

[80]Ibid., September 21, 1888; August 7, 1905. See also J. N. Lee, *Life. The Philosophy of its Origin and Preservation. A Brief Outline of the Fundamental Principles of Scientific Medicine. The Nature of Endemic Yellow Fever . . . with an Infallible Preventive and Cure for it, as well as the Epidemic Yellow Fever* . . . (New Orleans, 1883).

[81]*Picayune*, September 15, 1867; September 18, 1897.

[82]Ibid., August 6, 1905.

[83]Ibid., August 4, 6, 1905.

[84]Ibid., September 1, 1853; September 16, 1858; October 27, 1867.

[85]Ibid., September 7, 1858; see also John James Hayes, *Yellow Fever; Its Prevention and Cure* (New Orleans, 1858), 3, 6, 7, 43; J. J. Hayes, *Yellow Fever: A Treatise on its Cause, Nature, Prevention and Cure* . . . (New Orleans, 1879).

[86]*Picayune*, August 30, 1853.

[87]Ibid., September 7, 1858.

[88]*N. O. Med. News & Hosp. Gazette*, 5 (October, 1858): 549.

[89]T.H. Bache, *Some Practical Observations on Yellow Fever, published for the Use of Surgeons of the Volunteer Forces in the Department of the Gulf* (New Orleans, 1862), 13, 8-17.

[90]See Deléry, *Précis Historique de la Fièvre Jaune*, 149; and various board of health reports.

[91] *Report of the Committee . . . on the Yellow Fever Epidemic of 1873 at Shreveport*, 20-21.

[92] Smith, *Report of the Yellow Fever Epidemic of 1873, Shreveport, La.*, 6, 9.

[93] New Orleans Board of Health, *Official Report of the Deaths from Yellow Fever . . . 1878* (New Orleans, n.d.), 87, 90-95.

[94] Joseph Jones, "Treatment of Yellow Fever," *NOM&SJ*, new series, 7 (July, 1879): 30-32, 36, 44.

[95] Schmidt, "On the Pathology of Yellow Fever," 150.

[96] *NOM&SJ*, new series, 16 (July, 1888): 8-14.

[97] George M. Sternberg, *Report on the Etiology and Prevention of Yellow Fever* (Washington, D.C., 1890), 78-79. See also *Report of the Louisiana State Board of Health for 1881*, 207-8, for a description of mild treatment as the best treatment for yellow fever.

[98] *NOM&SJ*, 51 (October, 1898): 209. See also ibid., 50 (October, 1897): 247-48, 252-57, for Dr. T. S. Dabney's discussion of the traditional creole treatment and reasons for its enduring success.

[99] *Yellow Fever: Its Nature, Diagnosis, Treatment, and Prophylaxis, and Quarantine Regulations Relating Thereto*, by Officers of the U. S. Marine Hospital Service (Washington, 1898), reprinted in Rosenkrantz et al. eds., *Yellow Fever Studies*, 24.

[100] Ibid., 23-40.

[101] Touatre, *Yellow Fever*, 164-67, 173-202.

[102] Edmond Souchon, *Instructions to Laymen Why May Have to Manage Yellow Fever Cases in Default of a Physician. Also Recommendations to Physicians Inexperienced in the Treatment of Yellow Fever with Regard to the Use of Medicines* (New Orleans, 1898), 10-12, 14; *NOM&SJ*, 52 (July, 1899): 19.

[103] *NOM&SJ*, 58 (November, 1905): 403-4.

[104] Lucien F. Salomon, *The Treatment of Yellow Fever* (New Orleans, 1905), 1-7.

[105] *Picayune*, August 2, 1905.

[106] See Thomas P. Monath, "Yellow Fever: *Victor, Victoria?* Conqueror, conquest? Epidemics and research in the last forty years and prospects for the future," *American Journal of Tropical Medicine and Hygiene*, 45 (July, 1991): 1-43, for a review of outbreaks in the past few decades, the threat of yellow fever's reemergence in urban areas in South America, the problems of vector control, the advances in scientific knowledge of the virus and related matters, and an optimistic view that an effective antiviral therapy will eventually be found.

[107] Kerr, "The Clinical Aspects and Diagnosis of Yellow Fever," in Strode, ed., *Yellow Fever*, 417-22; see also 1987 *Merck Manual*, 15th ed., 193. P. E. C. Manson-Bahr, *Manson's Tropical Diseases*, 18th ed. (London, 1982), 266, 274, stated simply that there is no specific treatment and that yellow fever should be treated like other arbovirus diseases for which "nursing and general care are all-important." The 1925 edition of *Manson's* offered many suggestions but concluded that treatment was "more a matter of nursing than of drugs." (p. 174). As previously noted, the role of the nurse in yellow fever has long been a prominent theme in the literature. Marine Hospital Surgeon R. D. Murray in his 1898 article, although perhaps not unappreciative of the value of nursing, expressed a hostile view toward nurses, especially the new professional or trained nurse, who seemed always "at odds with the doctor." In his view, "The nurse should

have only sense enough to obey orders." *Yellow Fever: Its Nature, Diagnosis, Treatment, and Prophylaxis* . . . , 33. Some physicians felt threatened by women with knowledge, experience, and professional aspirations.

[108]G. Thomas Strickland, ed., *Hunter's Tropical Medicine*, 7th ed. (Philadelphia, 1991), 235; see also Brian Maegraith et al., *Adams & Maegraith: Clinical Tropical Diseases*, 9th ed. (Oxford, 1989), 423.

Chapter 14

[1]Ellis, "The New Orleans Yellow Fever Epidemic in 1878," 189.

[2]*NOM&SJ*, 7 (July, 1850): 67; La Roche, *Yellow Fever*, II, 25, 38.

[3]Ellis, "The New Orleans Yellow Fever Epidemic in 1878," 190. In discussing the psychological dimensions of yellow fever epidemics, Ellis also suggested that "acclimated" New Orleanians developed a "psychic resistance to suffering" by projecting responsibility for the disease on "insignificant others."

[4]La Roche, *Yellow Fever*, II, 64. During the yellow fever epidemic of 1839 in Mobile, fires destroyed one-third of the city, presumably set by unknown arsonists. Several years later, escaped slaves allegedly claimed that blacks had set the fires as part of a conspiracy to take over Mobile during the epidemic. No additional evidence supports their claim, and other explanations have been considered more plausible. Even so, the story suggests that blacks as well as whites thought of epidemics as offering an opportune time for action. See Harriet Amos, *Cotton City: Urban Development in Antebellum Mobile* (University, Ala., 1985), 124, 152.

[5]Savitt, *Medicine and Slavery*, 242-43; *Crescent*, August 11, 1853. Because of their resistance to the fever, blacks were recruited in Memphis during the terrible epidemics of the 1870s to augment a police force greatly diminished by disease and death. Rousey, "Yellow Fever and Black Policemen in Memphis," 357-74.

[6]Ellis, "The Southern Yellow Fever Epidemic of 1878," 21.

[7]See Jo Ann Carrigan, "Yellow Fever: The Scourge of the South," in Todd L. Savitt and James Harvey Young, eds., *Disease and Distinctiveness in the American South* (Knoxville, Tenn., 1988), 55-78.

[8]*NOM&SJ*, 10 (March, 1854): 603.

[9]Gayarré, *History of Louisiana*, IV, 636.

[10]Cable, *The Creoles of Louisiana*, 292.

[11]New Orleans *Daily Delta*, September 10, 1858.

[12]*NOM&SJ*, new series, 14 (June, 1887): 920.

[13]Waring, *Social Statistics of Cities*, 213.

[14]See Chapter 7 and 8 for discussion of "yellow fever panic" in the years after 1878. See also *NOM&SJ*, new series, 11 (September, 1883): ·228-29, for an editorial comment on the new wave of fear in response to yellow fever as a remarkable change in "public sentiment."

[15]William Dosite Postell, "The Medical Societies of Louisiana Prior to the War Between the States," *NOM&SJ*, 93 (August, 1940): 69-72.

16*NOM&SJ*, 10 (September, 1853): 279; (January, 1854): 566.

17Dr. O. H. Spencer to Nathaniel Evans, November 5, 13, 1808, Nathaniel Evans and Family Papers (Louisiana State University Archives, Baton Rouge).

18Duffy, ed., *Parson Clapp*, 106.

19Fenner, *Epidemic Yellow Fever*, 70; see also *Picayune*, August 23, 28, 1839; *NOM&SJ*, 10 (November, 1853): 387.

20Robinson, *Diary of a Samaritan*, 79-80.

21Ibid., 119, 259-60; Earl F. Niehaus, *The Irish in New Orleans, 1800-1860* (Baton Rouge, 1965), 32-33.

22[A. Walker], "History and Incidents of the Plague in New Orleans," *Harper's Magazine*, 7 (June-November, 1853): 806; Robinson, *Diary of a Samaritan*, 119, 259-60.

23Duffy, ed., *Parson Clapp*, 109.

24Joseph B. Stratton Diary, Joseph B. Stratton Papers (Louisiana State University Archives, Baton Rouge), November 22, 1853, January 18, 1854. The London *Times*, August 18, 1853, published a letter from an Episcopal minister in New Orleans to a friend in London, describing conditions and appealing for contributions to the Howard Association. The mortality was "unprecedented," he wrote, and "suffering exceeds anything I have ever witnessed." The minister had visited forty-one sick persons that day, expecting no more than a fourth of them to be alive the next day. "This morning I went into a lonely little hut, and there found the father dead, the mother hugging her babe, only four days old, to her breast, striving to nurse it, while the black vomit was actually streaming from her mouth." The woman died, and the minister took the infant and obtained a black woman "to be its mother."

25Walker, "History and Incidents of the Plague in New Orleans," 806; Stratton Diary, Janurary 18, 1854; Duffy, ed., *Parson Clapp*, 102-4; Autobiography, Emily Caroline Douglas Papers (Louisiana State University Archives, Baton Rouge), 318, 320-22.

26*Picayune*, July 31, 1905. See Chapter 9 for discussion of the clergy's role in the anti-mosquito campaign.

27*Crescent*, August 31, 1853.

28*Picayune*, August 24, 1853.

29Ibid., August 31, 1853.

30Ibid., September 2, 1853.

31*Bee*, November 3, 1841; New Orleans *Democrat*, October 2, 1878; *Picayune*, October 3, 1878.

32*Picayune*, October 7, 1897.

33Ibid., October 25, 1897.

34*American Missionary*, 59 (October, 1905): 242.

35Proceedings of the City Council of New Orleans, Vol. 3, Book 1, June 7, 1817 to December 29, 1818 (W.P.A. typescript, New Orleans Public Library): 40, 48-50; *Louisiana Courier*, September 8, 1819, August 28, 1820, September 6, October 2, 1822; *Picayune*, September 7, 1837, August 10, 1847.

36*DeBow's Review*, 15 (December, 1853): 629; *Crescent*, August 31, 1853; *Picayune*, August 29, 1858.

37*Gardner & Wharton's New Orleans Directory, for the Year 1858* ... (New Orleans, 1857), 389-90; see also *Bee*, October 16, 1858.

38*Bee*, October 20, 1867; *Picayune*, October 20, 1867.

39Blassingame, *Black New Orleans, 1860-1880*, 167-69.

40*Picayune*, September 14, 1878; Baton Rouge *Advocate*, November 29, 1878.

41Sister Mary Francis Borgia Hart, *Violets in the King's Garden: A History of the Sisters of the Holy Family of New Orleans* (New Orleans, 1976), 14, 55-57. Black or mulatto nurses were much in demand during yellow fever epidemics because they were believed to be immune and especially adept at treating yellow fever. See also Ketchum, "Yellow Fever in New Orleans," 137, n.170; Hildreth, "Early Red Cross," 56; Ellis, "The Yellow Fever Epidemic of 1878 in New Orleans," 191.

42*Picayune*, September 9, 1841, August 25, 1878; *Gardner & Wharton's New Orleans Directory for . . . 1858*, 389; Robinson, *Diary of a Samaritan*, 194-95.

43Robinson, *Diary of a Samaritan*, 194, 266.

44Ibid., 194-95; see also Duffy, *Medicine in Louisiana*, II, 205-9, 229-33; 503-7.

45Fortier, *Louisiana*, I, 515; Stuart O. Landry, "New Orleans' Predecessor of Red Cross," New Orleans *Times-Picayune*, Magazine Section, December 19, 26, 1937; Hildreth, "Early Red Cross," 49-75. As early as 1833, a group of young men had organized informally, agreeing to attend to each other and their acquaintances in the event of illness. When an epidemic occurred that year, they extended their aid to "many unfortunates." Inspired by their example, another band, the Society of Good Samaritans, was organized in 1837 to assist the indigent sick. Middle-aged gentlemen and well-established residents, the Samaritans obtained funds from the city government to pay for food and medicines and to hire nurses for those who applied for aid. A more active, youthful group was also formed in 1837 as the Young Men's Howard Association, relying on private donations, and vigorously and systematically seeking out the sick poor throughout the city. It is unclear whether the organizers included the same young men who had attracted notice by their service in 1833. During the next yellow fever epidemic in 1839, as the New Orleans outbreak began to subside, several Howards and Samaritans along with three physicians went to Mobile to assist the yellow fever sufferers in that city. After 1839, the Samaritan Society dissolved, some of its members later serving with the Howard Association, which continued its work and obtained a state charter in 1842. See *Report of the Howard Association of New Orleans, of Receipts, Expenditures, and Their Work in the Epidemic of 1878* . . . (New Orleans, 1878), 5-7; Robinson, *Diary of a Samaritan*, 17-18, 69; *Picayune*, September 21, 1839.

46Hildreth, "Early Red Cross," 51-52, 74-75 (quotation on 74); see also *Jewell's Crescent City Illustrated* (New Orleans, 1874), 44; Robinson, *Diary of a Samaritan*, 17-18, 72, 134-35, 280-85.

47This brief summary of the association's work is largely based on Hildreth's comprehensive article, "Early Red Cross," 49-75; and a contemporary account by a member of the Howards, Robinson's *Diary of a Samaritan*, 72, 125-26, 134-35, 166-67, 280-85, 321-22, and *passim*. See also Fenner, *Epidemic Yellow Fever*, 69-70; *Report of the Howard Association of New Orleans, Epidemic of 1853* (New Orleans, 1853), 3, 23-26; *Report of the Howard Association of New Orleans . . . 1878*, 17-24; Howard Association Memorandum Books, Addendum, 1878, John B. Vinet Papers (Louisiana State University Archives, Baton Rouge). In 1858, the Howard Association appealed only to local sources, attempting to collect only what was needed for that occasion. Sectional pride might also have been a factor. In September, 1858, under the caption, "Foreign aid declined," the *New York Times* quoted a letter from an officer of the Howard Association, published in the *Picayune*, refusing funds offered from Philadelphia and criticizing the YMCA for requesting aid from outsiders: "The Howard Association have the ability and the means to relieve all cases of distress, and, were they wanting, our own citizens would instantly subscribe any required amount. . . . I regard the application of the Young Men's Christian Association for foreign aid as wholly unwarranted, and an unjust reflection upon the proverbially liberal benevolence of our people." *New York Times*, September 21, 1858; see also Robinson, *Diary of a Samaritan*, 322.

[48]*Picayune*, August 31, September 5, 1878.

[49]For a more detailed treatment of the association's problems and its demise, see Hildreth, "Early Red Cross," 67-75; and *Report of the Howard Association of New Orleans . . . 1878*. See also Chapter 7 above for discussion of the complaint against the Howard and Peabody Associations in 1878 by the black relief organization of New Orleans. Similar dissatisfaction with the Howard Association and the Citizens Relief Committee also surfaced in Memphis that year. Both groups were charged with "favoritism and prejudice." Ellis, "The Southern Yellow Fever Epidemic of 1878," 21.

[50]*Picayune*, October 20, 1897; August 13, 1905. In its notice calling for contributions during the epidemic of 1905, the Charity Organization Society declared itself to be "fully organized, with permanent headquarters, perfected machinery, competent investigators, and an intimate knowledge of the poor of this City." Dr. Beverley Warner, the Episcopal minister serving as coordinator of the citizen voluntary organizations, attached a statement to the appeal supporting the work of the central agency and warning that "Emergencies like the present are rich opportunities for the charity 'grafters.' The misfortunes of the sick and poor are made the capital of the lazy and worthless." Warner believed the Charity Organization Society to be "better equipped than any other I know in New Orleans to deal with this important side of the volunteer work." Quoted in Boyce, *Yellow Fever Prophylaxis*, 32. See also Jackson, *New Orleans in the Gilded Age*, 194-95; and Keller, *Affairs of State*, 504.

[51]*DeBow's Review*, 15 (December, 1853): 626; Wharton Diary, August 28, October 1, 7, 1858; *Picayune*, August 29, 1858, September 4, 1867, October 3, 1905.

[52]*DeBow's Review*, 15 (December, 1853): 626; *Picayune*, September 24, 1897.

[53]*NOM&SJ*, 51 (October, 1898): 213; *Picayune*, October 28, 1905.

[54]*Picayune*, October 13, 1905.

[55]*American Missionary*, 59 (October, 1905): 236.

[56]*Report of the Board of Administrators of the Charity Hospital . . . for 1905*, 50, 52.

[57]*Picayune*, October 5, 15, 1905.

[58]Duffy, ed., *Parson Clapp*, 110. See also *NOM&SJ*, 4 (September, 1847): 275; *Bee*, September 16, 1841; *Picayune*, September 12, 1858, for more local praise of local benevolence.

[59]Perrin du Lac, *Travels*, 7.

[60]Robinson, *Diary of a Samaritan*, 162-63, 192-93, 196-97.

[61]*DeBow's Review*, 15 (December, 1853): 624. For discussion of the usual conditions of crime and disorder in the antebellum Crescent City, see Niehaus, *The Irish in New Orleans, 1800-1860*, 59-70; Rousey, "New Orleans Police, 1805-1889," 122-90.

[62]Shotgun quarantines and the 1897 riot in New Orleans have been discussed in Chapter 8.

[63] Walker, "History and Incidents of the Plague in New Orleans," 797.

[64] Rousey, "New Orleans Police, 1805-1889," 10, 12, 54, 57-58, 239-40.

[65] Proceedings of the New Orleans City Council, Vol. 3, Book 1, 1817-1818, 40; *DeBow's Review*, 15 (December, 1853): 615, 620; *Crescent*, August 11, 1853.

[66] Robinson, *Diary of a Samaritan*, 152.

[67] *Crescent*, August 11, 1853.

[68] *Report of the Louisiana State Board of Health for 1878*, 90-93.

[69] Proceedings of the City Council of New Orleans, Vol. 3, Book 1, 1817-1818, 32; Duffy, *Sword of Pestilence*, 71; *Picayune*, September 9, 1867; *Bee*, September 18, 1867.

[70] *DeBow's Review*, 15 (December, 1853): 627-28.

[71] *History of the Yellow Fever in New Orleans, During the Summer of 1853 with Sketches of the Scenes of Horror which Occurred during the Epidemic . . . by a Physician of New Orleans*, 98-99.

[72] Quoted in Rousey, "New Orleans Police, 1805-1889," 56.

[73] Kemp, ed., *Martin Behrman of New Orleans*, 131, 144.

[74] James Dugan, *Doctor Dispachemquic: A Story of the Great Southern Plague of 1878* (New Orleans, 1879).

[75] Dowler, "Tableau of the Yellow Fever of 1853," 62.

[76] Paul H. Hayne, "Dorothy—Gift of God. A Ballad of the New Orleans Plague of 1878" (undated pamphlet in Howard-Tilton Memorial Library, Tulane University, New Orleans); Henry Guy Carleton, "Andromeda Unchained" (1878 clipping in Howard-Tilton Memorial Library, New Orleans); J. F. Simmons, *The Welded Link, and Other Poems* (Philadelphia, 1881).

[77] Simmons, *The Welded Link*, 13-14; *Picayune*, September 22, 1878. Sample lines from Simmons (pp. 24, 32), which my friend Linda Ray Pratt, a poetry specialist, judged to be almost as "horrible" as the epidemic they purported to describe:

> 'Contagion' swept like wave of solid fire—
> Death in its train and desolation dire—
> O'er homes and hearthstones, towns and cities fair,
> And left its countless sad mementoes there.
> . . . .
>
> The busy hum was hushed on mart and street,
> The latter pressed alone by hurrying feet
> Of Good Samaritan or anxious nurse,
> Or—their work ended—overladen hearse.

Chapter 15

[1] Kendall, *History of New Orleans*, I, 132-33.

²Robinson, *Diary of a Samaritan*, 297-98.

³See for example, Latrobe, *Impressions*, 147; *Crescent*, June 22, 1853; *Picayune*, October 8, 1853, October 11, 1867; *Price-Current*, August 20, 27, October 1, 1853; *Bee*, October 22, 1858; Thomas C. Porteous to J. Levois, August-November, 1878, Thomas C. Porteous Letter Book; Smith & Son Company to Smith Company, September 3, October 3, November 14, 1839, October 17, 1840, October 22, 1841, T. Smith and Company Papers; Thomas W. Compton to Charles Mathews, July 4, 1856, Charles L. Mathews Family Papers (Louisiana State University Archives, Baton Rouge).

⁴*Bee*, October 22, 1858. The reference to yellow fever as "the chief drawback to our prosperity" was a common refrain in the writings of New Orleans journalists and physicians from the early 1800s through 1905.

⁵*Bee*, September 15, 1867; *Picayune*, October 11, 1867.

⁶Porteous to Levois, August 3, 1878, Thomas C. Porteous Letter Book.

⁷East, "Health and Wealth," 245-75. See also Porteous to R. Heydenreich, July 18, August 1, September 12, 1879; Porteous to E. Bourbon, July 22, September 2, 23, 1879, Thomas C. Porteous Letter Book, for effects of quarantine even when New Orleans had relatively few cases of yellow fever.

⁸*Picayune*, September 12, 1878.

⁹*DeBow's Review*, 6 (September, 1848): 226; see also J. C. Nott, "An Examination into the Health and Longevity of the Southern Sea Ports of the United States, with reference to the subject of Life Insurance," *Southern Journal of Medicine and Pharmacy*, 2 (March, 1847): 121, 145. According to Nott, anyone acclimated to the diseases of one of the following cities was safe from the fevers of all the others: Charleston, Savannah, Pensacola, Mobile, and New Orleans. He stated that yellow fever and other major causes of death attacked only the unacclimated non-native, that the lowest mortality was always among the better element, and that "it is only the better classes who apply for Life Insurance." He hoped his facts and tables would be taken into account by northern life insurance companies, as he could see no reason to charge more "on southern risks, where the applicants live in the seaport towns, and are acclimated, and if these companies will select faithful agents, and competent, honest, medical examiners."

¹⁰*Picayune*, August 31, September 1, 1839.

¹¹Ibid., July 26, 27, 28, 1878.

¹²Ibid., August 17, 1853; Robinson, *Diary of a Samaritan*, 271-72.

¹³Walter Prichard, ed., "Three Letters of Richard Claiborne to William Miller, 1816-1818," *Louisiana Historical Quarterly*, 24 (July, 1941): 739.

¹⁴Grace King, *New Orleans: The Place and the People* (New York, 1895), 287-88.

¹⁵*Crescent*, August 31, 1853.

¹⁶*Proceedings of the Board of Experts Authorized by Congress . . . 1878*, 31-35; Kelly, *Walter Reed and Yellow Fever*, 239-40.

¹⁷Simonds, "On the Sanitary Condition of New Orleans," 214-15, 237.

¹⁸*DeBow's Review*, 2 (December, 1846): 422; 4 (November, 1847): 400; 16 (February, 1854): 213.

¹⁹*NOM&SJ*, 2 (September, 1845): 129.

[20]Ibid., 3 (September, 1846): 274.

[21]Ibid., 5 (September, 1848): 261.

[22]Ibid., 6 (March, 1850): 666, 672, 676.

[23]Ibid., 7 (March, 1851): 591.

[24]E. H. Barton, "Report upon the Meteorology, Vital Statistics and Hygiene of the State of Louisiana," *Southern Medical Reports*, 2 (1850): 131, 141-43.

[25]Simonds, "On the Sanitary Condition of New Orleans," 242-43; see also *Daily Delta*, June 28, July 2, 3, 4, 9, 11, 12, 13, 18, 1850.

[26]*NOM&SJ*, 4 (November, 1852): 415-16.

[27]*Report of the Louisiana State Board of Health for 1855*, 6-7.

[28]Simonds, "On the Sanitary Condition of New Orleans," 237.

[29]Capers, *Occupied City*, 1. See also *Report on Population of the United States at the Eleventh Census: 1890*, Part I (Washington, D.C., 1895), 370-71, for New Orleans' ranking among the nation's cities from 1810 through 1890. According to the figures provided in the *1840 Census* itself, New Orleans was the fourth largest city. Some of the suburbs must have been included in the later calculations of changing rank over time.

[30]Quoted in Davis, *The Story of Louisiana*, 208.

[31]Ellis, "Businessmen and Public Health," 204-5.

[32]See Joy Jackson, *New Orleans in the Gilded Age: Politics and Urban Progress, 1880-1896* (Baton Rouge, 1969), 208-9. For a thorough analysis of the difficulties faced by antebellum southern cities, including disease, see David R. Goldfield, "Pursuing the American Urban Dream: Cities in the Old South," in Blaine A. Brownell and David R. Goldfield, eds., *The City in Southern History: The Growth of Urban Civilization in the South* (Port Washington, N. Y., 1977), 52-91.

[33]Noting the millions of dollars that disease cost antebellum New Orleans, David Goldfield suggested that the city's relative decline "as a major import-export center during the 1840s and 1850s might not have been solely a result of the diversion of the Mississippi River trade eastward." See his article, "The Business of Health Planning: Disease Prevention in the Old South," *Journal of Southern History*, 42 (November, 1976): 568-69. John Ellis stated flatly that it was not the "dispersion of trade" by railroad development nor was it the Civil War that caused New Orleans demographic and economic decline in the nineteenth century, but the "blighting consequences . . . of pestilence." ("Businessmen and Public Health," 204-5). I agree that the burden of recurring epidemics was a major cause of New Orleans' relative decline, and I suggest that the pestilence itself contributed to the diversion of commerce that injured the city.

[34]Jackson, *New Orleans in the Gilded Age*, 17-19, 209; Howard N. Rabinowitz, "Continuity and Change: Southern Urban Development, 1860-1900," in Brownell and Goldfield, eds., *The City in Southern History*, 103-4. Rabinowitz also noted the serious impact of yellow fever epidemics on Memphis and Mobile, both cities showing an absolute population decline in the 1870s. See also Don Harrison Doyle, "Urbanization and Southern Culture," in Orville Vernon Burton and Robert C. McMath, Jr., eds., *Towards a New South? Studies in Post-Civil War Southern Communities* (Westport, Conn., 1982), 14.

[35]*Proceedings of the Board of Experts Authorized by Congress . . . 1878*, 32-35; Ellis, "The New Orleans

Yellow Fever Epidemic in 1878," 195, 201.

[36]Latrobe, *Impressions*, 146.

[37]Robinson, *Diary of a Samaritan*, 122.

[38]*DeBow's Review*, 15 (December, 1853): 598.

[39]*Report of the Louisiana State Board of Health for 1873*, 74-75.

[40]*Picayune*, April 8, 1852; *Bee*, September 4, 1867.

[41]*Picayune*, July 26, August 19, 1853; *Delta*, August 10, 1858.

[42]*Picayune*, September 29, 1853.

[43]*Times-Democrat*, September 7, 1897; *Picayune*, October 13, 1897.

[44]*Report of the Louisiana State Board of Health for 1879*, 20-21.

[45]*Report of the Louisiana State Board of Health for 1881*, iv.

[46]*Reports and Papers, APHA, 1885*, 11 (Concord, N.H., 1886): 96.

[47]Stanford E. Chaillé, "Vital Statistics of New Orleans," *NOM&SJ*, 23 (January, 1870): 10.

[48]*Times-Democrat*, July 28, 1882.

[49]*City of New Orleans: The Book of the Chamber of Commerce and Industry* . . . (New Orleans, 1894), 17; see also "City of New Orleans" by John R. Ficklen, in *Art Work of New Orleans* (Chicago, 1895), 9.

[50]In the *Times-Democrat*, August 17, 1905, for example, one advertisement read: "Go North via Illinois Central. Absolutely no interruption on account of Quarantine." Fares were listed for Chicago, St. Louis, Louisville, Cincinnati, Denver, San Francisco, Niagara Falls, Saratoga, and Toronto. Many hotels and resorts also ran ads, including several in Chicago, West Virginia, Tennessee, and Yellowstone Park. Steamer lines offered special trips to New York, Philadelphia, and points in Florida. On August 20 the same paper carried additional resort ads—for Hot Springs, Arkansas, and locations in western North Carolina and the Adirondack Mountains of New York.

[51]*Picayune*, October 7, 19, 1905.

[52]In a list of the fifteen main causes of death in New Orleans during the years 1879-1903, compiled by the state board of health, yellow fever placed last. The three leading causes of mortality were tuberculosis, diarrheal disease, and heart disease, in that order. Ketchum, "Yellow Fever in New Orleans," 125, n. 24.

[53]*Louisiana Courier*, November 6, 1811; *Louisiana Gazette*, November 5, 1811.

[54]*NOM&SJ*, 15 (November, 1858): 733.

[55]*Crescent*, August 18, 1853.

[56]See Gillson, *Formative Years*, and *Progressive Years*, for a detailed history of the Louisiana State Board of Health. New Orleans' first comprehensive drainage, sewerage, and water supply systems were finally initiated and pushed to completion largely because of pressure resulting from yellow fever epidemics in 1897

and 1905. Matas, "A Yellow Fever Retrospect and Prospect," 468; Kendall, *History of New Orleans*, II, 525-26, 559, 575-79.

[57] *Reports and Papers, APHA, 1877-1878*, 4 (Boston, 1880): 206; Jones, *Medical and Surgical Memoirs*, III, pt. 1, p. 2.

[58] Gillson, *Progressive Years*, 56-57, 65, 74-75, 119-21, 132, 142-43, 165-66; Ketchum, "Yellow Fever in New Orleans," 58, 83-84, 91-94; Kohnke, "History of Maritime Quarantine in Louisiana against Yellow Fever," 175-79. By the 1890s New Orleans was second only to New York in tropical fruit imports. Jackson, *New Orleans in the Gilded Age*, 213-14.

[59] Minutes, Louisiana State Board of Health, Official Record Book, August, 1898-January, 1903 (History Room, Tulane Medical Library, New Orleans), February 18, April 1, 1902. See also Gillson, *Progressive Years*, 56.

[60] Minutes, Louisiana State Board of Health, February 18, 1902; see also August 10, 22, November 29, 1901.

[61] See Bruton, "The National Board of Health, 1879-1893"; Warner, "Local Control versus National Interest," 407-28; Carrigan, "The National Board of Health"; and Chapter 7 above.

[62] Kemp, ed., *Martin Behrman of New Orleans*, 132, 150.

BIBLIOGRAPHY

Primary Sources

ARCHIVES AND MANUSCRIPTS

Archives Nationales, Paris
    Letter from Louboey to the Minister, October 12, 1739. Colonies C13A, volume 24, folio 204, photocopy.

Center for Louisiana Studies, University of Southwestern Louisiana, Lafayette
    Hilliard-McVea Letters. Typescript copy from private collection of Mrs. Jac Chambliss, Lookout Mountain, Tennessee.

Darlington County Historical Society, Darlington, South Carolina
    Carrigan (William A.) Papers.

Howard-Tilton Memorial Library, Tulane University, New Orleans
    Ferdinand De Feriet Letters.
    New Orleans Board of Health. "Two-hundred and Fifteen Years of Sanitation in New Orleans," *Vox Sanitatis*, II (1933). Vertical File, Louisiana Collections.

Louisiana State Museum Library, New Orleans
    Documents of the City Council of New Orleans, 1823 to 1835, Record Book No. 4084. W. P. A. typescript.
    Records of the City Council of New Orleans, Book 4079, Document 259, October 21, 1796. W. P. A. trans. typescript.
    Records of the City Council of New Orleans and Documents Pertaining to the Government of Louisiana, 1800 to 1803, Book 4088. W. P. A. trans. typescript.
    Records of the City Council of New Orleans, 1815-1822, Book 4089. W. P. A. typescript.

Louisiana State University Archives, Baton Rouge
   Beraud (Joseph) Manuscript, "Guide Homeopathique," 1876.
   Bradford (David) Letters.
   Charles (Isaac H.) Letters.
   Claiborne (William C.C.) Letterbook, 1804-1805.
   Douglas (Emily Caroline) Papers, Autobiography.
   Evans (Nathaniel) Family Papers.
   Gove (A. D.) Letters.
   Jones (Joseph) Papers.
   McGrath (John) Scrapbook.
   McGuire (R. F.) Diary.
   Mathews (Charles L.) Family Papers.
   Pintard (John M.) Papers.
   Police Jury Minutes, Parishes of Acadia, Avoyelles, Caddo, Concordia, East Baton Rouge, East Feliciana, Iberville, Jefferson, Lafayette, Lafourche, Natchitoches, Rapides, St. Bernard, Terrebonne, and West Carroll. W. P. A. transcriptions of Parish Records of Louisiana.
   Pontalba (Joseph X.), "The Letters of Baron Joseph X. Pontalba to his Wife, 1796." W. P. A. trans. typescript.
   Porteous (Thomas C.) Letter Book.
   Smith (T.) & Company Papers.
   Stratton (Joseph B.) Papers.
   Town (Clarissa E. Leavitt) Diary.
   Vinet (John B.) Papers, Addendum.
   Wharton (Thomas K.) Diary.

New Orleans Public Library
   Coroner's Office, Record of Inquests and Views, 1844-1904.
   Digest of the Acts and Deliberations of the Cabildo, 1769-1808, A Record of the Spanish Government in New Orleans. W. P. A. typescript.
   Proceedings of the City Council of New Orleans, Vol. 3, Book 1, June 7, 1817, to December 29, 1818. W. P. A. typescript.
   Resolutions and Ordinances of the City Council of New Orleans, December 24, 1816, to February 19, 1821. W. P. A. typescript.

Rudolph Matas Library, Tulane University Medical Center, New Orleans
   Official Records, Louisiana State Board of Health, 1880s.

Scrapbooks, Louisiana State Board of Health.

Minutes, Louisiana State Board of Health, Official Record Book, 1898-1903.

PUBLIC DOCUMENTS

United States

Bache, Thomas Hewson. *Some Practical Observations on Yellow Fever: Published for the Use of Surgeons of the Volunteer Forces in the Department of the Gulf.* New Orleans: s.n., 1862.

Carter, Clarence E., ed. *The Territorial Papers of the United States*, Vol. IX, *The Territory of Orleans, 1803-1812*. Washington, D.C.: Government Printing Office, 1940.

Chaillé, Stanford E. *The Louisiana State Board of Health in its Annual Report for 1881 Versus the National Board of Health, Reply in Behalf of the Latter.* New Orleans: L. Graham & Son, 1882.

National Board of Health. *Annual Report of the National Board of Health.* Washington, D.C.: Government Printing Office, 1879-1886.

National Board of Health. *Bulletin of the National Board of Health*, 1879-1882.

Report of the Public Health and Marine-Hospital Service, 1905, 59th Cong., 1st sess., 1905, *House Documents*, Vol. 84, No. 320.

Report of the Public Health and Marine-Hospital Service, 1906, 59th Cong., 2nd sess., 1906-1907, *House Documents*, Vol. 49, No. 199.

Report on Population of the United States at the Eleventh Census: 1890, Pt. I. Washington, D.C.: Government Printing Office, 1895.

Rowland, Dunbar, ed. *Official Letter Books of William C. C. Claiborne, 1801-1816.* 6 Vols. Jackson, Miss.: Mississippi Department of Archives and History, 1917.

Sternberg, George M. *Report on the Etiology and Prevention of Yellow Fever*. Washington, D.C.: Government Printing Office, 1890.

United States Board of Experts. *Proceedings of the Board of Experts Authorized by Congress, to Investigate the Yellow Fever Epidemic of 1878: Meeting Held in Memphis, Tenn., December 26th, 27th, 28th, 1878*. New Orleans: L. Graham, 1878.

United States Marine-Hospital Service. *Report of the Commission of Medical Officers Detailed by Authority of the President to Investigate the Cause of Yellow Fever*. Washington, D.C.: Government Printing Office, 1899.

_____. *Yellow Fever: Its Nature, Diagnosis, Treatment, and Prophylaxis, and Quarantine Regulations Relating Thereto*, by Officers of the United States Marine Hospital Service. Washington, D.C., 1898. Reprinted in Barbara Gutmann Rosenkrantz, *et al.*, eds. *Yellow Fever Studies*. New York: Arno Press, 1977.

_____. *Annual Report of the Supervising Surgeon-General of the Marine-Hospital Service of the United States for the Fiscal Year 1897*. Washington, D.C.: Government Printing Office, 1899.

United States Public Health Service. *Annual Report of the Surgeon-General of the Public Health and Marine-Hospital Service of the United States for the Fiscal Year 1907*, 60th Cong., 1st sess., 1907-1908, *House Documents*, Vol. 83, No. 456.

United States Public Health Service. *Yellow Fever: Its Epidemiology, Prevention, and Control*. Lectures delivered at the United States Public Health Service School of Instruction by H. R. Carter, Senior Surgeon, USPHS. Washington, D.C., 1914. Reprinted in Barbara Gutmann Rosenkrantz, *et al.*, eds. *Yellow Fever Studies*. New York: Arno Press, 1977.

United States Surgeon General's Office. *Medical and Surgical History of the War of the Rebellion (1861-65)*, Pt. III, Vol. I. Washington, D.C.: Government Printing Office, 1888.

Waring, George E., Jr. "The Southern and Western States," *Report of the Social Statistics of Cities, Tenth Census, 1880*, XIX, pt. 2. Washington, D.C.: Government Printing Office, 1887.

Yellow Fever: A Compilation of Various Publications, 61st Cong., 3rd sess., 1910-1911, *Senate Documents*, Vol. 61, No. 822.

Louisiana

Acts Passed by the ... Legislature of the State of Louisiana ... , 1818, 1819, 1821, 1824, 1848, 1850, 1855, and 1858.

Acts Passed by the General Assembly of the State of Louisiana ... , 1870, 1876, 1877, 1878, 1882, 1884, and 1890.

Louisiana State Board of Health. *Investigation and Refutation of Certain Statements and Charges Made ... by the National Board of Health in Its Annual Report for the Year 1882*. New Orleans: Louisiana Board of Health, 1883.

_____. *Outbreak of Yellow Fever at Biloxi, Harrison County, Miss., and Its Relation to Interstate Notification*. New Orleans: Louisiana Board of Health, 1886.

_____. *The Sanitary Code, 1899*. New Orleans: Louisiana Board of Health, 1899.

New Orleans Board of Health. *Official Report of the Deaths from Yellow Fever, Alphabetically Arranged, Gives the Name, Nativity, Residence, and Date of Death of Each and Every One Who Died During the Terrible Epidemic of 1878. ...* New Orleans, n.d.

New Orleans Sanitary Commission. *Report of the Sanitary Commission of New Orleans on the Epidemic Yellow Fever, of 1853*. New Orleans:

New Orleans *Daily Picayune*, 1854.

Reports of the Board of Administrators of the Charity Hospital to the General Assembly of the State of Louisiana. 1897, 1905.

Reports of the Louisiana State Board of Health to the General Assembly of the State of Louisiana. 1855-1907.

NEWSPAPERS

Alexandria
   Louisiana Herald, 1820-1825.
   Red River Republican, 1847, 1853.

Baton Rouge
   Advocate, 1847, 1878, 1897.

Lake Providence
   Sentry, 1905.

London
   Times, 1853.

New Iberia
   Sugar Bowl, 1878, transcriptions.
   Weekly Iberian, 1906.

New Orleans
   Bee, 1829, 1833, 1837, 1839, 1841, 1847, 1858, 1867; *L'Abeille*, 1905.
   Daily Crescent, 1853.
   Daily Delta, 1850, 1853, 1858.
   Daily Picayune, 1837-1905.
   Daily True Delta, 1862.
   Democrat, 1878.
   Louisiana Courier, 1811, 1817, 1819, 1820-1825, 1827, 1829, 1832, 1833.
   Louisiana Gazette, 1804-1805, 1811, 1817, 1819, 1820, 1822, 1824.
   Price-Current and Commercial Intelligencer, 1837, 1841, 1843, 1853-

1855, 1858.
Times-Democrat, 1882, 1897, 1905.
Weekly Delta, 1853.
Weekly Louisianian, 1878.

New York
Times, 1856, 1858, 1897, 1905.

Plaquemine
Iberville South, 1867.

St. Francisville
Asylum and Feliciana Advertiser, 1821-1825.

Shreveport
Journal, 1897, 1905.

Thibodaux
Lafourche Comet, 1905.
Sentinel, 1878.

Vermillionville
Lafayette Advertiser, 1878.

PERIODICALS

Medical

Medical Repository (New York), 1797-1824.

Monthly Journal of Medicine (Hartford, Conn.), 1823-1825.

New Orleans Medical and Surgical Journal, 1844-1910.

New Orleans Medical News and Hospital Gazette, 1854-1861.

New Orleans Monthly Medical Register, 1851-1853.

Southern Medical Reports, 1849-1850.

General

American Missionary, 1878, 1905.

De Bow's Review, 1846-1880.

Niles' Weekly Register, 1811-1848.

CITY DIRECTORIES AND GUIDES

City of New Orleans: The Book of the Chamber of Commerce and Industry of Louisiana. . . . New Orleans: George W. Engelhardt, Publisher, 1894.

Cohen's New Orleans Directory, including Jefferson City, Carrollton, Gretna, Algiers, and McDonough, for 1854. New Orleans: New Orleans *Daily Picayune*, 1854.

Ficklen, John R. "City of New Orleans," *Art Work of New Orleans*. Chicago: W. H. Parish, 1895.

Gardner, Charles. *Gardner's New Orleans Directory, 1861.* . . . New Orleans: Gardner, 1861.

_____. *Gardner's New Orleans Directory, 1868.* . . . New Orleans: Gardner, 1868.

_____. *Gardner and Wharton's New Orleans Directory, for the Year 1858.* . . . New Orleans: Printed at E.C. Wharton's, 1857.

Gibson, John. *Gibson's Guide and Directory of the State of Louisiana and the Cities of New Orleans and Lafayette, 1838.* New Orleans: Gibson, 1838.

Jewell, Edwin L., ed. *Jewell's Crescent City Illustrated.* New Orleans:

Privately printed, 1874.

New Orleans Directory for 1842. . . . New Orleans: Pitts & Clarke, 1842.

Paxton, John Adams. *Paxton's New Orleans Directory and Register, 1822.* New Orleans: Benj. Levy, 1822.

Zacharie, James S. *New Orleans Guide, with Descriptions of the Routes to New Orleans, Sights of the City Arranged Alphabetically, and Other Information Useful to Travellers.* . . . New Orleans: F. F. Hansell & Brother, 1893.

BOOKS, PAMPHLETS, AND REPORTS

Atlanta Convention of the South Atlantic and Gulf States. *Uniform Regulations for the Management of Yellow Fever Epidemics. Unanimously Adopted and Recommended to the People, April 12, 1898. Revised at a Conference held in the City of New Orleans on February 9, 1899.* New Orleans: L. Graham & Son, 1899.

Bartlett, Elisha. *The History, Diagnosis, and Treatment of the Fevers of the United States.* 4th ed. Philadelphia: A. Clark, 1856.

Barton, Edward Hall. *Account of the Epidemic Yellow Fever, Which Prevailed in New Orleans during the Autumn of 1833.* Philadelphia: Joseph R.A. Skerrett, 1834.

_____. *An Address Before the Louisiana State Medical Society.* New Orleans: H. Spencer, 1851.

_____. *The Cause and Prevention of Yellow Fever, Contained in the Report of the Sanitary Commission of New Orleans.* Philadelphia: Lindsay and Blakiston, 1855.

_____. *Introductory Lecture on Acclimation, Delivered at the Opening of the Third Session of the Medical College of Louisiana.* New Orleans: Commercial Bulletin Printing, 1837.

Berquin-Duvallon. *Vue de la Colonie Espagnole du Mississippi ou des Provinces de la Louisiane . . . en l'année 1802.* Paris: Imprimerie Expeditive, 1803. Trans. by John Davis as *Travels in Louisiana and the Floridas, in the year, 1802.* . . . New York: I. Riley & Co., 1806.

Butler, Benjamin Franklin. *Autobiography and Personal Reminiscences of Major-General Benj. F. Butler: Butler's Book.* Boston: A. M. Thayer, 1892.

Carter, Henry Rose. *Yellow Fever: An Epidemiological and Historical Study of its Place of Origin.* Edited by Laura Armistead Carter and Wade Hampton Frost. Baltimore: Williams & Wilkins, 1931.

Cartier, A. J. F. *La Fièvre Jaune de la Nouvelle-Orléans.* Paris: J. B. Baillière *et fils*, 1859.

Chabert, Jean Louis. *Réflexions Médicales sur le Maladie Spasmodico-Lipyrienne des Pay Chauds Vulgairement Appelée Fièvre Jaune.* Nouvelle-Orléans: Ami des Lois, 1821.

Chisholm, Colin. *A Letter to John Haygarth . . . from Colin Chisholm . . . author of An Essay on the Pestilential Fever: Exhibiting Farther Evidence of the Infectious Nature of This Fatal Distemper in Granada, during 1793, 4, 5, and 6, and in the United States of America, from 1793 to 1805.* . . . London: J. Mawman, 1809.

Commercial and Statistical Almanac, Containing a History of the Epidemic of 1878, with the Best Known Remedies and Treatments of Yellow Fever. . . . New Orleans: F. F. Hamsell, 1879.

Deléry, François Charles. *Memoire sur l'Epidémie de Fièvre Jaune, qui a Regné à la Nouvelle-Orléans et dans les Campagnes pendant l'Année 1867.* New Orleans: Marchand, 1867.

_____. *Précis Historique de la Fièvre Jaune.* Nouvelle-Orléans: Imprimerie Franco-Américaine, 1859.

Dromgoole, John Parham. *Yellow Fever Heroes, Honors, and Horrors of*

1878. Louisville, Ky.: John P. Morton & Co., 1879.

Durac, D. *De La Fièvre Jaune et des Epidémies de 1853, 1854, et 1858 dans la paroisse Lafourche.* Nouvelle-Orléans: Imprimerie de l'Estafette du Sud, 1863.

Faget, Jean Charles. *Monographie sur le Type et la Spécificité de la Fièvre Jaune, Etablis avec l'Aide de la Montre et du Thermomètre.* Paris: Baillière, 1875.

Fenner, Erasmus Darwin. *History of the Epidemic Yellow Fever, at New Orleans, Louisiana, in 1853.* New York: Hall and Clayton, 1854.

Finlay, Carlos Juan. *El Mosquito Hipoteticamente Considerado como Agente de Transmision de la Fiebre Amarilla.* Habana: Imprenta la antilla, 1881.

Gazzo, John B. C. *Yellow Fever Facts as to its Nature, Prevention and Treatment.* New Orleans: Dunn, 1878.

Gros, Adrien Armand, et N. V. A. Gérardin. *Rapport fait a la Société Médicale sur la Fièvre Jaune qui a regné d'une Maniere Epidémique pendant l'Eté de 1817.* Nouvelle-Orléans: J. C. de St. Romes, 1818.

Hardenstein, Ernest. *The Epidemic of 1878 and its Homeopathic Treatment: A General History of the Origin, Progress, and End of the Plague in the Mississippi Valley.* New Orleans: J. S. Rivers, 1879.

Hayes, John James. *Yellow Fever: Its Nature, Cause, Prevention & Cure.* New Orleans: Rea's Rotary Press Office, 1858.

_____. *Yellow Fever: A Treatise on its Cause, Nature, Prevention and Cure....* New Orleans: T. H. Thomason, 1879.

Heustis, Jabez W. *Physical Observations and Medical Tracts and Researches, on the Topography and Diseases of Louisiana.* New York: T. and J. Swords, 1817.

History of the Yellow Fever in New Orleans, During the Summer of 1853, With Sketches of the Scenes of Horror Which Occurred during the Epidemic . . . by a Physician of New Orleans. Philadelphia and St. Louis: C. W. Kenworthy, 1854.

Holcombe, William H. *On the Treatment, Diet, and Nursing of Yellow Fever, for Popular Use.* New York: Boericks, n.d.

_____. *Yellow Fever and Its Homeopathic Treatment.* New York: W. Radde, 1856.

Holt, Joseph. *The Quarantine System of Louisiana, Methods of Disinfection Practiced. With Illustrations. An Addendum to the Report of the Committee on Disinfectants of the American Public Health Association. . . .* New Orleans: L. Graham, [1887].

_____. *Quarantine and Commerce. Their Antagonism Destructive to the Prosperity of City and State. A Reconciliation an Imperative Necessity. How This May be Accomplished. Remarks of the President of the Board of Health of the State of Louisiana, before the Representatives of the Exchanges and other Commercial Bodies. . . .* New Orleans: L. Graham & Son, [1884].

Homeopathic Relief Association of New Orleans. *Report . . . with Valuable Papers on Yellow Fever . . . 1878.* New Orleans: Nelson, [1878].

Howard Association of New Orleans. *Report of the Howard Association of New Orleans, Epidemic of 1853.* New Orleans: Sherman, 1853.

_____. *Report of the Howard Association of New Orleans, of Receipts, Expenditures, and Their Work in the Epidemic of 1878. . . .* New Orleans: Hyatt, 1878.

Jones, Joseph. *Medical and Surgical Memoirs, Containing Investigations on the Geographical Distribution, Causes, Nature, Relations and Treatment of Various Diseases.* 3 Vols. in 4. New Orleans: Clark & Hofeline, 1876-1890.

_____. *The Relation of Quarantine to Commerce in the Valley of the Mississippi River, During a Period of Eight Years, 1880-1887.* . . . New Orleans: L. Graham & Son, 1889.

La Roche, Réné. *Yellow Fever, Considered in its Historical, Pathological, Etiological and Therapeutical Relations.* . . . 2 Vols. Philadelphia: Blanchard & Lee, 1855.

Latrobe, Benjamin. *Impressions Respecting New Orleans, Diary and Sketches, 1818-1820.* Edited with introduction by Samuel Wilson, Jr. New York: Columbia University Press, 1951.

Lee, J. N. *Life. The Philosophy of its Origin and Preservation. A Brief Outline of the Fundamental Principles of Scientific Medicine. The Nature of Endemic Yellow Fever . . . with an Infallible, Preventive and Cure for it, as well as the Epidemic Yellow Fever.* . . . New Orleans: R. B. May, 1883.

Lyell, Charles. *A Second Visit to the United States of North America.* 2 Vols. New York: Harper & Bros., 1849.

McFarlane, J. S. *A Review of the Yellow Fever, Its Causes, etc., and an Interesting and Useful Abstract of Mortuary Statistics.* New Orleans: True Delta, 1853.

McGown, Thompson. *A Practical Treatise on the Most Common Diseases of the South: Exhibiting their Peculiar Nature and the Corresponding Adaptation of Treatment.* Philadelphia: Grigg, Elliot & Co., 1849.

Martineau, Harriet. *Retrospect of Western Travel.* 2 Vols. Cincinnati: U.P. James, 1838.

Milner, U. R. *Yellow Fever, not Imported, nor Contagious, but Indigenous, and Intrinsically Identical with our Paludal Fevers. Preventable by Well Determined and Wisely Executed Local Sanitary Measures. Quarantine a Wide-spread Calamity, and Should no Longer be Tolerated. A Lecture before the Academy of Sciences of New Orleans . . . 1879.* New Orleans: M. Jones Scott, 1880.

Olmsted, Frederick Law. *The Cotton Kingdom: A Traveller's Observations on Cotton and Slavery in the American Slave States.* Edited with introduction by Arthur M. Schlesinger. New York: Knopf, 1953.

Orleans Central Relief Committee. *Report of the Orleans Central Relief Committee to all Those who have so Generously Contributed to the Yellow Fever Sufferers of New Orleans, from the Great Epidemic of 1878.* New Orleans: Clark & Hofeline, 1879.

Orleans Parish Medical Society. *Circular of Information Addressed to the Medical Profession for Distribution Among Trained Nurses and Others Entrusted with the Care of Yellow Fever Patients.* New Orleans: Dameron-Pierson Co., 1905.

Perrin du Lac, François Marie. *Voyage dans les Deux Louisianes et chez les nations sauvages du Missouri, par les Etats-Unis, l'Ohio et les provinces qui le bordent, en 1801, 1802, et 1803. . . .* Paris: Capelle et Renard, 1805. Translated as *Travels Through the Two Louisianas . . . in 1801, 1802, and 1803.* London: J. G. Barnard, 1807.

Physico-Medical Society of New Orleans. *Report of the Committee of the Physico-Medical Society of New Orleans, on the Epidemic of 1820.* New Orleans: C.W. Duhy, 1821.

Reports and Papers of the American Public Health Association. Vols. 1-30. 1873-1905.

Robinson, William L. *The Diary of a Samaritan, By a Member of the Howard Association.* New York: Harper & Bros., 1860.

Salomon, Lucien F. *The Treatment of Yellow Fever.* New Orleans: [Author?], 1905.

Schmidt, Henry D. *The Pathology and Treatment of Yellow Fever, with Some Remarks upon the Nature of its Cause and its Prevention.* Chicago: Chicago Medical Press Association, 1881.

Shew, Joel. *The Water-Cure Manual: A Popular Work*. . . . New York: Fowlers and Wells, 1850.

Shreveport Medical Society. *Report of the Committee appointed by the Shreveport Medical Society on the Yellow Fever Epidemic of 1873 at Shreveport, Louisiana*. Shreveport: Simmons, 1874.

Sinclair, Harold. *The Port of New Orleans*. Garden City, N. Y.: Doubleday, Doran & Co., 1942.

Smith, Ashbel. *Yellow Fever in Galveston, Republic of Texas, 1839; An Account of the Great Epidemic, Together With a Biographical Sketch by Chauncey D. Leake, And Stories of the Men Who Conquered Yellow Fever*. Austin, Tex.: University of Texas Press, 1951.

Smith, Henry. *Report of the Yellow Fever Epidemic of 1873, Shreveport, Louisiana*. . . . New Orleans: Graham, 1874.

Société Médicale de la Nouvelle-Orléans. *Rapport publié au nom de la Société Médicale de la Nouvelle-Orléans sur la Fièvre Jaune, qui y a regné Epidémiquement, durant l'Eté et l'Automne de 1819*. Nouvelle-Orléans: James M'Karaher, 1820.

Souchon, Edmond. *Educational Points Concerning Yellow Fever*. . . . New Orleans: Palfrey, 1898.

_____. *Instructions to Laymen who may have to Manage Yellow Fever Cases in Default of a Physician. Also Recommendations to Physicians Inexperienced in the Treatment of Yellow Fever with Regard to the Use of Medicines*. New Orleans: L. Graham & Son, 1898.

_____. *Instructions to Medical Inspectors and to Health Officers for the Management of Yellow Fever*. New Orleans: L. Graham & Son, 1898.

Stoddard, Amos. *Sketches, Historical and Descriptive, of Louisiana*. Philadelphia: M. Carey, 1812.

Thomas, Pierre Frederic. *Essai sur la Fièvre Jaune d'Amérique, ou,*

Considerations sur les causes, les symptômes, la nature et le traitement de cette maladie, avec l'Histoire de l'Epidémie de la Nouvelle-Orléans en 1822. . . . Paris: Baillière, 1823.

Touatre, Just. *Yellow Fever: Clinical Notes by Just Touatre.* Trans. by Charles L. Chassaignac. New Orleans: New Orleans Medical and Surgical Journal, 1898.

Yellow Fever Statistics. Undated pamphlet. Tulane University Medical Library, New Orleans.

Articles

Agramonte, Aristides. "The Inside Story of a Great Medical Discovery," *Scientific Monthly* (December, 1915): 209-37. Reprinted in Barbara Gutmann Rosenkrantz, et al., eds. *Yellow Fever Studies.* New York: Arno Press, 1977.

Barton, Edward Hall. "Annual Report of the New Orleans Board of Health [1849]," *Southern Medical Reports*, 1 (1849): 77-106.

_____. "Sanitary Report of New Orleans, Louisiana," *Transactions of the American Medical Association*, 2 (1849): 591-610.

Beugnot, J. F. "An Essay on Yellow Fever," *New Orleans Medical Journal*, 1 (May, 1844): 1-28.

Billings, J. S. "National Public Health Legislation," *American Journal of the Medical Sciences*, 78 (October, 1879): 471-79.

Butler, Benjamin Franklin. "Some Experiences with Yellow Fever and its Prevention," *North American Review*, 147 (November, 1888): 528-41.

Cabell, James L. "A Review of the Operations of the National Board of Health," *Reports and Papers, American Public Health Association, 1882*, VIII:71-101.

Chaillé, Stanford E. "The Vital Statistics of New Orleans as Taught by the U. S. Census, 1880," *New Orleans Medical and Surgical Journal*, 33 (May, 1881): 1027-39.

_____. "Vital Statistics of New Orleans," *New Orleans Medical and Surgical Journal*, 23 (January, 1870): 1-65.

_____. "Acclimatisation, or Acquisition of Immunity from Yellow Fever," *New Orleans Medical and Surgical Journal*, new series, 8 (August, 1880): 101-36.

Cronkrite, Lyman. "An Inquiry into the Pathology and Treatment of Yellow Fever, as it Prevails at New Orleans at this Time, August, 1829," *Western Journal of the Medical and Physical Sciences*, 3 (1830): 367-93.

Dowler, Bennet. "Tableau of the Yellow Fever of 1853, with Topographical, Chronological and Historical Sketches of the Epidemics of New Orleans," *Cohen's New Orleans Directory . . . of 1854*. New Orleans, 1854.

Fenner, Erasmus Darwin. "Remarks on the Sanitary Condition of the City of New Orleans, during the period of Federal Military Occupation, from May 1862 to March 1866," *Southern Journal of the Medical Sciences*, 1 (May, 1866): 22-25.

_____. "Report on the Epidemics of Louisiana, Mississippi, Arkansas, and Texas in the year 1853," *Transactions of the American Medical Association*, 7 (1854): 421-553.

_____. "The Yellow Fever Quarantine at New Orleans," *Transactions of the American Medical Association*, 2 (1849): 623-34.

Finlay, Charles. "Yellow Fever: Its Transmission by Means of the Culex Mosquito," *American Journal of the Medical Sciences*, 92 (1886): 395-409.

Harris, Elisha. "Hygienic Experience in New Orleans during the War:

Illustrating the Importance of Efficient Sanitary Regulations," *Southern Journal of the Medical Sciences*, 1 (May, 1866): 25-37.

Hunt, Belle. "New Orleans, Yesterday and today," *Frank Leslie's Popular Monthly*, 31 (June, 1891): 641-45.

Jones, Joseph. "Yellow Fever Epidemic of 1878 in New Orleans," *New Orleans Medical and Surgical Journal*, new series, 6 (March, 1879): 683-715.

Kohnke, Quitman. "History of Maritime Quarantine in Louisiana against Yellow Fever," *New Orleans Medical and Surgical Journal*, 56 (September, 1903): 167-80.

LeHardy, J. C. "The Yellow Fever Panic," *Atlanta Medical and Surgical Journal*, 5 (1888-89): 605-16.

McMain, Eleanor. "Behind the Yellow Fever in Little Palermo: Housing Conditions Which New Orleans Should Shake Itself Free From Along With The Summer's Scourge," *Charities*, 15 (1905): 152-59.

Nott, J. C. "An Examination into the Health and Longevity of the Southern Sea Ports of the United States, with reference to the subject of Life Insurance," *Southern Journal of Medicine and Pharmacy*, 2 (March, 1847): 121-45.

_____. "Sketch of the Epidemic of Yellow Fever of 1847, in Mobile," *Charleston Medical Journal and Review*, 3 (January, 1848): 14-21. Reprinted in Barbara Gutmann Rosenkrantz, *et al.*, eds. *Yellow Fever Studies*. New York: Arno Press, 1977.

Randolph, Robert C. "Remarks on the Endemic Yellow Fever of New-Orleans during the summer and autumn of 1822," *Medical Repository* (New York), new series, 8 (1824): 165-72.

Reed, Walter. "The Propagation of Yellow Fever: Observations Based on Recent Researches," *Medical Record*, 60 (August 10, 1901): 201-9.

_____, et al. "The Etiology of Yellow Fever: A Preliminary Note," *Philadelphia Medical Journal*, 6 (October 27, 1900): 790-96.

Schmidt, Henry D. "On the Pathology of Yellow Fever. . .," *New York Medical Journal*, 29 (February, 1879): 113-56.

Simonds, J. C. "On the Sanitary Condition of New Orleans, as Illustrated by its Mortuary Statistics," *Southern Medical Reports*, 2 (1850): 204-46.

_____. "Report on the Hygienic Characteristics of New Orleans," *Transactions of the American Medical Association*, 3 (1850): 267-90.

_____. "The Sanitary Condition of New-Orleans, as Illustrated by its Mortuary Statistics," *Charleston Medical Journal and Review*, 6 (1851): 677-745.

Stark, James. "Vital Statistics of New Orleans," *Edinburgh Medical and Surgical Journal* (January, 1851): 130-44.

Toner, J. M. "Reports Upon Yellow Fever: The Distribution and Natural History of Yellow Fever as it has Occurred at Different Times in the United States," *Reports and Papers of the American Public Health Association, 1873*, 1 (1875): 359-84.

[Walker, A.] "History and Incidents of the Plague in New Orleans," *Harper's Magazine*, 7 (June-November, 1853): 797-806.

Waring, George E., Jr. "The National Board of Health," *Nation*, 29 (August 21, 1879): 123-24.

White, C. B. "The Yellow Fever Epidemic at New Orleans in 1878," *Reports and Papers of the American Public Health Association*, 7 (1881): 201-4.

FICTION AND POETRY

Carleton, Henry Guy. "Andromeda Unchained." New Orleans, 1878, clipping in Howard-Tilton Memorial Library, Tulane University.

New Orleans.

Dugan, James. *Doctor Dispachemquic: A Story of the Great Southern Plague of 1878*. New Orleans: Clark & Hofeline, 1879.

Hayne, Paul H. "Dorothy—Gift of God. A Ballad of the New Orleans Plague of 1878." Undated pamphlet in Howard-Tilton Memorial Library, Tulane University, New Orleans.

Simmons, J. F. *The Welded Link, and Other Poems*. Philadelphia: J. B. Lippincott & Co., 1881.

Secondary Works

BOOKS AND REFERENCE WORKS

Ackerknecht, Erwin H. *A Short History of Medicine*. Rev. ed. New York: Ronald Press, 1968.

_____, *Medicine at the Paris Hospital, 1794-1848*. Baltimore: Johns Hopkins Press, 1967.

Amos, Harriet. *Cotton City: Urban Development in Antebellum Mobile*. University, Ala.: University of Alabama Press, 1985.

Augustin, George. *History of Yellow Fever*. New Orleans: Searcy & Pfaff, Ltd., 1909.

Bean, William B. *Walter Reed: A Biography*. Charlottesville, Va.: University Press of Virginia, 1982.

Blassingame, John W. *Black New Orleans, 1860-1880*. Chicago: University of Chicago Press, 1973.

Boshell, Jorge, *et al. Yellow Fever: A Symposium in Commemoration of Carlos Juan Finlay*. Philadelphia: Jefferson Medical College, 1955.

Boyce, Sir Rubert William. *Yellow Fever Prophylaxis in New Orleans, 1905.* London: Williams & Norgate, [1906].

Brown, Richard D. *Modernization: The Transformation of American Life, 1600-1865.* New York: Hill and Wang, 1976.

Brownell, Blaine A., and David R. Goldfield, eds. *The City in Southern History: The Growth of Urban Civilization in the South.* Port Washington, N. Y.: Kennikat Press, 1977.

Burnet, Frank Macfarlane, and David O. White. *Natural History of Infectious Disease.* 4th ed. Cambridge, England: Cambridge University Press, 1972.

Burton, Orville Vernon, and Robert C. McMath, Jr., eds. *Toward a New South? Studies in Post-Civil War Southern Communities.* Westport, Conn.: Greenwood Press, 1982.

Cable, George W. *The Creoles of Louisiana.* New York: C. Scribner's Sons, 1884.

Capers, Gerald. *Occupied City: New Orleans Under the Federals, 1862-1865.* Lexington, Ky.: University of Kentucky Press, 1965.

Cassedy, James H. *American Medicine and Statistical Thinking, 1800-1860.* Cambridge, Mass.: Harvard University Press, 1984.

Chambers, Henry E. *A History of Louisiana.* 3 Vols. Chicago and New York: American Historical Society, 1925.

Claiborne, J. F. H. *Mississippi, As a Province, Territory and State: With Biographical Notes of Eminent Citizens.* Reprint ed. Baton Rouge, La.: Claitor's Publishing, 1964.

Clark, John G. *New Orleans, 1718-1812: An Economic History.* Baton Rouge, La.: Louisiana State University Press, 1970.

Davis, Edwin Adams, ed. *Plantation Life in the Florida Parishes of*

Louisiana, 1836-1846, as Reflected in the Diary of Bennet H. Barrow. New York: Columbia University Press, 1943.

_____. *The Story of Louisiana*. Vol. 1. New Orleans: J. F. Hyer Publishing Co., 1960.

Delaporte, François. *The History of Yellow Fever: An Essay on the Birth of Tropical Medicine*. Trans. by Arthur Goldhammer (Cambridge, Mass.: MIT Press, 1991).

Dubos, René, Jr. *Pasteur and Modern Science*. Garden City, N. Y.: Anchor Books, 1960.

Duffy, John. *Epidemics in Colonial America*. Baton Rouge, La.: Louisiana State University Press, 1953.

_____, ed. *Parson Clapp of the Strangers' Church of New Orleans*. Baton Rouge: Louisiana State University Press, 1957.

_____. *Sword of Pestilence: The New Orleans Yellow Fever Epidemic of 1853*. Baton Rouge, La.: Louisiana State University Press, 1966.

_____. *The Healers: A History of American Medicine*. Urbana, Ill.: University of Illinois Press, 1979.

_____, ed. *The Rudolph Matas History of Medicine in Louisiana*. 2 Vols. Baton Rouge, La.: Louisiana State University Press, 1958-1962.

Fortier, Alcée. *A History of Louisiana*. 4 Vols. New York: Manzi, Joyant & Co., 1904.

_____. *History of Louisiana*. Edited with commentary by Jo Ann Carrigan. 2nd ed. Vol II. Baton Rouge, La.: Claitor's Book Store, 1972.

_____. *Louisiana, Comprising Sketches of Parishes, Towns, Events, Institutions, and Persons, Arranged in Cyclopedic Order*. 3 Vols. Madison, Wis.: Century Historical Association, 1914.

Fox, John P., Carrie E. Hall, and Lila R. Elveback. *Epidemiology: Man and Disease*. New York: Macmillan, 1970.

Garrison, Fielding H. *John Shaw Billings: A Memoir*. New York: G. P. Putnam's Sons, 1915.

Gayarré, Charles. *History of Louisiana*. 4 Vols. Reprint ed. New Orleans: Pelican Press, 1965.

Gillson, Gordon E. *Louisiana State Board of Health: The Formative Years*. Baton Rouge: Louisiana State Board of Health, 1967.

_____. *Louisiana State Board of Health: The Progressive Years*. Baton Rouge: Louisiana State Board of Health, 1976.

Harre, Rom. *Great Scientific Experiments: Twenty Experiments That Changed Our View of the World*. New York: Oxford University Press, 1983.

Hart, Mary Francis Borgia. *Violets in the King's Garden: A History of the Sisters of the Holy Family of New Orleans*. New Orleans: Privately printed, 1976.

Hoffman, F. L. *Vital Statistics of New Orleans, 1787-1909*. New York: Author, 1913.

Huber, Leonard V., and Guy F. Bernard. *To Glorious Immortality: The Rise and Fall of the Girod Street Cemetery, New Orleans' First Protestant Cemetery*. New Orleans: Alblen Books, 1961.

Jackson, Joy J. *New Orleans in the Gilded Age: Politics and Urban Progress, 1880-1896*. Baton Rouge, La.: Louisiana Historical Association, 1969.

Kaufman, Martin. *Homeopathy in America: The Rise and Fall of a Medical Heresy*. Baltimore: Johns Hopkins Press, 1971.

Keller, Morton. *Affairs of State: Public Life in Late Nineteenth Century*

America. Cambridge, Mass.: Belknap Press of Harvard University Press, 1977.

Kelly, Howard A. *Walter Reed and Yellow Fever.* New York: McClure, Phillips & Co., 1906.

Kemp, John R., ed. *Martin Behrman of New Orleans: Memoirs of a City Boss.* Baton Rouge, La.: Louisiana State University Press, 1977.

Kendall, John Smith. *History of New Orleans.* 3 Vols. Chicago: Lewis Publishing Company, 1922.

King, Grace. *New Orleans: The Place and the People.* New York: Macmillan, 1895.

Kiple, Kenneth F., and Virginia Himmelsteib King. *Another Dimension to the Black Diaspora: Diet, Disease, and Racism.* Cambridge, England: Cambridge University Press, 1981.

Kuhn, Thomas S. *The Structure of Scientific Revolutions.* 2nd ed. Chicago: University of Chicago Press, 1970.

Leigh, Robert D. *Federal Health Administration in the United States.* New York: Harper & Brothers, 1927.

MacMahon, Brian, and Thomas F. Pugh. *Epidemiology: Principles and Methods.* Boston: Little, Brown & Co., 1970.

McNeill, William H. *Plagues and Peoples.* Garden City, N. Y.: Anchor Press, 1976.

Maegraith, Brian, and Alfred Robert Davies Adams. *Adams & Maegraith: Clincial Tropical Diseases.* 9th ed. Oxford: Boston Blackwell Scientific, 1989.

Manson, Patrick, *Manson's Tropical Diseases: A Manual of the Diseases of Warm Climates.* Edited by Philip H. Manson-Bahr. 8th ed. London: Cassell & Co., 1925.

Manson's Tropical Diseases. . . . Edited by Charles Wilcocks & P. E. C. Manson-Bahr. 17th ed. Baltimore: Williams & Wilkins Co., 1972.

Manson's Tropical Diseases. . . . Edited by P. E. C. Manson-Bahr. 18th ed. London: Bailliere Tindall, 1982.

Martin, François-Xavier. *The History of Louisiana, From the Earliest Period*. . . . Reprint ed. New Orleans: Pelican Press, 1963.

Merck Manual of Diagnosis and Therapy. Edited by Charles E. Lyght *et al*. 9th ed. Rahway, N. J.: Merck & Co., 1956.

Merck Manual. . . . Edited by Robert Berkow. 13th ed. Rahway, N. J.: Merck & Co., 1977.

Merck Manual. . . . Edited by Robert Berkow & Andrew Fletcher. 15th ed. Rahway, N. J.: Merck & Co., 1987.

Niehaus, Earl F. *The Irish in New Orleans, 1800-1860*. Baton Rouge, La.: Louisiana State University Press, 1965.

Parton, James. *General Butler in New Orleans*. New York: Mason Brothers, 1864.

Powell, John H. *Bring Out Your Dead: The Great Plague in Philadelphia in 1793*. Philadelphia: University of Pennsylvania Press, 1949.

Ravenel, Mazyck P., ed. *A Half-Century of Public Health*. New York: American Public Health Association, 1921.

Reinders, Robert C. *End of an Era: New Orleans, 1850-1860*. New Orleans: Pelican Publishing Company, 1964.

Robertson, James Alexander, trans. and ed. *Louisiana Under the Rule of Spain, France, and the United States, 1785-1807: Social, Economic, and Political Conditions of the Territory Represented in the Louisiana Purchase, as Portrayed in Hitherto Unpublished Contemporary Accounts*. . . . 2 Vols. Cleveland: A.H. Clarke Co., 1911.

Rosenberg, Charles E. *The Cholera Years: The United States in 1832, 1849, and 1866.* Chicago: University of Chicago Press, 1962.

Rosenkrantz, Barbara Gutmann et al., eds. *Yellow Fever Studies.* Public Health in America Series. New York: Arno Press, 1977.

Rothstein, William G. *American Physicians in the Nineteenth Century: From Sects to Science.* Baltimore: Johns Hopkins University Press, 1982.

Saucier, Corrine L. *History of Avoyelles Parish, Louisiana.* New Orleans: Pelican Publishing Co., 1943.

Savitt, Todd L. *Medicine and Slavery: The Diseases and Health Care of Blacks in Antebellum Virginia.* Urbana, Ill.: University of Illinois Press, 1978.

Schmeckebier, Laurence F. *The Public Health Service: Its History, Activities, and Organization.* Baltimore: Johns Hopkins University Press, 1923.

Shryock, Richard Harrison. *Medicine and Society in America: 1660-1860.* New York: New York University Press, 1960.

_____. *Medicine in America: Historical Essays.* Baltimore: Johns Hopkins University Press, 1966.

Shugg, Roger W. *Origins of Class Struggle in Louisiana: A Social History of White Farmers and Laborers during Slavery and After, 1840-1875.* Baton Rouge, La.: Louisiana State University Press, 1939.

Sitterson, J. Carlyle. *Sugar Country: The Cane Sugar Industry in the South, 1753-1950.* Louisville, Ky.: University of Kentucky Press, 1953.

Skowronek, Stephen. *Building a New American State: The Expansion of National Administrative Capacities, 1877-1920.* New York: Cambridge University Press, 1982.

Smillie, Wilson G. *Preventive Medicine and Public Health*. New York: Macmillan, 1946.

_____. *Public Health, Its Promise for the Future: A Chronicle of the Development of Public Health in the United States, 1607-1914*. New York: Macmillan, 1955.

Sontag, Susan. *Illness as Metaphor*. New York: Farrar, Straus and Giroux, 1978.

Spink, Wesley W. *Infectious Disease: Prevention and Treatment in the Nineteenth and Twentieth Centuries*. Minneapolis: University of Minnesota Press, 1978.

Straus, Robert. *Medical Care for Seamen: The Origins of Public Medical Service in the United States*. New Haven: Yale University Press, 1950.

Strickland, G. Thomas, ed. *Hunter's Tropical Medicine*. 7th ed. Philadelphia: W. B. Saunders, 1991.

Strode, George K., ed. *Yellow Fever*. New York: McGraw-Hill, 1951.

Strong, Richard P., ed. *Stitt's Diagnosis, Prevention and Treatment of Tropical Diseases*. 7th ed. 2 Vols. Philadelphia: The Blakiston Co., 1944.

Surrey, Nancy M. Miller. *The Commerce of Louisiana during the French Regime, 1699-1763*. Studies in the Social Sciences. New York: Columbia University Press, 1916.

Tinker, Edward Larocque. *Pen, Pills, and Pistols: A Louisiana Chronicle*. New York: American Society of the French Legion of Honor, 1934.

Vogel, Morris J. and Charles E. Rosenberg, eds. *The Therapeutic Revolution: Essays in the Social History of American Medicine*. Philadelphia: University of Pennsylvania Press, 1979.

Warner, John Harley. *The Therapeutic Perspective: Medical Practice, Knowledge, and Identity in America, 1820-1885*. Cambridge, Mass.: Harvard University Press, 1986.

White, Morton and Lucia. *The Intellectual Versus the City, from Thomas Jefferson to Frank Lloyd Wright*. Cambridge, Mass.: Harvard University Press, 1962.

Wiebe, Robert H. *The Search for Order, 1877-1920*. New York: Hill and Wang, 1967.

Williams, Ralph Chester. *The United States Public Health Service, 1798-1950*. Washington, D.C.: Commissioned Officers Association of the United States Public Health Service, 1951.

Winslow, Charles-Edward Amory. *The Conquest of Epidemic Disease: A Chapter in the History of Ideas*. Princeton, N. J.: Princeton University Press, 1943.

ARTICLES AND PARTS OF BOOKS

Aiken, John Gayle. "The Medical History of New Orleans." In *Standard History of New Orleans* . . . , edited by Henry Rightor. Chicago: Lewis Publishing Co., 1900.

Blake, John. "Yellow Fever in Eighteenth Century America," *Bulletin of the New York Academy of Medicine*, 44 (June, 1968): 673-86.

Bloch, Harry. "Yellow Fever in City of New York: Notes on Epidemic in 1798," *New York State Journal of Medicine*, 73 (October 15, 1973): 2503-5.

Carrigan, Jo Ann. "Yellow Fever in New Orleans, 1853: Abstractions and Realities," *Journal of Southern History*, 25 (August, 1959): 339-55.

_____. "Yellow Fever: The Scourge of the South." In *Disease and Distinctiveness in the American South*, edited by Todd L. Savitt and

James Harvey Young. Knoxville, Tenn.: University of Tennessee Press, 1988.

Del Regato, J. A. "Carlos Finlay and the Carrier of Death." Reprint from *Americas* (May, 1968).

Doyle, Don Harrison. "Urbanization and Southern Culture." In *Toward a New South? Studies in Post-Civil War Southern Communities*, edited by Orville Vernon Burton and Robert C. McMath, Jr. Westport, Conn.: Greenwood Press, 1982.

Duffy, John. "A Sidelight on Colonial Newspapers," *The Historian*, 18 (Spring, 1956): 230-48.

_____. "Yellow Fever in the Continental United States during the Nineteenth Century," *Bulletin of the New York Academy of Medicine*, 44 (June, 1968): 687-701.

East, Dennis, II. "Health and Wealth: Goals of the New Orleans Public Health Movement, 1879-84," *Louisiana History*, 9 (Summer, 1968): 245-75.

Ellis, John. "Businessmen and Public Health in the Urban South During the Nineteenth Century: New Orleans, Memphis, and Atlanta," *Bulletin of the History of Medicine*, 44 (May-June, 1970): 197-212; (July-August, 1970): 346-70.

_____. "The New Orleans Yellow Fever Epidemic in 1878: A Note on the Affective History of Societies and Communities," *Clio Medica*, 12 (1977): 189-216.

Farley, John. "The Social, Political, and Religious Background to the Work of Louis Pasteur," *Annual Review of Microbiology*, 32 (1978): 143-54.

Fossier, A. E. "Charles Aloysius Luzenberg, 1805-1848: A History of Medicine in New Orleans During the Years 1830 to 1848," *Louisiana Historical Quarterly*, 26 (January, 1943): 49-137.

Freedman, Ben. "The Establishment and Critical Points in the Early History of the Louisiana State Board of Health," 15-62. In *Biennial Report of the Louisiana State Board of Health, 1954-1955, Centennial Issue*. [Baton Rouge, 1956].

Geggus, David. "Yellow Fever in the 1790s: The British Army in Occupied Saint Domingue," *Medical History*, 23 (1979): 38-58.

Goldfield, David. "The Business of Health Planning: Disease Prevention in the Old South," *Journal of Southern History*, 42 (November, 1976): 557-70.

_____. "Pursuing the American Urban Dream: Cities in the Old South." In *The City in Southern History: The Growth of Urban Civilization in the South*, edited by Blaine A. Brownell and David R. Goldfield. Port Washington, N. Y.: Kennikat Press, 1977.

Goodyear, James D. "The Sugar Connection: A New Perspective on the History of Yellow Fever," *Bulletin of the History of Medicine*, 52 (Spring, 1978): 5-21.

Gorham, Frederic P. "The History of Bacteriology and Its Contribution to Public Health Work." In *A Half-Century of Public Health*, edited by Mazyck P. Ravenel. New York: American Public Health Association, 1921.

Gutman, Herbert G. "Work, Culture and Society in Industrializing America, 1815-1919," *American Historical Review*, 78 (June, 1973): 531-88.

Hildreth, Peggy Bassett. "Early Red Cross: The Howard Association of New Orleans, 1837-1878," *Louisiana History*, 20 (Winter, 1979): 49-75.

Honley, Steven Allen. "A History of the 1873 Yellow Fever Epidemic in Shreveport, Louisiana," *Journal of the North Louisiana Historical Association*, 13 (1982): 90-96.

Jensen, Richard. "Modernization and Community History," *Newberry*

Papers in Family and Community History. Photocopy. Chicago: Newberry Library, January, 1978.

Johnson, Howard Palmer. "New Orleans under General Butler," *Louisiana Historical Quarterly*, 24 (April, 1941): 434-536.

Jones, Jack Colvard. "The Feeding Behavior of Mosquitoes," *Scientific American*, 238 (June, 1978): 138-48.

Kiple, Kenneth F., and Virginia H. Kiple. "Black Yellow Fever Immunities, Innate and Acquired, as Revealed in the American South," *Social Science History*, 1 (Summer, 1977): 419-36.

Landry, Stuart O. "New Orleans' Predecessor of Red Cross," New Orleans *Times-Picayune*, Magazine Section, December 19, 26, 1937.

Leonard, Jonathan. "The Ghost of Yellow Jack," *Harvard Magazine* (March-April, 1981): 20-27.

Matas, Rudolph. "A Yellow Fever Retrospect and Prospect," *Louisiana Historical Quarterly*, 8 (July, 1925): 454-73.

Miciotto, R. J. "Shreveport's First Major Health Crisis: The Yellow Fever Epidemic of 1873," *Journal of the North Louisiana Historical Association*, 4 (1973): 111-18.

Monath, Thomas P. "Yellow Fever: Victor, Victoria? Conqueror, conquest? Epidemics and Research in the Last Forty Years and Prospects for the Future," *American Journal of Tropical Medicine and Hygiene*, 45 (July, 1991): 1-43.

Porteous, Laura L., trans. "Sanitary Conditions in New Orleans Under the Spanish Regime, 1799-1800," *Louisiana Historical Quarterly*, 15 (October, 1932): 610-17.

Postell, William Dosite. "The Medical Societies of Louisiana Prior to the War Between the States," *New Orleans Medical and Surgical Journal*, 93 (August, 1940): 65-74.

Prichard, Walter, ed. "Three Letters of Richard Claiborne to William Miller, 1816-1818," *Louisiana Historical Quarterly*, 24 (July, 1941), 729-43.

Purtilo, David T., and John L. Sullivan. "Immunological Bases for Superior Survival of Females," *American Journal of Diseases of Children*, 133 (December, 1979): 1251-53.

Rabinowitz, Howard N. "Continuity and Change: Southern Urban Development, 1860-1900." In *The City in Southern History: The Growth of Urban Civilization in the South*, edited by Blaine A. Brownell and David R. Goldfield. Port Washington, N. Y.: Kennikat Press, 1977.

Rousey, Dennis C. "Yellow Fever and Black Policemen in Memphis: A Post-Reconstruction Anomaly," *Journal of Southern History*, 51 (August, 1985): 357-74.

Scarpaci, Jean Anne. "Immigrants in the New South: Italians in Louisiana's Sugar Parishes, 1880-1910." In *American Workingclass Culture: Explorations in American Labor and Social History*, edited by Milton Cantor. Westport, Conn.: Greenwood Press, 1979.

Scramuzza, V. M. "Galveztown, A Spanish Settlement of Colonial Louisiana," *Louisiana Historical Quarterly*, 13 (October, 1930): 553-609.

Slosek, Jean. "*Aedes Aegypti* Mosquitoes in the Americas: A Review of Their Interactions with the Human Population," *Social Science and Medicine*, 23 (1986): 249-57.

Stepan, Nancy. "The Interplay between Socio-Economic Factors and Medical Science: Yellow Fever Research, Cuba and the United States," *Social Studies of Science*, 8 (1978): 397-423.

Tregle, Joseph G. "On That Word 'Creole' Again: A Note," *Louisiana History*, 23 (Spring, 1982): 193-98.

Trent, Josiah C., ed. "The Men Who Conquered Yellow Fever." In Ashbel

Smith. *Yellow Fever in Galveston, Republic of Texas, 1839: An Account of the Great Epidemic.* Austin, Tex.: University of Texas Press, 1951.

Warner, Margaret. "Hunting the Yellow Fever Germ: The Principle and Practice of Etiological Proof in Late Nineteenth-Century America," *Bulletin of the History of Medicine*, 59 (Fall, 1985): 361-82.

_____. "Local Control versus National Interest: The Debate over Southern Public Health, 1878-1884," *Journal of Southern History*, 50 (August, 1984): 407-28.

Whittington, G. P. "Rapides Parish, Louisiana—A History," *Louisiana Historical Quarterly*, 16 (July, 1933): 427-40 (4th part); (October, 1933): 628-38 (5th part).

Wood, Minter. "Life in New Orleans in the Spanish Period," *Louisiana Historical Quarterly*, 22 (July, 1939): 642-709.

Zimmerman, David. "The Mosquitos Are Coming . . . ," *Smithsonian*, 14 (June, 1983): 28-37.

UNPUBLISHED THESES, DISSERTATIONS, AND PAPERS

Bruton, Peter. "The National Board of Health, 1879-1893." Ph. D. dissertation, University of Maryland, 1974.

Carrigan, Jo Ann. "The National Board of Health, 1879-1893: A Significant Failure." Unpublished manuscript.

Doyle, Elisabeth Joan. "Civilian Life in Occupied New Orleans, 1862-65." Ph. D. dissertation, Louisiana State University, Baton Rouge, 1955.

Ellis, John. "The Southern Yellow Fever Epidemic of 1878." Unpublished manuscript.

Ketchum, Dana G. "Yellow Fever in New Orleans: A Study of the Decline in Incidence of Yellow Fever in the Crescent City from 1861 to 1905." M. A. thesis, John Hopkins University, Baltimore, 1983.

Langridge, Leland A. "Asiatic Cholera in Louisiana, 1832-1873." M. A. thesis, Louisiana State University, Baton Rouge, 1955.

Legan, Marshall Scott. "The Evolution of Public Health Services in Mississippi, 1865-1910." Ph. D. dissertation, University of Mississippi, 1968.

Rousey, Dennis. "The New Orleans Police, 1805-1889: A Social History." Ph. D. dissertation, Cornell University, 1978.

INDEX

A

Abolitionists, 337
Acadia Parish, La., 151, 152, 194
Acadians, 20, 191
acclimation, acclimated (see also "creolization"; Strangers' Disease; "unacclimated"), 46, 78, 249, 259; attitudes of, 10, 41, 335-36, 338-39, 351, 434n.3; described, 6, 236-39; and life insurance, 439n.9; and mosquitoes, 281, 282
advertisements (see also patent remedies), 322-24, 347, 375; "stegomyia wire," 176
Aedes aegypti, 201, 382nn.1, 2, 385n.29, 393n.71; anti-mosquito campaign, 168-69, 171-83, 198-203, 343-44; described, 281, 426n.54; origins, 12, 17; reinfestation, 427n.72; and sugar, 22, 44, 386n.4, 418n.24; as vector, 4-6, 93, 167, 264, 283-87
Africa, 12, 16-18, 26, 67, 332, 382n.2
African-Americans (see Blacks)
Agnes, Sister, 350
Agramonte, Aristides, 167, 278
alcohol, 235, 243, 293, 414n.49, 421n.29; in cupping, 303-4; wine and brandy as treatment, 296, 299, 319, 330
Alexandria, La.: in 1819, 51; in 1820s-1850s, 52, 53-54, 56, 73, 81, 389n.9, 396n.53, 397n.59; in 1860s-1890s, 101, 151, 158, 166; 1906 conference in, 200; antebellum population, 393n.77
Algiers, La., 53, 56, 73, 77, 81
American Medical Association, 250, 273
American Missionary Association, 121, 403n.30
American Public Health Association, 273, 286, 374, 378
Anglo-American immigrants, 1, 20, 36, 37
Anopheles mosquito, 286
Antoine, Father, 37
Archinard, John J., 278
Archinard, Paul E., 201, 278, 426n.50
Arkansas, 72, 125, 126, 150
Arkansas River, 72
Army of Tennessee Association, 123
Ascension Parish, La., 154, 194
Assumption Parish, La., 154, 194
Atchafalaya River, 78, 396n.57
Atlanta, Ga., 158; Regulations of 1898, 159
Attakapas Navigation Company, 102
attitudes toward yellow fever (see also social responses), 2, 3, 7, 41, 48; class and racial prejudice, 244, 253-55, 258-59, 335-37; demand for health legislation, 75, 360-61, 377-78, 380-81; during Civil War, 83-85; fear, 24, 115, 189, 367, 434n.14; medical proslavery argument, 67-68, 253-54; nativism, 11, 239-40, 258, 338; New Orleans' fatalism, 2, 30, 75, 237, 364-65; regional panic, 126, 130, 141, 149-56, 339, 352-53, 404n.50; sectional antagonisms, 336-37; urban-rural difference, 153, 156-57, 161-65, 335, 337-39; victim blaming, 10-11, 45, 239, 242-45, 336, 421n.31
Augusta, Ga., 52
Augustin, George, 9, 12, 196
Austin, Mother, 346
Austin, William, 401n.3
Avoyelles Parish, La., 194
Axson, A. F., 244

B

bacteriology (see germ theory)
Balize post, La., 14, 15
Banks, Nathaniel P., 89, 90, 91, 111
Barbados, 12
Barran, Pedro Dulcidio, 31
Bartlett, Elisha, 256-57
Barton, Edward Hall, 42, 256, 313, 374, 422n.45; 1849 Report, 251, 367; 1853 Sanitary Commission, 71, 218-19, 221, 224, 225, 267; on acclimation, 238; on causation, 418n.28; on treatment, 300, 308-9
Baton Rouge, La.: in 1817, 51; in 1820s-1850s, 52, 53, 56, 69, 73, 77, 81, 397n.59; in 1870s-1890s, 125, 151-52, 156, 158, 159, 166, 403n.27
Bayou Courtableau, 52, 73
Bayou Lafourche, 51, 52, 73, 138, 154, 191, 393n.71
Bayou Sara, La., 52, 53, 73, 81, 125, 396n.53
Bayou Teche, 52, 72, 73, 101, 126, 154, 393n.71, 396nn.42, 53, 397n.59
Beauperthuy, Louis Daniel, 282
Beauregard School, New Orleans, 147-49
Behan, Mrs. W. J., 175
Behrman, Martin, 171, 178, 195-96, 356, 381, 412n.14
Belden, James G., 318
Belize, 169
Bemis, Samuel, 132, 244
Benedict, N. B., 311
benevolence, 28, 69-70, 113, 351
benevolent associations and relief work (see also Howard Associations), 334, 344-46, 358; in 1878, 120-25, 362-63; in 1897, 155; in 1905, 187, 191-92; government action, 344, 349-50; in Memphis, 403n.30; Northern aid, 101, 124; physicians' charitable services, 340-41; U.S. Army, 107, 123-24, 404n.33
Berquin-Duvallon, 19, 235
Beugnot, J. F., 300-303, 304-6, 316
Bienville, Jean-Baptiste Le Moyne de, 14
Billings, John Shaw, 9, 273
Biloxi, Miss., 13, 20, 52, 72, 77, 142, 405n.57
Black River, 397n.59
Blacks (see also Africa; slavery), 35, 39, 46, 71, 303-4, 350; in 1860s-1870s, 100, 118, 121-25, 126, 403n.23, 403n.30, 437n.49; in 1905, 174-75, 176, 191, 192, 344; case fatality rates, 192, 255; gravediggers, 336, 354; mortality rate,

484

Saffron Scourge 485

1860-1880, 403n.25; mutual benefit associations, 122-23, 345; nurses, 436n.41; police, in Memphis, 403n.24; population, in New Orleans, 44, 412n.20; resistance to yellow fever, 26, 246, 253-56, 336, 385n.31; as sanitary police, 143
"black vomit" (see also symptoms), 47-48, 59-60, 229; treatment for, 330
Blanchard, Newton C., 178, 185, 190
blistering, 25, 68, 295-99, 305
bloodletting (see also cupping), 37, 307, 327-28; French v. American, 295-300; leeching, 303, 309; syncopal, 301-4, 429nn.17, 25
Boards of Health, see under name of location
Boston, Mass., 12, 250, 252, 253
Bowen, James, 90
Bowie, La., 158
Boyce, Rubert, 196
Brandreth's Vegetable Universal Pills, 319, 320
Brazil, 115, 135, 275-77
British and Foreign Medical Review, 304-6
"Bronze John" (see also yellow fever, labels and synonyms), 9, 98
Brownsville, Tex., 77, 405n.57
Bruns, Henry Dickson, 412n.12
Bunkie, La., 190
Buras Settlement, La., 125
burial practices (see also cemeteries; funerals), 63, 144
Butler, Benjamin Franklin, 83-94, 100, 172, 233, 398n.11

C

Cable, George Washington, 338
Caddo Parish, La., 194
Cairo, Ill., 125
Cajuns (see Acadians)
Calcasieu Parish, La., 152, 155, 184, 194
calentura, 384n.16
calomel, 11, 296-301, 304-5, 307, 309, 316, 327-29, 330, 331
Camp Hutton, La., 154
Canal-Louisiana Bank, 171
Canary Islands, 20
"Can't Get Away Club," 61
carbolic acid, 98, 100, 104-5, 263, 270, 399n.4, 400n.14, 406n.73
Carleton, Henry Guy, 357
Carmona y Valle, Manuel, 275, 276-77
Carondelet, Francisco Louis Hector, 21, 24, 28
Carondelet, Mme Francisco Louis Hector, 24
Carpenter, W. M., 214-15
Carroll, James, 167, 278
Carrollton, La., 53, 56, 81
Carter, Henry Rose, 6-7, 150, 152, 160, 202, 279-80, 286, 427n.67
Cartier, A. J. F., 267, 316
Cartwright, Samuel A., 240, 253, 254, 299-300
case fatality rates, 6-7, 382nn.3, 5, 410nn.50, 51; in 1897-1898, 158, 160, 409n.38; in 1905, 194, 195; black and white contrast, 192, 255; at Charity Hospital, 68; of Howard Ass'n, in 1867, 99, 400n.17
Catholic Relief Association, 123
causation, theories of (see also contagion; epidemic constitution; germ theory; miasma), 209; Gen. Butler's theory, 85; modes of living, 37, 38, 52, 242-44, 256
Cavalli, E., 412n.14
cemeteries (see also burial practices; funerals), 42, 62, 64, 138; described, 63, 66, 352, 354-55; and miasmata, 218; and records, 249-50, 376
Centerville, La., 72, 73, 81, 397n.59
Central Congregational Church, 344
Chabert, Jean, 212
Chaillé, Stanford E., 92, 140, 257; and Havana Commission, 274; and National Board of Health, 132; on theories, 249, 262, 264; on vital statistics, 250-51, 374-75
Charity Hospital, New Orleans, 29, 105, 147, 346, 353; in 1853, 59-60, 66, 68; and coffins, 363; experimentation at, 308, 310, 311; and filth, 224; pathologists, 276-77, 328; and "mosquito doctrine," 199; and quinine treatment, 304; research at, 268-69; statistics, 37, 46-47, 55
Charity Hospital Training School for Female Nurses, 350
Charity Organization Society, New Orleans, 155, 187, 350, 437n.50
Charles, Isaac H., 238, 239
Charleston, S.C., 3, 12, 16, 52, 75, 77, 136
Charleston Medical Journal, 310
Chassaignac, Charles, 201, 255-56
Chérot, Lassalinière, 328
Chisholm, Colin, 210-11
Cholera, 42, 90, 99-100, 189, 251, 400n.28
Choppin, Samuel, 114, 126-27, 135, 140, 368-69, 374, 378-79, 431n.64
cinchona (see quinine)
Cincinnati, Ohio, 106, 124, 125
cisterns, 93; oiling and screening, 168-69, 171-78, 180, 182, 183, 202-3, 412n.12
Citizens Auxiliary Sanitary Association, New Orleans, 128, 129, 272
Citizens Committee on Sanitation (1897), 145-46
Citizens Finance Committee (1905), 171, 176, 186
Civil War, 82-95, 133, 223, 233, 326, 335, 336, 370
Claiborne, William C. C., 32, 33, 36, 37, 234
Claiborne, Mrs. William C. C., 32, 36
Clapp, Theodore, 8, 41, 229, 316, 343, 351
class (see socio-economic class)
clergy, 108, 341-44, 355; 1873 deaths, in Shreveport, 109, 401n.41; 1905 crusade, 172, 174-75, 189, 190-91, 198, 255; Catholic Sisters, 187, 345-46; during Civil War, 83-84; permits for, 142-43; relief and care of the sick, 121, 435n.24
Clinton, La., 73, 81, 125, 156, 158
Cloutierville, La., 73, 81, 396n.53
Colored (Central) Sanitary Association, 175, 344
commerce (see also economic impact), 24, 373; damage to, 104, 115-16, 359, 360; decline of Miss. Valley trade, 48; with Latin America, 2,

6, 19, 93, 99, 118, 157, 158-59, 379; and quarantine, 138, 149-56, 368-69
commercial interests: concern with city image and interior trade, 128-29, 259, 362, 378; opposition to quarantine, 30, 38, 75, 78, 378-79, 405n.52; support for federal control, in 1905, 179-80; support for quarantine and health legislation, 197, 200, 380-81, 411n.4
Company of the Indies, 17
Concorde, La, 345
contagion, 207, 209; 19th cent. views on, 212, 218-19, 224-26, 229-30, 262; and quarantine, 212-14
contagionists, 72, 209, 212-13, 230
"contingent contagion," 212, 218-19, 226, 229
Cooke, T. A., 53, 225-26, 267-68, 307, 338
Corbin, Henry Adams, 403n.23
Costa Rica, 379
Coushatta, La., 111, 166
Covington, La., 53, 56, 73, 81
Craighead, E. B., 375-76
creole immunity, doctrine (myth) of, 11, 117, 119, 237, 245-46, 249, 259, 424n.26
creoles, 39, 46, 63, 243, 346; acquired immunity, 6, 23, 26, 29; defined, 422n.33; and Gen. Butler, 89; and mosquito bites, 281, 282; physicians and treatment, 68, 117, 249, 292, 318, 330
creolization (see also acclimation), 237, 238, 259, 335, 420n.6
Crescent City Ice Company, 363
crime, during epidemics, 107-8, 352
Cronkrite, Lyman, 299-300
Crossman, A. D., 62, 67, 219, 368
Cuba (see also Carlos Finlay; Reed Commission), 22, 249, 275, 283-88; refugees from, 35-36, 115; as source of disease, 18, 157
cultural impact of yellow fever, 334-58; humor, 84, 355-57; poetry, 357, 438n.77
cupping (see also bloodletting), 303-4, 307, 309, 327, 329-30, 429n.25

D

Dallas, Tex., 110
Dalton, S. W., 316
Dalzell, W. T. D., 108
Dames de la Providence, 346
Darby's Prophylactic Fluid, 321
Day, R. H., 328
death rates (see case fatality rates; mortality)
DeBow's Review, 18, 251, 352, 363, 366, 371
Deléry, Charles, 246, 247
Delhi, La., 125, 166
Delille, Henriette, 345-46
Delta, La., 125, 166
Democratic party, 111, 195, 377
dengue fever, 7, 105-6, 130, 142, 236, 407n.2
Department of the Gulf, 89, 327
Devron, John, 191
diagnostic confusion, 7, 11, 13, 36-37, 117, 130-31, 200-2, 236-37, 246, 275, 416n.81; theory of blending fevers, 47-48, 265-67

diet and yellow fever, 235, 414n.49, 421n.29; ethnic foods, 188-89, 243, 421n.31
disinfection (see also fumigation; germ theory; "Maritime Sanitation"): in 1867, 97-98, 99-100; in 1870s, 104-5, 113, 127, 129, 270-71; in 1897, 142-43, 145-46; commercial products, 321; and Gen. Butler, 88; methods of, 399n.4, 400n.14; at quarantine station, 114, 126-27, 134-37, 375, 379, 406n.73; "scientific and modem," 159, 196-97
Doctor Dispachemquic: A Story of the Great Southern Plague of 1878, 356-57
Donaldsonville, La., 51, 52, 56, 73, 81, 125, 166, 325
Dowell, Greensville, 282
Dowler, Bennet, 18, 281, 312, 357; on acclimation, 237, 240; on causation, 230, 232; statistics, 39, 58, 73, 422n.45; on treatment, 309, 315
Dowler, Morton, 222-23, 254-55, 309, 317-18
Drake, Daniel, 19
Duffy, John, 71
Dugan, James, 356-57
Durac, D., 231-32, 309
Dutch immigrants, 53

E

"Eanes, a colored man," cupper, 303-4
East Baton Rouge Parish, La., 194
East Carroll Parish, La., 192, 194, 195
East Feliciana Parish, La., 166
economic impact of yellow fever (see also commerce), 239-41, 381; in 1878, 117-18, 127-29, 365, 370; New Orleans' "chief drawback," 49, 360, 361, 368, 374-76, 439n.4; decline of Memphis and Mobile, 440n.34; disruption and diversion of trade, 43-44, 154-55, 359, 360, 361-62, 368-70; long-range costs, 365-70, 440n.33; profiteering, 363-64; unemployment, 154-55, 187, 362-63
Edinburgh Medical and Surgical Journal, 253
Elks Club, 356
Ellis, John, 115, 127
Emily B. Souder (ship), 114-15, 401n.3
emetics, 25, 295, 297, 299, 306, 309
Emory, W. H., 107
"epidemic constitution of the atmosphere," 67, 208, 209, 417n.6; 19th-cent. views of, 210-12, 217-20; challenged, 232
epidemics (see also name of town and state): comparison of, 159-62; definition of, 410n.53; as defined in 19th-cent. New Orleans, 34, 48-49, 58-59, 74, 98, 399n.8; varied perceptions of, 161-62
epidemiology of yellow fever, 4-7, 23-24, 79, 118-20, 134; Carter's "extrensic incubation," 279-80; theories, 207-10, 262-64
Era Club, 175
Eudes, Mr., 310
experimentation, 431n.58; attempted blood transfusion, 311; with "black vomit," 229; at Charity Hospital, 310, 311, 315, 431n.64; fear

Saffron Scourge 487

of, 431n.60; with mosquitoes and humans, 283-87; on prostitutes, 310
extrensic incubation, 279-80, 286, 427n.67

F

Faget, Charles A., 199-200, 269
Faget, Jean Charles, 246, 248, 249, 269-70
Faget's sign, 269-70, 424n.26
Federation of Women's Clubs, 200
Fenner, Erasmus Darwin, 19, 46-47, 48, 59-60, 61-62, 71, 340; on causation, 217-18, 219; and experimentation, 311, 315; on "second attacks," 236; on susceptibility, 242, 253; on treatment, 303, 304, 306, 307-8; on unity of fevers, 266-67; on wartime health measures, 90-92
Feriet, Ferdinand de, 388n.21
Finlay, Carlos, 97, 134, 167, 261, 283-85, 286, 287, 290, 426n.62, 427n.67
Firemen's Charitable Association, New Orleans, 345
Firemen's Relief Committee, 124
First Street A. M. E. Church, 175
"floating population," 235, 240, 241, 250, 251
Florence Peters (ship), 99
Florida (see also town names), 125, 130
fomites, 168, 199, 225, 226, 258, 262, 264; disproved by Reed Commission, 287
Fontainebleau, La., 154
Fonvergne, Gabriel, 23, 25, 210
Formento, Felix, 143, 145, 160, 176
Fort Assumption, 14
Fort Saint Philip, 86
Fortier, Alcée, 13, 160
Franklin, La., 52, 56, 72, 73, 77, 81, 102, 156, 157-58, 396n.53
Free Persons of Color, 35
Freire, Domingos, 275-76, 277
French Colonial Louisiana, yellow fever in, 12-18
French immigrants, 44
French Market, 87, 104, 169, 191
French Quarter, 86
French Revolution, 16, 21
French West Indian refugees in New Orleans, 1, 20, 22, 35-36
fumigation (see also disinfection; "Maritime Sanitation"): in 1867, 99-100; in 1897, 143, 157; in 1905, 177, 180, 183, 190-91, 193, 197-98, 200; in 1906, 200-1; of freight, and mail, 150, 155, 164, 187, 380; at quarantine station, 78; with sulphur, 105, 174, 262-63; with tar and gun powder, 67, 263
funerals (see also burial practices; cemeteries), 41, 242, 342; cost of, 117; processions, 62, 107, 354, 355

G

Galen, 207-8
Galveston, Tex., 52, 72, 75, 77, 102, 126, 136, 405n.57
Gálvez, Bernardo de, 28

Gayarré, Charles, 14, 239, 338
Gayoso de Lemos, 36, 388n.26
Geddings, H. D., 278, 285, 329, 330
Georgia (see also town names), 150
Gérardin, N. V. A., 38, 211
germ theory (see also disinfection), 120, 128, 421n.30, 425n.41; in late 19th cent., 263-64, 270-74, 279; animalcules and cryptogamia, 221-22, 224-26, 262; and disinfection, 97, 105, 141, 150, 272; hunting yellow fever germ, 134, 274-78, 287; and therapeutics, 330; "virus," 419n.53
Germans, German immigrants, 53, 187, 311, 345, 353; in 1822, 40, 45; in 1853, 60, 62, 69, 71, 394n.3; antebellum increase, 44, 223; and "mode of living," 37, 60, 239, 243, 336; mortality, 235-36
Gillson, Gordon, 137
Gorgas, William C., 168, 287
Grand Army of the Republic, 123
Grand Ecore, La., 81
Grant, Ulysses S., 107
Grassi, G. P., 286
Greenwood, La., 166
Gretna, La., 77, 81, 125, 166
Gros, Adrien Armand, 38, 211
Guadeloupe, 17, 35, 328
Guatemala, 379
Guiteras, John, 150, 151
Gulfport, Miss., 414n.61

H

Hahnemann, Samuel, 317, 318
Hamilton, John M., 132
Hammond, La., 125, 166
Harrison, John, 216, 236, 293, 294-95, 303, 304, 366
Harrisonburg, La., 81
Havana, Cuba (see also Carlos Finlay; Reed Commission): Gorgas in, 168, 287-88; and quarantine, 135, 158, 413n.39; research in, 274, 276, 277, 289; as a source of fever, 12, 17, 19, 21, 110, 114, 115
Havana Royal Academy of Medical, Physical, and Natural Sciences, 283
Hayes, J. J., 325
Hayes, Rutherford B., 370
Hayne, Paul H., 357
Hebrew Benevolent Association, 123
"heroic" practice (see treatment)
Herrick, S. S., 272
Heustis, Jabez, 211, 235, 265-66, 298-99
Hilliard, Robert, 102-3
Holcombe, William, 230, 314, 318
Holt, Joseph, 135-37, 140, 257, 374, 375, 406n.73, 412n.12
Holt's Prescription and Remedies for Yellow Fever, 319
Homeopathic Relief Association, New Orleans, 124, 318, 432n.75
homeopathy, 282, 315-19, 426n.58, 432n.73
Honduras, 379
Hort, William P., 366

hospitals (see also Charity Hospital), 90, 218, 334, 344, 353, 354; emergency hospitals in 1905, 173, 189, 193, 200, 350; Howard Ass'n infirmaries, 68-69, 293-94, 348, 352, 395n.25; mob action against, 146-49, 190; at quarantine station, 78, 114
Houma, La., 158, 166
Houston, Tex., 52, 72, 77
Howard, B. B., 143
Howard, John, 347
Howard Association, of New Iberia, 102
Howard Association, of New Orleans (see also benevolent associations; hospitals), 334-35, 344, 346-50, 358; in 1840s-1850s, 46, 61, 68-69, 303, 395n.25; in 1867, 101, 102, 103, 400n.17; in 1873, 106; in 1878, 120-24, 348-49, 358, 403n.30; criticism of physicians, 341, 364; origins of, 45, 436n.45; and newspaper policy, 371; sectarian and black complaints against, 121-25, 348, 403n.30, 437n.49; sectionalism and, 436n.47; therapies, 293-94, 325
Howard Association, of Shreveport, 106, 107, 109
Humboldt, Dr., 276
Hunt, Thomas, 304
hydropathy, 315-16, 319

I

Iberia Benevolent Association, 345
Iberia Parish, La., 194
Iberville, Pierre Le Moyne, Sieur d', 384n.21
Iberville Parish, La., 154, 194
Illinois, 125, 154
Illinois Central Railroad, 184
immigrants (see Anglo-American; Dutch; French; German; Irish; Italian)
immigration: 18th-early 19th cent. to New Orleans, 35-36; antebellum increase, in New Orleans, 44, 48, 235-36, 364-65; decline of, 118-19, 223, 241-42, 409n.48; disruption by Civil War, 94, 370
"importationists v. local causationists," 38-39, 54, 72-73, 75-76, 79, 90-94, 104, 209-10, 224
insurance: life, 363, 439n.9; sickness and burial (mutual aid societies), 69, 334, 345
Irion, Clifford H., 200, 201
Irish, Irish immigrants, 187, 311, 345, 353; in 1822, 40, 45; in 1853, 60, 62, 69, 71, 394n.3; antebellum increase, 44, 223; and "mode of living," 37, 60, 239, 243, 293, 336; mortality, 235-36
irregular practice (see homeopathy; hydropathy)
Isleños, 20
Italian Relief Committee, 187
Italian Societies, League of, 187, 412n.14
Italians, Italian immigrants: in 1897, 137, 144, 164, 259, 431n.60; in 1905 New Orleans, 165, 169-70, 173, 176, 179, 187-89, 193; migratory labor force, 154, 409n.32, 410n.56; and "mode of living," 37, 104, 243, 336; New Orleans slum area, 413n.46; and spread of yellow fever, 171, 190-91, 193

J

Jackson, La., 158, 166
Jackson, Miss., 405n.57, 409n.34
Jacksonville, Fla., 405n.57
Jamaica, 22, 35, 206
Janvier, Charles, 171, 186
Jeanerette, La., 101, 166, 396n.53
Jefferson, Thomas, 32, 34, 35, 389n.13
Jefferson Parish, La., 154, 194, 195
Jeunes Amis, Les, 345
Johns Hopkins University, Medical School, 272
Jones, Hamilton, 149, 173
Jones, J. L., 175
Jones, James, 267-68
Jones, Joseph, 13, 18, 140; in 1878, 114-15, 116-17, 127; and laboratory research, 268-69; and La. State Board of Health, 114-15, 135, 374, 379, 405n.52; opposition to National Board of Health, 132, 406n.63; on treatment, 328
Judge Baker's plantation, 396nn.42, 53

K

Kane, W. J., 147
Kenner, La., 190
Kentucky, 125
Key West, Fla., 91, 136, 405n.57
King, Grace, 364
King William's War, 16
Koch, Robert, 97, 207, 263, 271-72, 275, 278, 330
Kohnke, Quitman, 181, 332; anti-mosquito campaign, 168-69, 170, 171, 172, 174-76, 198, 288; on federal control, 178-79; on quarantine, 157, 379
Kuhn, Thomas, 423n.4, 427n.71

L

Labadieville, La., 125, 138, 166
Ladies Benevolent Society, 346
Ladies Physiological Society, 122, 346
Lafayette, La., 101, 102, 126, 151, 166, 404n.41
Lafayette (suburb of New Orleans), La., 47, 50, 53, 56
Lafayette Cemetery, 62
Lafayette Parish, La., 194
Lafourche Parish, La., 154, 186, 191, 194, 195, 309, 328
Lake Borgne, 185
Lake Charles, La., 101, 151, 155, 158, 166
Lake Pontchartrain, 27, 32, 40, 53, 73, 88, 154, 185; quarantine station, 78, 396n.57
Lake Providence, La., 73, 81, 125, 166, 190, 192, 193
Lambert, P. A., 215, 266, 303
LaRoche, René, 229-30
Latrobe, Benjamin, 39, 280-81, 370-71, 390n.29
Lazard, Jules, 195
Lazear, Jesse W., 167, 286
League of Italian Societies, 187, 412n.14
LeBeuf, Louis G., 174, 412n.12

Leeville, La., 191-92
Lewis, P. H., 214, 301
Littell's Liquid Sulphur, 321
Liverpool School of Tropical Medicine, 196
local causationists (see importationists; miasma)
Londonderry Lithia Water, 322
Longley's Western Indian Panacea, 319
Louboey, Henri de, 15, 18
Louisiana Naval Brigade, 185-86
Louisiana State Board of Health, 2, 374; 1867 disinfection, 99-100, 400n.14; in 1870s-1880s, 104-5, 113, 114, 117-18, 134-37; in 1897, 142-46, 155, 156, 157, 198, 411n.4; in 1898, 158, 331; in 1905, 170, 184, 188, 193, 200, 201, 372; in 1906, 200-202; established, 76, 230-31, 378; on germ theory, 231, 270-71, 278; opposition to National Board of Health, 96, 132, 380; and quarantine, 77-80, 82-83, 127, 262, 368-69; on Reed Commission, 168, 288; reorganizations, 90, 97, 163
Louisiana State Medical Society, 288
Louisianian, 403n.23
Lutcher, La., 158
Luzenberg, Charles A., 301, 303, 429nn.17, 25
Lyell, Charles, 281

M

McDonoughville, La., 77, 81
McEnery, Samuel D., 135
McFarlane, J. S., 67, 219-20, 223, 240
McGown, Thompson, 305
Mackie, J. M., 304
McMain, Eleanor, 189, 413n.46
Madison, James, 37
Madison Parish, La., 192, 194, 195
Madisonville, La., 53, 56, 73, 81
Mal de Siam, 9, 13-17, 18, 383n.9
malaria, 14, 114, 130, 142, 268
Mandeville, La., 53, 56
Mansfield, La., 111, 166
Manson, Patrick, 427n.67
"Maritime Sanitation," 135-37, 159, 406n.73
Marshall, Tex., 110, 111
Martineau, Harriet, 241
Martinique, 17
Masdevall, Dr., 24, 297
Masons, 344
Massie, J. C., 216-17
Matas, Rudolph, 169, 173, 202, 284, 331
Medical College of Louisiana, 216, 221, 236, 293, 366
medical profession, 90-91, 133, 326; and acclimation, 245, 249; concern with costs of yellow fever, 129-30, 366-69, 376; on contagion theory, 207, 213, 215, 217, 224, 230; during epidemics, 62, 339-41; French v. American, 37-38, 49-50, 68, 340; on germ theory, 141, 270, 274; on "mosquito doctrine," 168, 288; and therapeutic theory, 294-95
Medical Repository, 210
Medico-Chirurgical Society of Louisiana, 215, 300, 301, 303

Memphis, Tenn., 14, 138, 381; in 1873, 105, 111; in 1878, 126, 128, 255, 362-63, 403nn.24, 30; in 1879, 129, 132, 398n.1
Merchants and Manufacturers Association, 200
Mercier, Armand, 249
mercurials (see also calomel), 300; poisoning, 297
Mexican War, 46, 48
Mexico, 275-77, 368, 375
miasma, "noxious effluvia," 23, 36, 67, 105, 146, 207-8; 1850s debates on, 217-20; Barton on, 418n.28; challenged, 222-24, 231-32, 282, 283; described, 218; as dominant theory, 208-12, 215-17, 265, 267, 378; Gen. Butler on, 87; and germ theory, 97, 221-22, 263, 273, 421n.30
Milner, U. R., 270
Mississippi (see also town names), 72, 125, 130, 362; in 1897, 150, 154, 156, 157; in 1905-1906, 170, 173, 184-85, 186, 201
Mississippi Board of Health, 150, 160
Mississippi River, 13, 21, 27, 51, 72, 125, 359, 362, 397n.59
Mississippi River Quarantine Station, 78, 99, 103, 114, 135-37, 157, 203, 204-5, 213, 379
Missouri, 125
Mobile, Ala., 3, 156, 170, 214, 301, 381; 18th-cent. epidemics in, 13, 18; in 1839, 52, 434n.4; in 1850s, 72, 75, 77; Josiah Nott of, 224, 282; quarantine in, 126, 136-37, 157
Monette, J. W., 214, 215
Monroe, La., 106, 110, 126
Montevideo, Uruguay, 278
Morales, Juan Ventura, 23, 24
Morgan City, La., 124, 125
Morgan Steamship Lines, 379
Morgan's Louisiana and Texas Railroad and Steamship Company v. the Board of Health of the State of Louisiana, 135
Morrow, La., 158
mortality, causes of, in New Orleans: in 1879-1903, 441n.52; during Civil War, 92
mortality in New Orleans (see also case fatality rates), 161-62, 374-75; in 1796, 25-26, 387n.15; in 1800-1820s, 31, 39-40; in 1830s-1840s, 41-42, 46-47, 48, 391n.38; in 1850s, 58, 63, 74, 76, 77, 374-75; in 1853, 61, 62, 63, 69, 70-71; in 1860s-1870s, 82-83, 89, 90, 98-99, 101, 116-17, 127, late 19th century, 96, 103, 104, 129-30, 156, 159, 402n.19; in 1905, 194-95; Simond's statistics, 249-53, 365-66, 367, 420n.12, 422n.45 (see also list of tables)
mosquito doctrine, 173-75, 196, 198-99, 200, 287-88, 351, 375, 379, 416n.76
mosquitoes (see also *Aedes aegypti*), 1, 16, 19, 256, 280-88; Finlay's hypothesis, 97, 134, 261, 283-85; fumigation and, 67, 79, 100, 137, 263, 379; Nott on, 225, 282; unusual presence noted during epidemic, 42, 61, 209
Mouton, Guildmaire, 201-2, 416n.81
Murray, R. D., 329, 330, 433n.107
Mutual Benevolent Relief Association, 122-23

N

Napoleon, Ark., 72
Napoleonville, La., 125, 166
Nassau, Bahamas, 86, 89, 398n.11
Natchez, Miss., 51, 52, 72, 77, 126, 299, 341, 414n.61
Natchitoches, La., 52, 53, 56, 73, 81, 152, 393n.71
Natchitoches Parish, La., 194
National Board of Health, 96, 113, 127-28; duties and operations, 130-33; opposition to, 132-33, 180, 380, 406n.63
National Conference of State Boards of Health, 128
New Iberia, La., 52, 56, 81, 104, 166, 397n.59; in 1867, 101-3; in 1878, 124, 126; 1906 case in, 201-2, 416n.81
New Orleans: first appearance of yellow fever in, 13-19; Fourteenth Ward in, 172; Fourth District of, 59, 60, 62, 66, 147-48; myth of salubrity, 30, 49, 249-53, 367; reputation as unhealthy, 49, 82, 104; Second District of, 104, 345; Third District of, 345; Third Ward in, 147-48; yellow fever as "chief drawback" of, 374-81 (For specific epidemics, see table of contents)
New Orleans Auxiliary Sanitary Association, 128, 129, 272
New Orleans Board of Health, 71, 168, 172, 177, 213, 367; 1849 Report, 251-53
New Orleans Board of Trade, 153
New Orleans Chamber of Commerce, 127, 145, 362, 375
New Orleans City Council, 62, 74, 87, 90, 102, 177-78, 186, 218
New Orleans Health Association, 176
New Orleans Medical News and Hospital Gazette, 245-46, 309, 311, 326
New Orleans Medical and Surgical Journal, 3, 53, 101, 242, 255, 329; established in 1844, 49, 65, 214, 300; on germs, 271, 272, 275-77, 278; on impact of epidemics, 59, 239, 366, 368; on mosquitoes, 168, 169, 287-88; on quinine, 305, 308
New Orleans and Northeastern Railroad, 184
New Orleans, Opelousas and Great Western Rail Road, 102
New Orleans Polyclinic, 255
New Orleans School of Medicine, 102
New York, N.Y., 12, 16, 75, 101, 125, 210, 252, 386n.3
newspaper policy, 33-34, 37, 40-41, 46, 349, 364-65, 370-73, 389nn.10, 12; in 1853, 60-61, 70; in 1878, 113-14; on medical advice, 321, 325-26; commercial pressure on, 370-72; criticism of local quarantines, 153-54; criticism of officials, 42-43, 59, 62, 97, 156, 249; opposition to federal quarantine, 203; praising New Orleans health, 10, 42, 103, 360; small town, 51-52, 53-54; support for 1905 crusade, 171-72, 173, 180, 196, 198, 288; support for quarantine and sanitation, 75-76, 143, 145; urban-rural difference, 150, 151-52, 163, 337, 372; victim-blaming, 39, 243-44

Nicaragua, 379
Nicholls, Francis T., 343
Norfolk, Va., 75
Nott, Josiah C., 224-25, 226, 227, 282, 283, 309, 310-11
nurses, 98, 190, 199, 325; blacks in demand as, 336, 346, 436n.41; and Howard Ass'n., 69, 102, 106, 122; instructions for, 173, 331; misbehavior of, 352, 356; pay of, 395n.25; sent by state health board, 191, 193; Sisters of Charity, 102, 346; training school for, 350-53
nursing, importance of, 245, 293, 400n.17, 433n.107; in French creole tradition, 68, 292, 296, 309, 319, 327; and powers of nature, 307, 308; with symptomatic treatment, 11, 327, 328, 329, 332

O

Ocean Springs, Miss., 137, 142, 157
Odd Fellows, 344
Ohio, 125
Old River, 73
Olliphant, Samuel R., 143, 150, 156
Olmsted, Frederick Law, 73
Opelousas, La., 51-53, 56, 73, 81, 101, 102, 151, 166
opium, 296, 297, 298, 299, 304, 306, 308, 309, 318, 319
Orleans, Territory of, 32-37
Orleans Central Relief Committee, 123-24
Orleans Dramatic Association, 106
Orleans Parish, La., 185, 194, 195
Orleans Parish Medical Society, 168, 169, 171, 172, 173, 174, 178, 179, 270, 331
orphans, orphan asylums, 68, 69, 107, 353, 362
Orto, Arturo Dell, 412n.14
Orwood, Miss., 279
Ouachita River, 73, 397n.59

P

Page, Fred B., 325
Paincourtville, La., 81, 125, 166
Panama Canal, 288
Papini, Charles, 412n.14
Paris, France, 115, 268, 278
Paroli, Reverend, 173
Pass Christian, Miss., 77
Pasteur, Louis, 97, 207, 263, 271, 272, 330
patent remedies, 319-21
Patomo, Anthony, 412n.14
Patterson, La., 73, 81, 125, 156, 190, 191, 255, 396nn.45, 53, 397n.59
Peabody Subsistence Association, 122-25, 348, 403n.30, 414n.61
Pearl River, 185
Pensacola, Fla., 3, 18, 40, 72, 75, 136, 405n.57
Perrin du Lac, 32, 351
Perry, Alfred, 105, 406n.73
Philadelphia, Pa., 12, 16, 106, 238-39, 252-53; in

1790s, 23, 24, 29, 208, 210, 280, 386n.3; in 1850s, 70, 75
Physico-Medical Society, 212, 299, 340, 390n.27
Pickwick Dispensary, 124
Pierce, Franklin, 69
Plaquemine, La., 52, 53, 56, 73, 77, 81, 101, 125, 158, 166, 397n.59
Plaquemines Parish, La., 81, 159, 166, 194, 396n.53
Pointe Coupée District, La., 21
Pointe Coupée Parish, La., 81, 397n.59
police, 105, 110, 144, 352, 353, 403n.24; at isolation hospital, in 1897, 148-49; on relief, in 1878, 124-25; sanitary police, in 1897, 142-43, 353
politics and yellow fever, 376-81; first state health board, 378
Polk, Leonidas, 342-43
Ponchatoula, La., 125, 166
Pontalba, Joseph Xavier de, 21, 23-28, 210, 234
"popular health conferences," 200
population of Louisiana: in 1803-1810, 35-36; main cities in 1890, 410n.54; of Spanish La., 20
population of New Orleans, 369, 440n.29; 18th-early 19th cent., 17, 26, 31, 385n.30, 387nn.15, 16; antebellum, 44-45, 71, 339, 394n.3; late 19th cent., 161, 402n.19, 410n.54; in 1905, 169, 412n.20
Port Barre, La., 104
Port Eads, La., 125
Port Hudson, La., 52, 56, 125, 166
Porteous, Thomas C., 115, 116
Potter's Field, New Orleans, 354-55
preventive measures (see also disinfection; quarantine; sanitary improvements), 2-3, 24; Jefferson's plan, 34-35
Priessnitz, Vincent, 316
Protection Hose Fire Company, 347
Protestant Episcopal Diocese of Louisiana, 342
Protestants, 26, 28, 69, 342
Puerto Cortez, 169
Pullman Strike of 1894, 154

Q

quarantine legislation: in 1818-1825, 38, 212-14; in 1855, 75-76, 230-31, 396n.57; 1858 revision, 78-79; 1876 revision, 127; federal, in 1879, 131; house flags required, 145
quarantines (see also commerce; contagion; railroads; shotgun quarantines), 75-79, 103-4, 134-39, 169, 193-94; during Civil War, 83, 85-86, 90, 91, 93-94; federal activity in, 131-34, 204-5, 381; house quarantine, in 1897, 142-45, 410n.51; interstate, 149-56, 183-86; loopholes for fruit trade, 137, 157, 158, 378, 379; opposition to, 77-79, 143-45, 405n.52; passenger detention, 180, 184, 413n.39; ship detention, 127, 135-36; stations, 396n.57; 1905 La.-Miss. conflict, 185-86
quarantines, local, 72-73, 411n.4; in 1870s, 106, 108, 115-16, 125-28; in 1880s-1890s, 130, 149-56, 157, 159; in 1905, 184, 414n.51
quinine, 327, 328, 329, 387n.10; abortive treatment, 304-6, 307-8, 309; cinchona, 24-25, 296, 297, 298, 299

R

Radway's Ready Relief, Regulating Pills and Resolvent, 320
railroads (see also quarantine): bridge burning, 110, 155, 352, 409n.34; inspection and certification, 150, 152, 154, 157, 180, 184, 380; and New Orleans' decline, 369-70, 375; and quarantine, 106, 110, 128, 149-56, 408n.19; relief trains, 106, 362; support for National Board of Health, 133; and unemployment, 362-63; vio-lence and threats against, 151-52, 352-53; and 1906 case, 201
Randolph, Robert, 45
Rapides Parish, La., 194
Rayne, La., 151-52
Reconstruction, 96-111, 133, 255, 326, 336
Red River, 51, 52, 53, 73, 110, 111, 125, 393n.71, 397n.59
Reed Commission (see also U.S. Army Commission), 168, 261, 280, 286, 287, 288, 379
Reed, Walter, 4, 134, 167, 261, 278, 280, 286, 291, 427n.67
refugees, West Indian, 1, 20, 35-36
regional health agencies, 128, 131
Riddell, John L., 221-22, 224, 225, 228, 232
Rio de Janeiro, Brazil, 135, 275
Robertson, Thomas Bolling, 213
Robinson, William L., 293-94, 352
Rockefeller Foundation, International Health Division of, 382n.2
Roosevelt, Theodore, 178, 195-96
Ross, Ronald, 286, 427n.67
Rush, Benjamin, 208-10, 265, 266, 280, 292, 296, 298, 299, 301

S

Saint Bernard Parish, La., 125, 166, 185-86, 194
St. Charles Hotel, 355
Saint Charles Parish, La., 159, 166, 194
Saint-Domingue, 15-17, 22, 35
Saint Francisville, La., 51, 52, 53, 56, 73, 81
Saint James Parish, La., 166, 194
Saint John the Baptist Parish, La., 81, 125, 166, 194, 195
Saint Louis, Mo., 125
Saint Martinville, La., 52, 56, 81, 101, 166, 397n.59
Saint Mary Parish, La., 72, 75, 81, 157, 166, 190, 194, 195, 396n.53
Saint Tammany Parish, La., 194
Saint Vincent de Paul Society, 123
Salomon, Lucien F., 331
Sanarelli, Guiseppe, 277-79, 285-86, 426n.50
Sanitary Commission of New Orleans, 71, 221, 224, 225, 267
Sanitary Council of the Mississippi Valley, 128
sanitary improvements (see also disinfection; fumigation), 145-46, 159, 196; arguments for,

367-68, 370, 376; during Civil War, 85, 87-94; factors retarding, 50-51, 112; "Maritime Sanitation," 134-37; public utilities, 441n.56; after 1905, 202-3
sanitation, lack of, in New Orleans: late 18th-early 19th cent., 23, 30, 31, 32, 50, 212; 1850s-1860s, 59, 60, 85, 87-88, 92, 97, 218-20, 223-24; late 19th cent., 145-46, 343, 353; topographical problems, 32
Santo Domingo, 19
Sardis, Miss., 357
Sauvolle, 13
Savannah, Ga., 3, 52, 75, 77
Schaeuble, Paul, 191
Schmidt, E. F., 102
Schmidt, Henry D., 273-74, 328
schools and colleges: 1905 crusade in, 176-77, 351; effect of yellow fever on, 350-51
"Science," and modernity, 159, 196-99
scientific research, 128, 221-22; clinical work, 269-70; federal funding for, 131, 134; laboratory work, 268-69, 271-72, 275; on mosquitoes, 283-87; new paradigms, 260-61, 272
Scotti, Rev. P., 412n.14
Scruggs, R. L., 308
Second Baptist Church, New Orleans, 175
Second District Infirmary, New Orleans, 293
Shakespeare Club, 102, 106
Sheridan, Philip S., 98
Ship Island, 132, 157
shotgun quarantines, 72, 110, 149-54, 163, 352-53, 369
Shreveport, La., 73, 81, 101, 166; in 1873, 104, 105, 106-11, 327; quarantines, 125-26, 150, 151, 152, 193-94
Sicilian immigrants, 104, 164, 188, 189, 410n.56
Simmons, Judge J. F., 357
Simonds, J. C., 250, 251-52, 365-66, 367-68, 369, 374, 420n.12, 422n.45
Sisters of Charity, 102, 148, 199, 340, 346
Sisters of the Holy Family, 345-46
Sisters of the Sacred Heart, 187
Slaughter, La., 158
slavery, 16, 17, 18; fears of potential slave rebellions, 33, 336, 389n.9, 434n.4; medical pro-slavery argument, 67-68, 253-54, 337
smallpox, 28, 92, 145, 225, 400n.28
small towns (see also attitudes; local quarantines; newspaper policy): in 1850s, 72-74; in 1867, 101-3; in 1873, 106-11; in 1897, 157; in 1905, 190-95; demand health legislation, 378; impact of epidemics on, 2, 337-38; scarcity of records, 3, 53
Smith, A. C., 170, 188
Smith, Henry, 327
social responses to yellow fever, 27, 41; in 1796, 28-29; in 1853, 70; diversions and humor, 27-28, 84; epidemic conditions, 334-35, 351-53; flight from city, 27, 40, 45, 60, 62, 115, 351, 367, 441n.50; professionalism and expertise, 197-99; resistance to health measures, in 1897, 143-45, 146-49, 151-52, 153, 156-57, 163-64; resistance to health measures, in 1905, 170,

188-89, 190-91; urban-rural differences, 163-65, 195
Société Médicale, 38, 39, 211-12, 280, 297, 298, 340
Society of Good Samaritans, 436n.45
socio-economic class, 234, 335-36, 367-68; "better element" and disease, 46-47, 112, 115, 118-20, 245; class elitism, 239-40, 258-59; class resentment and protest, 144, 146-49; laboring classes and disease, 77, 107, 362-63; of nurses, 352; and relief ass'ns, 70; Potter's Field, 354-55; poverty and disease, 44-47, 60, 101, 120-25, 187, 239-40, 242-45, 339, 421n.30
Sontag, Susan, 10, 11
Souchon, Edmond, 158, 160, 170, 181, 184, 190, 200, 331
Souder (see *Emily B. Souder*)
Southern Chemical Works, New Orleans, 320
Southern Cotton Growers, 200
Southern Express Company, 106
Southern Pacific Railroad, 150-51, 155, 184, 201, 365, 375
Spanish-American War, 134, 167, 261
Spanish Louisiana, yellow fever in, 17-19, 20-31, 384n.16
specificity, doctrine of, 265-70, 326, 384n.17, 388n.26, 430n.52
Stark, James, 253
Steamboatmen's Relief Association, 124
steamboats, 1, 44, 51, 72, 362
Stegomyia mosquito (see *Aedes aegypti*)
Sternberg, George M., 274, 277-79, 285, 328
Stillman, Truman, 320
Straight University, 350
Strangers' Disease (see also acclimation; "unacclimated"), 9-11, 27, 29, 32-33, 37, 44-45, 115, 119, 120, 234-42, 383n.11; during Civil War, 82
Stratton, Joseph B., 341
"sugar connection," 22, 44, 72, 99, 385n.29, 386n.4, 392n.48, 393n.71, 418n.24
sugar plantations, 20-21, 190, 396n.42, 409n.32, 410n.56, 413n.46; labor for, 154, 155, 380
Sugar Planters Association of Louisiana, 200
sulphur, sulphurous oxide gas (see also fumigation), 98, 100, 136, 137, 174, 177, 263, 406n.73, 409n.48
symptoms of yellow fever (see also "black vomit"), 7-8, 59-60, 246, 267, 275, 301, 319; symptomatic treatment, 331-32

T

Tallulah, La., 192, 193, 255
Tampa, Fla., 52, 136, 405n.57
Tangipahoa, La., 125, 166
Tangipahoa Parish, La., 194
Taylor, Miss., 279
telegraph, 105, 106, 107, 153, 158, 201, 349
telephones, 183, 197
Tennessee (see also town names), 125, 150, 154
Tensas Parish, La., 194
Terrebonne Parish, La., 154, 194, 195

Saffron Scourge 493

Texas (see also town names), 110, 111, 130, 150, 365, 375; in 1905-1906, 170, 184-85, 201
Texas and Pacific Railroad, 106, 108, 110, 150, 151, 184
therapeutic discourse, 428n.1, 430n.44
therapeutic nihilism, 430n.52
thermometer, 269-70, 424n.27
Thibodaux, La., 51, 52, 56, 73, 81, 125, 166, 191, 396n.53
Thomas, Pierre F., 45, 212
Thomson, Samuel, 315
Tichenor, G. H., 321
Tichenor's Antiseptic, 321
Touatre, Just, 157, 269, 279, 330
Tougaloo University, 350
transportability: concept of, 224-26, 229, 231, 262, 264
treatment of yellow fever, 24-25, 292-333; abortive plans, 302-6; creole method, 68, 292, 318, 328, 330; diversity, 293-94, 306, 315; "expectant," 300, 306, 319, 326-27, 332; French v. American practice, 37-38, 292, 295-300, 317; "heroic," 11, 68, 296-98, 300-6, 307, 309, 316, 319-20; individualized therapeutics, 292, 294-95; new drugs, anti-pyretics, 329, 330, 331
Trenton, La., 73, 81, 110
Trinity Episcopal Church, New Orleans, 172
Tuck, W. J., 267-68
Tulane University, 262, 350, 374, 375

U

Ulloa, Antonio de, 18
"unacclimated," 23, 26, 40, 48, 84, 85, 339, 340
Union Francaise, L', 124
Union Sulphur Company, Lake Charles, 177
United Fruit Company, 379
United Laborer's Benevolent Association, 345
United States Army, 123, 278, 328, 404n.33
United States Army Commission (see also Reed Commission), 4, 97, 134, 167, 280, 285-87
United States Army Medical Corps, 9, 134, 261, 272, 273
United States Congress, 127, 131, 133, 203, 276, 277, 370, 380
United States Department of Agriculture, 272
United States Mail, postoffices, 110, 128, 150, 153, 155, 163, 184-85, 353, 380
United States Marine Corps, 37
United States (Public Health and) Marine Hospital Service, 114, 158, 169, 201; 1905 campaign, 170, 171, 173, 178-83, 186, 193, 196-98, 415n.74; opposition to National Board of Health, 132; origin and expansion of, 133-34, 203, 380-81, 408n.21, 411n.6; railway inspection service, 150-52, 154, 155-56, 157; research, 278-79, 285; on yellow fever treatment, 329, 330
United States Supreme Court, 135
unity of fevers: concept of, 265-68; blending fevers, 47-48, 267

V

vaccination (inoculation) for yellow fever, 382n.2; false claims of, 275-77
Vardaman, James K., 185
Vaughan, John, 280
Venezuela, 282, 321
Vera Cruz, Mex., 48, 135
veratrum viride, 431n.63; experimentation with, 311, 315
Vermilionville, La. (see also Lafayette, La.), 126
Vernon Parish, La., 194
Vicksburg, Miss., 44, 52, 72, 77, 125, 414n.61
Vidalia, La., 73, 81
Ville Platte, La., 104
Villeré, Jacques, 212, 213
Vinton, La., 184
virus, 12, 22, 261, 419n.53; current knowledge about, 332-33; filterable, 263, 264, 287
voluntary associations (see also benevolent associations): 1905 crusade, 172-77, 183; "Cleaning Day," in 1897, 146

W

Warner, Beverley, 172, 174, 176, 177, 412n.12, 437n.50
Wasdin, Eugene, 278, 285
Washington, D.C., 98, 124, 166, 170, 195
Washington, La., 52, 56, 73, 81, 101, 103, 166, 396n.53
Washington, Miss., 214
Waterproof, La., 81, 318
Webster, Noah, 208-10, 265
West Baton Rouge Parish, La., 154
West Feliciana Parish, La., 166
West Indies, 13, 99, 214; epidemics of 1790s, 20, 296, 385n.26; and New Orleans' "mal de Siam," 15-18; and quarantine, 224, 368; spread of disease by refugees from, 20, 35-36
Western Union Telegraph Company, 106, 150
Whig party, 377
White, C. B., 120
White, Joseph H., 170, 171, 180, 181, 183, 184, 196-98, 203
Wholesale Grocery Merchants Association, 191
Wilkinson, J. B., 305
Wilmington, Del., 280
Wilson, La., 158, 166
Woman's League, 175, 176, 413n.46
women: in 1796 epidemic, 24, 27-28; Catholic Sisters, 102, 148, 187, 199, 341, 345-46; resistance to yellow fever, 256-58; as trained nurses, 350, 433n.107; in voluntary ass'ns, 122, 175-76, 200, 345-46
Woodville, Miss., 77, 301
World Exposition of 1884-1885, 277
Wyman, Walter, 178, 278, 329

Y

yellow fever: African origins, 11-12, 256; arrival in colonial New Orleans, 13-19; black resistance to, 26, 246, 253-56, 336, 385n.31; continuing presence in Africa and Latin America, 332-33; decline of, 159-60, 409n.48; epidemiology of, 4-7, 23-24, 79, 118-20, 134, 207-10, 262-64, 279-80; jungle and urban forms, 5, 382n.2; labels and synonyms, 8-11, 383n.9; as national problem, 131-34, 370, 372, 380-81; symptoms of, 7-8, 59-60, 246, 267, 275, 301, 319; victims described, 6, 11, 37, 46, 115, 118-20, 187-89, 234-49, 258-59 (For specific epidemics, see town names or table of contents)

Yellow Fever Commission (U.S., 1879), 274, 276-78, 289

"yellowoid," 160

Young Female Benevolent Association, 345

Young Men's Christian Association, 122, 123, 344, 436n.47

Young Men's Crescent and Star Benevolent Association, 345

Yucatan, Mex., 12

www.ingramcontent.com/pod-product-compliance
Lightning Source LLC
Chambersburg PA
CBHW021136080526
44588CB00008B/88